D1779966

INTERNATIONAL ENCYCLOPEDIA OF
PHARMACOLOGY AND THERAPEUTICS

Sponsored by the International Union of Pharmacology (IUPHAR)
(Chairman: B. Uvnäs, Stockholm)

Executive Editor: G. Peters, Lausanne

Section 41

PHARMACOLOGY OF THE ENDOCRINE SYSTEM AND RELATED DRUGS: THE NEUROHYPOPHYSIS

Section Editors:

H. HELLER
Bristol, U.K.

B. T. PICKERING
Bristol, U.K.

Volume I

EDITORIAL BOARD

D. BOVET, *Rome*
A. S. V. BURGEN, *Cambridge*
J. CHEYMOL, *Paris*
C. HEYMANS, *Ghent*

G. B. KOELLE, *Philadelphia, Pa.*
G. PETERS, *Lausanne*
C. RADOUCO-THOMAS, *Quebec*
V. V. ZAKUSOV, *Moscow*

CONSULTING EDITORS

S. V. ANICHKOV, *Leningrad*
A. ARIËNS, *Nijmegen*
B. B. BRODIE, *Bethesda, Md.*
F. VON BRÜCKE, *Vienna*
A. CERLETTI, *Basle*
C. CHAGAS, *Rio de Janeiro*
K. K. CHEN, *Indianapolis, Ia.*
SIR HENRY DALE, *London*
P. DI MATTEI, *Rome*
J. C. ECCLES, *Canberra*
V. ERSPARMER, *Parma*
C. FORTIER, *Quebec*
A. GOLDIN, *Bethesda, Md.*
R. HAZARD, *Paris*
P. HOLTZ, *Frankfurt am Main*
J. JACOB, *Paris*
K. KAMIJO, *Tokyo*
A. G. KARCZMAR, *Chicago, Ill.*
C. A. KEELE, *London*
P. KUBIKOWSKI, *Warsaw*
H. KUMAGAI, *Tokyo*
L. LASAGNA, *Baltimore, Md.*
C. D. LEAKE, *San Francisco, Cal.*

L. LENDLE, *Göttingen*
A. LESPAGNOL, *Lille*
J. LEVY, *Paris*
G. LILJESTRAND, *Stockholm*
A. LOUBATIÈRES, *Montpellier*
O. H. LOWRY, *St. Louis, Miss.*
G. MARDOÑES, *Santiago*
W. MODELL, *New York, N. Y.*
B. MUKERJI, *Lucknow*
M. NICKERSON, *Winnipeg*
H. RAŠKOVA, *Prague*
M. ROCHA E SILVA, *São Paulo*
E. ROTHLIN, *Basle*
C. F. SCHMIDT, *Johnsville, Md.*
P. STERN, *Sarajevo*
E. TRABUCCHI, *Milan*
J. TREFOUEL, *Paris*
S. UDENFRIEND, *Bethesda, Md.*
B. UVNÄS, *Stockholm*
F. G. VALDECASES, *Barcelona*
P. WASER, *Zurich*
A. D. WELCH, *New Haven, Conn.*
B. YAMADA, *Kyoto*

INTERNATIONAL ENCYCLOPEDIA OF
PHARMACOLOGY AND THERAPEUTICS

Pharmacology of the Endocrine System and Related Drugs: The Neurohypophysis

VOLUME I

CONTRIBUTORS

L. A. Branda
Barbara M. Ferrier
B. K. Follett
S. J. Folley
R. Hall
H. Heller
K. Jayasena

G. S. Knaggs
H. D. Lauson
A. Leaf
K. Lederis
R. A. Munsick
G. Peters
B. T. Pickering

Françoise Roch-Ramel
H. Sachs
G. W. G. Sharp
M. W. Smith
G. W. Theobald

PERGAMON PRESS
OXFORD · LONDON · EDINBURGH · NEW YORK
TORONTO · SYDNEY · PARIS · BRAUNSCHWEIG

Pergamon Press Ltd., Headington Hill Hall, Oxford
4 & 5 Fitzroy Square, London W.1
Pergamon Press (Scotland) Ltd., 2 & 3 Teviot Place, Edinburgh 1
Pergamon Press Inc., Maxwell House, Fairview Park, Elmsford, New York 10523
Pergamon of Canada Ltd., 207 Queen's Quay West, Toronto 1
Pergamon Press (Aust.) Pty. Ltd., 19a Boundary Street, Rushcutters
Bay, N.S.W. 2011, Australia
Pergamon Press S.A.R.L., 24 rue des Écoles, Paris 5e
Vieweg & Sohn GmbH, Burgplatz 1, Braunschweig

Copyright © 1970
Pergamon Press Ltd.

All Rights Reserved. No part of this publication
may be reproduced, stored in a retrieval system,
or transmitted, in any form or by any means,
electronic, mechanical, photocopying, recording
or otherwise, without the prior permission of
Pergamon Press Ltd.

First edition 1970

Library of Congress Catalog Card No. 69-18527

Printed in Hungary

08 013220 0

CONTENTS

LIST OF CONTRIBUTORS   vii

INTRODUCTION: NOMENCLATURE OF NEUROHYPOPHYSIAL HORMONES AND RELATED PEPTIDES   ix
H. Heller and B. T. Pickering, Bristol

CHAPTER 1.   REMARKS ON THE HISTORY OF NEUROHYPOPHYSIAL RESEARCH   1
H. Heller, Bristol

CHAPTER 2.   CHEMISTRY OF NEUROHYPOPHYSIAL HORMONES AND THEIR SYNTHETIC ANALOGUES   19
L. A. Branda and B. M. Ferrier, Montevideo

CHAPTER 3.   THE DISTRIBUTION OF VERTEBRATE NEUROHYPOPHYSIAL HORMONES AND ITS RELATION TO POSSIBLE PATHWAYS FOR THEIR EVOLUTION   59
H. Heller and B. T. Pickering, Bristol

CHAPTER 4.   ASPECTS OF THE RELATIONSHIPS BETWEEN THE CHEMICAL STRUCTURE AND BIOLOGICAL ACTIVITY OF THE NEUROHYPOPHYSIAL HORMONES AND THEIR SYNTHETIC STRUCTURAL ANALOGUES   81
B. T. Pickering, Bristol

CHAPTER 5.   STORAGE OF NEUROHYPOPHYSIAL HORMONES AND THE MECHANISM FOR THEIR RELEASE   111
K. Lederis, Bristol and K. Jayasena, Peradeniya

CHAPTER 6.   BIOSYNTHESIS OF THE NEUROHYPOPHYSIAL HORMONES   155
H. Sachs, Cleveland, Ohio

CHAPTER 7.   ESTIMATION OF NEUROHYPOPHYSIAL HORMONES IN BODY FLUIDS   173
M. W. Smith, Cambridge

CHAPTER 8.	(a) RENAL EFFECTS OF POSTERIOR PITUITARY PEPTIDES AND THEIR DERIVATIVES *G. Peters and F. Roch-Ramel, Lausanne*	229
	(b) PHYSIOLOGICAL AND PHARMACOLOGICAL EFFECTS OF NEUROHYPOPHYSIAL HORMONES AND THEIR SYNTHETIC ANALOGUES: UTERINE ACTION *R. A. Munsick, New Mexico*	279
	(c) PHYSIOLOGICAL AND PHARMACOLOGICAL EFFECTS: MAMMARY ACTION *S. J. Folley and G. S. Knaggs, Reading*	295
CHAPTER 9.	EFFECTS OF NEUROHYPOPHYSIAL HORMONES AND THEIR SYNTHETIC ANALOGUES ON LOWER VERTEBRATES *B. K. Follett, Leeds*	321
CHAPTER 10.	CELLULAR MODE OF ACTION OF VASOPRESSIN *A. Leaf and G. W. G. Sharp, Boston, Mass.*	351
CHAPTER 11.	FATE OF THE NEUROHYPOPHYSIAL HORMONES *H. D. Lauson, New York, N. Y.*	377
CHAPTER 12.	CLINICAL PHARMACOLOGY	
	(a) OXYTOCIN *G. W. Theobald, London*	399
	(b) VASOPRESSIN *R. Hall, Newcastle upon Tyne*	423
AUTHOR INDEX		447
SUBJECT INDEX		469

LIST OF CONTRIBUTORS

BRANDA, LUIS A. Laboratory of Polypeptides, Service of Obstetrical Physiology, Faculty of Medicine, Montevideo, Uruguay.

FERRIER, BARBARA M. Laboratory of Polypeptides, Service of Obstetrical Physiology, Faculty of Medicine, Montevideo, Uruguay.

FOLLETT, B. K. Department of Zoology, University of Leeds, Leeds 2, England

FOLLEY, S. J. National Institute for Research in Dairying, Shinfieldl Reading, England.

HALL, REGINALD. Department of Medicine, Royal Victoria Infirmary, Newcastle upon Tyne 1, England.

HELLER, H. Department of Pharmacology, University of Bristol, Bristo, 8, England.

JAYASENA, K. Department of Pharmacology, Faculty of Medicine, University of Ceylon, Peradeniya, Ceylon.

KNAGGS, G. S. National Institute for Research in Dairying, Shinfieldl Reading, England.

LAUSON, HENRY D. Department of Physiology, Albert Einstein College of Medicine, Yeshiva University, New York, N. Y., U.S.A.

LEAF, ALEXANDER. Department of Medicine, Massachusetts Genera, Hospital, Boston, Mass., U.S.A.

LEDERIS, K. Department of Pharmacology, University of Bristol, Bristol 8, England.

MUNSICK, ROBERT A. Department of Obstetrics and Gynecology, University of New Mexico, Albuquerque, New Mexico, U.S.A.

PETERS, GEORGES. Department of Pharmacology, University of Lausanne, Lausanne, Switzerland.

PICKERING, B. T. M. R. C. Group for Research in Neurosecretion, Department of Pharmacology, University of Bristol, Bristol 8, England.

ROCH-RAMEL, FRANÇOISE. Department of Pharmacology, University of Lausanne, Lausanne, Switzerland.

SACHS, HOWARD. Department of Physiology, Western Reserve University School of Medicine, Cleveland, Ohio, U.S.A.

SHARP, GEOFFREY W. G. Department of Medicine, Massachusetts General Hospital, Boston, Mass., U.S.A.

SMITH, M. W. Agricultural Research Council Institute of Animal Physiology, Babraham, Cambridge, England.

THEOBALD, G. W. Obstetric Unit, University College Hospital, London, England.

INTRODUCTION
NOMENCLATURE OF NEUROHYPOPHYSIAL HORMONES AND RELATED PEPTIDES

H. Heller and B. T. Pickering

Department of Pharmacology, University of Bristol, Bristol, England

THE nomenclature of neurohypophysial hormones and their synthetic analogues, and indeed of other biologically active peptides, lacks uniformity. There are really two problems. Firstly the trivial or laboratory names of these peptides and secondly their generic chemical names. The mammalian hormones were called oxytocin and vasopressin long before their chemical constitution was known and these "laboratory names" were assigned by du Vigneaud and his colleagues to the nonapeptides whose structure they had determined. Similar trivial names were subsequently given to other naturally-occurring peptides in this series and to some of their synthetic analogues, e.g. vasotocin and oxypressin. The use of these trivial names is by now so common that they have been retained throughout this monograph. Objections have been raised from time to time against the use of the name vasopressin, since it describes a pharmacological rather than a physiological action of the hormone, and to ADH since the antidiuretic hormone of birds, for example, is arginine vasotocin. However, it was felt that provided it is understood that ADH refers to a mammalian antidiuretic principle (i. e. arginine or lysine vasopressin) contributors to this monograph should not be restricted in the use of either of these terms.

In numerous cases the full or abbreviated chemical name has to be used, and in these cases it has to be decided in what way an amino acid change in the molecule should be indicated. This problem has been considered by the IUPAC-IUB Commission of Biochemical Nomenclature who have issued tentative rules for naming amino acid and peptide derivatives *(Biochem. J.* **102**, 23–27 (1967) and **104,** 17–19 (1967)). It is proposed to follow these recommendations throughout this monograph. The rules state that in a polypeptide of trivial name, X, if the qth amino acid is replaced by another residue, the semitrivial name of the modified polypeptide is [q-new amino acid]-X and the abbreviated form is [Abc^q]X. For example [8-citrulline]-vasopressin or [Cit^8]-vasopressin. It follows from this that the naturally occurring vasopressins, for example, are written [8-arginine]-vasopressin and [8-lysine]-vasopressin.

CHAPTER 1

REMARKS ON THE HISTORY OF NEUROHYPOPHYSIAL RESEARCH

H. Heller

*Department of Pharmacology,
University of Bristol, Bristol, England*

THE pituitary gland was well known to Galen as an anatomical entity and was so called because it was assumed to act as a filter or trap for the slime or *pituita*—the waste material excreted by the brain—which was then supposed to be conducted from the gland to the nasopharynx. This ancient concept of the pituitary as a gland of external secretion survived well into the eighteenth century (see Rolleston, 1936), but the celebrated author of the *Cerebri Anatome,* Thomas Willis (1664), seems to have rejected it since he wrote: "The ramification of the carotids into a reticulated plexus shows ... that the blood ... before it is led into the cerebrum takes some part of the superfluous serum of the pituitary gland and instils another part into the various shoots to be led back towards the heart." This explanation—as Harvey Cushing (1932) has pointed out—bears a curious resemblance to the concept of internal secretion, even though it was based on a factual misconception.

Recognition that the glandula pituitaria consists of two parts seems to have arisen at about the same period. For example, Thomas Willis seems to distinguish two lobes (but note that no division is shown in the plates of his *Cerebri Anatome),* and is followed in this view by Vieussens (1684) and Winslow (1723). The Venetian anatomist Santorini (1724), however, appears to have been the first who recognized that the anterior part of the gland was not a continuation of the infundibulum. By 1766 the distinction between pars anterior and pars posterior is clearly made by A. von Haller in his *Elementa Physiologiae Corporis Humani* (1766), or to quote William Cullen's (1779) translation of the same author's *Primae Lineae Physiologiae* (1767): "This (the pituitary glandule) is compressed on both sides, simple, of uncertain structure; in the anterior part almost round, and of reddish colour; the posterior part less, cinereous, broad transversely, covered with the pia mater of the brain: it lies upon the proper impression of the sella turcica, and seems to be a kind of appendix to the brain."

The nineteenth century saw very little progress in research on the neurohypophysis (as it came to be called after Soemmering in 1778 had introduced the term hypophysis as an alternative to "pituitary gland") probably because, when studied with ordinary methods of fixation and staining, the posterior lobe has a rather nondescript appearance. As late as 1889, for example, A. Macalister described the pituitary as "probably the rudiments of an archaic sense organ". The first and decisive advance—foreshadowing recognition of the physiological significance of the neurohypophysis—was made by Oliver and Schäfer (1895) who showed that the intravenous injection of an extract of the whole pituitary produced a rise in blood pressure. Shortly afterwards Howell (1898) proved that the pressor principle stemmed from the posterior lobe. Since then progress has been rapid and the directions it has taken will, for convenience of description, be described under the following headings: (1) morphology of the hypothalamo-neurohypophysial system; (2) chemistry of the active principles; (3) pharmacological action and biological function of the neurohypophysial hormones; (4) clinical use of neurohypophysial hormones.

MORPHOLOGICAL ASPECTS

Bundles of non-myelinated nerve-fibers entering the posterior lobe through the pituitary stalk were first described by Ramon y Cajal (1894) in two-day-old mice and later by Tello in 1912. Further studies showed that most of these fibers were derived from the supraoptic and paraventricular nuclei in higher vertebrates (Pines, 1925a, b; Greving, 1926) and the preoptic nuclei of lower vertebrates (Meyer, 1935).

Besides nerve fibers and their endings, the neurohypophysis contains glial elements (Retzius, 1894; Berkeley, 1894). Bucy in 1930 reported that these glial cells differed from the astrocytes and oligodendroglia of the adjacent brain and introduced the term pituicyte. Romeis (1940), who adopted this name, distinguished four types of pituicytes in man, one of which he compared with glandular cells and called adenopituicytes. He followed Bucy in the belief that these modified glial cells secreted the neurohypophysial hormones, a view which seemed to be supported by the observations of Gersh (1939) who claimed that osmiophilic granules accumulated in the pituicytes of rats deprived of water. However,

Gersh's findings could not be confirmed by Hickey, Hare and Hare (1941), or de Robertis and Primavesi (1942). Selye and Hall (1943) and Chambers (1945) described mitotic changes in the pituicytes of dehydrated rats, but it has been pointed out by Green (1947) that mitosis might have been due to unspecific stress. The functional significance of the pituicytes is thus obscure, but it should perhaps be noted that it has been stressed in a recent electron microscopic investigation (Lederis, 1965) that their processes often extend to the immediate vicinity of blood vessels, apparently ending near or in the perivascular space.

Another morphological feature of the posterior lobe and the neural stalk, described as early as 1908 by Herring, was the basophilic colloid masses or droplets which subsequently became known as "Herring bodies". Herring himself regarded them as cells derived from the adenohypophysis and his view was supported by Cushing and Goetsch (1910), but was contested by Carlson and Martin (1911) and Maurer and Lewis (1922). Some of the early investigators (e.g. Cushing and Goetsch, 1910; Collin, 1928) assumed also that the colloid droplets might represent the hormones of the neurohypophysis and this view became acceptable as concepts about the function of the neurohypophysial neurones began to change. Beginning with a description of hypothalamic neurones in a bony fish, *Phoxinus laevis*, in 1928 and continuing with investigations in other vertebrates including man, E. Scharrer developed the concept of neurosecretion, that is of nerve cells which, like other neurones in the central nervous system, show Nissl substance and neurofibrils but which, in addition, contain secretory material (for reference see Scharrer and Scharrer, 1954). Between the years 1930 to 1935 Scharrer then developed the concept that it was these neurones which had an endocrine function. This view was shared by Roussy and Mossinger (1934) but did at that time not gain general acceptance (see e.g. Ranson and Magoun 1939). The situation changed dramatically when Bargmann (1949) applied Gomori's (1941) staining method with chrome-hematoxylin-phloxine to the hypothalamo-neurohypophysial system. By this technique secretory neurones stain selectively and can be traced from the perikaryon in a hypothalamic nucleus to the nerve-ending in the posterior lobe, and it is seen that the Herring bodies are probably nothing but swellings in the course of individual nerve fibers. Bargmann assumed from the very first that the neurosecretory material containing the neurohypophysial hormones was formed in the nuclear cells and was transported to the posterior lobe from which the hormones are released. He and his co-workers (Ortmann, 1951; Hild and Zetler, 1953a, b) then showed in the subsequent years that the amounts of Gomori-positive material and antidiuretic activity in the hypothalamo-neurohypophysial complex are correlated and that, when the pituitary stalk is severed, neurosecretory material accumulates rostral to the cut (Hild, 1951; Hild and Zetler, 1953a). The new concept of the function of the hypothalamo-neurohypophysial system was summarized in a joint publication by Bargmann and Scharrer (1951) in which they postulated that "the pars nervosa of the vertebrate hypophysis stores but does not produce the stainable material which it contains. This material originates in the neurosecretory cells of the nuclei supraopticus and paraventricularis in the higher vertebrates and the homologous nucleus preopticus in the lower vertebrates; it passes to the pars nervosa by way of the hypothalamo-hypophysial tracts."

Further selective staining methods, useful for the light microscopical study of the hypothalamo-neurohypophysial complex and other neurosecretory systems, were the aldehyde-fuchsin method elaborated by Gabe (1953), the performic acid-Alcian blue method introduced by Adams and Sloper (1956), and the pseudoisocyanine reaction developed by Sterba (1961, 1964).

Numerous investigators have by now studied the hypothalamo-neurohypophysial system with the electron microscope and have shown that its ultrastructure is similar from the elasmobranch fishes (see Knowles, 1965) to man (Lederis, 1965). Two kinds of subcellular granules are recognized. One ranging in diameter up to 120 nm, called the "elementary granules" by Bargmann and Knoop (1957), was suspected from the start to contain the neurohypophysial hormones. Another family of smaller granules (about 60 nm, was originally called "synaptic", but this interpretation which was only based on morphological features has been contested (see Holmes and Knowles, 1960; Knowles, 1963; Lederis, 1963, 1965).

That the "elementary granules" contain vasopressin and oxytocin (and in the case of a teleost fish vasotocin, Lederis, 1962) has been verified by isolation of these subcellular entities by differential centrifugation and estimation of the hormone content of the fractions (Schiebler, 1952; Pardoe and Weatherall, 1955; Lederis and Heller, 1960; Heller and Lederis, 1962; Weinstein, Malamed and Sachs, 1961; LaBella, Beaulier and Reiffenstein, 1962; Barer, Heller and Lederis, 1963). It has also been shown by Ginsburg and Ireland (1966) that the distribution of neurophysin, the protein carrier of the active peptides in subcellular fractions, is essentially similar to that of the hormones.

CHEMICAL ASPECTS

Dudley (1919, 1923) found that the pressor and the oxytocic activities of posterior lobe extracts could be separated by extraction with butanol and he concluded in his paper of 1923 that "the uterine stimulant and pressor principles are two distinct chemical substances". In collaboration with H. H. Dale (Dale and Dudley, 1921) he studied the effect of proteolytic enzymes on these active principles, the results laying the foundation for the recognition that they are polypeptides. Further progress in the purification of the active principles was made when Kamm *et al.* (1928) and Stehle and Fraser (1935) introduced methods of separation by fractional precipitation from organic solvents. The procedure used by Kamm and his colleagues yielded a pressor fraction containing 160 units/mg and an oxytocic fraction of 300 units/mg. Kamm *et al.* estimated that each fraction was contaminated with 2–5% of the other hormone, but since it is now known (Munsick, Sawyer and van Dyke, 1960) that oxytocin has some "intrinsic" pressor-antidiuretic and vasopressin some oxytocic activity, it seems likely that the separation was complete though the products still contained some inert material. However, Kamm also prepared an oxytocic extract containing 500 units/mg, i.e. a preparation with the same potency as that of synthetic oxytocin.

Du Vigneaud and his colleagues (du Vigneaud, 1954/55) applied the technique of counter-current distribution to the isolation of oxytocin and vasopressin from fractions prepared according to Kamm *et al*. More recently the neurohypophysial hormones have been prepared by methods employing partly electrophoresis on a cellulose column (Porath, 1957), partly partition chromatography (Condliffe, 1955) and partly ion-exchange chromatography (Acher, Light and du Vigneaud, 1958). A method utilizing the specific binding of the hormones to neurophysin has also been successfully used for the isolation of the hormones of the ox and the pig (Acher, Light and du Vigneaud, 1958) and of other mammals including men. The use of non-homologous neurophysin for the preparation of non-mammalian hormones may, however, be hazardous since apparently vasopressin may be introduced into neurohypophysial extracts of species in which it normally does not occur (Munsick, 1964).

The structure of oxytocin was simultaneously and independently determined by du Vigneaud *et al.* (1953) and by Tuppy and Michl (1953). The same year saw the establishment of the structure of the vasopressin in ox neurohypophysial extracts (arginine vasopressin) by du Vigneaud, Lawler and Popenoe (1953). Popenoe, Lawler and du Vigneaud (1952) had already found previously that the vasopressin of the pig contained lysine instead of arginine, thus furnishing the first example of the polymorphism of a neurohypophysial hormone (see Heller and Spickett, 1966). The synthesis of oxytocin followed in 1953-4 (du Vigneaud, Lawler and Popenoe, 1953), and that of arginine vasopressin in 1954 (du Vigneaud, Gish and Katsoyannis, 1954).

Comparisons of potency ratios obtained by bioassay techniques, of non-mammalian neurohypophysial extracts with the same ratios of mammalian gland extracts showed early (Heller, 1941a, b; Lazo-Wasem and Weisel, 1952) that non-mammalian pituitaries contained active principles related to but different from oxytocin and vasopressin. This technique of pharmacological characterization, in the refinement of which W. H. Sawyer and H. B. van Dyke were especially prominent, was substantially aided by the introduction of a simple paper chromatographic method for the separation and partial purification of very small quantities of neurohypophysial peptides (Heller and Lederis, 1958). Establishment of pharmacological spectra of activity, usually by a combination of chromatographic and bioassay procedures, led not only to the discovery of several new neurohypophysial hormones, but also—from the comparison with the profiles of synthetic analogues—to the tentative identification of several new hormones (see Chapter 3).

The discovery of these new neurohypophysial principles was much aided by the synthesis and pharmacological characterization of an extensive series of oxytocin analogues by a number of distinguished chemists amongst whom the names of Boissonnas, du Vigneaud, Rudinger and Šorm are particularly prominent (see Chapter 4). Their researches had the additional important result that structure–action relationships of this family of biologically active peptides are by now better explored than those of any other group of protein hormones (see Chapter 4).

PHARMACOLOGICAL ACTION AND BIOLOGICAL FUNCTION

It was apparent from the earliest work with mammalian posterior pituitary extracts that they exerted a variety of actions. As already mentioned, Oliver and Schäfer (1895) discovered the blood pressure raising effect in mammals. Dale in 1906 and 1909 showed that they contracted the uterus, and Ott and Scott in 1910 were the first to report the milk ejection effect of posterior pituitary extract. Farini and von der Velden, both in 1913, demonstrated their antidiuretic effect in man, Paton and Watson (1912) described the blood pressure-lowering action of undifferentiated neurohypophysial extracts in birds, and Brunn (1921) showed that mammalian posterior pituitary extracts injected into frogs produced water retention—the so-called "Brunn" or "water balance" (Heller, 1941b) effect.

These investigations were subsequently extended—mainly by Herring (1913), Hogben and de Beer (1925) and Heller (1941a, b, 1942)—to extracts of non-mammalian neurohypophysial tissue and it could be shown that, qualitatively speaking, all vertebrate classes contain active principles which have the same biological effects as extracts of mammalian posterior lobes. Much work has also been expended—and is still being expended—on the problem of the physiological significance of these effects. Since administration of posterior pituitary extracts (or snuff) to patients suffering from diabetes insipidus reduced their excessive urine output to normal proportions, it was evident from the start that the pressor-antidiuretic principle (vasopressin) was normally involved in the regulation of water metabolism. Verney (1926), in experiments on the isolated head–kidney preparation, showed subsequently that the antidiuretic hormone had a renal site of action, and the same author (Verney, 1947) demonstrated that a small increase in plasma osmotic pressure led to a release of vasopressin from the neurohypophysis. These investigations led to the concept (see Chapter 8a) that water reabsorption by the mammalian renal tubule is under the control of the antidiuretic hormone and that this control is released when the plasma osmotic pressure falls as a result of fluid ingestion, the blood dilution leading to an inhibition of vasopressin secretion accompanied by the quick disappearance of the circulating hormone whose very short half-life has been demonstrated by Ginsburg and Heller (1953) and others (see Chapter 11).

The vascular action of vasopressin has, until recently, been regarded as an experimental artefact, mainly because antidiuretic effects can be produced without a demonstrable change in glomerular filtration rate. However, the suggestion has recently been made that effects of the hormone on the blood vessels of the renal medulla may be concerned in the physiological antidiuretic mechanism (Kramer, Thurau and Deetjén, 1960; Lilienfield, Maganzini and Bauer, 1961).

The demonstration that the injection of neurohypophysial extracts caused milk ejection in various species including man (Schäfer, 1913) suggested the possibility that the posterior pituitary plays a physiological role in the process of suckling. The first clear support for this concept derived probably from the work of Gaines (1915) who concluded that milk ejection was caused by a direct effect of posterior pituitary extract on muscular elements in the mammary gland. Ely and Petersen (1941) showed subsequently in cows that oxytocin was more effective than vasopressin in stimulating milk-ejection and postulated that the former hormone was normally concerned in the galactobolic reflex. The next advance was the demonstration (Gomez, 1939; Harris and Jacobsohn, 1952; Benson and Cowie, 1956) that milk production can be maintained in hypophysectomized animals but that the litters die unless posterior pituitary extracts are given to the mothers. Further understanding of the complex interrelationship between the mammary gland, the hypothalamus and the posterior pituitary is due to the work of Andersson (1951) Harris (1958) and Cross (1961) which in the aggregate firmly established the physiological significance of oxytocin in milk-ejection.

In contrast, the precise role of oxytocin in parturition is still controversial (see Chapter 12a) although there is little doubt that considerable amounts of oxytocin are released from the neurohypophysis during labor, as demonstrated by records of milk ejection or increased intra-mammary pressure during labor (see e.g. Gunther, 1948; Cross, 1959) and measurements of the oxytocin concentration in the blood of parturient animals and women (Fitzpatrick and Walmsley, 1962, 1965; Folley and Knaggs, 1965; Coch et al., 1965).

The problem of the significance of the neurohypophysis in parturition cannot be divorced from the question of the interaction of the ovarian hormones and oxytocin on the uterine muscle, a question to which much work has been devoted during the last 40 years. Dixon and Marshall (1924) seem to have been the first who suggested a relation between the state of the ovary in pregnancy and the activity of the posterior pituitary lobe. They postulated that the "ovarian secretion which at other times activates the (posterior) pituitary is inhibited or else neutralized by the secretion coming from the corpus luteum. At the close of pregnancy, when the corpora lutea are in an advanced stage of involution, the normal secretory activity is once more produced, and the pituitary is excited to secrete in greater quantity." However, their assumptions were based on experimental results (attempt to assay oxytocic activity of neurohypophysial origin in the cerebrospinal fluid) which in the light of later methodological progress must be considered invalid (see van Dyke and Kraft, 1927, and van Dyke, 1936).

The real basis to many concepts on the cause of the variations in uterine activity at the end of pregnancy was laid by the pioneer work of Knaus (1926) who showed that the sensitivity of the rabbit uterus to posterior pituitary extracts is low at the beginning of pregnancy but increases from the 18th day onwards to achieve its height on the 29th day of gestation. Knaus (1928) showed subsequently (see also Knaus, 1953) that this behavior of the pregnant rabbit uterus could be linked with the secretory activity of the corpus luteum, or, in other words, that progesterone inhibited the action of oxytocin until, at term, this progesterone block was withdrawn to leave the myometrium under the dominance of oestrogen and highly sensitive to oxytocin. This mechanism appears also to operate in other species than the rabbit but there are others (for reference see Fitzpatrick, 1966) in which there is some doubt whether progesterone withdrawal is the terminating event of pregnancy.

Compared with the great effort spent on the clarification of the physiological significance of the posterior pituitary in mammals, inquiries into the effects of the neurohypophysial hormones in non-mammalian vertebrates have been relatively scanty (see Chapter 9).

THE CLINICAL USE OF POSTERIOR PITUITARY HORMONES

Posterior pituitary extract would seem to have been first put to clinical use by W. Blair Bell who published his observations in 1909. The possibility of an "oxytocic" action of these extracts occurred to him independently of H. H. Dale. To quote his own words (Blair Bell, 1909): "Three years ago it occurred to me, while working on the physiology of the female genital organs, to try, among other things, the influence of the extract of the infundibular body on uterine contractions. I wrote to Messrs. Burroughs Wellcome and Co. for a supply and they very courteously put me in communication with Mr. H. H. Dale who made for me a large quantity for intravenous injection. At the same time he informed me that he had already found that the infundibular extract caused uterine contractions." Blair Bell then proceeded to inject Dale's preparation into pregnant women and in two cases of Caesarian section observed that "the uterus contracted into a blanched ball and only relaxed subsequently to a moderate degree". He did, however, at least initially, not use the extract in protracted labor but reported on its efficacy in post-partum hemorrhage. It seems to have been Hofbauer in 1911 who first used posterior pituitary extracts to increase uterine activity in labor. In 1927 Bourne and Burn concluded that the intramuscular injection of "the comparatively small dose of two units (of posterior pituitary extract) is sufficient in the majority of women in labor to produce a definite and sometimes striking effect on the strength and frequency of uterine contractions. In most instances the effect persisted for the whole period of observation..."
In 1948, however, G. W. Theobald (Theobald et al. 1948) pointed out that the amounts of posterior pituitary extract given to parturient women were in no proportion to the minimum doses of antidiuretic hormone which produced an inhibition of urine flow. He and his colleagues showed that the administration of posterior pituitary extract by intravenous drip

in a dilution between 1:5000 and 1:10,000 increased both the frequency and the intensity of the uterine contractions in cases of uterine inertia. The use of highly purified natural oxytocin or of synthetic oxytocin is obviously a further advantage of this technique since vascular or antidiuretic effects are thus avoided.

Early investigators of the actions of posterior pituitary extracts (Magnus and Schäfer, 1901; Schäfer and Herring, 1908) described a diuretic effect in anaesthetized animals which they either explained by "a specific stimulation of the renal cells" (Sharpey-Schäfer, 1926) or ascribed to vascular effects (Houghton and Merrill, 1908; Knowlson and Silverman, 1918). It was only when F. Farini and R. von den Velden, both in 1913, tried the extracts in unanaesthetized human subjects that the antidiuretic action was discovered. Farini's report appeared in the number of the *Gazzetta degli Ospedali* published on September 11, 1913 and was therefore two months earlier than that of von den Velden which was published in a number of the *Berliner Klinische Wochenschrift* dated November 10, 1913. Farini's first case was a young woman with a positive Wassermann reaction with a daily urine volume of 5−6 l. of a specific gravity of 1000−1002. Treatment of the patient with injections of Pituitrin, Parke, Davis and Co. (200 mg posterior lobe/ml) led Farini to the following conclusion: "...dirò solo che ogni interruzione della cura segno una rapida ascesa nella diuresi ed ogni sua ripresa un repentino abbassamento della curva urinaria..."

This conclusion is borne out by a chart which shows the patient's daily urine output during four months. Similar results were obtained in a second patient whose daily urine volume of 7.5−8.0 l. was decreased by Pituitrin to 2 l. Von den Velden (1913) showed not only −− like Farini —that posterior pituitary extracts controlled the urine flow in patients with diabetes insipidus, but he demonstrated also an inhibitory effect on water diuresis in healthy men thus providing the first indication of the physiological significance of the neurohypophysis for the metabolism of water.

Another advance in the treatment of diabetes insipidus was the introduction of nasal insufflation of posterior pituitary powder (Rutledge and Rynearson, 1939) and that of the long-acting preparation of Pitressin Tannate in oil (Greene and January, 1940).

The field covered in this short review is so great that many reports of considerable historical interest had to be omitted. Moreover, the choice of references was undoubtedly influenced by the greater familiarity of the writer with certain aspects of the subject. An unqualified apology is, therefore, tendered for omissions.

REFERENCES

BOOKS, REVIEWS, AND MONOGRAPHS

Cross, B. A. (1959). Neurophysial control of parturition. *Endocrinology of Reproduction.* Lloyd, C. W. (ed.). Academic Press, New York.

Cross, B. A. (1961). Neural control of lactation. *Milk: the Mammary Gland and Its Secretion.* Konn, S. K. and Cowie, A. T. (eds.). Academic Press, London.

Cushing, H. (1932). *Papers relating to the Pituitary Body, Hypothalamus and Parasympathetic Nervous System.* Charles C. Thomas, Springfield.

du Vigneaud, V. (1954/55). Hormones of the posterior pituitary gland; oxytocin and vasopressin. *The Harvey Lectures,* Series L, pp. 1–26.

Fitzpatrick, R. J. (1966). The posterior pituitary gland and the female reproductive tract. *The Pituitary Gland.* Harris, G. W. and Donovan, B. T. (eds.). Butterworths, London.

Fitzpatrick, R. J. and Walmsley, C. F. (1965). The release of oxytocin during parturition. *Advances in Oxytocin.* Pinkerton, J. H. M. (ed.). Pergamon Press, Oxford.

Heller, H. and Lederis, K. (1962). Characteristics of isolated neurosecretory vesicles from mammalian neural lobes. In *Neurosecretion, Mem. Soc. Endocr.,* **12**: 35–50.

Heller, H. and Spickett, S. G. (1966). The polymorphism of the neurohypophysial hormones. In *Endocrine Genetics, Mem. Soc. Endocr.,* **15**: 89–106.

Knaus, H. (1953). *Die Physiologie der Zeugung des Menschen.* W. Maudrich, Wien.

Knowles, F. G. W. (1963). Techniques in the study of neurosecretion. *Techniques in Endocrine Research.* Eckstein, P. and Knowles, F. G. W. (eds.). Academic Press, London.

Macalister, A. (1889). *Textbook of Human Anatomy.* C. Griffin, London.

Ranson, S. W. and Magoun, H. W. (1939). The hypothalamus. *Ergbn. Physiol.,* **41**: 56–163.

Rolleston, H. D. (1936). *The Endocrine Organs in Health and Disease,* with an historical review. Oxford University Press, London.

Romeis, B. (1940). Hypophyse. *Handbuch der mikroskopischen Anatomie des Menschen.* Möllendorf, W. V. (ed.). Bd. 6, Tl. 3. Springer, Berlin.

Santorini, G. D. (1724). *Observationes Anatomicae.* Gysberg Langerak, Leyden.

Scharrer, E. and Scharrer, B. (1954). Neurosekretion. *Handbuch der mikroskopischen Anatomie des Menschen.* Bargmann, W. (ed.). Bd. 6, Tl. 5. Springer, Berlin.

Sharpey-Schafer, E. (1926). *The Endocrine Organs.* Longmans, London.

van Dyke, H. B. (1936). *The Physiology and Pharmacology of the Pituitary Body.* Vol. 1. University of Chicago Press, Chicago.

Vieussens, R. (1684). *Neurographia Universalis.* J. Certe, Lyons.

von Haller, A. (1766). *Elementa Physiologiae Corporis Humani.* Vol. IV. Grasset et soc., Lausanne.

von Haller, A. (1779). *First Lines of Physiology.* Cullen, W. (trans.). Charles Elliott, Edinburgh.

von Soemmering, S. T. (1778). *Dissertio de basi encephali et originibus nervorum.* A. Vandenhoeck, Göttingen.

Willis, T. (1664). *Cerebri Anatome: Cui accessit nervorum descriptio et usus.* J. Flesher, London.

Winslow, J. B. (1723). *An Anatomical Exposition of the Structure of the Human Body.* Douglas, G. (trans.). Ware et soc., London.

ORIGINAL PAPERS

ACHER, R., LIGHT, A. and DU VIGNEAUD, V. (1958). Purification of oxytocin and vasopressin by way of a protein complex. *J. Biol. Chem.*, **233**: 116–120.

ADAMS, C. W. M. and SLOPER, J. C. (1956). The hypothalamic elaboration of the posterior pituitary principles in man, the rat and dog. Histochemical evidence derived from the performic acid—Alcian blue reaction for cystine. *J. Endocr.*, **13**: 221–228.

ANDERSSON, B. (1951). Some observations on the neurohormonal regulations of milk ejection. *Acta Physiol. Scand.*, **23**: 1–7.

BARER, R., HELLER, H. and LEDERIS, K. (1963). The isolation, identification and properties of the hormonal granules of the neurohypophysis. *Proc. Roy. Soc. B*, **158**: 388–416.

BARGMANN, W. (1949). Über die neurosekretorische Verknüpfung von Hypothalamus und Neurohypophyse. *Z. Zellforsch. mikrosk. Anat.*, **34**: 610–634.

BARGMANN, W. and KNOOP, A. (1957). Elektronmikroskopische Beobachtungen an der Neurohypophyse. *Z. Zellforsch. mikrosk. Anat.*, **46**: 242–254.

BARGMANN, W. and SCHARRER, E. (1951). The site of origin of the hormones of the posterior pituitary. *Amer Scient.*, **39**: 255–259.

BENSON, G. K. and COWIE, A. T. (1956). Lactation in the rat after hypophysial posterior lobectomy. *J. Endocr.*, **14**: 54–65.

BERKELEY, H. J. (1894). The finer anatomy of the infundibular region of the cerebrum, including the pituitary gland. *Brain*, **17**: 515–547.

BLAIR BELL, W. (1909). The pituitary body and the therapeutic value of the infundibular extract in shock, uterine atony and intestinal paresis. *Brit. Med. J.*, **ii**: 1609–1613.

BOURNE, A. and BURN, J. H. (1927). The dosage and action of pituitary extract and of ergot alkaloids on the uterus in labour, with a note on the action of adrenaline. *J. Obstet. Gynaec. Brit. Empire*, **35**: 249–272.

BRUNN, F. (1921). Beitrag zur Kenntniss der Wirkung von Hypophysenextrakten auf den Wasserhaushalt des Frosches. *Z. ges. exp. Med.*, **25**: 170–175.

BUCY, P. C. (1930). The pars nervosa of the bovine hypophysis. *J. Comp. Neurol.*, **50**: 505–519.

CAJAL, S. R. y. (1894). Algunas contribuciones al conocimiento de los ganglios del encéfalo. *An. Soc. exp. Hist. nat. 2 ser.*, **23**: 195–237.

CARLSON, A. J. and MARTIN, L. M. (1911). Contribution to the physiology of lymph. XVII. The supposed presence of the secretion of the hypophysis in the cerebrospinal fluid. *Amer. J. Physiol.*, **29**: 64–75.

CHAMBERS, G. H. (1945). Changes in the rat's posterior pituitary following sodium chloride administration. *Anat. Rec.*, **92**: 391–399.

COCH, J. A., BROVETTO, J., CABOT, H. M., FIELITZ, C. A. and CALDEYRO-BARCIA, R. (1965). Oxytocin-equivalent activity in the plasma of women in labor and during the puerperium. *Amer. J. Obstet. Gynec.*, **91**: 10–17.

COLLIN, R. (1928). Étude histophysiologique du complexe tubero-infundibulo-pituitaire. *Archs. Morph. gén. exp.*, **28**: 1–100.

CONDLIFFE, P. G. (1955). Partition chromatography of oxytocin and vasopressin. *J. Biol. Chem..* **216**: 455–464.

CUSHING, H. and GOETSCH, E. (1910). Concerning the secretion of the infundibular lobe of the pituitary body and its presence in the cerebrospinal fluid. *Amer. J. Physiol.*, **27**: 60–86.

DALE, H. H. (1906). On some physiological actions of ergot. *J. Physiol., Lond.*, **34**: 163–206.
DALE, H. H. (1909). The action of extracts of the pituitary body. *Biochem. J.*, **4**: 427–447.
DALE, H. H. and DUDLEY, H. W. (1921). On the pituitary active principles and histamine. *J. Pharmac. Exp. Ther.*, **18**: 27–42.
DE ROBERTIS, E. and PRIMAVESI, L. (1942). Citología de la neurohipófisis de la rata despues de la privación de agua y de la inyección de pitresina. *Revta. Soc. argent. Biol.*, **18**: 363–366.
DIXON, W. E. and MARSHALL, F. H. A. (1924). The influence of the ovary on pituitary secretion; a probable factor in parturition. *J. Physiol., Lond.*, **49**: 276–288.
DUDLEY, H. W. (1919). Some observations on the active principles of the pituitary gland. *J. Pharmac. Exp. Ther.*, **14**: 295–312.
DUDLEY, H. W. (1923). On the active principles of the pituitary gland. *J. Pharmac. Exp. Ther.*, **21**: 103–122.
DU VIGNEAUD, V., GISH, D. T. and KATSOYANNIS, P. G. (1954). A synthetic preparation possessing biological properties associated with arginine vasopressin. *J. Amer. Chem. Soc.*, **76**: 4751–4752.
DU VIGNEAUD, V., LAWLER, H. C. and POPENOE, A. (1953). Enzymatic cleavage of glycinamide from vasopressin and a proposed structure for the pressor-antidiuretic hormone of the posterior pituitary. *J. Amer. Chem. Soc.*, **75**: 4880–4881.
DU VIGNEAUD, V., RESSLER, C., SWANN, J. M., ROBERTS, C. W., KATSOYANNIS, P. C and GORDON, S. (1953). The synthesis of an octapeptide amide with the hormone activity of oxytocin. *J. Amer. Chem. Soc.*, **75**: 4870–4880.
ELY, F. and PETERSEN, W. E. (1941). Factors involved in the ejection of milk. *J. Dairy Sci.*, **24**: 211–223.
FARINI, F. (1913). Diabete insipido éd opoterapia ipofisaria. *Gazz. Osp. Clin.*, **34**: 1135–1139.
FITZPATRICK, R. J. and WALMSLEY, C. F. (1962). The concentration of oxytocin in bovine blood during parturition. *J. Physiol., Lond.*, **163**: 13–14P.
FOLLEY, S. J. and KNAGGS, G. S. (1965). Levels of oxytocin in the jugular vein blood during parturition. *J. Endocr.*, **33**: 301–315.
GABE, M. (1953). Sur quelques applications de la coloration par la fuchsine-paraldéhyde. *Bull. Microsc. Appl.*, **3**: 153–162.
GAINES, W. L. (1915). A contribution to the physiology of lactation. *Amer. J. Physiol.*, **38**: 285–312.
GERSH, J. (1939). Structure and function of parenchymatous glandular cells in the neurohypophysis of the rat. *Amer. J. Anat.*, **64**: 407–443.
GINSBURG, M. and HELLER, H. (1953). The clearance of injected vasopressin from the circulation and its fate in the body. *J. Endocr.*, **9**: 283–291.
GINSBURG, M. and IRELAND, M. (1966). The role of neurophysin in the transport and release of neurohypophysial hormones. *J. Endocr.*, **35**: 289–298.
GOMEZ, E. T. (1939). Relations of the posterior hypophysis in the maintenance of lactation in hypophysectomised rats. *J. Dairy Sci.*, **22**: 488.
GOMORI, G. (1941). Observations with differential stains on human islets of Langerhans. *Amer. J. Path.*, **17**: 395–406.
GREEN, J. D. (1947). Some aspects of the anatomy and function of the pituitary gland, with a special reference to the neurohypophysis. *Alexander Blair Hosp. Bull.*, **6**: 128–142.

GREENE, J. A. and JANUARY, L. E. (1940). Efficacy of pellets of posterior hypophysis and of pitressin in oil in diabetes insipidus. *Proc. Soc. Exp. Biol. Med.*, **44**: 217–218.

GREVING, R. (1926). Beiträge zur Anatomie der Hypophyse und deren Funktion. II. *Z. ges. Neurol. Psychiat.*, **104**: 466–479.

GUNTHER, M. (1948). The posterior pituitary and labour. *Brit. Med. J.*, **i**: 567.

HARRIS, G. W. (1958). The central nervous system, neurohypophysis and milk ejection. *Proc. Roy. Soc.*, **B149**: 336–353.

HARRIS, G. W. and JACOBSOHN, D. (1952). Functional grafts of the anterior pituitary gland. *Proc. Roy. Soc.*, **B139**: 263–276.

HELLER, H. (1941a). The distribution of the pituitary antidiuretic hormone throughout the vertebrate series. *J. Physiol., Lond.*, **99**: 246–256.

HELLER, H. (1941b). Differentiation of a (amphibian) water balance principle from the antidiuretic principle of the posterior pituitary gland. *J. Physiol., Lond.*, **100**: 125–141.

HELLER, H. (1942). The posterior pituitary principles of a species of reptile *(Tropidonotus natrix)*, with some remarks on the comparative physiology of the posterior pituitary gland generally. *J. Physiol., Lond.*, **101**: 317–326.

HELLER, H. and LEDERIS, K. (1958). Paper chromatography of small amounts of vasopressin and oxytocin. *Nature, Lond.*, **182**: 1231–1232.

HERRING, P. T. (1908). The histological appearance of the mammalian pituitary body. *Quart. J. Exp. Physiol.*, **1**: 121–159.

HERRING, P. T. (1913). Further observations upon the comparative anatomy and physiology of the pituitary body. *Quart. J. Exp. Physiol.*, **6**: 281–285.

HICKEY, R. C., HARE, K. and HARE, R. S. (1941). Some cytological and hormonal changes in the posterior lobe of the rat's pituitary after water deprivation and Stalk section. *Anat. Rec.*, **81**: 319–331.

HILD, W. (1951). Experimentell-morphologische Untersuchengen über das Verhalten der "Neurosekretorischen Bahn" nach Hypophysenstieldurchtrennungen, Eingriffen in den Wasserhaushalt und Belastung der Osmoregulation. *Virchows Arch. path. Anat. Physiol.*, **319**: 526–546.

HILD, W. and ZETLER, G. (1953a). Experimenteller Beweis für die Entstehung der sog. Hypophysenhinterlappenwirkstoffe im Hypothalamus. *Pflügers Arch. ges. Physiol.*, **257**: 169–201.

HILD, W. and ZETLER, G. (1953b). Über die Funktion des Neurosekrets im Zwischenhirn-Neurohypophysensystem als Trägersubstanz für Vasopressin, Adiuretin und Oxytocin. *Z. exp. Med.*, **120**: 236–243.

HOFBAUER, J. (1911). Hypophysenextract als Wehenmittel. *Zentbl. Gynäk.*, **35**: 137–141.

HOGBEN, L. and DE BEER, G. R. (1925). Studies on the pituitary. VI. Localisation and phyletic distribution of active materials. *Quart. J. Exp. Physiol.*, **15**: 163–176.

HOLMES, R. L. and KNOWLES, F. G. W. (1960). "Synaptic vesicles" in the neurohypophysis. *Nature, Lond.*, **185**: 710–711.

HOUGHTON, E. M. and MERRILL, C. H. (1908). The diuretic action of adrenalin and the active principle of the pituitary gland. *J. Amer. Med. Ass.*, **51**: 1849–1854.

HOWELL, W. H. (1898). The physiological effects of extracts of the hypophysis cerebri and infundibular body. *J. Exp. Med.*, **3**: 245–258.

KAMM, O., ALDRICH, T. B., GROTE, I. W., ROWE, L. W. and BUGBEE, E. P. (1928). The active principles of the posterior lobe of the pituitary gland. I. The demonstration of the presence of two active principles. II. The separation of the two active principles and their concentration in the form of potent solid preparations. *J. Amer. Chem. Soc.*, **50**: 573–601.

KNAUS, H. (1926). The action of pituitary extract upon the pregnant uterus of the rabbit. *J. Physiol., Lond.*, **61**: 383–397.
KNAUS, H. (1928). Zur Ursache des Geburtseintrittes. *Münch. med. Wschr.*, **75**: 553–556.
KNOWLES, SIR F. (1965). Evidence for a dual control by neurosecretion of hormone synthesis and hormone release in the pituitary of the dogfish *Scyliorhinus stellaris*. *Phil. Trans. Roy. Soc., Ser.* **B249**: 435–456.
KNOWLTON, F. P. and SILVERMAN, A. C. (1918). The action of pituitary extract on the kidney. *Amer. J. Physiol.*, **47**: 1–12
KRAMER, K., THURAU, K. and DEETJÉN, P. (1960). Hämodynamik des Nierenmarks I. Capilläre Passagezeit, Blutvolumen, Durchblutung, Gewebshäematokrit und O_2-Verbrauch des Nierenmarks *in situ*. *Pflügers Arch. ges. Physiol.*, **270**: 251–269.
LABELLA, F., BEAULIER, C. and REIFFENSTEIN, R. (1962). Evidence for the existence of separate vasopressin and oxytocin-containing granules in the neurohypophysis. *Nature, Lond.*, **193**: 173–174.
LAZO-WASEM, E. A. and WEISEL, G. F. (1952). The comparative effects of fish and beef pituitary extracts on the retention of water by frogs. *Biol. Bull. Mar. Biol. Lab., Woods Hole*, **102**: 25–29.
LEDERIS, K. (1962). Isolation of hormone containing particles from the neurohypophysis of the cod *(Gadus morrhua)*. *Biochem. J.* **84**: 27P.
LEDERIS, K. (1963). A preliminary report on the ultrastructure of the human neurohypophysis. *J. Endocr.*, **27**: 133–135.
LEDERIS, K. (1965). An electron microscopical study of the human neurohypophysis. *Z. Zellforsch. mikrosk. Anat.*, **65**: 847–868.
LEDERIS, K. and HELLER, H. (1960). Intracellular storage of vasopressin and oxytocin in the posterior pituitary lobe. *Proc. 1st. Inter. Congr. Endocr. Acta Endocr., Copenh.* Suppl. **51**, 115–116.
LILIENFIELD, L. S., MAGANZINI, H. G. and BAUER, M. H. (1961). Blood flow in the renal medulla. *Circulation Res.*, **9**: 614–617.
MAGNUS, R. and SCHÄFER, E. A. (1901). The action of pituitary extracts upon the kidney. *J. Physiol., Lond.*, **27**: IX–X.
MAURER, S. and LEWIS, D. (1922). The structure and differentiation of the specific elements of the pars intermedia of the hypophysis of the domestic pig. *J. Exp. Med.*, **36**: 141–156.
MEYER, W. C. (1935). Phylogenetische Ableitung des Nucleus supraopticus vom Nucleus paraventricularis. *Dt. Z. NervHeilk*, **46**: 65–74.
MUNSICK, R. A. (1964). Neurohypophysial hormones of chickens and turkeys. *Endocrinology*, **75**: 104–112.
MUNSICK, R. A., SAWYER, W. H. and VAN DYKE, H. B. (1960). Avian neurohypophysial hormones: pharmacological properties and tentative identification. *Endocrinology*, **66**: 860–871.
OTT, I. and SCOTT, J. C. (1910). The action of infundibulin upon the mammary secretion. *Proc. Soc. Exp. Biol. Med.* **8**: 48–49.
OLIVER, G. and SCHÄFER, E. A. (1895). On the physiological action of extracts of the pituitary body and certain other glandular organs. *J. Physiol., Lond.*, **18**: 277–279.
ORTMANN, R. (1951). Über experimentelle Veränderungen der Morphologie des Hypophysen-Zwischenhirnsystems und die Beziehung der sog. "Gomorisubstanz" zum Adiuretin. *Z. Zellforsch. mikrosk. Anat.*, **36**: 92–140.
PARDOE, A. V. and WEATHERALL, M. (1955). Intracellular localization of oxytocic and vasopressor substances in the pituitary glands of rats. *J. Physiol., Lond.*, **127**: 201–212.

PATON, D. N. and WATSON, A. (1912). The actions of pituitrin, adrenaline and barium on the circulation of the bird. *J. Physiol., Lond.*, **44**: 413–424.
PINES, I. L. (1925a). Über die Innervation der Hypophysis cerebri, I. Mitt. *J. Psychol. Neurol., Lpz.*, **32**: 80–88.
PINES, I. L. (1925b). Über die Innervation der Hypophysis cerebri, II. Mitt. *Z. ges. Neurol. Psychiat.*, **104**: 466–479.
POPENOE, A., LAWLER, H. C. and DU VIGNEAUD, V. (1952). Partial purification and amino acid content of vasopressin from hog posterior pituitary glands. *J. Amer. Chem. Soc.*, **74**: 3713.
PORATH, J. (1957). Application of zone electrophoresis and cellulose in exchange chromatography to the fractionation of posterior pituitary hormones. *Ark. Kemi*, **11**: 259–274.
RETZIUS, G. (1894). Die Neuroglia des Gehirns beim Menschen und bei Säugetieren. *Biol. Unters.*, **6**: 21–24.
ROUSSY, G. and MOSINGER, M. (1934). Étude anatomique et physiologique de l'hypothalamus. *Revue neurol.*, **41**: 848–888.
RUTLEDGE, D. I. and RYNEARSON, E. H. (1939). Diabetes insipidus: treatment by insufflation of powdered posterior pituitary substance. *Proc. Staff Meet. Mayo Clin.* **14**, 443–446.
SCHÄFER, E. A. (1913). On the effect of pituitary and corpus luteum extracts on the mammary gland in the human subject. *Quart. J. Exp. Physiol.*, **6**: 17–19.
SCHÄFER, E. A. and HERRING, P. T. (1908). I. The action of pituitary extracts upon the kidney. *Phil. Trans. Roy. Soc., Ser.* **B199**: 29.
SCHARRER, E. (1928). Die Lichtempfindlichkeit blinder Elritzen. I. Untersuchungen über das Zwischenhirn der Fische. *Z. vergl. Physiol.*, **7**: 1–28.
SCHIEBLER, T. H. (1952). Cytochemische und elektronenmikroskopische Untersuchungen an granulären Fraktionen der Neurohypophyse des Rindes. *Z. Zellforsch. mikrosk. Anat.*, **36**: 563–576.
SELYE, H. and HALL, C. E. (1943). Further studies concerning the actions of sodium chloride on the pituitary. *Anat. Rec.*, **86**: 579–583.
STEHLE, R. L. and FRASER, A. M. (1935). The purification of the pressor and oxytocic hormones of the pituitary gland and some observations on the chemistry of the products. *J. Pharmac. Exp. Ther.*, **55**: 136–151.
STERBA, G. (1961). Fluoreszenzmikroskopische Untersuchungen über die Neurosekretion beim Bachneunauge. *Z. Zellforsch. mikrosk. Anat.*, **55**: 763–789.
STERBA, G. (1964). Grundlagen des histochemischen und biochemischen Nachweises von Neurosekret (= Trägerprotein der Oxytozine) mit Pseudozyanin. *Acta histochem.*, **17**: 268–292.
TELLO, F. (1912). Algunas observaciones sobre la histología de la hipófisis humana. *Trab. Lab. Invest. biol. Univ. Madr.*, **10**: 145–184.
THEOBALD, G. W., GRAHAM, A., CAMPBELL, J., GANGE, P. D. and DRISCOLL, W. J. (1948). The use of post-pituitary extract in physiological amounts in obstetrics. *Brit. Med. J.*, **i**: 123–127.
TUPPY, H. and MICHL, H. (1953). Über die chemische Struktur des Oxytocins. *Mh. Chem.*, **84**: 1011–1020.
VAN DYKE, H. B. and KRAFT, A. (1927). The role of the hypophysis in the initiation of labor. *Amer. J. Physiol.*, **82**: 84–90.
VERNEY, E. B. (1926). The secretion of pituitrin in mammals, as shown by perfusion of the isolated kidney of the dog. *Proc. Roy. Soc. B*, **99**: 487–517.

VERNEY, E. B. (1947). The antidiuretic hormone and the factors which determine its release. *Proc. Roy. Soc. B*, **135**: 25–106.
VON DEN VELDEN, R. (1913). Die Nierenwirkung von Hypophysenextrakten beim Menschen. *Berl. klin. Wschr.*, **50**: 2083–2086.
WEINSTEIN, H., MALAMED, S. and SACHS, H. (1961). Isolation of vasopressin-containing granules from the neurohypophysis of the dog. *Biochim. Biophys. Acta*, **50**, 386–389.

CHAPTER 2

CHEMISTRY OF NEUROHYPOPHYSIAL HORMONES AND THEIR SYNTHETIC ANALOGUES

Luis A. Branda* and Barbara M. Ferrier*

*Laboratory of Polypeptides,
Service of Obstetrical Physiology,
Faculty of Medicine, Montevideo, Uruguay*

UNTIL recently there has been an understandable reticence on the part of workers in the field to treat the neurohypophysial hormones as compounds capable of examination by classical chemical methods, beyond those necessary to establish their structure. The hormones occur naturally in very small amounts, and their isolation from the glands is a lengthy and enormously expensive task. The methods of synthesis of the compounds now worked out make them more available but still not readily accessible compounds. This inaccessibility has meant that much of the knowledge of the chemical nature of the hormones has been collected in the course of studies directed to other ends, principally to establish their structure. Therefore to give an account of their chemistry it is most convenient to describe the elucidation of their structure and their synthesis before attempting to present the most significant of the somewhat isolated and unrelated pieces of information which have been otherwise gathered on their chemical nature.

DETERMINATION OF THE STRUCTURE OF OXYTOCIN AND THE VASOPRESSINS

This problem was taken up in 1932 by du Vigneaud, who followed it to its conclusion in the successful synthesis of oxytocin in 1953 (du Vigneaud *et al.*, 1953c, 1954), of lysine-vasopressin in 1957 (du Vigneaud *et al.*, 1957) and of arginine-vasopressin in 1958 (du Vigneaud *et al.*, 1958).

* Present address: Department of Biochemistry, McMaster University, Hamilton, Ontario, Canada.

Before 1932 there existed some evidence that the hormones were sulfur-containing, polypeptide-like substances of rather low molecular weight. A vital early experiment was the treatment of partially purified oxytocin with cysteine (Sealock and du Vigneaud, 1935), a procedure which inactivates insulin by rupture of disulfide linkages. Oxytocin was not inactivated.* However, when cysteine-treated oxytocin was treated with benzyl-chloride, a reagent which has no effect on oxytocin itself, inactivation occurred. These results gave strong evidence that the sulfur in oxytocin existed in the form of a disulfide linkage, which is cleaved to the dithiol on treatment with cysteine. The thiol groups are benzylated by benzyl chloride and thus re-oxidation to oxytocin is precluded.

The introduction of countercurrent distribution (Craig, 1944) as a laboratory technique facilitated the purification of partially purified hormone fractions (Livermore and du Vigneaud, 1949). The oxytocin obtained after countercurrent distribution between secondary-butyl alcohol and 0.05% acetic acid appeared, by the criterion of its behavior on countercurrent distribution, to be a pure compound. This preparation of oxytocin was found (Pierce and du Vigneaud, 1950a) by chromatography of an acid hydrolysate on a starch column (Moore and Stein, 1949) to contain 8 amino acids: aspartic acid, cystine, glutamic acid, glycine, isoleucine, leucine, proline and tyrosine, and ammonia, the amino acids being present in equimolar proportions and there being 3 moles of ammonia for each mole of any one amino acid. Oxytocin extracted from either beef or pig glands had the same composition. The molecular weight of the purified oxytocin was found to be about 1000 which is compatible with a monomer composed of the quoted amino acids in peptide linkage and the ammonia in amide linkage (Pierce and du Vigneaud, 1950b). More extensive countercurrent distribution did not result in any change in composition. From the countercurrent-purified material a crystalline flavianate was obtained (Pierce *et al.*, 1952).

When one of the pressor fractions obtained from beef posterior pituitary lobes was submitted to countercurrent distribution between n-butyl alcohol and 0.1 M aqueous *p*-toluenesulfonic acid, highly purified vasopressin was obtained (Turner *et al.*, 1951a). When an acid hydrolysate of this preparation was analyzed, the vasopressin was seen to have the same composition as oxytocin, with the exception that the amino acids leucine and isoleucine of oxytocin were replaced by arginine and phenylalanine

* In this chapter, the expression "inactivation" in reference to the neurohypophysial hormones, is used to mean loss of the biological activities which are characteristic of the hormones; i.e. the oxytocic, milk-ejecting, avian vasodepressor, vasoconstrictor and the antidiuretic activities.

in vasopressin. A similar isolation and analysis of a pressor fraction from pig pituitary glands showed that this pressor principle differed from that from beef in that it contained lysine instead of arginine (Popenoe *et al.*, 1952). The two distinct vasopressins were therefore called arginine-vasopressin and lysine-vasopressin. The molecular weight of the vasopressins was assumed to be very close to that of oxytocin since it was known from diffusion studies that the hormones were of approximately the same molecular size.

Of the amino acids known to occur in oxytocin only cystine is oxidized by performic acid (Toennies and Homiller, 1942). The oxidation results in cleavage of the disulfide linkage with the formation of two sulfonic acid groups. The treatment of oxytocin with performic acid did not cause the liberation of cysteic acid or of cysteamide, thus showing that the cystine or cystinamide did not occupy a terminal position in the molecule i.e. both half cystines were involved in peptide linkage. No more than one product could be detected. An acid hydrolysate of performic acid-treated oxytocin was shown to possess the pattern of amino acids characteristic of oxytocin except that 2 moles of cysteic acid were present for each mole of cystine in oxytocin (Mueller *et al.*, 1951).

The sulfur present in oxytocin can be removed by treatment with Raney nickel (Turner *et al.*, 1951b). This results in the replacement of the cystine residue in the original molecule by 2 residues of alanine. No evidence was obtained that more than one desulfurized product was formed, further indicating that the cystine had been involved in a cyclic structure.

In subsequent studies (Mueller *et al.*, 1953) oxytocin was oxidized with bromine water under such conditions that it could be expected that the disulfide group would be oxidatively cleaved to a disulfonic acid and the aromatic ring of the tyrosine residue would be brominated. This reaction was found to yield at least two products, of which one gave dibromotyrosine and cysteic acid in equimolar amounts on hydrolysis, and the other gave cysteic acid, leucine, isoleucine, proline, glutamic acid, aspartic acid, glycine and ammonia, with the amino acids in the ratio 1:1, and the ammonia to each amino acid ratio 3:1. When performic acid-oxidized oxytocin was treated with bromine water, two fragments were isolated with the same amino acid and ammonia composition as those obtained from bromine-water treated oxytocin. The possibility that the cleavage of oxytocin into the two fragments was the result of the action of performic acid was discarded when it was shown that each of the possible small fragments (tyrosyl-cysteic acid and β-sulfoalanyltyrosine) was readily separable from performic acid-oxidized oxytocin (Ressler *et al.*, 1953).

The small fragment obtained from the bromine water treatment was identified as β-sulfoalanyl-dibromotyrosine, since after reaction with 2,4-dinitrofluorobenzene (DNFB, Sanger's reagent), no cysteic acid was identified in the hydrolysate. Treatment of the large fragment with DNFB caused the disappearance of isoleucine in the hydrolysate, showing that the only amino group to be liberated by the action of bromine water was that of the isoleucine residue. On the other hand, isoleucine did not have a free amino group in the performic acid-oxidized oxytocin molecule.

These results showed that the N-terminal sequence of oxytocin is hemicystinyl-tyrosyl-isoleucyl-, that only this one of the two half-cystine residues in oxytocin bears a free amino group, and that the disulfide group of the cystine residue is involved in a cyclic structure.

The determination of the sequence of the remaining amino acids was done by partial hydrolysis studies on oxytocin, desulfurized oxytocin, performic acid oxidized-oxytocin and on the large fragment resulting from the bromine–water treatment of performic acid-oxidized oxytocin, and by a sequence of modified phenylisothiocyanate (Edman) degradations (du Vigneaud *et al.*, 1953 d). A partial structure was established as: cysteinyl-tyrosyl-isoleucyl-glutamyl-aspartyl-cysteinyl-prolyl-leucyl-glycine.

Oxytocin, when hydrolyzed in 1 N hydrochloric acid at 90–100° for 1 hr, loses 1 mole of ammonia (Taylor and du Vigneaud, 1953). When the product of this hydrolysis was submitted to the thiohydantoin carboxyl end-group determination, glycine was shown to have borne a free carboxyl group. By the same test, oxytocin was shown to contain no free carboxyl group (du Vigneaud *et al.*, 1953d). It was also shown that oxytocin is not inactivated or cleaved by carboxypeptidase (Taylor and du Vigneaud, 1953). Thus one of the three ammonia molecules liberated from oxytocin on hydrolysis must exist in the hormone in glycinamide. The other two moles of ammonia were assumed to be located on the β- and γ-carboxyl groups of the aspartic acid and glutamic acid residues respectively. That glutamine and asparagine did occur in the hormone, rather than their isomers was supported by degradative evidence from hydrolysis with papain (Lawler *et al.*, 1954). With these and the further assumptions that all peptide linkages are α, that no small fragment of the molecule had escaped detection in the analyses, and that none of the analytical techniques had caused rearrangements of the molecule, the structure of oxytocin was proposed as the heterodetic cyclic polypeptide amide I (Fig. 1).

It was not long before the validity of this structure was proved by the synthesis of oxytocin.

The same structure was arrived at and proposed independently by Tuppy and Michl (Tuppy, 1953; Tuppy and Michl, 1953), on the basis of some of the earlier findings from du Vigneaud's laboratory together with their own sequence determinations after partial hydrolysis of oxytocin by acid and by a crystalline proteinase from *B. subtilis*.

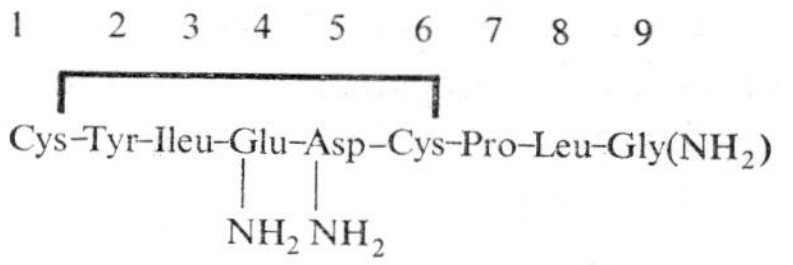

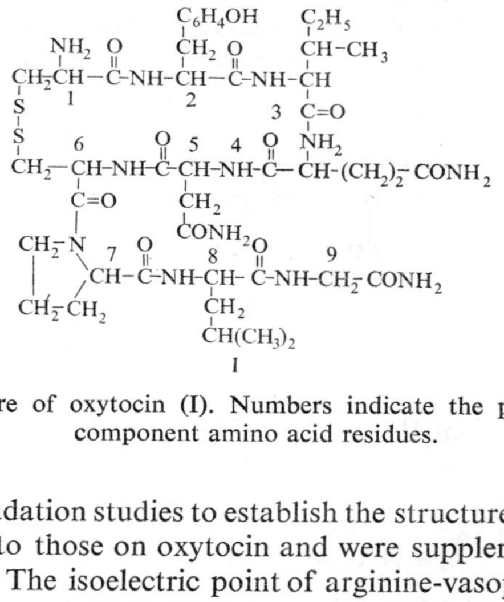

$$\begin{array}{c} 1\quad 2\quad 3\quad 4\quad 5\quad 6\quad 7\quad 8\quad 9 \\ \overline{\text{Cys-Tyr-Ileu-Glu-Asp-Cys}}\text{-Pro-Leu-Gly(NH}_2\text{)} \\ \quad\quad\quad\quad | \quad | \\ \quad\quad\quad\quad \text{NH}_2\;\text{NH}_2 \end{array}$$

FIG. 1. Structure of oxytocin (I). Numbers indicate the positions of the component amino acid residues.

Chemical degradation studies to establish the structure of the vasopressins were similar to those on oxytocin and were supplemented by enzymatic degradation. The isoelectric point of arginine-vasopressin was shown to be 10.85 (Cohn *et al.*, 1941; Taylor *et al.*, 1953), whereas that of oxytocin is 7.7 (Kunkel *et al.*, 1953). This difference can be fully accounted for by the presence of the free guanidino group of arginine in the molecule of arginine-vasopressin. Performic acid oxidation of vasopressin gave an apparently homogeneous product with two cysteic acid residues in place of the cystine residue in the original material. Sanger's technique for the determination of free amino groups was applied to vasopressin and to performic acid-oxidized vasopressin. Performic acid-oxidized vasopressin was treated with bromine water and was also submitted to Edman degradation. From the results of these studies (Popenoe and du Vigneaud, 1953, 1954) and of enzymic degradation (Lawler and du Vigneaud, 1953) a partial sequence was obtained:

cysteinyl-tyrosyl-phenylalanyl-glutamyl-aspartyl-cysteinyl-prolyl-arginyl-glycine.

However, the sequence of the proline, arginine and glycine residues was still in doubt. Trypsin and a crystalline enzyme from *Aspergillus oryzae* released glycinamide from arginine-vasopressin, to leave a fragment containing all the other amino acids. Since only peptide bonds involving the carboxyl group of arginine or lysine are known to be cleaved by trypsin, the C-terminal sequence can be established as -prolyl-arginyl-glycine. Furthermore, the fragment of arginine-vasopressin, which was left after the loss of glycinamide, loses urea under attack by arginase, an enzyme which has no action on the intact hormone (du Vigneaud *et al.*, 1953a).

All these results allowed the structure of arginine-vasopressin to be formulated as the heterodetic cyclic polypeptide amide II (Fig. 2).

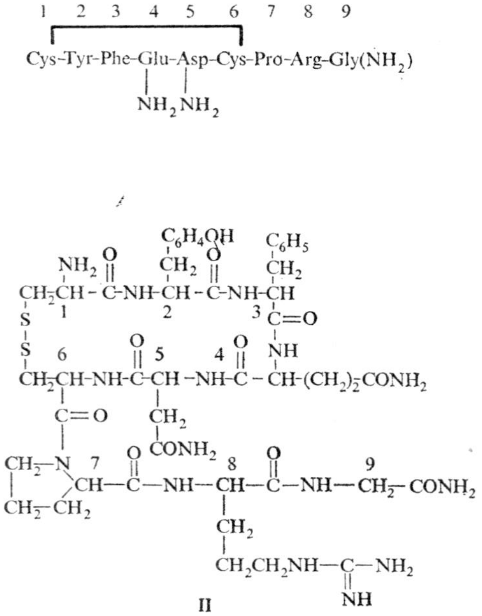

$$\text{1 2 3 4 5 6 7 8 9}$$
$$\overline{\text{Cys-Tyr-Phe-Glu-Asp-Cys}}\text{-Pro-Arg-Gly(NH}_2\text{)}$$
$$\text{NH}_2 \text{ NH}_2$$

FIG. 2. Structure of arginine-vasopressin (II). Numbers indicate positions of the component amino acid residues.

The same conclusions with respect to the structure of arginine-vasopressin were reached independently by Acher and Chauvet (1953, 1954).

Lysine-vasopressin is also hydrolysed by trypsin with the release of glycinamide (du Vigneaud et al., 1953a) and its structure was therefore assumed to be similar to that of arginine-vasopressin with the substitution of a residue of lysine for that of arginine and to be the heterodetic cyclic polypeptide amide III (Fig. 3).

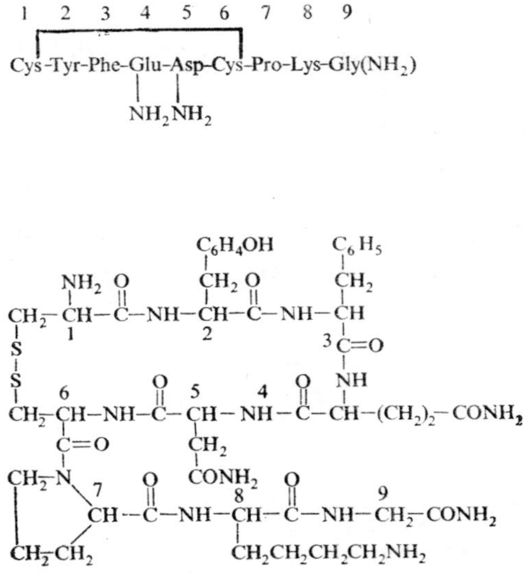

$$\begin{array}{c} 1 \quad 2 \quad 3 \quad 4 \quad 5 \quad 6 \quad 7 \quad 8 \quad 9 \\ \overline{\text{Cys-Tyr-Phe-Glu-Asp-Cys}}\text{-Pro-Lys-Gly(NH}_2) \\ \quad\quad\quad\quad\quad | \quad | \\ \quad\quad\quad\quad\text{NH}_2\text{NH}_2 \end{array}$$

FIG. 3. Structure of lysine-vasopressin (III). Numbers indicate positions of the component amino acid residues.

The same assumptions as those made in formulating the structure of oxytocin were also made in the case of the vasopressins, and conclusive proof of the correctness of the structures was achieved by synthesis.

SYNTHESIS OF OXYTOCIN

The approach to the synthesis of oxytocin made by du Vigneaud and his collaborators (Fig. 4) was based on prior observations on its behavior. Benzyl chloride had been shown to cause inactivation of cysteine-treated oxytocin (Sealock and du Vigneaud, 1935) whereas cysteine treatment alone did not cause inactivation. These results were interpreted to mean that cysteine did cause a reduction of the disulfide group in oxytocin to give the open-chain dithiol, but that reoxidation by air rapidly took place, reforming the disulfide bond and thus regenerating oxytocin. This reoxidation is precluded by the benzylation of the two thiol groups in the reduced compound. Another experiment gave further evidence that oxy-

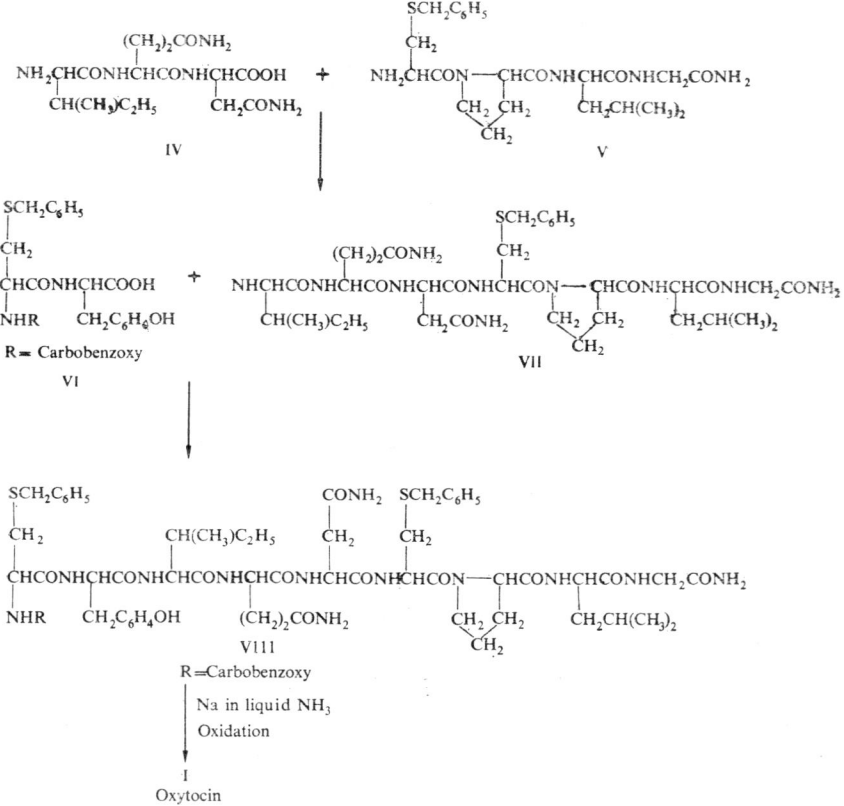

FIG. 4. Synthesis of oxytocin (du Vigneaud et al., 1953c, 1954).

tocin can be readily reduced and regenerated. Oxytocin in liquid ammonia solution was treated with sodium and then with benzyl chloride. The product, which on amino acid analysis was shown to consist of 2 residues of S-benzyl-cysteine and the 7 other amino acid residues of oxytocin, was redissolved in liquid ammonia and reduced with sodium. Subsequent oxidation yielded oxytocin. It therefore appeared that if S,S'-dibenzyloxytoceine* could be synthesized, then oxytocin could be prepared from it. It was also known that amino-protecting carbobenzoxy groups could be removed by the action of sodium in liquid ammonia. As a result of these considerations, it was decided to attempt the synthesis of N-carbobenzoxy-S,S'-dibenzyl-oxytoceine, the nonapeptide amide derivative VIII (Fig. 4). This was accomplished by coupling the tetrapeptide amide S-benzyl-cysteinyl-prolyl-leucyl-glycinamide (V) with isoleucyl-glutaminyl-asparagine (IV) and by condensing the resulting heptapeptide amide (VI) with N-carbobenzoxy-S-benzyl-cysteinyl-tyrosine (VII). Established methods of peptide synthesis were used. Then the protected nonapeptide amide in liquid ammonia was treated with sodium to effect the cleavage of the benzyl and carbobenzoxy groups and the product of this reaction was oxidized without isolation, by aeration of a dilute aqueous solution at pH 6.5. Biological activities characteristic of oxytocin were detected in the solution after aeration. Oxytocin was isolated from this solution by countercurrent distribution. The synthetic material was not distinguishable from natural oxytocin on comparison of their physical, chemical and biological properties (du Vigneaud et al., 1953c, 1954).

Details of several other syntheses of oxytocin have been published subsequently. In all, the final step involves the oxidation of oxytoceine, which however, is synthesized in various ways. Bodanszky and du Vigneaud (1959b) built it up by adding one amino acid residue at a time from the carboxamide-terminal end by the use of the protected amino acid p-nitrophenyl esters. Other syntheses were accomplished by suitable assembly of peptide fragments and with the use of a variety of protecting groups (e.g. Boissonnas et al., 1955; Rudinger et al., 1956; Bodanszky and du Vigneaud, 1959a; Beyerman et al., 1959; Photaki, 1966; Jošt, 1966; Guttmann, 1966). To obtain oxytocin, the protecting groups of the protected nonapeptide amide precursor were removed and the dithiol so produced was oxidized to give the cyclic disulfide. The cleavage of the protecting groups has most frequently been achieved by the action of sodium in liquid ammonia. Refluxing trifluoroacetic acid has been used by Sakakibara et al. (1965) to remove N-carbobenzoxy and S-methoxybenzyl groups, but some hydrolysis of the amide bonds resulted and the yield of oxytocin, as determined by biological assay, was consequently low. Velluz et al. (1956) used the trityl group to protect the amino and mercapto groups. The amino-protecting trityl group was removed by treatment with 5 N hydrochloric acid in acetic acid and the mercapto groups were liberated by the action of 10 N hydrochloric acid in methylene chloride.

---

* It has been suggested that S,S'-dihydrooxytocin and S,S'-dihydrovasopressin be called oxytoceine and vasopresseine respectively (du Vigneaud et al., 1960a).

Anhydrous hydrogen fluoride has also been used as a cleaving agent (Sakakibara and Shimonishi, 1965) and it has been found that potassium can replace sodium in the original method of reduction in liquid ammonia solution (Boissonnas and Huguenin, 1965). For oxidation of oxytoceine to oxytocin, aeration has been the method of choice. Countercurrent distribution has commonly been used for the purification of the oxytocin so obtained. More recently partition chromatography on Sephadex has proved to be equally efficient (Yamashiro, 1964).

SYNTHESIS OF LYSINE-VASOPRESSIN

Material with the biological properties of lysine-vasopressin was first synthesized in 1953. Du Vigneaud, Popenoe and Roeske used a route closely parallel to that of the original synthesis of oxytocin; however the yield was too low to allow for adequate identification of the biologically active material. In a different approach (Fig. 5), a protected nonapeptide derivative (XI) was synthesized by du Vigneaud et al. (1957) by the condensation of N-tosyl-S-benzyl-cysteinyl-tyrosyl-phenylalanyl-glutaminyl-asparagine (IX) and S-benzyl-cysteinyl-prolyl-N^ε-tosyl-lysyl-glycinamide (X). In this case the tosyl group was chosen to protect the amino group because of its superior stability during some of the synthetic steps. The free nonapeptide amide was obtained by the action of sodium in liquid ammonia, and oxidation to the disulfide-containing hormone was achiev-

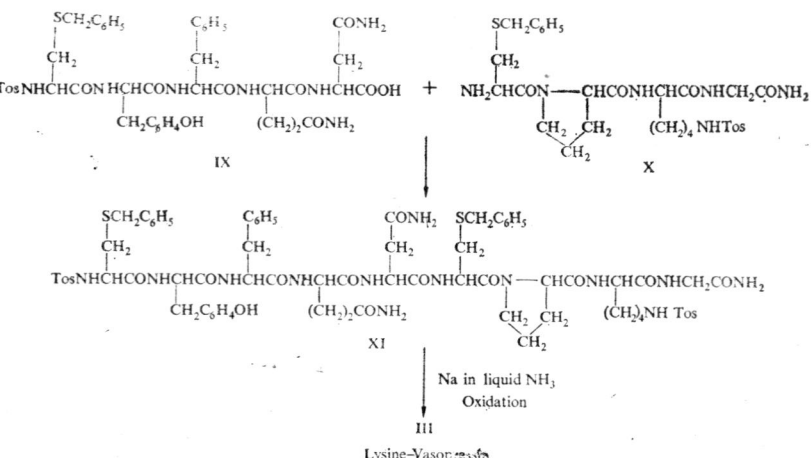

FIG. 5. Synthesis of lysine-vasopressin (du Vigneaud et al., 1957).

ed by aeration of a dilute solution at pH 6.5–6.8. The lysine-vasopressin was isolated by countercurrent distribution and electrophoresis. Some of the steps of this synthesis of lysine-vasopressin were modified by Meienhofer and du Vigneaud (1960) who obtained the protected lysine-vasopresseine (XI) in crystalline form. Further modifications were also introduced into the subsequent stages of reduction, oxidation and purification. After oxidation the solution containing the synthetic hormone was desalted by the use of Amberlite resin IRC-50 (XE-64) and the product was purified by the technique of ion-exchange chromatography. In later syntheses of lysine-vasopressin Boissonnas and Huguenin (1960) and Zaoral (1965b) assembled protected vasopresseines by the combination of different peptide fragments, while Bodanszky et al. (1960) added amino acid residues to ethyl glycinate in a stepwise fashion by the use of carbobenzoxy-amino acid p-nitrophenyl esters, and purified their synthetic lysine-vasopressin by cellulose-block electrophoresis, countercurrent distribution or ion-exchange chromatography.

SYNTHESIS OF ARGININE-VASOPRESSIN

In their first attempts to prepare this compound, du Vigneaud and his coworkers (1954) applied the method used in the synthesis of lysine-vasopressin (1957). Reduction of the nonapeptide derivative, followed by

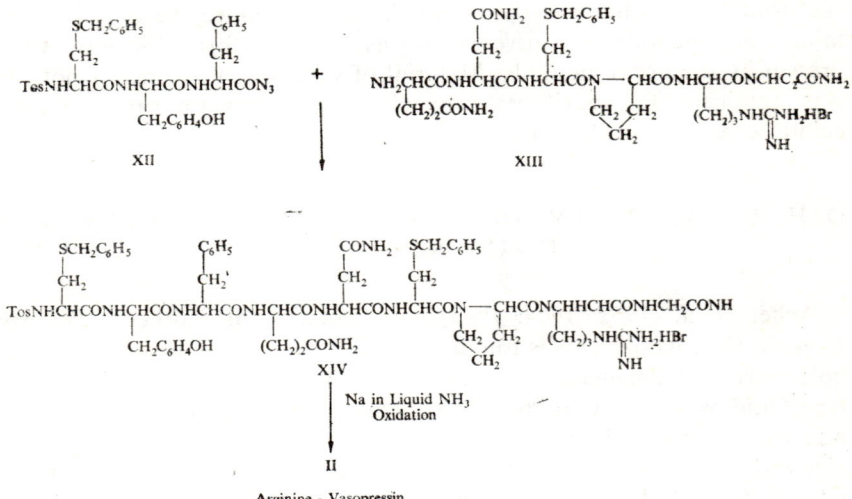

FIG. 6. Synthesis of arginine-vasopressin (du Vigneaud et al., 1958).

oxidative aeration of the free nonapeptide amide gave material which possessed vasopressor activity but to a considerably lower degree than the natural hormone. A more active product with a vasopressor potency similar to that of the natural arginine-vasopressin was obtained (du Vigneaud et al., 1958) when the nonapeptide derivative (XIV) (Fig. 6) was synthesized by the coupling of glutaminyl-asparaginyl-S benzyl-cysteinyl-prolyl-arginyl-glycinamide monohydrobromide (XIII) with the azide of N-tosyl-S-benzyl-cysteinyl-tyrosyl-phenylalanine (XII). The crude synthetic product obtained after cleavage of the protecting groups by sodium in liquid ammonia followed by air-oxidation was subjected to countercurrent distribution and then to cellulose-block electrophoresis. The improvement seen in the second method of synthesis is ascribed to the fact that it precludes the possibility of the formation of anhydro peptides which can result when asparagine is the C-terminal residue in a peptide bond-forming coupling reaction (Gish et al., 1956; Katsoyannis et al., 1958). The anhydro compounds are not readily separable from the parent compounds.

Other synthetic methods of arriving at protected arginine-vasopresseine by assembly of peptide fragments have been reported (e.g. Studer and du Vigneaud, 1960; Huguenin and Boissonnas, 1962; Studer, 1963). Bodanszky et al. (1964) synthesized N-carbobenzoxy-S-benzyl-cysteinyl-tyrosyl-phenylalanyl-glutaminyl-asparaginyl-S-benzyl-cysteinyl-prolyl-N^δ-phthalyl-ornithyl-glycinamide by the p-nitrophenyl ester stepwise method. This compound was treated with hydrazine to remove the phthalyl group and the ornithine residue was then guanylated to produce the arginine-containing nonapeptide derivative which was then transformed into the vasopressin by the usual methods. Material of very high vasopressor potency was obtained after purification by chromatography on carboxymethyl cellulose and Sephadex G-25.

OTHER NATURALLY OCCURRING NEUROHYPOPHYSIAL HORMONES (FIG. 7)

Acher et al. (1962, 1964, 1965) have isolated three other hormones. Isotocin (ichthyotocin) was found in some bony fishes and was shown to be [4-serine, 8-isoleucine]-oxytocin (XV). Mesotocin was obtained from frogs and was shown to be [8-isoleucine]-oxytocin (XVI). Glumitocin was isolated from the neurohypophysis of some cartilagenous fish species and was shown to be [4-serine, 8-glutamine]-oxytocin. Isotocin (Guttmann, 1962; Jöhl et al., 1963) and mesotocin (Jaquenoud and Boissonnas, 1961) have been synthesized by the general methods applied to the synthesis of oxytocin; appropriate nonapeptide derivatives were synthesized by assembly of peptide fragments, and the dithiols produced by removal of the protecting groups were oxidized to give the disulfide-containing hormones.

Arginine-vasotocin (XVIII) was synthesized by Katsoyannis and du Vigneaud (1958) in the course of studies directed to the elucidation of struct-

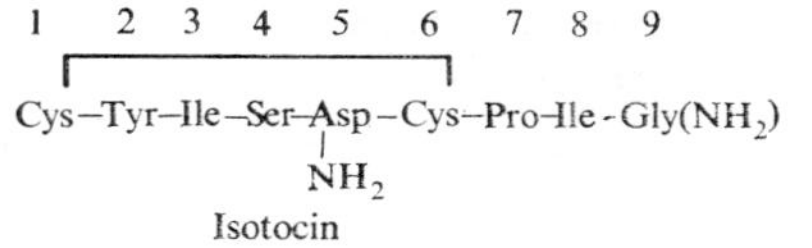

```
              1   2    3    4    5    6   7    8   9
              ┌─────────────────────────┐
XV            Cys—Tyr—Ile—Ser—Asp—Cys—Pro—Ile-Gly(NH₂)
                              │
                             NH₂
                         Isotocin


              ┌─────────────────────────┐
XVI           Cys—Tyr—Ile—Glu—Asp—Cys—Pro—Ile—Gly(NH₂)
                          │    │
                         NH₂  NH₂
                         Mesotocin


              ┌─────────────────────────┐
XVII          Cys—Tyr—Ile—Ser—Asp—Cys—Pro—Glu—Gly (NH₂)
                              │              │
                             NH₂            NH₂
                         Glumitocin


              ┌─────────────────────────┐
XVIII         Cys—Tyr—Ile—Glu—Asp—Cys—Pro—Arg—Gly(NH₂)
                          │    │
                         NH₂  NH₂
                      Arginine - vasotocin
```

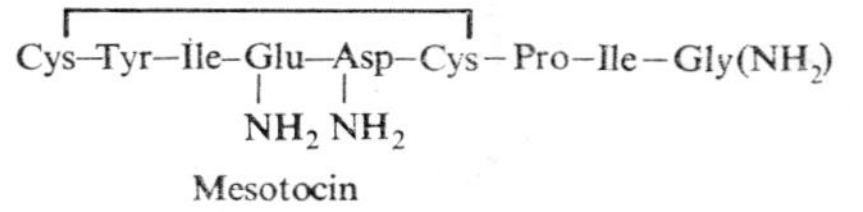

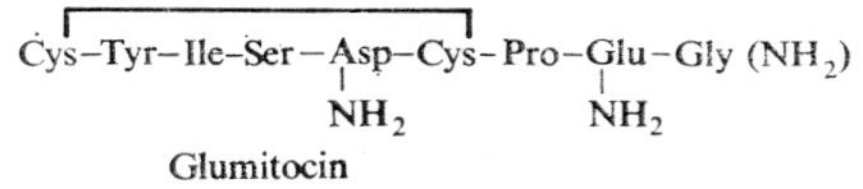

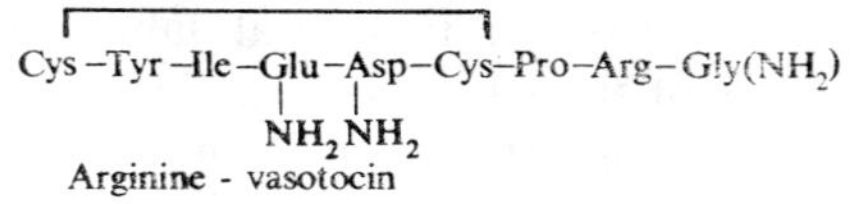

FIG. 7. Naturally occurring neurohypophysial hormones other than oxytocin, arginine-vasopressin and lysine-vasopressin.

ure-activity relationships in oxytocin and the vasopressins. Vasotocin was the name given to compounds possessing the ring of oxytocin and the side chain of a vasopressin (oxypressin, a synthetic compound (Katsoyannis, 1957), is correspondingly made up of the ring of vasopressin and the side chain of oxytocin)*. Subsequent to its synthesis, arginine-

---

* It has been suggested (Walter and du Vigneaud, 1966b) that the ring of oxytocin may be referred to as the *tocin* ring and that of vasopressin as the *pressin* ring.

vasotocin was found to be widely distributed in non-mammalian vertebrates (Acher *et al.*, 1960, 1961; Chauvet *et al.*, 1960a; Heller and Pickering, 1960; Rasmussen and Craig, 1961). The synthesis accomplished by Katsoyannis and du Vigneaud followed a method used for a successful synthesis of arginine-vasopressin (du Vigneaud *et al.*, 1958). The nonapeptide derivative *N*-carbobenzoxy-S-benzyl-cysteinyl-tyrosyl-isoleucyl-glutaminyl-asparaginyl-S-benzyl-cysteinyl-prolyl-arginyl-glycinamide was prepared by reacting the protected amino-terminal tripeptide azide with the protected carboxyl-terminal hexapeptide amide. The hormone was obtained by reduction with sodium in liquid ammonia followed by oxidation by air. It was purified by countercurrent distribution and electrophoresis. Huguenin and Boissonnas (1962) prepared a nonapeptide derivative with a tosylated terminal amino group in their synthesis of arginine-vasotocin. Bodanszky *et al.* (1964) guanylated a nonapeptide amide precursor to [8-ornithine]-vasotocin, to give the corresponding arginine-containing compound, using the method employed by them for the synthesis of arginine-vasopressin.

Perks and Sawyer (1965) have discussed the structure [3-serine, 8-isoleucine]-oxytocin for a peptide isolated from the ray. This compound was synthesized by standard methods (Klieger and Schröder, 1965).

ANALOGUES OF THE NEUROHYPOPHYSIAL HORMONES

After the structures of the neurohypophysial hormones were established by synthesis, there began in several laboratories the systematic synthesis of analogues of these hormones and the comparison of their biological activities with those of the parent hormones. It is hoped that eventually this approach will give an understanding of the relationships between the remarkable biological activities possessed by the hormones and their molecular structures. Up to the present, although what must be the largest series of analogues of natural products has been collected, progress to the desired end has been slow. The complexity of the structure-activity relationships has thereby been emphasized; but the attempts continue.

Appropriate analogues of the cyclic peptide hormones have been prepared in the hope of determining the importance of the size of the 20-membered ring present in the hormones, of the relative position and character of the constituent amino acids, and of the spatial arrangement of the constituents of the molecule. Reviews have been published which list the analogues prepared up till the end of 1964 (Meienhofer, 1962; Schwartz and Livingston, 1964; Law, 1965; Schröder and Lübke, 1966). In Table 1 we list the analogues whose syntheses have been reported subsequently.

Usually the synthesis of the analogues has been achieved by methods used for the synthesis of the hormones. However, Rudinger and Jošt (1964) were obliged to depart from the established paths when they prepared the lactam of tyrosyl-isoleucyl-glutaminyl-asparaginyl-S-(3-carboxypropyl)-cysteinyl-prolyl-leucyl-glycinamide (XXI, Fig. 8), in which one of the sulfur atoms in the disulfide group of deamino-oxytocin was replaced by a methylene group. In deamino-oxytocin ([1-β-mercaptopropionic acid]-oxytocin) the free amino group at position 1 of oxytocin

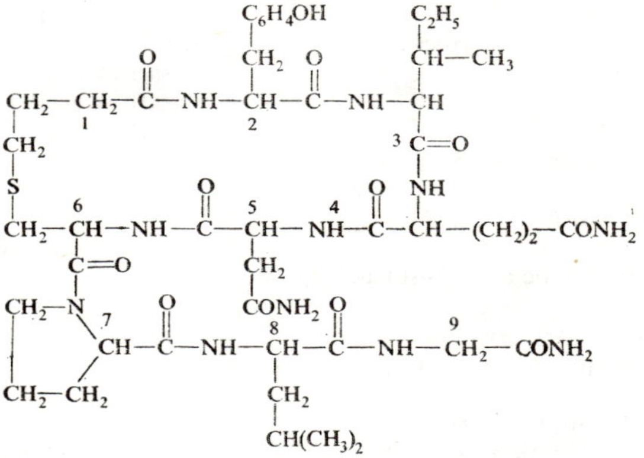

FIG. 8. Structure of "deamino-1-carba-oxytocin" (XXI).

has been replaced by an atom of hydrogen. It possesses biological activities characteristic of oxytocin to a very high degree. The analogue XXI must closely resemble deamino-oxytocin in its topochemical properties since the two compounds differ only in that XXI contains CH_2-S in place of S-S in deamino-oxytocin. This synthesis proved to be very important since it showed that the presence of a disulfide group is not essential for the manifestation of biological activity. This so called "carba" analogue (XXI) of deamino-oxytocin also possesses several of the biological activities of oxytocin to a considerable degree. In the synthesis (Fig. 9) the protected octapeptide amide (XIX) was reduced with sodium in liquid ammonia and alkylated with tertiary-butyl-4-iodobutyrate. The t-butyl ester group was hydrolyzed with acid and the resulting peptide derivative (XX) was cyclized by treatment with N-ethyl-5-phenylisoxazolium-3'-sulfonate (Reagent K) (Woodward et al., 1961).

TABLE 1

SYNTHESES OF ANALOGUES OF OXYTOCIN AND VASOPRESSIN REPORTED SUBSEQUENT TO THOSE LISTED BY SCHRÖDER AND LÜBKE (1966), LAW (1965), SCHWARTZ AND LIVINGSTON (1964), AND MEIENHOFER (1962).

OXYTOCIN
Modifications at position 1

[1-Hemi-D-cystine]-oxytocin	Yamashiro et al. (1966a)
[1-Mercaptoacetic acid]-oxytocin	Jarvis and du Vigneaud (1967)
[1-β-Mercaptobutyric acid]-oxytocin	Schulz and du Vigneaud (1966b)
[1-D-β-Mercaptobutyric acid]-oxytocin	Schulz and du Vigneaud (1966b)
[1-γ-Mercaptobutyric acid]-oxytocin	Jarvis et al. (1965)
[1-Penicillamine]-oxytocin	Schulz and du Vigneaud (1966a)
[1-D-Penicillamine]-oxytocin	Schulz and du Vigneaud (1966a)
[1-Deaminopenicillamine]-oxytocin	Schulz and du Vigneaud (1966a)
Glycyl-glycyl-oxytocin	Kasafírek et al. (1965)
D-Leucyl-oxytocin	Kasafírek et al. (1965)
Leucyl-leucyl-oxytocin	Kasafírek et al (1965)
Phenylalanyl-oxytocin	Kasafírek et al. (1965)
Prolyl-oxytocin	Kasafírek et al. (1965)

Modifications at positions 1 and 2

Deamino-[2-isoleucine]-oxytocin ([1-β-Mercaptopropionic acid, 2-isoleucine]-oxytocin)	Branda et al. (1967)
Deamino-[2-D-tyrosine]-oxytocin ([1-β-Mercaptopropionic acid, 2-D-tyrosine]-oxytocin)	Drabarek and du Vigneaud (1965)

Modifications at positions 1 and 4

Deamino-4-decarboxamido-oxytocin ([1-β-Mercaptopropionic acid, 4-α-aminobutyric acid]-oxytocin)	Branda et al. (1966)
Deamino-[4-valine]-oxytocin ([1-β-Mercaptopropionic acid, 4-valine]-oxytocin)	du Vigneaud et al. (1966)
[1-Mercaptoacetic acid, 4-β-alanine]-oxytocin	Jarvis et al. (1967)

Modifications at positions 1 and 5

Deamino-[5-valine]-oxytocin ([1-β-Mercaptopropionic acid, 5-valine]-oxytocin)	Walter and Schwartz (1966)

Modifications at positions 1 and 6

Oxytoceine (S,S'-Dihydro-oxytocin)	Yamashiro et al. (1966b)
Deamino-oxytoceine ([1-β-Mercaptopropionic acid]-S,S'-dihydro-oxytocin)	Yamashiro et al. (1966b)
[1,6-Selenocystine]-oxytocin	Frank (1964)
Deamino-[1,6-Selenocystine]-oxytocin	Walter and du Vigneaud (1966a)
Deamino-[6-hemi-selenocystine]-oxytocin	Walter and du Vigneaud (1965)

Modifications at positions 1 and 7

Deamino-[7-D-proline]-oxytocin ([1-β-Mercaptopropionic acid, 7-D-proline]-oxytocin)	Ferraro and du Vigneaud (1966)

Modifications at positions 1 and 8
Deamino-[8-alanine]-oxytocin   Walter and du Vigneaud (1966b)
([1-β-Mercaptopropionic acid, 8-alanine]-oxytocin)
Deamino-[8-ornithine]-oxytocin   Huguenin (1966)
([1-β-Mercaptopropionic acid, 8-ornithine]-oxytocin)
Modifications at positions 1, 2 and 4
Deamino-deoxy-4-decarboxamido-oxytocin   Branda and du Vigneaud (1966b)
([1-β-Mercaptopropionic acid, 2-phenylalanine-4-α-aminobutyric acid]-oxytocin)
Modifications at positions 1, 2 and 8
Deamino-deoxy-[8-ornithine]-oxytocin   Huguenin (1966)
([1-β-Mercaptopropionic acid, 2-phenylalanine, 8-ornithine]-oxytocin)
Modifications at positions 1, 4 and 8
Deamino-isotocin   Klieger and Schröder (1965)
([1-β-Mercaptopropionic acid, 4-serine, 8-isoleucine]-oxytocin)
Modifications at positions 1, 2, 3, 4, 5, 6, 7, 8 and 9
D-Oxytocin   Flouret and du Vigneaud (1965)
Modifications at position 2
[2-Isoleucine]-oxytocin   Branda *et al.* (1967)
[2-D-Tyrosine]-oxytocin   Drabarek and du Vigneaud (1965)
Modifications at positions 2 and 4
2-Deoxy-4-decarboxamido-oxytocin   Branda and du Vigneaud (1966b)
([2-Phenylalanine, 4-α-aminobutyric acid]-oxytocin)
Modifications at positions 2 and 8
Deoxy-[8-ornithine]-oxytocin   Huguenin (1964)
([2-Phenylalanine, 8-ornithine]-oxytocin)
Modifications at position 3
[3-Cyclohexylglycine]-oxytocin   Eisler *et al.* (1966)
[3-D-Cyclohexylglycine]-oxytocin   Eisler *et al.* (1966)
[3-Cyclopentylglycine]-oxytocin   Eisler *et al.* (1966)
[3-Diethylalanine]-oxytocin   Eisler *et al.* (1966)
[3-*O*-Methylthreonine]-oxytocin   Chimiak and Rudinger (1965)
Modifications at positions 3 and 8
[3-Serine, 8-isoleucine]-oxytocin   Klieger and Schröder (1965)
Modifications at position 4
[4-β-Alanine]-oxytocin   Manning and du Vigneaud (1965a)
4-Deamido-oxytocin   Photaki and du Vigneaud (1965)
([4-Glutamic acid]-oxytocin)
[4-D-Glutamine]-oxytocin   Dutta and Anand (1965), Dutta *et al.* (1966a)
[4-Glycine]-oxytocin   Fosker and Law (1965)
[4-Valine]-oxytocin   du Vigneaud *et al.* (1966)
Modifications at positions 4 and 5
[4-D-Glutamine, 5-D-asparagine]-oxytocin   Dutta *et al.* (1966a)

Modifications at position 5
[5-D-Asparagine]-oxytocin — Dutta et al. (1966a)
[5-Valine]-oxytocin — Walter and Schwartz (1966)
Modifications at position 6
[6-Hemi-D-cystine]-oxytocin — Manning and du Vigneaud (1965b)
[6-Hemi-selenocystine]-oxytocin — Walter and du Vigneaud (1965)
Modifications at position 7
[7-Hydroxyproline]-oxytocin — Bespalova et al. (1966); Dutta et al. (1966b)
[7-Pipecolic acid]-oxytocin — Bespalova et al. (1966)
[7-D-Proline]-oxytocin — Ferraro and du Vigneaud (1966)
Modifications at position 8
[8-Alanine]-oxytocin — Jaquenoud (1965); Walter and du Vigneaud (1966b)
[8-α-Aminobutyric acid]-oxytocin — Jaquenoud (1965)
[8-Glycine]-oxytocin — Jaquenoud (1965)
Modifications at position 9
[9-Alanine]-oxytocin — Dutta et al. (1966b)
[9-β-Alanine]-oxytocin — Dutta and Anand (1965); Dutta et al. (1966b)

9-Deamido-oxytocin ([9-Glycine]-oxytocin) — Dutta et al. (1966b); Ferrier and du Vigneaud (1966)
9-Decarboxamido-oxytocin — Branda and du Vigneaud (1966a)

VASOPRESSIN
Modifications at position 1
Deamino-arginine-vasopressin ([1-β-Mercaptopropionic acid]-arginine-vasopressin) — Huguenin and Boissonnas (1966)
Glycyl-lysine-vasopressin — Zaoral and Šorm (1965)
Glycyl-glycyl-lysine-vasopressin — Kasafírek et al. (1966)
Glycyl-glycyl-glycyl-lysine-vasopressin — Kasafírek et al. (1966)
Glycyl-prolyl-lysine-vasopressin — Kasafírek et al. (1966)
Leucyl-lysine-vasopressin — Kasafírek et al. (1966)
Leucyl-leucyl-lysine-vasopressin — Kasafírek et al. (1966)
Phenylalanyl-lysine-vasopressin — Kasafírek et al. (1966)
Prolyl-lysine-vasopressin — Kasafírek et al. (1966)
Sarcosyl-glycyl-lysine-vasopressin — Kasafírek et al. (1966)
Tryptophyl-lysine-vasopressin — Kasafírek et al. (1966)
Tyrosyl-lysine-vasopressin — Kasafírek et al. (1966)
Modifications at positions 1 and 2
Deamino-deoxy-arginine-vasopressin ([1-β-Mercaptopropionic acid, 2-phenylalanine]-arginine-vasopressin) — Stürmer et al (1965); Huguenin and Boissonnas (1966)
Glycyl-[2-O-methyl-tyrosine]-lysine-vasopressin — Zaoral and Šorm (1965)
Modifications at positions 1 and 6
Dethio-arginine-vasopressin ([1-Alanine, 6-alanine]-arginine-vasopressin) — Huguenin and Guttmann (1965)
Deamino-dethio-arginine-vasopressin ([1-Propionic acid, 6-alanine]-arginine-vasopressin) — Huguenin and Guttmann (1965)
Dethio-lysine-vasopressin — Huguenin and Guttmann (1965)

([1-Alanine, 6-alanine]-lysine-vasopressin)
Deamino-dethio-lysine-vasopressin   Huguenin and Guttmann (1965)
([1-Propionic acid, 6-alanine]-lysine-vasopressin)
Modifications at positions 1 and 8
Deamino-[8-alanine]-vasopressin   Walter and du Vigneaud (1966b)
([1-β-Mercaptopropionic acid, 8-alanine]-vasopressin;
Deamino-[8-alanine]-oxypressin)
Deamino-[8-ornithine]-vasopressin   Huguenin (1966)
([1-β-Mercaptopropionic acid, 8-ornithine]-vasopressin)
Modifications at positions 1, 2 and 8
Deamino-deoxy-[8-ornithine]-vasopressin   Huguenin (1966)
([1-β-Mercaptopropionic acid, 2-phenylalanine, 8-ornithine]-vasopressin)
Modifications at position 2
[2-O-Propyl-tyrosine]-lysine-vasopressin   Zaoral et al. (1965)
Modifications at positions 2 and 8
Deoxy-[8-ornithine]-vasopressin   Huguenin (1964)
([2-Phenylalanine, 8-ornithine]-vasopressin)
Modifications at position 4
[4-Asparagine]-lysine-vasopressin   Zaoral (1965)
Modifications at position 8
[8-D-Arginine]-vasopressin   Zaoral et al. (1966)
[8-D-Lysine]-vasopressin   Zaoral et al. (1966)
[8-α,γ-Diaminobutyric acid]-vasopressin   Zaoral and Šorm (1966a)
[8-D-α,γ-Diaminobutyric acid]-vasopressin   Zaoral and Šorm (1966b)
[8-Thialysine]-vasopressin   Hermann and Zaoral (1965)
([8-[3-(2-aminoethyl)thio]-alanine]-vasopressin)

Other analogues which do not contain a disulfide group are the 21-membered ring-containing [1,6-djenkolic acid]-oxytocin and [1,6-djenkolic acid]-lysine-vasopressin, in which the S-S group of the hormones has been replaced by S-CH$_2$-S. Highly purified natural oxytocin and lysine-vasopressin were reduced with sodium in liquid ammonia and then treated with stoichiometric amounts of methylene dichloride to form the S-CH$_2$-S bridge (Schwartz, I. L., Howard, J. D., and Livingston, L. M., personal communication).

In the synthesis of analogues several modifications have been introduced at the stage of oxidation of the dithiol compounds to give the cyclic disulfide structures. It was found that in the oxidation by aeration to give deamino-oxytocin the yields were very low, and subsequently potassium ferricyanide was used successfully as the oxidizing agent in this preparation (du Vigneaud et al., 1960b; Hope et al., 1962). It has generally been found that aeration as a method of oxidation to give 1-deamino analogues is not satisfactory. The oxidation is slow and considerable amounts of insoluble material are formed. 1,2-Diiodoethane (Yamashiro et al.,

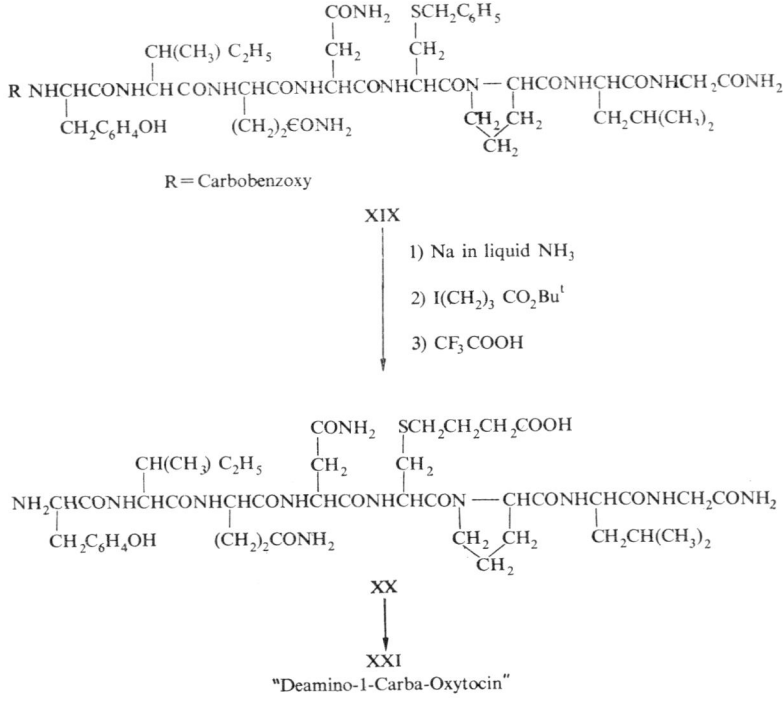

FIG. 9. Synthesis of "deamino-l-carba-oxytocin".

1966a) and hydrogen peroxide (Huguenin and Boissonnas, 1966) have also been used as oxidizing agents in the synthesis of analogues.

For the purification of analogues the techniques of countercurrent distribution, partition chromatography on Sephadex, electrophoresis, and ion-exchange chromatography have been used. Schneider and du Vigneaud (1962), were able to separate oxytocin from its diastereoisomer, [8-D-leucine]-oxytocin, by the use of countercurrent distribution. Further evidence of the sensitivity of this technique and of partition chromatography on Sephadex was given by Yamashiro et al. (1966a), who applied them to the separation of the diastereoisomers, oxytocin and [1-hemi-D-cystine]-oxytocin which were prepared simultaneously by the oxidation of DL-cysteinyl-tyrosyl-isoleucyl-glutaminyl-asparaginyl-cysteinyl-prolyl-leucyl-glycinamide.

From a chemical viewpoint, among the most interesting analogues recently prepared have been D-oxytocin, the enantiomer of the hormone

(Flouret and du Vigneaud, 1965), the "carba" analogue of Rudinger and Jošt (1964) which has already been mentioned, and several in which selenium replaces one or more of the sulfur atoms in oxytocin, or in its deamino analogue. Frank (1964) prepared [1,6-selenocystine]-oxytocin, and Walter and du Vigneaud (1965, 1966a) prepared [6-hemi-selenocystine]-oxytocin, 1-deamino-[6-hemi-selenocystine]-oxytocin, and 1-deamino-[1,6-selenocystine]-oxytocin. All were prepared with the use of selenocystine derivatives by methods that had been applied in the synthesis of oxytocin. The selenium analogues, which are highly potent, may prove to be useful in biological investigations into the mode of action and metabolism of the hormones.

SOME PROPERTIES OF THE HORMONES AND THEIR ANALOGUES

Neurohypophysial hormones in highly purified form are amorphous solids. They have so far resisted attempts to obtain them in crystalline form, although the crystalline flavianate (Pierce et al., 1952) and p-hydroxy-azobenzene-p'-sulfonate (Bodanszky and du Vigneaud, 1959) of oxytocin have been prepared. The successful crystallization of several analogues of oxytocin will yield, it is hoped, considerable information about their molecular arrangement. The homologous compounds deamino-oxytocin ([1-β-mercaptopropionic acid]-oxytocin) and [1-γ-mercaptobutyric acid]-oxytocin were originally crystallized from 1 N acetic acid (Jarvis and du Vigneaud, 1964) and were subsequently both found to be crystallizable from water (Ferrier et al., 1965; Jarvis et al., 1965). Deamino-4-decarboxamido-oxytocin has also been crystallized fuom water (Branda et al., 1966). Deamino-oxytocin has the 20-membered ring which occurs in oxytocin, whereas its homologue [1-γ-mercaptobutyric acid]-oxytocin, as a result of the formal introduction of a methylene group at position 1 adjacent to the disulfide group, has a 21 membered ring. These two analogues are of particular significance in the attempt to relate biological activity to molecular structure, since deamino-oxytocin has several of the activities of oxytocin to an even higher degree than the hormone itself (Hope et al., 1962; Ferrier et al., 1965), whereas [1-γ-mercaptobutyric acid]-oxytocin is practically inactive (Jarvis et al., 1965). Low and Chen (1966) have published some X-ray crystallographic data which include cell dimensions and space groups of the wet and dry form of deamino-oxytocin and of the dry form of [1-γ-mercaptobutyric acid]-oxytocin. The cell dimensions and intensity distribution in the principal planes of both forms of deamino-oxytocin and the dry form of [1-γ-mercaptobutyric acid]-oxytocin are remarkably similar, a finding which suggests that although the two analogues are so strikingly different in biological activity, they do not differ greatly in their molecular conformations in crystalline form.

Crystalline deamino-oxytocin was found to be remarkably stable to heat, as assessed by biological activity (Ferrier et al., 1965). Material of unchanged activity could be obtained in crystalline form from a melt.

The rate at which a molecule diffuses through a membrane depends largely on its molecular volume, shape and degree of solvation and thus also on its flexibility and charge distribution, and ultimately on its chemical structure. Information about these molecular features has been gained by Craig and his coworkers in dialysis studies with the use of calibrated membranes and the thin film dialysis technique. For molecules of the same molecular weight, the more compact the shape, the faster the rate of diffusion. It has therefore been possible to derive some information about the shape of oxytocin, vasopressin and some of their analogues from their relative diffusion rates (Craig and Konigsberg, 1961; Craig, 1964; Craig et al., 1964), since they are all of approximately the same molecular weight. Lysine-vasopressin diffuses considerably more slowly than oxytocin. It has been shown that where there is more than one charge spaced appropriately on a peptide chain, charge interaction will strongly affect the conformation. In the case of vasopressin the basic group in position 8 in the side chain will be repelled by the basic group (NH_2) at position 1 in the ring, thus causing the side chain to be extended. That the nature of the side chain determines this is shown by the fact that [8-histidine]-vasopressin and [8-lysine]-vasotocin both dialyze at a rate similar to vasopressin, whereas deamino-lysine vasopressin diffuses at a rate similar to that of oxytocin and deamino-oxytocin. Oxytocin is much more compact, near to minimal diffusion size, with the chain folded closer to the ring. The dimer of oxytocin also appears to be a compact molecule, probably due to some degree of folding. Deamino-oxytocin diffuses at much the same rate as oxytocin, showing that in the case of oxytocin the amino group of the half-cystine residue at position 1 is not involved in major shape-determining interactions.

It appears that in oxytocin small changes in the ring may greatly influence its diffusional properties. The rate of diffusion of [8-D-leucine]-oxytocin does not differ markedly from that of oxytocin, whereas [1-hemi-D-cystine]-oxytocin, in which the configuration about the α-carbon of the half-cystine residue at position 1 has been changed, diffuses considerably more slowly, as does [1-hemi-homocystine]-oxytocin in which the ring has been enlarged by one methylene unit. Deamino-oxytocin and *N*-carbamoyl-oxytocin dialyze at similar rates. This further suggests that the ring of 20 atoms may be the principal rate determining unit in this case.

These dialysis studies have been done in dilute acidic solutions and different molecular shapes have been assigned to oxytocin and vasopressin on the basis of the possibility of repulsion between the amino group at position 1 and the basic group at position 8 in vasopressin. However, at physiological pH these conformational differences may not exist since the amino group at position 1 in the hormones has an unusually low pK value (6.3) and would thus be nucleophilic at pH 7.4.

Oxytocin and vasopressin appear to be stored in the neurohypophysis in the form of a protein complex. This complex, usually called the van Dyke protein, can be extracted from the neurohypophysis under mild conditions (van Dyke et al., 1942) and can subsequently be dissociated by dialysis against acetic acid, electrodialysis, countercurrent distribution, precipitation of the protein component by trichloroacetic acid (Acher et al., 1956; Acher and Fromageot, 1957) and gel filtration on Sephadex G-25 with the use of 0.1 N formic acid as eluent (Lindner, Elmquist and Porath, 1958; Hope et al., 1963; Frankland et al., 1966). The protein, named neurophysin (Chauvet et al., 1960b), has been shown to consist of at least 4 fractions all of which are capable of binding oxytocin and vasopressin (Breslow and Abrash, 1966). The complex may be reconstituted from its protein and polypeptide components. A complex from a purified protein fraction and oxytocin and vasopressin has been obtained in crystalline form (Hollenberg and Hope, 1966). The van Dyke protein obtained from sheep pituitaries can be dissociated by trichloroacetic acid, the components purified by chromatography, and then reconstituted, where upon 90% of the original biological activity is restored to the complex (Chauvet et al., 1960b). Neurophysin in solution has been used for the isolation and purification of oxytocin and vasopressin (Takabatake and Sachs, 1964), and a new modification in its use for the purification of vasopressin has recently been described (Portanova and Sachs, 1967). Neurophysin is coupled to cellulose and the cellulose-neurophysin is used as a specific adsorbent for the hormone which can subsequently be eluted.

Ginsburg and Ireland (1965) have found that up to 7 moles of oxytocin or 4 moles of arginine-vasopressin may be bound to each mole of neurophysin. However, Breslow and Abrash (1966) have more recently reported from results of thin film dialysis studies that a maximum of 2 moles of oxytocin are bound to each mole of protein, with an apparent intrinsic binding constant of 1.8×10^5. The addition of oxytocin or lysine-vasopressin in equivalent amounts to neurophysin results in the binding of equal amounts of the two hormones. When a mixture of equivalent proportions of the hormones is added, the total amount of polypeptide bound remains the same, each hormone making up half of the total. Thus it appears that the affinities of oxytocin and lysine-vasopressin for neurophysin are essentially the same, and that their binding is competitive at identical sites.

The nature of the binding in the complex has aroused considerable interest. The bonds appear to be electrostatic in nature. That the free amino group of the half cystine residue at position 1 in the hormone is involved, has been convincingly stated on the basis of the fact that deamino-oxytocin does not bind to neurophysin (Stouffer et al., 1963; Breslow and Abrash, 1966). The study of the binding of other analogues of oxytocin to neurophysin has given more information about which factors in the polypeptide molecules may influence their binding (Breslow and Abrash, 1966). Stereochemical factors are obviously important since the enantiomer of oxytocin does not bind to neurophysin. It appears that the nature of the amino acid residue at position 2 is very important and that the existence of the possibility of $\pi-\pi$ interactions between the aromatic ring at position 2 in oxytocin with suitable groups in the protein may facilitate binding. These conclusions were reached when it was shown that [2-glycine]-oxytocin does not detectably bind to neurophysin, whereas the binding constants of 2-deoxy-oxytocin ([2-phenylalanine]-oxytocin) and oxytocin are of the same order. [1-Hemi-homocystine]-oxytocin, in which a methylene group has been formally introduced at position 1, adjacent to the disulfide group, has a binding constant which is not distinguishable from that of oxytocin. Furthermore, [2-isoleucine]-oxytocin, which would permit hydrophobic interactions but preclude $\pi-\pi$ interactions at position 2 of the peptide, does not bind to neurophysin. However, topochemical factors must also be involved since [2-D-tyrosine]-oxytocin does not bind. The nature of the amino acid residue at position 3 in oxytocin is also important since replacement of the isoleucine residue in the hormone by a glycine residue in [3-glycine]-oxytocin significantly reduces the binding capacity, whereas [4-glycine]-oxytocin binds almost as well as oxytocin.

From the fact that the neurophysin-hormone reaction is pH dependent (Ginsburg and Ireland, 1964) and from the results of titration studies (Breslow and Abrash, 1966) it is suggested that a bond is formed between the protonated amino group at position 1 in the hormone and an unprotonated carboxyl group in the protein. It is also suggested that the importance of the residues at positions 2 and 3 may lie in their possible ability to provide a non-polar environment for such an electrostatic bond and so enhance its strength. However, some of the results of the studies of the binding of analogues of oxytocin make it clear that other factors must be involved. Breslow and Abrash make the point that the combination of neurophysin with polypeptide hormones provides an unusually simple system for the study of protein-protein interactions. A further point may be added that this study is a good example of the powerful possibilities which exist when a range of analogues of natural products is at hand.

In studies which are among the most revealing about the chemical nature of oxytocin and vasopressin, Yamashiro et al. (1965), found that another compound was gradually formed when an aqueous acetone solution of oxytocin was allowed to stand for a few days. The compound was chromatographically distinct from oxytocin and similar to a by-product of the oxidation of oxytoceine by the Weygand reagent (1,2-diiodoethane in 60% aqueous acetone). It was subsequently proved that the new compound is a condensation product of oxytocin and acetone with elementary and amino acid analyses corresponding to an isopropylidene-oxytocin. The formation of "acetone-oxytocin" could be followed polarimetrically (the optical rotation of the solution becomes less negative) or from a parallel fall in avian vasodepressor activity. Acetone-oxytocin in solution decomposes slightly at room temperature, but in solid form it is a stable compound and may be a very satisfactory form in which to store oxytocin, since the hormone can be quantitatively regenerated from it by treatment with 0.25% acetic acid at 90° for 30 min. Similar results were obtained when the reaction of acetone with lysine vasopressin was examined (Yamashiro et al., 1967)

Work is under way to establish the structure of the "acetone-hormone" compounds. It is suspected that the free amino group at position 1 in the polypeptides is involved, since deamino-oxytocin and deamino-lysine-vasopressin appear not to react with acetone. The 2,2-dimethyl-4-imidazolidinone and the 5-amino-2,2-dimethyloxazolidine appear likely possibilities for the structures. Evidence gained from the examination of model compounds favors the former in which an isopropylidine moiety bridges the nitrogen of the amino group at position 1 and the nitrogen of the peptide bond between the half cystine residue at position 1 and the tyrosine residue at position 2.

Another reaction in which the free amino group at position 1 in oxytocin and lysine-vasopressin may be involved is the formation of 1:1 complexes with cupric ions. This is thought to be so since neither N-acetyl-lysine-vasopressin nor deamino-oxytocin form copper complexes. The phenolic hydroxyl group of the tyrosine residue is not involved since a copper complex is formed by 2-deoxy-oxytocin ([2-phenylalanine]-oxytocin) (Breslow, 1961; Campbell et al., 1963). The four ligands of the cupric ion appear to be attached to the terminal amino group and to three peptide or amide bonds.

The reactivities of the amino group at position 1 and the phenolic hydroxyl group at position 2 in oxytocin have been demonstrated by their carbamylation (Smyth, 1965). The O-carbamyl group at position 2 in N,O-dicarbamyloxytocin undergoes slow hydrolysis at pH 7.4 at 37° to give N-carbamyloxytocin.

The S,S'-dihydro-derivatives of oxytocin and of vasopressins—oxytoceine and vasopresseines—are key intermediates in the synthesis of the hormones but are not isolated during the synthesis. Evidence for the formation of oxytoceine by the action of excess cysteine on oxytocin was presented by Sealock and du Vigneaud (1935). It has proved to be a refractory compound due to its very ready oxidation in air. Yamashiro et al. (1966b), found that it could be isolated by partition chromatography on Sephadex at 0° with the use of a solvent acidified with strong acid (e. g. trifluoracetic acid) containing a metal complexing agent (EDTA). The compound so obtained was not detectably contaminated by oxytocin.

Deamino-oxytoceine was also prepared. It is more resistant to oxidation than is oxytoceine, as was already suspected from the fact that oxidation conditions which are satisfactory in the synthesis of oxytocin, give poor yields of deamino-oxytocin (Hope et al., 1962).

In order to determine whether oxytoceine possessed some of the biological activities of oxytocin, it was necessary to find conditions under which the reduced compound was stable in solution. The thiol content of a solution of 2 μg/ml of oxytoceine in a 0.9% sodium chloride solution containing 0.25% acetic acid and 10^{-4}M EDTA (pH 2.97) remained unchanged for 24 hours. This solution had a significant avian vasodepressor activity. The responses were lower and more protracted than those to oxytocin and this suggests that the dithiol compound may be oxidized to the disulfide-containing oxytocin *in vivo*.

During the oxidation of dithiol-containing polypeptides to give the corresponding disulfides, cyclic dimers of parallel or antiparallel structures (Fig. 10), or linear higher polymers may be formed. The formation of higher polymers is minimal in dilute solution. The relative proportion in which monomer and dimers are formed depends on the concentration of the solution and the distance between the two mercaptoamino acid residues in the peptide chains (Heaton et al., 1956). Experiments with cysteinyl-(glycyl)$_n$-cysteine show that optimal monomer formation occurs in the hexapeptide (n=4) to give a 20-membered ring. Thus the formation of the 20-membered ring-containing oxytocin and vasopressin is probably favored over their dimeric forms. However, it does appear that dimers of the hormones are produced to some extent during isolation from their natural source, when the monomers are kept in dilute alkaline solution (Ressler, 1959), during synthesis of the hormones, and on storage. The structure of a dimer of lysine-vasopressin obtained by repeated lyophilization from weakly basic solutions (Schally

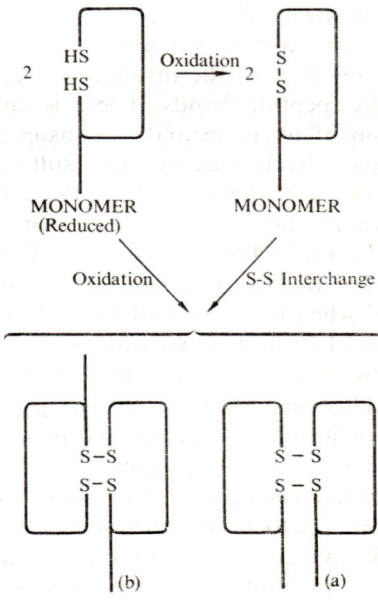

FIG. 10. Parallel (a) and antiparallel (b) dimers formed from cyclic disulfides.

and Guillemin, 1964) has been established (Schally and Barrett, 1965). That the compound was dimeric was shown by using thin film dialysis to determine its molecular weight, and that it was cyclic was shown by the absence of detectable sulfhydryl groups. That the dimer was of a cyclic antiparallel structure was ingeniously established by the examination of the products of chymotryptic hydrolysis. The enzyme chymotrypsin preferentially hydrolyzes peptide bonds on the carboxyl side of aromatic amino acid residues. The composition of fragments so produced by hydrolysis of lysine-vasopressin dimer were only compatible with an antiparallel cyclic structure.

The disulfide group of oxytocin and the vasopressins, as described earlier, can be reversibly reduced to give the dithiol compound (Gordon and du Vigneaud, 1953) by a variety of reagents including thiol-containing compounds such as cysteine, thioglycolic acid, and glutathione (Sealock and du Vigneaud, 1935; Dicker and Greenbaum, 1958). It can be oxidized by performic acid to give the disulfonic acid (Mueller et al., 1951; Popenoe and du Vigneaud, 1953) and it can be replaced by hydrogen atoms by the action of Raney nickel to give dethio-oxytocin ([1,6-dialanyl]-oxytocin, Turner et al., 1951b) and dethio-vasopressin ([1,6-dialanyl]-vasopressin, Fong et al., 1964).

The ring of the hormones can be cleaved by several methods other than by reduction or removal of the disulfide bridge, or by simple chemical hydrolysis of the peptide bonds. There is considerable chemical interest in the reaction of oxytocin and the vasopressins with bromine water. This reagent oxidatively cleaves the disulfide group to give the disulfonic acid, it brominates the aromatic ring of the tyrosine residue, and subsequently cleaves the tyrosyl-isoleucyl or tyrosyl-phenylalanyl bonds (Mueller et al., 1953; Popenoe and du Vigneaud, 1953). That bromination of the aromatic ring of tyrosine does not in itself cause fragmentation was proved when two atoms of bromine were introduced into the ring in performic acid-oxidized oxytocin (i.e. the disulfonic acid derivative) without otherwise altering the molecule detectably (Ressler and du Vigneaud, 1954). This was achieved by carrying out the bromination in glacial acetic acid or in dilute aqueous hydrobromic acid. The brominated product was subsequently fragmented by the action of bromine water. However, when halogenation of the ring of the tyrosyl residue in performic acid-oxidized oxytocin was precluded by previously converting the phenolic hydroxyl group into its dinitrophenyl ether, bromine water had no action on the molecule. It therefore appears that the presence of the bromine atoms in the tyrosyl residue facilitates the subsequent cleavage of the peptide bond involving its carboxyl group.

In certain analogues it has been found that cleavage of some peptide bonds by acidic hydrolysis is less easy than is generally the case. It was found to be necessary to prolong the hydrolysis of [4-valine]-oxytocin, deamino-[4-valine]-oxytocin (du Vigneaud et al., 1966), [2-isoleucine]-oxytocin and deamino-[2-isoleucine]-oxytocin (Branda et al., 1967), in order to complete the cleavage of the isoleucyl-valyl and isoleucyl-isoleucyl bonds. It had previously been found (Harfenist, 1953) that the isoleucyl-valyl bond in insulin is difficult to hydrolyze.

As with many biologically important compounds, the effects of radiation on lysine-vasopressin have been examined. Almost complete loss of biological activity results and the destruction of amino acids occurs. Cystine is the most susceptible amino acid. The inactivation occurs more rapidly in air than in nitrogen, probably due to the chemical action of ozone (Odell et al., 1966).

The enzymic destruction of oxytocin and the vasopressins has received some attention. The half-lives of the hormones in the body are short largely due to inactivation in the tissues, particularly the liver and kidneys. There is evidence that the hormones are first reduced to the dithiol form by the action of a glutathione-requiring transhydrogenase and subsequently degraded by aminopeptidase action (Rychlík, 1964; Bartošek et al., 1964). During pregnancy a new cystinaminopeptidase called "oxytocinase" appears in the blood of primates. This oxytocinase inactivates oxytocin by cleavage of the peptide bond between the half-cystine residue at position 1 and the tyrosine residue at position 2 (Tuppy and Nesvadba, 1957). The open chain polypeptide which results, tyrosyl-isoleucyl-glutaminyl-asparaginyl-S-(S-cysteine)-cysteinyl-prolyl-leucyl-glycinamide has been independently synthesized, by oxidizing a mixture of the octapeptide, tyrosyl-isoleucyl-glutaminyl-asparaginyl-cysteinyl-prolyl-leucyl-glycinamide and cysteine (Ferrier and Branda, 1966).* Deamino-oxytocin, lacking a free amino group, is not inactivated or degraded by plasma oxytocinase (Golubow et al., 1963).

It is clear that in biological studies, isotopically labelled hormones may yield much information about the function, action and fate of the hormones in the body, and several preparations have been described. Random labelling of oxytocin and lysine-vasopressin by exposure to tritium gas according to the method of Wilzbach (1957) has been attempted. Oxytocin of somewhat lowered biological activity and low specific radioactivity was obtained (du Vigneaud et al., 1962), and the yield of tritiated lysine vasopressin was extremely low (Fong et al., 1959). When Fong and coworkers (1960) applied a modified Wilzbach procedure to the tritiation of arginine-vasopressin their product had high specific radioactivity and the full biological activity of the hormone. A specifically labelled oxytocin was prepared by incorporating tritium labelled leucine in the total synthesis (du Vigneaud et al., 1962). This oxytocin has been used to demonstrate the effectiveness of countercurrent distribution as a means to separate oxytocin from its diastereoisomers [1-hemi-D-cystine]-oxytocin and [8-D-leucine]-oxytocin. Carlsson and Sjöholm (1966) have achieved the syn-

---

* Sjöholm (1964) has reported that the degradation proceeds somewhat differently in that the molecule is first attacked at the tyrosyl-isoleucyl bond and that at least the first three N-terminal amino acid residues are cleaved. However, the oxytocinase preparation with which Sjöholm worked was considerably less pure than that of Tuppy.

thesis of specifically tritiated oxytocin and lysine-vasopressin by the *p*-nitrophenyl ester stepwise method with the incorporation of a tritiated tyrosine residue. A specific tritiation of oxytocin itself has been described by Agishi and Dingman (1965). Oxytocin was treated with iodine to yield an iodinated product containing 1 mole of iodine for each mole of the hormone. Catalytic tritiation subsequently gave two tritiated peptides, one of which, on purification, had the biological potency of oxytocin, the other appeared to be polymeric. Much less successful were attempts (Gilliland and Prout, 1965a) to prepare a radioiodinated oxytocin by iodination of oxytocin by the method used to label human growth hormone. At least 7 products were obtained only one of which corresponded to oxytocin.

A recent development in the field of the posterior pituitary peptide hormones has been the demonstration of their ability to provoke the production of specific antibodies, both when the hormones are administered alone or in conjugation with larger protein molecules. The first evidence that the production of antibodies can be induced by natural octapeptides without prior conjugation was presented by Gilliland and Prout (1965b). That the administration of oxytocin to rabbits produced specific antibodies was shown by the subsequent association of ^{131}I-oxytocin and the γ-globulin of immune rabbit serum, and by the demonstration by autoradiography of ^{131}I-oxytocin in the precipitin arc of the γ-globulin. The association was inhibited by oxytocin but not by lysine-vasopressin.

Holländer *et al.* (1966) demonstrated the formation in rabbits of antibodies to oxytocin or vasopressin which prior to administration had been conjugated to rabbit serum albumin, by the action of a water-soluble carbodiimide. The antibody to oxytocin-albumin seems to inactivate oxytocin, but lysine-vasopressin is not inactivated by the antibody to its albumin-conjugate. Bashore (1967) has developed a complement fixation test for the immunoassay of oxytocin with the use of oxytocin-albumin antibodies. Permutt *et al.* (1966) have also produced lysine-vasopressin-albumin antibodies. In studies on the inhibition of the ^{125}I- or ^{131}I-lysine-vasopressin immunoprecipitation reaction they found that unlabelled lysine-vasopressin as an inhibitor could be detected in quantities as low as 15 pg. To inhibit the reaction equally, 1.4 times as much arginine-vasopressin, 3.3 times as much [2-phenylalanine]-lysine-vasopressin and 4000 times as much oxytocin were needed. Bovine or human serum albumin did not inhibit the immunoprecipitation reaction.

Roth *et al.* (1966) have found antibodies to vasopressin in one man who was receiving the hormone as treatment of diabetes insipidus.

It is apparent that for many purposes, the series of oxytocin, the vasopressins, and their analogues can provide a valuable model system. Vision may be cleared far beyond the confines of the subject of the neurohypophysial hormones by further study of their chemical, biochemical, physiological and pharmacological behavior.

REFERENCES

BOOKS, REVIEWS, AND MONOGRAPHS

ACHER, R. and FROMAGEOT, C. (1957). The relationships of oxytocin and vasopressin to active proteins of posterior pituitary origin. In *The Neurohypophysis* pp. 39–48. Heller, H. (ed.). Butterworths London.
LAW, H. D. (1965). Polypeptides of medicinal interest. In *Progr. Med. Chem.* Vol. 4, pp. 86–154. Ellis, G. P., and West, G. B. (eds.). Butterworths, London.
MEIENHOFER, J. (1962). Synthesis of biologically active peptides. *Chimia*, 16: 385–414.
RYCHLÍK, I. (1964). Inactivation of oxytocin and vasopressin by tissue enzymes: a basis for the design of analogues. *Oxytocin, Vasopressin and their Structural Analogues* pp. 153–162. Rudinger, J. (ed.). Proc. 2nd Int. Pharmacol. Meeting, Pergamon Press, Oxford.
SCHRÖDER, E. and LÜBKE, K. (1966). *The Peptides* 1st ed., pp. 320–335, 366–375. Academic Press, New York and London.
SCHWARTZ, I. L. and LIVINGSTON, L. M. (1964). Cellular and molecular aspects of the antidiuretic action of vasopressins and related peptides. *Vitamins and Hormones* Vol. 22, pp. 261–358. Harris, R. S., Wool, I. G., and Loraine, J. A. (eds.).
STOUFFER, J. E., HOPE, D. B. and DU VIGNEAUD, V. (1963). Neurophysin, oxytocin and desamino-oxytocin. In *Perspectives in Biology* pp. 75–80. Cori, C. F., Foglia, V. G., Leloir, L. F. and Ochoa, S. (eds.). Elsevier, Amsterdam.

ORIGINAL PAPERS

ACHER, R. and CHAUVET, J. (1953). Structure of ox vasopressin. *Biochim. Biophys. Acta*, 12: 487–488.
ACHER, R. and CHAUVET, J. (1954). Structure of ox vasopressin. *Biochim. Biophys. Acta*, 14: 421–429.
ACHER, R., CHAUVET, J., CHAUVET, M. T. and CREPY, D. (1962). The neurohypophysial hormones of fish: isolation of a vasotocin from the bib *(Gadus Luscus L.)*. *Biochim. Biophys. Acta*, 51: 419–420.
ACHER, R., CHAUVET, J., CHAUVET, M.T. and CREPY, D. (1961). Isolation of a new neurohypophysial hormone, isotocin, present in bony fishes. *Biochim. Biophys. Acta*, 58: 624–625.
ACHER, R., CHAUVET, J., CHAUVET, M. T. and CREPY, D. (1964). Phylogeny of the neurohypophysial peptides: isolation of mesotocin (Ileu$_8$-oxytocin) from the frog, intermediary between the Ser$_4$-Ileu$_8$-oxytocin of the bony fishes and the oxytocin of the mammals. *Biochim. Biophys. Acta*, 90: 613–615.
ACHER, R., CHAUVET, J., CHAUVET, M. T. and CREPY, D. (1965). Phylogeny of the neurohypophysial peptides: isolation of a new hormone, glumitocin (Ser$_4$-Gln$_8$-oxytocin) present in a cartilagenous fish, the ray. *Biochim. Biophys. Acta*, 107: 393–396.

ACHER, R., CHAUVET, J., LENCI, M. T., MOREL, F. and MAETZ, J. (1960). Presence of a vasotocin in the neurohypophysis of the frog (*Rana esculenta* L.). *Biochim. Biophys. Acta*, **42**: 379–380.

ACHER, R., CHAUVET, J. and OLIVRY, G. (1956). Existence of a single posterior hypophysis hormone. I. Relations between oxytocin, vasopressin and van Dyke's protein from ox posterior hypophysis. *Biochim. Biophys. Acta*, **22**: 421–427.

AGISHI, Y.. and DINGMAN, J. F. (1965). Specific tritiation of oxytocin by catalytic deiodination. *Biochem. Biophys. Res. Commun.*, **18**: 92–97.

BARTOŠEK, I., PLIŠKA, F., RYCHLÍK, I. and ŠORM, F. (1964). The inactivation of oxytocin in the liver. Proteolytic degradation. *Prob. Evolyutsionnoi i Tekhn. Biokhim.*, *Akad. Nauk. S.S.S.R., Inst. Biokhim.*, pp. 276–286.

BASHORE, R. A. (1967). Immunoassay of oxytocin. *Obstet. Gynecol.*, **29**: 431.

BESPALOVA, J. D., KAUROV, O. A., MARTINOV, V. F., NATOCHIN, J. V., TITOV, M. I. and SHAKHMATOVA, E. I. (1966). New analogues of oxytocin: [7-L-pipecolic acid] -oxytocin and [7-L-hydroxyproline]-oxytocin. *Vestn. Leningrad. Univ., Ser. Fiz. Khim.*, **21**: 157–159.

BEYERMAN, H. C., BONTEKOE, J. S. and KOCH, A. C. (1959). Synthesis of oxytocin. *Rec. Trav. Chim.*, **78**: 935–946.

BODANSZKY, M. and DU VIGNEAUD, V. (1959a). An improved synthesis oxytocin. *J. Amer. Chem. Soc.*, **81**: 2504–2507.

BODANSZKY, M. and DU VIGNEAUD, V. (1959b). A method of synthesis of long peptide chains using a synthesis of oxytocin as an example. *J. Amer. Chem. Soc.*, **81**: 5688–5691.

BODANSZKY, M. and DU VIGNEAUD, V. (1959c). A new crystalline salt of oxytocin. *Nature, Lond.*, **184**: 981–982.

BODANSZKY, M., MEIENHOFER, J. and DU VIGNEAUD, V. (1960). Synthesis of lysine-vasopressin by the nitrophenyl ester method. *J. Amer. Chem. Soc.*, **82**: 3195–3198.

BODANSZKY, M., ONDETTI, M. A., BIRKHIMER, C. A. and THOMAS, P. L. (1964). Synthesis of arginine-containing peptides through their ornithine analogs. Synthesis of arginine vasopressin, arginine vasotocin, and L-histidyl-L-phenylalanyl-L-arginyl-L-tryptophylglycine. *J. Amer. Chem. Soc.*, **86**: 4452–4459.

BOISSONNAS, R. A. and HUGUENIN, R. L. (1960). Synthesis of Lys^8-oxytocin (lysine-vasotocin) and a new synthesis of lysine-vasopressin. *Helv. Chim. Acta*, **43**: 182–190.

BOISSONNAS, R. A. and HUGUENIN, R. L. (1965). A new polypeptide. Pat. Fr. 1,396,607; *Chem. Abstr.*, **63**: 13412^c.

BOISSONNAS, R. A., GUTTMANN, S., JAQUENOUD, P.-A. and WALLER, J. P. (1955). A new synthesis of oxytocin. *Helv. Chim. Acta*, **38**: 1491–1501.

BRANDA, L. A. and DU VIGNEAUD, V. (1966a). Synthesis and pharmacological properties of 9-decarboxamido-oxytocin. *J. Med. Chem.*, **9**: 169–172.

BRANDA, L. A. and DU VIGNEAUD, V. (1966b). Deoxy-4-decarboxamido-oxytocin and deamino-deoxy-4-decarboxamido-oxytocin. *J. Biol. Chem.*, **241**: 4051–4054.

BRANDA, L. A., DRABAREK, S. and DU VIGNEAUD, V. (1966). The synthesis and pharmacological properties of deamino-4-decarboxamido-oxytocin (1-β-mercaptopropionic acid-4-α-aminobutyric acid-oxytocin). *J. Biol. Chem.*, **241**: 2572–2575.

BRANDA, L. A., HRUBY, V. and DU VIGNEAUD, V. (1967). 2-isoleucine-oxytocin and deamino-2-isoleucine-oxytocin: their synthesis and some of their pharmacological activities. *Molec. Pharmac.*, **3**: 248–253.

BRESLOW, E. (1961). Cupric ion complexes of oxytocin and 2-phenylalanine-oxytocin. *Biochim. Biophys. Acta*, **53**: 606–609.

BRESLOW, E. and ABRASH, L. (1966). The binding of oxytocin and oxytocin analogues by purified bovine neurophysins. *Proc. Nat. Acad. Sci. U.S.A.*, **56**: 640–646.

CAMPBELL, B. J., CHU, F. S. and HUBBARD, S. (1963). Reactions of cupric ion with lysine-vasopressin and acetyllysine-vasopressin. *Biochemistry*, **2**: 764–769.

CARLSSON, L. and SJÖHOLM, I. (1966). Synthesis of tritium labelled oxytocin and lysine-vasopressin. *Acta Chem. Scand.*, **20**: 259–260.

CHAUVET, J., LENCI, M. T. and ACHER, R. (1960a). Presence of two vasopressins in chicken neurohypophysis. *Biochim. Biophys. Acta*, **38**: 571–573.

CHAUVET, J., LENCI, M. T. and ACHER, R. (1960b). Oxytocin and vasopressin of the sheep. Reconstitution of an active hormone-complex. *Biochim. Biophys. Acta*, **38**: 266–272.

CHIMIAK, A. and RUDINGER, J. (1965). Amino acids and peptides. LIII. Synthesis and some biological properties of 3-*O*-methyl-threonine-oxytocin. *Colln. Czech. Chem. Commun.*, **30**: 2592–2599.

COHN, M., IRVING, G. W. JR. and DU VIGNEAUD, V. (1941). The amphoteric nature of the pressor principle of the posterior lobe of the pituitary gland. *J. Biol. Chem.*, **137**: 635–642.

CRAIG, L. C. (1944). Identification of small amounts of organic compounds by distribution studies. II. Separation by countercurrent distribution. *J. Biol. Chem.*, **155**: 519–534.

CRAIG, L. C. (1964). Differential dialysis. *Science, N.Y.* **144**: 1093–1099.

CRAIG, L. C. and KONIGSBERG, W. H. (1961). Dialysis studies. III. Modification of pore size and shape in cellophane membranes. *J. Phys. Chem.*, **65**: 166–172.

CRAIG, L. C., HARFENIST, E. J. and PALADINI, A. C. (1964). Dialysis studies. VII. Behaviour of angiotensin, oxytocin and vasopressin. *Biochemistry*, **3**: 764–769.

DICKER, S. E. and GREENBAUM, A. L. (1958). The destruction of the antidiuretic activity of vasopressin by SH active compounds. *J. Physiol., Lond.*, **141**: 107–116.

DRABAREK, S. and DU VIGNEAUD, V. (1965). 2-D-tyrosine-oxytocin and 2-D-tyrosine-deamino-oxytocin, diastereoisomers of oxytocin and deamino-oxytocin. *J. Amer. Chem. Soc.*, **87**: 3974–3978.

DUTTA, A. S. and ANAND, N. (1965). Synthesis of 9-β-alanine-oxytocin and 4-D-glutamine-oxytocin. *Indian J. Chem.*, **3**: 232–233.

DUTTA, A. S., ANAND, N. and KAR, K. (1966a). Synthesis and pharmacological activity of 4-D-glutamine-oxytocin; 5-D-asparagine-oxytocin and 4-D-glutamine-5-D-asparagine-oxytocin. *J. Med. Chem.*, **9**: 497–499.

DUTTA, A. S., ANAND, N. and KAR, K. (1966b). Synthesis and pharmacological activity of 7-L-hydroxyproline-oxytocin, 9-β-alanine-oxytocin, 9-L-alanine-oxytocin and 9-deamido-oxytocin. *Indian J. Chem.*, **4**: 488–492.

DU VIGNEAUD, V., BARTLETT, M. F. and JÖHL, A. (1957). The synthesis of lysine-vasopressin. *J. Amer. Chem. Soc.*, **79**: 5572–5575.

DU VIGNEAUD, V., FITT, P. S., BODANSZKY, M. and O'CONNELL, M. (1960a). Synthesis and some pharmacological properties of a peptide derivative of oxytocin: glycyl-oxytocin. *Proc. Soc. Exp. Biol. Med.*, **104**: 653–656.

DU VIGNEAUD, V., FLOURET, G. and WALTER, R. (1966). Synthesis and some biological properties of 4-valine-oxytocin and deamino-4-valine-oxytocin. *J. Biol. Chem.*, **241**: 2093–2096.

DU VIGNEAUD, V., GISH, D. T., KATSOYANNIS, P. G. and HESS, G. P. (1958). Synthesis of the pressor-antidiuretic hormone, arginine-vasopressin. *J. Amer. Chem. Soc.*, **80**: 3355–3358.

DU VIGNEAUD, V., LAWLER, H. C. and POPENOE, E. A. (1953a). Enzymatic cleavage of glycinamide from vasopressin and a proposed structure for this pressor-antidiuretic hormone of the posterior pituitary. *J. Amer. Chem. Soc.*, **75**: 4880.

DU VIGNEAUD, V., POPENOE, E. A. and ROESKE, R. (1953b). Reported in a footnote to du Vigneaud, V., Lawler, H. C. and Popenoe, E. A. (1953a).

DU VIGNEAUD, V., RESSLER, C., SWAN, J. M., ROBERTS, C. W. and KATSOYANNIS, P. G. (1954). The synthesis of oxytocin. *J. Amer. Chem. Soc.*, **76**: 3115–3121.

DU VIGNEAUD, V., RESSLER, C., SWAN, J. M., ROBERTS, C. W., KATSOYANNIS, P. G. and GORDON, S. (1953c). The synthesis of an octapeptide amide with the hormonal activity of oxytocin. *J. Amer. Chem. Soc.*, **75**: 4879–4880.

DU VIGNEAUD, V., RESSLER, C. and TRIPPETT, S. (1953d). The sequence of amino acids in oxytocin with a proposal for the structure of oxytocin. *J. Biol. Chem.*, **205**: 949–957.

DU VIGNEAUD, V., SCHNEIDER, C. H., STOUFFER, J. E., MURTI, V. V. S., AROSKAR, J. P. and WINESTOCK, G. (1962). Tritiation of oxytocin by the Wilzbach method and the synthesis of oxytocin from tritium-labelled leucine. *J. Amer. Chem. Soc.*, **84**: 409–413.

DU VIGNEAUD, V., WINESTOCK, G., MURTI, V. V. S., HOPE, D. B. and KIMBROUGH, R. D. JR. (1960b). Synthesis of 1-β-mercaptopropionic acid-oxytocin (desamino-oxytocin), a highly potent analogue of oxytocin. *J. Biol. Chem.*, **235**: PC64–PC66.

EISLER, K., RUDINGER, J. and ŠORM, F. (1966). Amino acids and peptides. LXV. Analogues of oxytocin with isoleucine replaced by L-diethylalanine, L-cyclopentylglycine, and L- and D-cyclohexylglycine. *Colln. Czech. Chem. Commun.*, **31**: 4563–4580.

FERRARO, J. J. and DU VIGNEAUD, V. (1966). 7-D-proline-oxytocin and its deamino analog. Diastereoisomers of oxytocin and deamino-oxytocin. *J. Amer. Chem. Soc.*, **88**: 3847–3850.

FERRIER, B. M. and BRANDA, L. A. (1966). Degradation of oxytocin by oxytocinase: synthesis of the peptide expected as the first product. *Proc. 3rd Int. Pharmacological Congr., São Paulo, Brazil*, July 1966, Abstract No. 454.

FERRIER, B. M. and DU VIGNEAUD, V. (1966). 9-Deamido-oxytocin, an analog of the hormone containing a glycine residue in place of the glycinamide residue. *J. Med. Chem.*, **9**: 55–57.

FERRIER, B. M., JARVIS, D. and DU VIGNEAUD, V. (1965). Deamino-oxytocin: its isolation by partition chromatography on Sephadex and crystallization from water, and its biological activities. *J. Biol. Chem.*, **240**: 4264–4266.

FLOURET, G. and DU VIGNEAUD, V. (1965). The synthesis D-oxytocin, the enantiomer of the posterior pituitary hormone, oxytocin. *J. Amer. Chem. Soc.*, **87**: 3775–3776.

FONG, C. T. O., SCHWARTZ, I. L., POPENOE, E. A., SILVER, L. and SCHOESSLER, M. A. (1959). On the molecular bonding of lysine vasopressin at its renal receptor site. *J. Amer. Chem. Soc.*, **81**: 2592–2593.

FONG, C. T. O., SILVER, L., CHRISTMAN, D. R. and SCHWARTZ, I. L. (1960). The mechanism of action of the antidiuretic hormone, vasopressin. *Proc. Nat. Acad. Sci. U.S.A.*, **46**: 1273–1277.

FONG, C. T. O., SILVER, L. and LOUIE, D. D. (1964). Necessity of the disulfide bond of vasopressin for antidiuretic activity. *Biochem. Biophys. Res. Commun.*, **14**: 302–306.

FOSKER, A. P. and LAW, H. D. (1965). Oxytocin and 4-glycine-oxytocin. *J. Chem. Soc.*, **1965**: 4922–4929.

FRANK, W. (1964). Synthesis of selenium-containing peptides. III. Diseleno-oxytocin. *Hoppe-Seyler's Z. Physiol. Chem.*, **339**: 202–213.

FRANKLAND, B. T. B., HOLLENBERG, M. D., HOPE, D. B. and SCHACTER, B. A. (1966).

Dissociation of oxytocin and vasopressin from their carrier protein by chromatography on Sephadex G-25. *Brit. J. Pharmac. Chemother.*, **26**: 502–510.

GILLILAND, P. F. and PROUT, T. E. (1965a). Immunologic studies of octapeptides. I. Radioiodination of oxytocin. *Metab. Clin. Exptl.*, **14**: 912–917.

GILLILAND, P. F. and PROUT, T. E. (1965b). Immunologic studies of octapeptides. II. Production and detection of antibodies to oxytocin. *Metab. Clin. Exptl.*, **14**: 918–923.

GINSBURG, M. and IRELAND, M. (1964). Binding of vasopressin and oxytocin to protein in extracts of bovine and rabbit neurohypophysis. *J. Endocrinol.*, **30**: 131–145.

GINSBURG, M. and IRELAND, M. (1965). The preparation bovine neurophysin and the estimation of its maximum capacity to bind oxytocin and arginine-vasopressin. *J. Endocrinol.*, **32**: 187–198.

GISH, D. T., KATSOYANNIS, P. G., HESS, G. P. and STEDMAN, R. J. (1956). Unexpected formation of anhydro compounds in the synthesis of asparaginyl and glutaminyl peptides. *J. Amer. Chem. Soc.*, **78**: 5954.

GOLUBOW, J., CHAN, W. Y. and DU VIGNEAUD, V. (1963). Effect of human pregnancy serum on avian depressor activities of oxytocin and desamino-oxytocin. *Proc. Soc. Exp. Biol. Med.*, **113**: 113–115.

GORDON, S. and DU VIGNEAUD, V. (1953). Preparation of S,S'-dibenzyloxytocin and its reconversion to oxytocin. *Proc. Soc. Exp. Biol. Med.*, **84**: 723–725.

GUTTMANN, S. (1962). Synthesis of Ser^4-Ile^8-oxytocin, a possible hypophysial hormone of certain fish (isotocin). *Helv. Chim. Acta*, **45**: 2622–2627.

GUTTMANN, S. (1966) Synthesis of glutathione and oxytocin using a new thiol protecting group. *Helv. Chim. Acta*, **49**: 83–96.

HARFENIST, E. J. (1953). The amino acid composition of insulin isolated from beef, pork and sheep glands. *J. Amer. Chem. Soc.*, **75**: 5528–5533.

HEATON, G. S., RYDON, H. N. and SCHOFIELD, J. A. (1956). Polypeptides. III. Oxidation of peptides of cysteine and glycine. *J. Chem. Soc.*, **1956**: 3157–3168.

HELLER, H. and PICKERING, B. T. (1960). Identification of a new neurohypophysial hormone. *J. Physiol. Lond.*, **152**: 56P–57P.

HERMANN, P. and ZAORAL, M. (1965). Amino acids and peptides. LVI. Synthesis of thialysine^8-vasopressin. *Colln. Czech. Chem. Commun.*, **30**: 2817–2826.

HOLLÄNDER, L. P., FRANZ, J. and BERDE, B. (1966). An attempt to produce antibodies to oxytocin and vasopressin. *Experientia*, **22**: 325–333.

HOLLENBERG, M. D. and HOPE, D. B. (1966). Crystallization of a purified protein fraction from posterior lobes of pituitary gland in the presence of vasopressin and oxytocin. *J. Physiol. Lond.*, **185**: 51P–52P.

HOPE, D. B., MURTI, V. V. S. and DU VIGNEAUD, V. (1962). A highly potent analogue of oxytocin, desamino-oxytocin. *J. Biol. Chem.*, **237**: 1563–1566.

HOPE, D. B., SCHACTER, B. A. and FRANKLAND, B. T. B. (1963). Dissociation of oxytocin, vasopressin and neurophysin by gel filtration. *Biochem. J.*, **93**: 7P.

HUGUENIN, R. L. (1964). Synthesis of Phe^2-Orn^8-vasopressin and Phe^2-Orn^8-oxytocin. Two analogues of vasopressin with selective pressor activity. *Helv. Chim. Acta*, **47**: 1934–1941.

HUGUENIN, R. L. (1966). Synthesis of desamino^1-Orn^8-vasopressin, of desamino^1-Phe^2-Orn^8-vasopressin, of desamino^1-Ile^3-Orn^8-vasopressin (= desamino^1-Orn^8-oxytocin), and of desamino^1-Phe^2-Ile^3-Orn^8-vasopressin (= desamino^1-Phe^2-Orn^8-oxytocin). *Helv. Chim. Acta*, **49**: 711–725.

HUGUENIN, R. L. and BOISSONNAS, R. A. (1962). Synthesis of Phe^2-arginine-vasopressin and of Phe^2-arginine-vasotocin and a new synthesis of arginine-vasopressin and arginine-vasotocin. *Helv. Chim. Acta*, **45**: 1629–1643.

HUGUENIN, R. L. and BOISSONNAS, R. A. (1966). Synthesis of desamino^1-Arg^8-vasopressin and desamino^1-Phe^2-Arg^8-vasopressin. Two analogues possessing a higher and more selective antidiuretic activity than that of the natural vasopressins. *Helv. Chim. Acta*, **49**: 695–705.

HUGUENIN, R. L. and GUTTMAN, S. (1965). Synthesis of Ala^1-Ala^6-Arg^8-vasopressin and Ala^1-Ala^6-Lys^8-vasopressin and of (desamino-Ala)^1-Ala^6-Arg^8-vasopressin and (desamino-Ala)^1-Ala^6-Lys^8-vasopressin. *Helv. Chim. Acta*, **48**: 1885–1898.

JAQUENOUD, P.-A. (1965). Synthesis of Gly^8-oxytocin, Ala^8-oxytocin and But^8-oxytocin. *Helv. Chim. Acta*, **48**: 899–911.

JAQUENOUD, P.-A. and BOISSONNAS, R. A. (1961). Synthesis of isoleucine^8-oxytocin and valine^8-oxytocin. Two analogues of oxytocin modified in the side chain. *Helv. Chim. Acta*, **44**: 113–122.

JARVIS, D. and DU VIGNEAUD, V. (1964). Crystalline deamino-oxytocin. *Science, N.Y.* **143**: 545–548.

JARVIS, D. and DU VIGNEAUD, V. (1967). The effect of decreasing the size of the ring present in deamino-oxytocin by one methylene group on its biological properties: the synthesis of 1-mercaptoacetic acid-oxytocin. *J. Biol. Chem.*, **242**: 1768–1771.

JARVIS, D., FERRIER, B. M. and DU VIGNEAUD, V. (1965). The effect of increasing the size of the ring present in deamino-oxytocin by one methylene group on its biological properties: the synthesis of 1-γ-mercaptobutyric acid-oxytocin. *J. Biol. Chem.*, **240**: 3553–3557.

JARVIS, D., MANNING, M. and DU VIGNEAUD, V. (1967). 1-mercaptoacetic acid-4-β-alanine-oxytocin. *Biochemistry*, **6**: 1223–1225.

JÖHL, A., HARTMANN, A. and RINK, H. (1963). Synthesis of Ser^4-Ile^8-oxytocin (Isotocin). *Biochim. Biophys. Acta*, **69**: 193–195.

JOŠT, K. (1966). Amino acids and peptides. LXI. A new synthetic route to oxytocin and vasopressin suitable for the preparation of analogues modified at position 6. *Colln. Czech. Chem. Commun.*, **31**: 2784–2793.

KASAFÍREK, E., JOŠT, K., RUDINGER, J. and ŠORM, F. (1965). Amino acids and peptides. LIV. Synthesis of further extended-chain analogues of oxytocin. *Colln. Czech. Chem. Commun.*, **30**: 2600–2608.

KASAFÍREK, E., RÁBEK, V., RUDINGER, J. and ŠORM, F. (1966). Amino acids and peptides. LXVI. Synthesis of ten extended chain analogues of lysine-vasopressin. *Colln. Czech. Chem. Commun.*, **31**: 4587–4591.

KATSOYANNIS, P. G. and DU VIGNEAUD, V. (1958). Arginine-vasotocin, a synthetic analogue of the posterior pituitary hormones containing the ring of oxytocin and the side chain of vasopressin. *J. Biol. Chem.*, **233**: 1352–1354.

KATSOYANNIS, P. G., GISH, D. T., HESS, G. P. and DU VIGNEAUD, V. (1958). Synthesis of two protected hexapeptides containing the N-terminal and C-terminal sequences of arginine-vasopressin. *J. Amer. Chem. Soc.*, **80**: 2558–2562.

KIMBROUGH, R. D. JR., and DU VIGNEAUD, V. (1961). Lysine-vasotocin, a synthetic analogue of the posterior pituitary hormones containing the ring of oxytocin and the side chain of vasopressin. *J. Biol. Chem.*, **236**: 778–780.

KLIEGER, E. and SCHRÖDER, E. (1965). Peptide synthesis. XXXVIII. Synthesis of Ser^3-Ileu^8-oxytocin and deamino-Ser^4-Ileu^8-oxytocin (Desamino-isotocin). *Tetrahedron Letters*, **1965**: 2067.

KUNKEL, H. G., TAYLOR, S. P. JR. and DU VIGNEAUD, V. (1953). Electrophoretic properties of oxytocin. *J. Biol. Chem.*, **200**: 559–564.

LAWLER, H. C. and du VIGNEAUD, V. (1953). Enzymatic evidence for the intrinsic oxytocic activity of the pressor-antidiuretic hormones. *Proc. Soc. Exp. Biol. Med.*, **84**: 114–116.

LAWLER, H. C., TAYLOR, S. P. JR., SWAN, J. M. and DU VIGNEAUD, V. (1954). Presence of glutamine and asparagine in enzymatic hydrolysates of oxytocin and vasopressin. *Proc. Soc. Exp. Biol. Med.*, **87**: 550–552.

LINDNER, E. B., ELMQVIST, A. and PORATH, J. (1959). Gel filtration as a method of purification of protein-bound peptides exemplified by oxytocin and vasopressin. *Nature, Lond.*, **184**: 1565–1566.

LIVERMORE, A. H. and DU VIGNEAUD, V. (1949). Preparation of high potency oxytocic material by the use of counter-current distribution. *J. Biol. Chem.*, **180**: 365–373.

LOW, B. W. and CHEN, C. C. H. (1966). Deamino-oxytocin and 1-γ-mercaptobutyric acid-oxytocin. X-ray crystallographic data. *Science, N.Y.* **151**: 1552–1553.

MANNING, M. and DU VIGNEAUD, V. (1965a). 4-β-alanine-oxytocin: an oxytocin analog containing a twenty-one-membered disulfide ring. *Biochemistry*, **4**: 1884–1887.

MANNING, M. and DU VIGNEAUD, V. (1965b). 6-hemi-D-cystine-oxytocin, a diastereoisomer of the posterior pituitary hormone, oxytocin. *J. Amer. Chem. Soc.*, **87**: 3978–3982.

MEIENHOFER, J. and DU VIGNEAUD, V. (1960). Preparation of lysine-vasopressin through a crystalline protected nonapeptide intermediate and purification of the hormone by chromatography. *J. Amer. Chem. Soc.*, **82**: 2279–2282.

MOORE, S., and STEIN, W. H. (1949). Chromatography of amino acids on starch columns. Solvent mixtures for the fractionation of protein hydrolysates. *J. Biol. Chem.*, **178**: 53–77.

MUELLER, J. M., PIERCE, J. G., DAVOLL, H. and DU VIGNEAUD, V. (1951). The oxidation of oxytocin with performic acid. *J. Biol. Chem.*, **191**: 309–313.

MUELLER, J. M., PIERCE, J. G. and DU VIGNEAUD, V. (1953). Treatment of performic acid-oxidized oxytocin with bromine water. *J. Biol. Chem.*, **204**: 857–860.

ODELL, W. D., SWAIN, R. W., BOWERS, C. Y. and SCHALLY, A. V. (1966). Radiation inactivation of purified lysine-vasopressin. *Experientia*, **22**: 1–6.

PERKS, A. M. and SAWYER, W. H. (1965). A new neurohypophysial principle in the elasmobranch, *Raia ocellata*. *Nature, Lond.*, **205**: 154–156.

PERMUTT, M. A., PARKER, C. W. and UTIGER, R. D. (1966). Immunochemical studies with lysine-vasopressin. *Endocrinology*, **78**: 809–814.

PHOTAKI, I. (1966). New synthesis of oxytocin using S-acyl-cysteines as intermediates. *J. Amer. Chem. Soc.*, **88**: 2292–2299.

PHOTAKI, I. and DU VIGNEAUD, V. (1965). 4-Deamido-oxytocin, an analog of the hormone containing glutamic acid in place of glutamine. *J. Amer. Chem. Soc.*, **87**: 908–913.

PIERCE, J. G. and DU VIGNEAUD, V. (1950a). Preliminary studies on the amino acid content of a high potency preparation of the oxytocic hormone of the posterior lobe of the pituitary gland. *J. Biol. Chem.*, **182**: 359–366.

PIERCE, J. G. and DU VIGNEAUD, V. (1950b). Studies on high potency oxytocic material from beef posterior pituitary lobes. *J. Biol. Chem.*, **186**: 77–84.

PIERCE, J. G., GORDON, S. and DU VIGNEAUD, V. (1952). Further distribution studies on the oxytocic hormone of the posterior lobe of the pituitary gland and the preparation of an active crystalline flavianate. *J. Biol. Chem.*, **199**: 929–940.

POPENOE, E. A. and DU VIGNEAUD, V. (1953). Degradative studies on vasopressin and performic acid-oxidized vasopressin. *J. Biol. Chem.*, **205**: 133–143.

POPENOE, E. A. and DU VIGNEAUD, V. (1954). A partial sequence of amino acids in performic acid-oxidized vasopressin. *J. Biol. Chem.*, **206**: 353-360.

POPENOE, E. A., LAWLER, H. C. and DU VIGNEAUD, V. (1952). Partial purification and amino acid content of vasopressin from hog posterior pituitary glands. *J. Amer. Chem. Soc.*, **74**: 3713.

PORTANOVA, R. and SACHS, H. (1967). A specific adsorbent for vasopressin: the purification of labeled hormone. *Endocrinology*, **80**: 527-529.

RASMUSSEN, H. and CRAIG, L. (1961). The isolation of arginine-vasotocin from fish pituitary glands. *Endocrinology*, **68**: 1051-1055.

RESSLER, C. (1959). Inactivation of oxytocin suggesting peptide denaturation. *Science, N.Y.* **128**: 1281-1282.

RESSLER, C. and DU VIGNEAUD, V. (1954). Bromination of performic acid-oxidized oxytocin. *J. Biol. Chem.*, **211**: 809-814.

RESSLER, C., TRIPPETT, S. and DU VIGNEAUD, V. (1953). Free amino groups of performic acid-oxidized oxytocin and of its cleavage products formed by treatment with bromine water. *J. Biol. Chem.*, **204**: 861-869.

ROTH, J., GLICK, S. M., KLEIN, L. A. and PETERSEN, M. J. (1966). Specific antibody to vasopressin in man. *J. Clin. Endocrinol. Metab.*, **26**: 671-675.

RUDINGER, J., and JOŠT, K. (1964). A biologically active analogue of oxytocin not containing a disulfide group. *Experientia*, **20**: 570-571.

RUDINGER, J., HONZL, J. and ZAORAL, M. (1956). Syntheses in the oxytocin field. III. An alternative synthesis of oxytocin. *Chem. Listy*, **50**: 288-295.

SAKAKIBARA, S. and SHIMONISHI, Y. (1965). New method for releasing oxytocin from fully protected nonapeptides using anhydrous hydrogen fluoride. *Bull. Chem. Soc. Japan*, **38**: 1412-1413.

SAKAKIBARA, S., NOBUHARA, Y., SHIMONISHI, Y. and KIYOI, R. (1965). Synthesis of oxytocin. *Bull. Chem. Soc. Japan*, **38**: 120-123.

SCHALLY, A. V. and BARRETT, J. F. (1965). Configuration of a lysine-vasopressin dimer. *J. Amer. Chem. Soc.*, **87**: 2497-2499.

SCHALLY, A. V. and GUILLEMIN, R. (1964). Some biological and chemical properties of a lysine-vasopressin dimer. *J. Biol. Chem.*, **239**: 1038-1041.

SCHNEIDER, C. H. and DU VIGNEAUD, V. (1962). Synthesis of D-leucine-oxytocin, a biologically active diastereoisomer of oxytocin, and demonstration of its separability from oxytocin upon countercurrent distribution. *J. Amer. Chem. Soc.*, **84**: 3005-3008.

SCHULZ, H. and DU VIGNEAUD, V. (1966a). Synthesis of 1-L-penicillamine-oxytocin, 1-D-penicillamine-oxytocin, and 1-deaminopenicillamine-oxytocin, potent inhibitors of the oxytocic response of oxytocin. *J. Med. Chem.*, **9**: 647-650.

SCHULZ, H. and DU VIGNEAUD, V. (1966b). The effect of replacing one of the hydrogens of the β-carbon of the β-mercaptopropionic acid residue in deamino-oxytocin by a methyl group on its oxytocic and avian vasodepressor activity. *J. Amer. Chem. Soc.*, **88**: 5015-5017.

SEALOCK, R. R. and DU VIGNEAUD, V. (1935). Studies on the reduction of pitressin and pitocin with cysteine. *J. Pharmacol. Exp. Therap.*, **54**: 433-447.

SJÖHOLM, I. (1964). Enzymatic inactivation of oxytocin. *Acta Chem. Scand.*, **18**: 889-898.

SMYTH, D. G. (1965). Reactions of cyanate with amino and hydroxyl groups. Application to oxytocin. *Acta Chim. Acad. Sci. Hung.*, **44**: 197-204.

STUDER, R. O. (1963). Comparison of synthetic and natural arginine-vasopressin. *Helv. Chim. Acta*, **46**: 421-425.

STUDER, R. O., and DU VIGNEAUD, V. (1960). Synthetic work related to arginine-vasopressin. *J. Amer. Chem. Soc.*, **82**: 1499–1501.
STURMER, E., HUGUENIN, R. L., BOISSONNAS, R. A. and BERDE, B. (1965). Desamino-Phe^2-Arg^8-vasopressin, a peptide with a highly selective antidiuretic activity. *Experientia*, **21**: 583–585.
TAKABATAKE, Y. and SACHS, H. (1964). Vasopressin biosynthesis. III. *In vitro* studies. *Endocrinology*, **75**: 934–942.
TAYLOR, S. P. JR. and DU VIGNEAUD, V. (1953). Unpublished data, quoted in DU VIGNEAUD, V., RESSLER, C. and TRIPPETT, S. (1953d).
TAYLOR, S. P. JR., DU VIGNEAUD, V. and KUNKEL, H. G. (1953). Electrophoretic studies of oxytocin and vasopressin. *J. Biol. Chem.*, **205**: 45–53.
TOENNIES, G. and HOMILLER, R. P. (1942). Oxidation of amino acids by hydrogen peroxide in formic acid. *J. Amer. Chem. Soc.*, **64**: 3054–3056.
TUPPY, H. (1953). Amino acid sequence in oxytocin. *Biochim. Biophys. Acta*, **11**: 449–450.
TUPPY, H. and MICHL, H. (1953). The chemical structure of oxytocin. *Mh. Chem.*, **84**: 1011–1020.
TUPPY, H. and NESVADBA, H. (1957). Aminopeptidase activity of the serum of pregnant women, and its ability to inhibit oxytocin. *Mh. Chem.*, **88**: 977–988.
TURNER, R. A., PIERCE, J. G. and DU VIGNEAUD, V. (1951a). The purification and the amino acid content of vasopressin preparations. *J. Biol. Chem.*, **191**: 21–28.
TURNER, R. A., PIERCE, J. G. and DU VIGNEAUD, V. (1951b). The desulfuration of oxytocin. *J. Biol. Chem.*, **193**: 359–361.
VAN DYKE, H. B., CHOW, B. F., GREEP, R. O. and ROTHEN, A. (1942). Isolation of a protein from the pars neuralis of the ox pituitary with constant oxytocic, pressor and diuresis-inhibiting activities. *J. Pharmacol. Exp. Therap.*, **74**: 190–209.
VELLUZ, L., AMIARD, G., BARTOS, J., COFFINET, B. and HEYMÈS, R. (1956). Access to synthetic oxytocin by the aid of S,N-trityl intermediates. *Bull. Soc. Chim. France*, **1956**: 1464–1467.
WALTER, R. and DU VIGNEAUD, V. (1965). 6-Hemi-L-selenocystine-oxytocin and 1-Deamino-6-hemi-L-selenocystine-oxytocin, highly potent isologs of oxytocin and 1-Deamino-oxytocin. *J. Amer. Chem. Soc.*, **87**: 4192–4193.
WALTER, R. and DU VIGNEAUD, V. (1966a). 1-Deamino-1,6-L-selenocystine-oxytocin, a highly potent isolog of 1-Deamino-oxytocin. *J. Amer. Chem. Soc.*, **88**: 1331.
WALTER, R. and DU VIGNEAUD, V. (1966b). 8-Alanine-oxytocin, 8-alanine-oxypressin, and their deamino analogs. Their synthesis and some of their pharmacological properties. *Biochemistry*, **5**: 3720–3727.
WALTER, R. and SCHWARTZ, I. L. (1966). 5-Valine-oxytocin and Deamino-5-valine-oxytocin. Synthesis and some pharmacological properties. *J. Biol. Chem.*, **241**: 5500–5503.
WILZBACH, K. E. (1957). Tritium-labelling by exposure of organic compounds to tritium gas. *J. Amer. Chem. Soc.*, **79**: 1013.
WOODWARD, R. B., OLOFSON, R. A. and MAYER, H. (1961). A new synthesis of peptides. *J. Amer. Chem. Soc.*, **83**: 1010–1012.
YAMASHIRO, D. (1964). Partition chromatography of oxytocin on "Sephadex". *Nature, Lond.*, **201**: 76–77.
YAMASHIRO, D., AANNING, H. L. and DU VIGNEAUD, V. (1965). Inactivation of oxytocin by acetone. *Proc. Nat. A. Acad. Sci. U.S.A.*, **54**: 166–171.
YAMASHIRO, D., GILLESSEN, D. and DU VIGNEAUD, V. (1966a). Simultaneous synthesis 1-hemi-D-cystine-oxytocin and oxytocin and separation of the diastereoisomers

by partition chromatography on Sephadex and by countercurrent distribution. *J. Amer. Chem.Soc.*, **88**: 1310–1313.

YAMASHIRO, D., GILLESSEN, D. and DU VIGNEAUD, V. (1966b). Oxytoceine and Deamino-oxytoceine. *Biochemistry*, **5**: 3711–3720.

YAMASHIRO, D., HAVRAN, R. T., AANNING, H. L. and DU VIGNEAUD, V. (1967). Inactivation of lysine-vasopressin by acetone. *Proc. Nat. Acad. Sci. U.S.A.*, **57**: 1058–1061.

ZAORAL, M. (1965). Amino acids and peptides. L. Synthesis of Asp(NH$_2$)^4-lysine-vasopressin; a new synthesis of lysine-vasopressin. *Colln. Czech. Chem. Commun.*, **30**: 1853–1868.

ZAORAL, M. and ŠORM, F. (1965). Amino acids and peptides. LV. Synthesis of Gly-Cys^1-lysine-vasopressin and Gly-Cys^1-Tyr (Me)^2-lysine-vasopressin. *Colln. Czech. Chem. Commun.*, **30**: 2812–2816.

ZAORAL, M. and ŠORM, F. (1966a). Amino acids and peptides. LIX. Synthesis of L-DAB^8-vasopressin. *Colln. Czech. Chem. Commun.* **31**: 90–97.

ZAORAL, M. and ŠORM, F. (1966b). Amino acids and peptides. LX. Synthesis of D-DAB^8-vasopressin. *Colln. Czech. Chem. Commun.*, **31**: 310–314.

ZAORAL, M., KOLC, J. and ŠORM, F. (1966). Synthesis of D-Arg^8 and D-Lys^8-vasopressin *Colln. Czech. Chem. Commun.*, **31**: 382–383.

ZAORAL, M., RUDINGER, J. and ŠORM, F. (1965). Preparation of a derivative of vasopressin. Pat. Fr. M 2793 (1964); *Chem. Abstr.*, **62**: 14822^d.

CHAPTER 3

THE DISTRIBUTION OF VERTEBRATE NEUROHYPOPHYSIAL HORMONES AND ITS RELATION TO POSSIBLE PATHWAYS FOR THEIR EVOLUTION

H. Heller and B. T. Pickering

*M.R.C. Group for Research in Neurosecretion,
Department of Pharmacology,
University of Bristol, Bristol, England*

THE neurohypophysial hormones consist of a family of closely related polypeptides. Some of these have been chemically identified (Table 1) and the occurrence of others is suggested from pharmacological studies. All the hormones whose structure have been elucidated have the same pattern. They consist of a chain of nine amino acids with a disulfide bridge between residues 1 and 6. It seems likely that other hormones whose existence is known but which are not as yet chemically identified have a similar structure since, for example, they are inactivated by sodium thioglycollate, a reagent which cleaves disulfide bridges. For the sake of simplicity, irrespective of evolutionary aspects, the identified hormones will be referred to as derivatives of oxytocin. If this is done one arrives at a series of peptides which differ from oxytocin either by one or by two amino acid substitutions (Table 1). All the substitutions so far known are in positions 3, 4 or 8.

Neurohypophyses from representatives of all vertebrate classes and most of their important subgroups have by now been analysed so that a tentative scheme of distribution of the hormonal peptides can be attempted (Table 2). Inspection of Table 2 suggests that certain hormones, or combinations of hormones, are characteristic of taxonomic groups. For instance, the vasopressins have only been found in mammals. Moreover, all mammalian species (of which about 30 have been investigated) elaborate either arginine vasopressin or lysine vasopressin or both. Simi-

Pharmacology of the Endocrine System

TABLE 1. THE CHEMICAL STRUCTURES OF THE NEUROHYPOPHYSIAL HORMONE SO FAR CHARACTERIZED

CyS. Tyr. Ile. Glu(NH$_2$). Asp(NH$_2$). CyS. Pro. Leu. Gly(NH$_2$)

(Oxytocin, OXY)

CyS. Tyr. Phe. Glu(NH$_2$). Asp(NH$_2$). CyS. Pro. Lys. Gly(NH$_2$)

[3-Phenylalanine, 8-Lysine]-oxytocin
(Lysine vasopressin, LVP)

CyS. Tyr. Phe. Glu(NH$_2$). Asp(NH$_2$). CyS.. Pro. Arg. Gly(NH$_2$)

[3-Phenylalanine, 8-Arginine]-oxytocin
(Arginine Vasopressin, AVP)

CyS. Tyr. Ile. Glu(NH$_2$). Asp(NH$_2$). CyS. Pro. Arg. Gly(NH$_2$)

[8-Arginine]-oxytocin
(Arginine Vasotocin, AVT)

CyS. Tyr. Ile. Glu(NH$_2$). Asp(NH$_2$). CyS. Pro. Ile. Gly(NH$_2$).

[8-Isoleucine]-oxytocin
(Mesotocin, MST)

CyS. Tyr. Ile. Ser. Asp(NH$_2$). CyS. Pro. Ile. Gly(NH$_2$)

[4-Serine, 8-Isoleucine]-oxytocin
(Ichthyotocin, isotocin, ICT)

CyS. Tyr. Ile. Ser. Asp(NH$_2$). CyS. Pro. Glu(NH$_2$). Gly(NH$_2$)

[4-Serine, 8-Glutamine]-Oxytocin
(Glumitocin, GLT)

TABLE 2. PHYLETIC DISTRIBUTION OF NEUROHYPOPHYSIAL HORMONES

Vertebrate class and sub-class	Hormones detected*
Mammalia	
Eutheria	LVP, AVP, OXY.
Metatheria	AVP, OXY.
Prototheria	AVP, OXY.
Aves	
Neornithes	OXY, AVT.
Reptilia	
Lepidosauria	OXY, AVT, MST.
Amphibia	
Anura	OXY, AVT, MST.
Urodela	AVT, MST
Choanichthyes (lungfishes)	
(Dipnoi)	OXY, AVT, MST.
Actinopterygii (other bony fishes)	
(Teleostei)	AVT, ICT.
(Holostei)	AVT, ?ICT.
(Chondrostei)	AVT, ?ICT.
(Paleoniscoidei)	AVT, ?MST.
Elasmobranchii	
Bradyodonti	?OXY, AVT, ?MST.
Selachii	AVT, GLT, X
Cyclostomata	
(Petromyzontia)	AVT.
(Myxinoidea)	AVT.

* Key: LVP, lysine vasopressin; AVP, arginine vasopressin; OXY, oxytocin; AVT, arginine vasotocin; MST, mesotocin; ICT, ichthyotocin; GLT, glumitocin; X, unidentified peptide(s).

larly [4-serine, 8-isoleucine]-oxytocin (ichthyotocin or isotocin) has only been found in bony fishes. However, the lower vertebrates have been much less thoroughly investigated than the mammals and the occurrence of this hormone in other taxonomic groups can, therefore, not be rigidly excluded. [4-Serine, 8-glutamine]-oxytocin (Glumitocin) seems to be restricted to selachian elasmobranchs. In contrast, there are also neurohypophysial peptides which are widely distributed. In fact, it seems that [8-arginine]-oxytocin (vasotocin) occurs in all vertebrate classes except the mammals and it may be the only hormone occurring in cyclostomes. [8-Isoleucine]-oxytocin (mesotocin) and oxytocin apparently occur also in several subdivisions of the vertebrate phylum. The former has been pharmacologically characterized in lungfishes, in amphibians and in reptiles and is probably also present in other fishes. Oxytocin seems to be distributed in a similar manner, with the addition that it occurs also in birds and mammals. It seems that both oxytocin and mesotocin may be present in some cold-blooded vertebrates (for example the snake, *Naja naja*, certain amphibians and some lungfishes).

PHARMACOLOGICAL CHARACTERIZATION OF NEUROHYPOPHYSIAL HORMONES

The occurrence of two separate hormones (oxytocin and vasopressin) in mammalian posterior pituitary extracts was established in the 1920's by Dudley (1920, 1923) and Kamm *et al.* (1928) and long-known pharmacological properties of these extracts could be attributed to one or the other of these principles. The same pharmacological actions as those of mammalian posterior pituitary extracts (i.e. the effect on the uterus, the blood pressure and the kidneys) were known to be also exerted by non-mammalian extracts. Mammalian extracts were also shown (see Chapter 1) to produce water retention in amphibians. When non-mammalian extracts were assayed by this test, it was found (Heller, 1941) that their amphibian water-retaining potency in terms of equi-pressor, equi-antidiuretic and equi-oxytocic doses of mammalian extracts was greater than that of vasopressin and oxytocin. It was thus demonstrated that non-mammalian neurohypophyses elaborate a hormone—or hormones—different from those of mammals. This method of establishing potency ratios of a series of pharmacological actions has since been frequently applied to the discovery and characterization of neurohypophysial hormones. The careful work of Sawyer, Munsick and van Dyke (1959) established the ratios of pharmacological activities of neurohypophysial extracts of a number of other non-mammalian vertebrates and compared them with those of synthetic analogues of oxytocin and vasopressin which had by then been prepared by du Vigneaud and his colleagues. In this way they found that the potency ratios obtained with chicken neurohypophysial extracts were similar to those of the synthetic peptide [8-arginine]-oxytocin (Katsoyannis and du Vigneaud, 1958). These findings were a major step in the identification of the first non-mammalian neurohypophysial hormone. Even better results can be obtained when this technique is applied to partially purified hormones, and a further refinement is obtained by extending the number of bioassay methods applied. The assay methods in current use and their limits of sensitivity are shown in Table 3. The introduction of perhaps the most useful potency ratio arose from the obser-

TABLE 3. ASSAY METHODS USED IN THE CHARACTERIZATION OF NEUROHYPOPHYSIAL HORMONES

Method	Abbreviation	Preparation used	Sensitivity in terms of μg pure oxytocin (OXY) or arginine vasopressin (AVP)
Mammalian pressor	V.P.	Rat blood pressure	2.5×10^{-3} (AVP)
Mammalian antidiuretic	A.D.H	Rat antidiuresis	2×10^{-5} (AVP)
Avian depressor	F.V.D.	Chicken blood pressure	2×10^{-2} (OXY)
Oxytocic	R.U.	Stilboestrol-sensitized rat uterus	5×10^{-4} (OXY)
Milk ejection	M.E.	Lactating guinea pig or rabbit	10^{-3} (AVP)
Natriferic	N.F.	Frog or toad bladder	10^{-3} (Frog, OXY) (Toad, AVP)
Amphibian water balance	W.B.	Amphibian bladder or skin	10^{-3} (Frog, OXY) (Toad, AVP)

vation of Munsick (1960) that the oxytocic activities of several synthetic analogues, relative to the International Standard Powder, are potentiated when magnesium ions are present in the organ bath.

The "pharmacological spectra" of the peptides known to occur naturally are given in Table 4. Attempts at differentiating the profile of potency ratios of one peptide from that of another have to take account of the fact that the calculation of each potency ratio compounds the errors of the two assay methods concerned. Hence a sufficient number of assays of *each type* must be available to submit the results to the specific statistical treatment for the evaluation of differences between ratios. Even with this precaution it can be seen that some of the hormones yield one or another potency ratio which is highly characteristic. For instance Fig. 1 shows that the ratio

$$\frac{\text{frog bladder activity}}{\text{rat uterus activity}}$$

of [8-arginine]-oxytocin (vasotocin) is exceptionally high as also is the ratio

$$\frac{\text{rat antidiuretic activity}}{\text{rat uterus activity}}$$

TABLE 4. POTENCY RATIOS FOR NEUROHYPOPHYSIAL HORMONES RELATIVE TO THEIR RAT UTERUS ACTIVITY IN THE ABSENCE OF MAGNESIUM IONS**

Hormone \ Activity*	R.U. with Mg^{2+}	M.E.	F.V.D.	V.P.	ADH	NF†	W.B.
Oxytocin	0.9	0.8	1.0	0.006	0.002	1.0	1.0
[Phe³, Lys⁸]-Oxytocin	2.5	10.2	5.6	54	33	1.1	0.4
[Phe³, Arg⁸]-Oxytocin	2.3	5.7	4.7	44	44	3.6	2.5
[Arg⁸]-Oxytocin	1.9	2.2	2.3	2.0	1.6	14.7	910
[Ile⁸]-Oxytocin	1.3	1.1	2.1	0.04	0.003	2.1	3.7
[Ser⁴, Ile⁸]-Oxytocin	2.8	2.5	2.1	0.0003	0.005	0.03	0.04
[Ser⁴, Glu(NH₂)⁸]-Oxytocin	10‡						

* The abbreviations are those defined in Table 3.
** Many of the ratios are taken from Sawyer (1965).
† Calculated from Morel and Bastide (1964).
‡ Acher, Chauvet, Chauvet and Crepy (1965b).

for arginine vasopressin. Other potency ratios may be close to the limits of discrimination but may be very valuable heuristically. For instance, the discrepancy between the uterus/frog bladder ratio of a peptide found in bony fishes and oxytocin led to the postulate of a hitherto unknown neurohypophysial peptide (Heller et al., 1961) which was subsequently chemically identified (Acher et al., 1962) as [4-serine-8-isoleucine]-oxytocin (ichthyotocin). Similarly the chicken vasodepressor/rat uterus potency ratio for an amphibian principle led to the discovery (Follett and Heller, 1963a) of [8-isoleucine]-oxytocin (mesotocin). Although these potency ratios are very useful for the differentiation of peptides and have been of importance in the discovery of new hormones, they are not acceptable as criteria for absolute identification since apparently characteristic values for ratios may be shared by several nonapeptides.

SEPARATION AND PURIFICATION OF NEUROHYPOPHYSIAL HORMONES

Crude extracts are usually prepared by boiling neurohypophysial homogenates briefly (3–10 min) in dilute acetic acid (usually 0.05N), though it may be advisable for some purposes to extract for longer periods in the cold. When oxytocin and vasopressin were obtained in a pure state it became clear that many of their biological activities overlapped. Thus

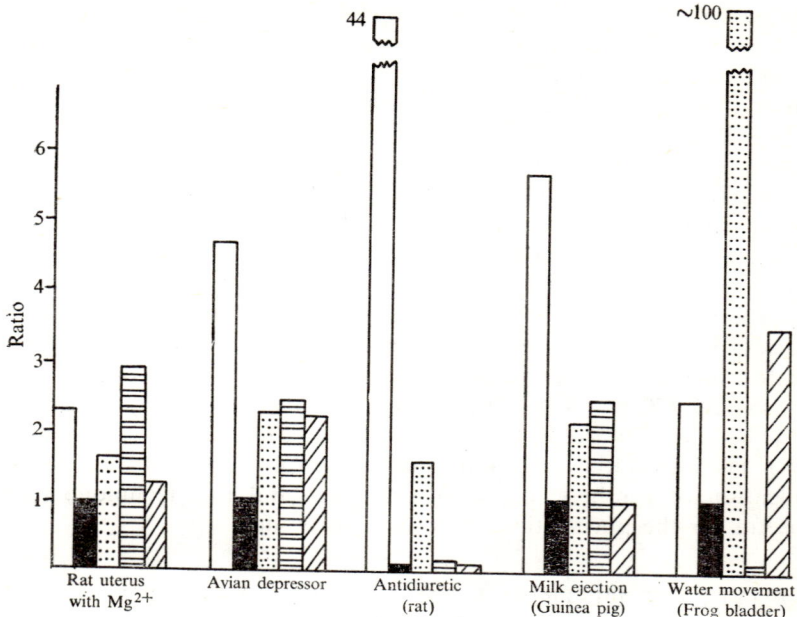

Fig. 1. The "pharmacological spectra" of some of the neurohypophysial hormones. The potency ratios are relative to the action of the hormones on the isolated rat uterus in the absence of Mg^{2+} ions. ☐, Arginine vasopressin; ■, oxytocin; ▦, arginine vasotocin [arg⁸]-oxytocin; ▤, ichthyotocin ([ser⁴−ile⁸]-oxytocin); ▧, mesotocin ([ile⁸]-oxytocin).

in order to characterize unknown hormones by establishing potency ratios it is essential to separate the active principles in neurohypophysial extracts if more than one hormone is present. The method to be adopted depends on the amount of material at ones disposal. If only a few or a single gland is available, separation by paper (Heller and Lederis, 1958) or thin-layer (Ferguson, 1965) chromatography in the solvent system butan-1-ol/acetic acid/water (4:1:5 or 6:2:2) is at present the method of choice. The active principles are eluted in a fluid which is suitable for immediate use in bioassay; the recovery is usually 30−50%.

When larger amounts of material are available, however, one may attempt to obtain the hormones as pure peptides and submit them to chemical analysis. The neurohypophysial hormones can be obtained as an active protein complex, the "van Dyke protein" (van Dyke et al., 1942) by precipitation with sodium chloride. Acher, Light and du Vigneaud (1958) prepared the complex as the first stage in the purification of neurohypophysial hormones of pigs and oxen. The complex was dissociated with trichloroacetic acid which precipitated the inactive protein (neurophysin) and left the free peptide hormones in solution. The oxytocin and vasopressin present in solution were then separated by ion exchange chromatography on the resin Amberlite CG-50. A similar procedure was used by Heller and Pickering (1961) for the isolation of arginine vasotocin from the pituitary gland of a marine teleost fish, *Pollachius virens*.

As an alternative to precipitation, the active protein complex may be separated from free peptides by exclusion chromatography on Sephadex pH 5.8 (Lindner, Elmqvist and Porath, 1959) and then resolved into its protein and hormonal peptide components by chromatography on Sephadex at low pH (0.1 N acetic acid). Further purification of the hormones prepared in this way can be achieved by ion-exchange chromatography on Amberlite CG50 (Acher, Light and du Vigneaud, 1958) or carboxymethyl cellulose (Ward and Guillemin, 1957). More recently, Yamashiro (1964) has introduced partition chromatography on Sephadex for the purification of synthetic oxytocin analogues and this technique might be useful for the purification of natural hormones.

PHYLETIC DISTRIBUTION OF NEUROHYPOPHYSIAL HORMONES

Mammals.

More species have been investigated in mammals than any other class of vertebrates (Table 5). By pharmacological methods oxytocin has been characterized in all these species and it has been chemically identified in

TABLE 5. NUMBER OF SPECIES IN WHICH NEUROHYPOPHYSIAL HORMONES HAVE BEEN INVESTIGATED

	Pharmacologically characterized	Chemically identified
Cyclostomes	3	—
Elasmobranchs	8	3
Actinopterygians	12	5
Dipnoi	3	—
Amphibians	5	1
Reptiles	4	1
Birds	4	1
Mammals	31	6

the neurohypophyses of the ox (du Vigneaud, Ressler and Trippett, 1953; Tuppy, 1953), the pig (du Vigneaud et al., 1953), man (Light and du Vigneaud, 1958), the sheep (Chauvet, Lenci and Acher, 1960a), the horse (Acher, Chauvet and Lenci, 1959) and the whale (Chauvet, Chauvet and Acher, 1963). All mammalian neurohypophyses seem also to contain vasopressin but it had already been shown in 1952 by du Vigneaud (Popenoe, Lawler and du Vigneaud, 1952) that ox glands contained [8-arginine]-vasopressin and pig glands [8-lysine]-vasopressin. These three peptides are the only neurohypophysial hormones which, so far, have been found in mammals.

The pig is a member of the artiodactyls or even-toed ungulates which are comprised of the three groups of the pig-like animals (Suiformes), the ruminants (Ruminantia) and the camel-like animals (Tylopoda). The results of an investigation, by a combination of chromatographic and multiple bio-assay techniques of 7 pig-like species, 8 species of the ruminants and both subgroups of the tylopods suggest that [8-lysine]-vasopressin is characteristic of the Suiformes (Heller and Lederis, 1960; Ferguson et al., 1962; Ferguson and Heller 1965). So far, lysine vasopressin alone has been found in glands of the domestic pig and hippopotamus, but both vasopressins were occasionally found in a single gland of the European wild boar, the warthog, the giant forest hog and the peccary. Recent unpublished work of D. R. Ferguson suggests that the neurohypophysis of the collared peccary contains either arginine vasopressin only or a mixture of both hormones, while those of the white-lipped peccary contain either lysine vasopressin alone or again a mixture of both hormones.

Birds.

Only four species of birds have so far been investigated, namely the chicken, the turkey, the Japanese quail and the pigeon. Oxytocin and [8-arginine]-oxytocin (vasotocin) have been isolated from chicken neurohypophysis and chemically identified (Acher, Chauvet and Lenci, 1960). Chromatographic and pharmacological evidence has been presented for the occurrence of the same two peptides in glands of turkeys, Japanese quails and pigeons (Munsick, Sawyer and van Dyke, 1960; Heller and Pickering, 1961; Munsick, 1964; Follett and Farner, 1966). The occurrence of arginine vasopressin in chicken neurohypophysial extracts (Chauvet, Lenci and Acher, 1960b) has not been confirmed (Munsick, 1964).

Reptiles.

Vasotocin has been chromatographically and pharmacologically characterized in several reptilian species in which oxytocin-like peptides were also detected (Sawyer, Munsick and van Dyke, 1961; Heller and Pickering, 1961; Munsick, 1966). Chemical investigations of the neurohypophysial hormones of a species of snake *(Naja naja)* confirmed the presence of vasotocin and suggests that the oxytocin-like component is a mixture of oxytocin and [8-isoleucine]-oxytocin (Pickering, 1967). The presence of both oxytocin-like peptides in single snake glands has not been demonstrated but is a distinct possibility.

Amphibians.

The distribution of active peptides in amphibians seems to be much the same as that in reptiles. Vasotocin has been isolated (Acher *et al.*, 1960) from one species of frog *(Rana esculenta)* and appears also to occur in other anuran and in urodele amphibians (Sawyer, Munsick and van Dyke, 1961; Heller and Pickering, 1961; Follett and Heller 1964a). [8-Isoleucine]-oxytocin has been isolated from *R. esculenta* by Acher *et al.*, (1964) and recently (Acher *et al.*, 1967) from the toad *(Bufo bufo)* as well, but the same group of workers had obtained evidence for the presence of two oxytocin-like hormones in the former species (Morel *et al.*, 1961). The results of the chromatographic and pharmacological investigations of Follett and Heller (1964a) in a number of amphibians, while compatible with the occurrence of [8-isoleucine]-oxytocin, suggested also that more than one oxytocin-like hormone might be present in these species. Moreover, Munsick (1966) has recently shown that the neurohypophysis of another species of frog *(R. pipiens)* contains oxytocin.

Lungfishes.

The lungfishes are of special interest since they may be regarded as an evolutionary bridge between the fishes and the tetrapods. Only three species survive, namely the African lungfish *(Protopterus)*, the Australian lungfish *(Neoceratodus)* and the South American lungfish *(Lepidosiren)*. Neurohypophysial extracts of all these forms have been studied and vasotocin has been found in each. The oxytocin-like principles are characteristic of those of the tetrapods rather than those of other bony fishes in that [8-isoleucine]-oxytocin and oxytocin seem to occur in *Protopterus* (Follett and Heller, 1962, 1963b, 1964a; Sawyer and van Dyke, 1963). The oxytocin-like principles in the other lungfishes may also be a mixture, but [8-isoleucine]-oxytocin seems to predominate in *Neoceratodus* (Follett and Heller, 1963b, 1964a), and oxytocin appears to be the major peptide in *Lepidosiren* (Pickering and McWatters, 1966). A proviso which is of special importance for the lungfishes is that very few glands have been investigated from each species.

Bony fishes.

The division of bony fishes *(Osteichthyes)* contains besides the lungfishes two other subclasses, the *Brachiopterygii* which are usually regarded as descendants of the primitive paleoniscoids, and the much more numerous group of the ray-finned fishes or Actinopterygians. Only one species of the *Brachiopterygii* the African bichir *(Polypterus senegalus)* has been investigated, and preliminary analysis of this rare fish suggests that its neurohypophysis contains vasotocin (Sawyer and van Dyke, 1963; Follett and Heller 1964b) and an oxytocin-like principle which may be [8-isoleucine]-oxytocin (Sawyer and van Dyke, 1963).

The Actinopterygians are usually divided into three superorders, the *Chondrostei, Holostei* and *Teleostei* of which the *Teleostei* are considered to be the more advanced. Follett and Heller (1964b) found evidence for the occurrence of [8-arginine]-oxytocin in the pituitary extracts of representative species from all members of these groups. Whenever a second active principle was detected in actinopterygian neurohypophysial extracts it had the chromatographic and pharmacological characteristics of [4-serine, 8-isoleucine]-oxytocin (ichthyotocin) which has also been chemically identified in the teleosteans pollack, Boston hake, cod, whiting pout and carp (Acher *et al.*, 1965a). However, extracts of chondrostean glands and of the holostean *Polyodon* contained little or no ichthyotocin. This need not necessarily be a taxonomic characteristic since Sawyer and Pickford (1963) have shown that the occurrence of ichthyotocin in the pituitary glands of another fish *Fundulus heteroclitus* depends on the time of the year at which the animals are caught.

Elasmobranch fishes.

The neurohypophysial hormones of the large group of cartilaginous fishes *(Elasmobranchii)* are still under investigation. An oxytocic principle which has not been detected elsewhere has been isolated from *Raia clavata* and shown to be [4-serine-8 glutamine]-oxytocin, glumitocin (Acher *et al.*, 1965b). It has so far not been detected in pituitary extracts from the other group of elasmobranchs, the *Holocephali,* or in a primitive selachian, the shark *Hexanchus* (Heller, 1966). Small amounts of [8-arginine]-oxytocin (vasotocin) have also been detected in many elasmobranch species (Sawyer, 1965). One group of workers have chromatographic and pharmacological indications for the occurrence of more than one oxytocin-like principle in elasmobranch pituitary extracts (Heller and Pickering, 1961; Heller and Roy, 1965), whereas other investigators have been unable to find more than one (Perks and Dodd, 1963; Perks and Sawyer, 1965; Chauvet *et al.*, 1965).

The cyclostomes.

The cyclostomes which are the most primitive of surviving vertebrates are the earliest forms with a distinct *pars nervosa*. Pituitary extracts from species from both subgroups of these jawless vertebrates, the lampreys *(Petromyzon marinus* and *Lampetra fluviatilis)* and the hagfishes *(Myxine glutinosa)* have been investigated and [8-arginine]-oxytocin (vasotocin) was the only neurohypophysial hormone detected (Sawyer, Munsick and van Dyke, 1959; Follett and Heller, 1964b; Sawyer, 1965).

MOLE RATIOS OF HORMONES IN THE NEUROHYPOPHYSIS

When considering the distribution of neurohypophysial hormones it is of interest to study not only the variation of the primary structure of the peptides, but also the relative proportions of the several hormones which may be present in the hypothalamo-neurohypophysial system of a species. These ratios may be considered with reference to three sites: the hypothalamus, the gland itself and perhaps most importantly the blood, since this proportion is the one in which the hormones are presented to the target organs. All these ratios are subject to variation because of varying rates of synthesis in the hypothalamus, varying rates of release from the neurohypophysis and differential uptake from the blood by the tissues. In spite of this there is sufficient evidence to show that the ratio in the gland is maintained relatively constant and that, moreover, the gland ratio is characteristic of the species (Follett, 1963; Ferguson and Heller 1965). For instance the absolute amount of vasopressin and oxytocin in the neurohypophysis of the female rat varies during the estrus cycle, but the ratio of the two hormones seems to be constant at each stage (Heller and Lederis, 1959; König and Böttcher, 1966). It would appear that this ratio is of genetic significance since its value is not only constant for a given species but also characteristic of larger taxonomic groups such as orders and suborders. This feature is well documented in mammals (Ferguson and Heller, 1965) in which, for example, the mean arginine vasopressin to oxytocin ratio in the order of *Marsupialia* is 4.4, and 0.72 in the order *Perissodactyla*. Similarly it would seem that there may even be characteristic differences between suborders, e.g. a mean of 1.3 in ruminants as compared with 3.4 in tylopods, both suborders of the artiodactyls.

If it is assumed that these ratios are genetically determined, there are two mechanisms by which they may be established. First, hormones may be synthesized in separate neurones (Heller, 1961; Sokol and Valtin, 1967), when the proportion of vasopressin- to oxytocin-producing neurones would determine the mole ratio of the products. Secondly, if both vasopressin and oxytocin are synthesized in the same neurone, this ratio would be determined by a control system of genes which regulates their production. Since there is ample evidence for the differential release of the hormones, there must be a feedback system to stimulate resynthesis of one or other hormone in order to maintain the ratio at the genetically determined level. While this mechanism appears to work under physiological conditions it may break down under pathological conditions of severe stress, for instance in extreme dehydration (Hild and Zetler, 1953).

It seems likely that the mole ratio of neurohypophysial hormones may also be a taxonomic characteristic in non-mammals. For example the mean mole ratio has been calculated to be 2.8 in teleost fishes and 7.2 in amphibians (Follett, 1963). The absolute values for such ratios, however, may be subject to modification since their calculation requires a knowledge of the specific activities of the hormones in question and these are either not available or may be subject to increase with improved methods of peptide synthesis.

EVOLUTION OF NEUROHYPOPHYSIAL HORMONES

The study of the distribution of neurohypophysial hormones throughout the various vertebrate classes leads naturally to the question of their evolution. As already mentioned only one neurohypophysial hormone —arginine vasotocin—has been detected in both groups of the most primitive forms of vertebrates, the jawless fishes (Agnatha). It has, therefore, been tentatively assumed by all workers in the field that vasotocin is the most primitive neurohypophysial hormone. This assumption can only be accepted with the proviso that it is always precarious to argue from a negative result. It applies with special emphasis to the neurohypophysial hormones since there may be hormones in existence which do not react in the assay systems which are currently used for their identification. Evidently, such "silent hormones" may be present not only in the cyclostomes but also in any other vertebrate group. However, notwithstanding the possibility of "silent hormones" in cyclostomes, vasotocin would still remain a very primitive hormone.

Variations in the neurohypophysial hormones may be discussed from three standpoints, namely in terms of their phyletic distribution, in terms of the function which they exert in the various taxonomic groups and in terms of their "feasibility" as products of simple mutations with regard to the genetic code. A combination of these approaches has been taken by the various groups of workers who have proposed evolutionary schemes.

Sawyer (1965), who has mainly considered the distribution of the hormones, points out that oxytocin occurs as early as in the holocephalean elasmobranchs and in the *Dipnoi*, and that it therefore "may have arisen from vasotocin amongst the agnathous ancestors of the early jawed fishes, or in the jawed ancestors of both the cartilaginous and bony fishes". In this view mesotocin, ichthyotocin and glumitocin would be derivatives of oxytocin.

Acher *et al.* (1965c), who consider the function of the hormones in proposing an evolutionary scheme, suggest that there have been two lines of development. They consider vasotocin to be a primitive form of the vasopressins, both hormones being concerned with salt and water metabolism. They then propose a second line of hormones concerned with reproductive functions in which ichthyotocin may be regarded as a primitive form of oxytocin with mesotocin as an intermediate between the two. However, there is very little evidence to support the assumption that hormones like ichthyotocin or mesotocin play a role in the reproductive processes of the animals in which they occur. In fact, so far as the effect on the oviduct is concerned, it would appear that vasotocin is more potent in those species of birds (Munsick, Sawyer and van Dyke, 1960), reptiles (LaPointe, 1967) and amphibians (Heller, Ferreri and Leathers, 1967) which have been studied.

If the neurohypophysial hormones are a series in which differences arise from point mutations, it should be possible to clarify evolutionary relationships, at least to some extent, by inspection of the code used in protein synthesis for the translation of genetic information into amino acid sequences. The amino acid sequences of seven (Table 1) hormones are known and two groups of workers (Heller and Spickett, 1967; Vliegenhart and Versteeg, 1967) have examined the steps by which one peptide might arise from another as the result of a single base change in the DNA of the gene. The simplest issue is the conversion of arginine vasopressin to lysine vasopressin. [8-Lysine]-vasopressin (LVP) has been found in the neurohypophysis of the Suiformes and evidence that this hormone is genetically related to [8-arginine]-vasopressin (AVP) is afforded by the observation (Ferguson and Heller, 1965) that some individuals in some species of *Suina* may secrete lysine vasopressin alone, some arginine vasopressin alone and others both, thus probably representing the two homozygotes and the heterozygote for the two lines. This mutation from AVP to LVP could arise from a single base change in the messenger RNA which acts as the template in the biosynthesis of the hormone, namely the replacement of guanine by adenine in the triplet coding for arginine resulting in a triplet coding for lysine. In the version of the messenger RNA code described by Nirenberg *et al.* (1965) this would be effected by conversion of the arginine triplet AGA or AGG to the lysine triplet AAA or AAG. Similarly, arginine vasopressin can be considered to have arisen in its turn from arginine vasotocin by a single base change. This interconversion requires the change of a codon for isoleucine into one for phenylalanine and this can be represented as the mutation AUC or AUU → UUC or UUU. Thus both of the mammalian vasopressins could be derived from the "primitive" hormone arginine vasotocin (Fig. 2).

The derivation of the oxytocin-like hormones is a problem of greater complexity. All the oxytocin-like hormones, oxytocin, mesotocin, ichthyotocin and glumitocin have been found in one or other of the fishes but since both ichthyotocin and glumitocin would require at least two changes in the molecule of AVT rather than the one needed for either oxytocin or mesotocin, the choice of the developmentally earlier peptide would seem to be between the latter two. Indeed, it may be significant that both oxytocin and mesotocin appear to be present in the more primitive bony fishes like *Polypterus*, and cartilaginous fishes like *Hexanchus*. Both peptides have been found in the lungfishes which are, in some ways, a very primitive group but are also related to the amphibians in which again both hormones occur. However, the question of which is the older of these two peptides cannot be answered from their taxonomic distribution since both peptides have been found in very primitive forms. Can a solution of this problem be found from an examination of the genetic code? Can both peptides be derived from AVT by a single mutation? Here again one runs into problems since one amino acid may be coded for by several triplets, the so called degeneracy of the code. Arginine, for example, can be coded for by three triplet pairs and from one of these couples (CGA or CGG), CUA or CUG can be derived to give leucine which would result in a change from AVT → oxytocin. However, this codon pair was not the one used in the derivation of the vasopressins above where AGA or AGG was used. Oxytocin cannot be derived in one stage from vasotocin if this latter codon is used for arginine, but mesotocin can—by the mutation AGA or AGG → AUA being a change from Arg → Ile. This does not necessarily mean that mesotocin is more primitive, since oxytocin could arise from vasotocin if there were a prior mutation in the arginine codon from AGA or AGG → GGA or CGG perhaps during gene duplication. Mesotocin and oxytocin themselves are interconvertible by a single step mutation. The two other peptides found in fishes, ichthyotocin and glumitocin would, in this interpretation, be regarded as being derived from the more primitive hormones by multiple mutations.

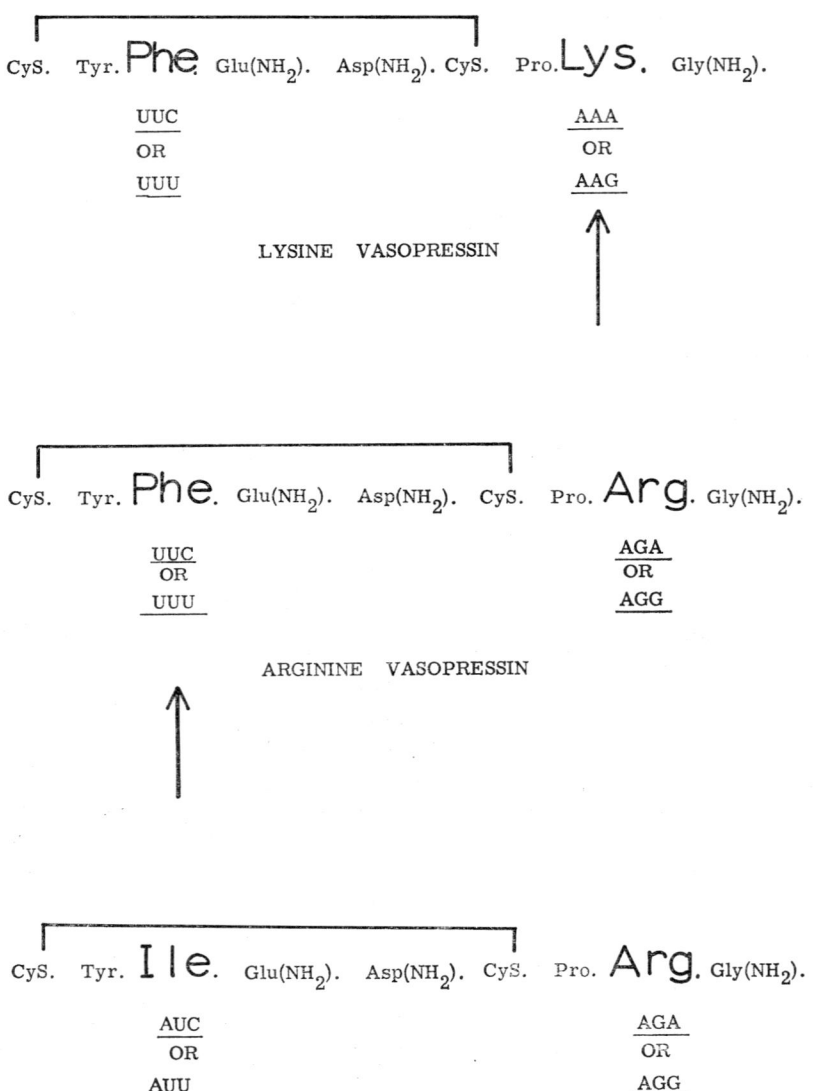

FIG. 2. The evolution of lysine vasopressin from arginine vasopressin, and of the latter from arginine vasotocin, by single base mutations. The triplets shown beneath the amino acids are according to the messenger-RNA code of Nirenberg et al. (1965).

GENERAL CONSIDERATIONS

A study of the evolution of neurohypophysial hormones is clearly of more than intrinsic interest. They are only one example of a family of homologous polypeptides with similar biological properties. Species-specific differences in amino acid composition of other polypeptide hormones are well known (e.g. insulin, adrenocorticotrophin and melanocyte-stimulating hormones)—but the only investigated series that spans the entire vertebrate phylum is that of the neurohypophysial hormones. That this is so, is due to the simplicity of their chemical structure which results in the fact that the substitution of any one amino acid produces quantitative changes in their pharmacological activities (see next chapter). In contrast the substitution of several amino acids in a larger peptide as for example, ACTH (39 amino acids) may have little or no effect on its biological potency if these substitutions are outside the "active center" (Li, 1962).

Mutational changes in polypeptide hormones might also be of clinical importance. For example, familial diabetes insipidus of hypothalamic origin is very likely due to an inability to synthesize vasopressin. This is suggested from observations (Valtin, Sawyer and Sokol, 1965) on a strain of rats with hereditary hypothalamic diabetes insipidus whose neurohypophyses have been shown to be devoid of vasopressin. This pathological condition could arise either from gene deletion or from a simple mutation resulting in the synthesis of a peptide with an altered amino acid sequence and little or no antidiuretic activity. The same etiology may apply to other endocrine diseases.

REFERENCES

BOOKS, REVIEWS, AND MONOGRAPHS

HELLER, H. (1961). Occurrence, storage and metabolism of oxytocin. *Oxytocin.* Caldeyro-Barcia, R. and Heller, H. (eds.). Pergamon Press, Oxford.

HELLER, H. and LEDERIS, K. (1959). The neurohypophysis during the estrous cycle, pregnancy and lactation. *Recent Progress in the Endocrinology of Reproduction.* Lloyd, C. W. (ed.). Academic Press, New York.

HELLER, H. and SPICKETT, S. G. (1967). The polymorphism of the neurohypophysial hormones. *Mem. Soc. Endocr.*, **15**: 89–106.

LI, C. H. (1962). Synthesis and biological properties of ACTH peptides. *Recent Prog. Horm. Res.*, **18**: 1–32.

MOREL, F. and BASTIDE, F. (1964). Relationship between the structure of several analogues of oxytocin and their natriferic activity *in vitro*. *Oxytocin, Vasopressin and Their Structural Analogues* vol 10. pp. 47-55. Rudinger, J. (ed.). Proc. 2nd Int. Pharmacol. Meeting, Pergamon Press, Oxford.

ORIGINAL PAPERS

ACHER, R., CHAUVET, J. and LENCI, M. T. (1959). Purification et structure de l'ocytocine et de la vasopressine du cheval. *Biochim. Biophys. Acta*, **31**: 545-548.

ACHER, R., CHAUVET, J. and LENCI, M. T. (1960). Isolement de l'ocytocine du poulet. *Biochim. Biophys. Acta*, **38**: 344-345.

ACHER, R., CHAUVET, J., CHAUVET, M. T. and CREPY, D. (1962). Isolement d'une nouvelle hormone neurohypophysaire, l'isotocine, présente chez les poissons osseux. *Biochim. Biophys. Acta*, **58**: 624-625.

ACHER, R., CHAUVET, J., CHAUVET, M. T. and CREPY, D. (1964). Phylogenie des peptides neurohypophysaires: isolement de la mesotocine (Ileu$_8$-ocytocine) de la grenouille, intermédiare entre la Ser$_4$-Ileu$_8$-ocytocine des poissons osseux et l'ocytocine des mammifères. *Biochim. Biophys. Acta*, **90**: 613-615.

ACHER, R., CHAUVET, J., CHAUVET, M. T. and CREPY, D. (1965a). Caractérisation des hormones neurohypophysaires d'un poisson osseux d'eau douce, la carpe *(Cyprinus carpio)*. Comparaison avec les hormones des poissons osseux marine. *Comp. Biochem. Physiol.*, **14**: 245-254.

ACHER, R., CHAUVET, J., CHAUVET, M. T. and CREPY, D. (1965b). Phylogénie des peptides neurohypophysaires: isolement d'une nouvelle hormone, la glumitocine (Ser$_4$-Gln$_8$-ocytocine) présente chez un poisson cartilagineux, la raie *(Raia clavata)*. *Biochim. Biophys. Acta*, **107**: 393-396.

ACHER, R., CHAUVET, J., CHAUVET, M. T. and CREPY, D. (1965c). Les hormones neurohypophysaires des vertébrés. Variations des structures au cours de l'évolution. *Ann. Endocrinol., Paris*, **26**: 662-669.

ACHER, R., CHAUVET, J., CHAUVET, M. T. and CREPY, D. (1967) Les hormones neurohypophysaires des amphibiens: isolement et caractérisation de la mésotocine et de la vasotocine chez le crapaud *(Bufo bufo)*. *Gen. comp. Endocrinol.*, **8**: 337-343.

ACHER, R., CHAUVET, J., LENCI, M. T., MOREL, F. and MAETZ, J. (1960). Présence d'une vasotocine dans la neurohypophyse de la grenouille *(Rana esculenta)*. *Biochim. Biophys. Acta*, **42**: 379-380.

ACHER, R., LIGHT, A. and DU VIGNEAUD, V. (1958). Purification of oxytocin by way of a protein complex. *J. Biol. Chem.*, **233**: 116-120.

CHAUVET, J., CHAUVET, M. T. and ACHER, R. (1960). Les hormones neurohypophysaires des mammifères: isolement et caractérisation de l'ocytocine et de la vasopressine de la baleine *(Balaenoptera physalus)*. *Bull. Soc. Chim. Biol.*, **45**: 1369-1378.

CHAUVET, J., LENCI, M. T. and ACHER, R. (1960a). L'ocytocine et la vasopressine du mouton: reconstitution d'un complex hormonal actif. *Biochim. Biophys. Acta*, **38**: 266-272.

CHAUVET, J., LENCI, M. T. and ACHER, R. (1960b). Présence de deux vasopressines dans la neurohypophyse du poulet. *Biochim. Biophys. Acta*, **38**: 571-573.

CHAUVET, J., CHAUVET, M. T., BEAUPAIN, D. and ACHER, R. (1965). Les hormones neurohypophysaires des raies: comparaison des hormones du pocheteau blanc *(Raia batis)* et de la raie bouclée *(Raia clavata)*. *C. R. Séanc. Acad. Sci. Paris*, **261**: 4234-4236.

DUDLEY, H. W. (1920). Some observations on the active principles of the pituitary gland. *J. Pharmacol., Exp. Ther.*, **14**: 295–312.
DUDLEY, H. W. (1923). On the active principles of the pituitary gland. *J. Pharmacol., Exp. Ther.*, **21**: 103–122.
VAN DYKE, H. B., CHOW, B. F., GREEP, R. O. and ROTHEN, A. (1942). The isolation of a protein from the pars neuralis of ox pituitary with constant oxytocic, pressor and diuresis-inhibiting activities. *J. Pharmacol., Exp. Ther.*, **74**: 190–209.
FERGUSON, D. R. (1965). Separation of mammalian neurohypophysial hormones by thin-layer chromatography. *J. Endocrin.*, **32**: 119–120.
FERGUSON, D. R. and HELLER, H. (1965). Distribution of neurohypophysial hormones in mammals. *J. Physiol. Lond.*, **180**: 846–863.
FERGUSON, D. R., HELLER, H., LEDERIS, K. and PICKFORD, M. (1962). The distribution of neurohypophysial hormones in Suiformes. *Gen. Comp. Endocrin.*, **2**: 605.
FOLLETT, B. K. (1963). Mole ratios of the neurohypophysial hormones in the vertebrate neural lobe. *Nature, Lond.*, **198**: 693–694.
FOLLETT, B. K. and FARNER, D. S. (1966). The effects of daily photoperiod on gonadal growth, neurohypophysial hormone content, and neurosecretion in the hypothalamo-neurohypophysial system of the Japanese quail *(Coturnix coturnix japonica)*. *Gen. Comp. Endocrin.*, **7**: 111–124.
FOLLETT, B. K. and HELLER, H. (1962). The neurohypophysial hormones of the African lungfish *(Protopterus aethiopicus)*. *Gen. Comp. Endocrin.*, **2**: 606–607.
FOLLETT, B. K. and HELLER, H. (1963a). Pharmacological comparison between the teleost neurohypophysial hormone, ichthyotocin, and synthetic 4-ser, 8-ileu oxytocin. *Biochem. Pharmacol.*, **12**, Suppl. p. 183.
FOLLETT, B. K. and HELLER, H. (1963b). Pharmacological characteristics of neurohypophysial hormones of lungfishes and amphibians. *Nature, Lond.*, **199**: 611–612.
FOLLETT, B. K. and HELLER, H. (1964a). The neurohypophysial hormones of lungfishes and amphibians. *J. Physiol. Lond.*, **172**: 92–106.
FOLLETT, B. K. and HELLER, H. (1964b). The neurohypophysial hormones of bony fishes. *J. Physiol. Lond.*, **172**: 74–91.
HELLER, H. (1941). Differentiation of a (amphibian) water balance principle from the antidiuretic principle of the posterior pituitary gland. *J. Physiol. Lond.*, **100**: 125–141.
HELLER, H. (1966). The hormone content of the vertebrate hypothalamo-neurohypophysial system. *Brit. Med. Bull.*, **22**: 227–231.
HELLER, H., FERRERI, E. and LEATHERS, D. H. G. (1967). The effect of neurohypophysial hormones on the amphibian oviduct. *J. Endocrin.*, **37**: xxxix.
HELLER, H. and LEDERIS, K. (1958). Paper chromatography of small amounts of vasopressins and oxytocins. *Nature, Lond.*, **182**: 1231–1232.
HELLER, H. and LEDERIS K. (1960). Posterior pituitary hormones of the hippopotamus. *J. Physiol., Lond.* **151**: 47–49P.
HELLER, H. and PICKERING, B. T. (1961). Neurohypophysial hormones of non-mammalian vertebrates. *J. Physiol. Lond.*, **155**: 98–114.
HELLER, H., PICKERING, B. T., MAETZ, J. and MOREL, F. (1961). Pharmacological characterisation of the oxytocic peptides in the pituitary of a marine teleost fish *(Pollachius virens)*. *Nature, Lond.*, **191**: 670–671.
HELLER, H. and ROY, B. P. (1965). Elasmobranch neurohypophysial hormones. *J. Physiol. Lond.*, **177**: 50–51P.
HILD, W. and ZETLER, G. (1953). Experimenteller Beweis für die Entstehung der sog.

Hypophysenhinterlappenwirkstoffe im Hypothalamus. *Pflügers Arch. ges. Physiol.*, **257**: 169–201.

KAMM, O., ALDRICH, T. B., GROTE, I. W., ROWE, L. W. and BUGBEE, E. P. (1928). The active principles of the posterior lobe of the pituitary gland. *J. Am. Chem. Soc.*, **50**: 573–601.

KATSOYANNIS, P. G. and DU VIGNEAUD, V. (1958). Arginine vasotocin, a synthetic analogue of the posterior pituitary hormones containing the ring of oxytocin and the side chain of vasopressin. *J. Biol. Chem.*, **233**: 1352–1354.

KÖNIG, A. and BÖTTCHER, D. (1966). Der Hormongehalt des Hypophysenhinterlappens während des Sexualcyclus von Wistar-Ratten. *Archiv. für Gynäkologi*, **203**: 485–490.

LAPOINTE, J. L. (1967). Oviducal responses to neurohypophysial hormones in the placental lizard, *Klauberina riversiana*. *Gen. comp. Endocrin.*, **9**: 467.

LIGHT, A. and DU VIGNEAUD, V. (1958). On the nature of oxytocin and vasopressin from human pituitary. *Proc. Soc. Exp. Biol. Med., N.Y.*, **98**: 692–696.

LINDNER, E. B., ELMQVIST, A. and PORATH, J. (1959). Gel filtration as a method of purification of protein-bound peptides exemplified by oxytocin and vasopressin. *Nature, Lond.*, **184**: 1565–1566.

MOREL, F., MAETZ, J., ACHER, R., CHAUVET, J. and LENCI, M. T. (1961). A natriferic principle other than arginine vasotocin in the frog neurohypophysis. *Nature, Lond.*, **190**: 828–829.

MUNSICK, R. A. (1960). Effect of magnesium ion on the response of the rat uterus to neurohypophysial hormones and analogues. *Endocrinology*, **66**: 451–457.

MUNSICK, R. A. (1964). Neurohypophysial hormones of chickens and turkeys. *Endocrinology*, **75**: 104–112.

MUNSICK, R. A. (1966). Chromatographic and pharmacologic characterization of the neurohypophysial hormones of an amphibian and a reptile. *Endocrinology*, **78**: 591–599.

MUNSICK, R. A., SAWYER, W. H. and VAN DYKE, H. B. (1960). Avian neurohypophysial hormones: pharmacological properties and tentative identification. *Endocrinology*, **66**: 860–871.

NIRENBERG, M., LEDER, P., BERRIFIELD, M., BRIMACOMBE, R., TRUPIN, J., ROFFMAN, F. and O'NEAL, C. (1965). RNA codewords and protein synthesis VII. On the general nature of the RNA code. *Proc. Natn. Acad. Sci., U. S. A.*, **53**: 1161–1168.

PERKS, A. M. and DODD, M. H. I. (1963). Evidence for a neurohypophysial principle in the pituitary gland of certain elasmobranch fishes. *Gen. Comp. Endocrin.*, **3**: 286–299.

PERKS, A. M. and SAWYER, W. H. (1965). A new neurohypophysial principle in an elasmobranch *Raia ocellata*. *Nature, Lond.*, **205**: 154–156.

PICKERING, B. T. (1967). The neurohypophysial hormones of a reptile species, the cobra *(Naja naja)*. *J. Endocrin.*, **39**: 285–294.

PICKERING, B. T. and MCWATTERS, S. (1966). Neurohypophysial hormones of the South American lungfish *Lepidosiren paradoxa*. *J. Endocrin.*, **36**: 217–218.

POPENOE, E. A., LAWLER, H. C. and DU VIGNEAUD, V. (1952). Partial purification and amino acid content of vasopressin from hog posterior pituitary glands. *J. Am. Chem. Soc.*, **74**: 3713.

SAWYER, W. H. (1965). Active principles from a cyclostome *(Petromyzon marinus)* and two cartilaginous fishes *(Squalus acanthias* and *Hydrolagus collei)*. *Gen. Comp. Endocrin.*, **5**: 427–439.

SAWYER, W. H. and VAN DYKE, H. B. (1963). Principles resembling oxytocin in neurohypophyses of fishes. *Fedn. Proc. Fedn. Am. Socs. Exp. Biol.*, **22**: 386.

SAWYER, W. H., MUNSICK, R. A. and VAN DYKE, H. B. (1959). Pharmacological evidence for the presence of arginine vasotocin in neurohypophysial extracts from cold-blooded vertebrates. *Nature, Lond.*, **184**: 1464.

SAWYER, W. H., MUNSICK, R. A. and VAN DYKE, H. B. (1961). Evidence for the presence of arginine vasotocin (8-arginine oxytocin) and oxytocin in neurohypophysial extracts from amphibians and reptiles. *Gen. Comp. Endocrin.*, **1**: 30–36.

SAWYER, W. H. and PICKFORD, G. E. (1963). Neurohypophysial principles of *Fundulus heteroclitus*: characteristics and seasonal changes. *Gen. Comp. Endocrin.*, **3**: 439–445.

SOKOL, H. W. and VALTIN, H. (1967). Evidence for the Synthesis of oxytocin and vasopressin in separate neurons. *Nature, Lond.*, **214**: 314–316.

TUPPY, H. (1953). The amino acid sequence in oxytocin. *Biochim. Biophys. Acta*, **11**: 449–450.

VALTIN, H., SAWYER, W. H. and SOKOL, H. W. (1965). Neurohypophysial principles in rats homozygous and heterozygous for hypothalamic diabetes insipidus (Brattleboro strain). *Endocrinology*, **77**: 701–706.

DU VIGNEAUD, V., RESSLER, C. and TRIPPETT, S. (1953). The sequence of the amino acids in oxytocin with a proposal for the structure of oxytocin. *J. Biol. Chem.*, **205**: 949.

VLIEGENTHART, J. F. G. and VERSTEEG, D. H. G. (1967). The evolution of the vertebrate neurohypophysial hormones in relation to the genetic code. *J. Endocrin.*, **38**: 3–12.

WARD, D. N. and GUILLEMIN, R. (1957). A simple method for the preparation of highly purified vasopressin. *Proc. Soc. Exp. Biol. Med., N.Y.*, **96**: 568–570.

YAMASHIRO, D. (1964). Partition chromatography of oxytocin on Sephadex. *Nature, Lond.*, **201**: 76–77.

CHAPTER 4

ASPECTS OF THE RELATIONSHIPS BETWEEN THE CHEMICAL STRUCTURE AND BIOLOGICAL ACTIVITY OF THE NEUROHYPOPHYSIAL HORMONES AND THEIR SYNTHETIC STRUCTURAL ANALOGUES

B. T. Pickering

M.R.C. Group for Research in Neurosecretion,
Department of Pharmacology,
University of Bristol

INTRODUCTION

A host of peptides is now available, some occurring naturally, others purely synthetic, which are structural analogues of the mammalian neurohypophysial hormones oxytocin and vasopressin. These hormones are active to a greater or lesser extent in a number of biological assay systems (Table 1) and there is thus great scope for the study of the effects of changes in chemical structure on biological activity. Much has already been written on indications of the structure–action relationships of these peptides in review articles (Sawyer, 1961; Rudinger and Jošt, 1964; Schwartz and Livingston, 1964; Berde and Boissonnas, 1966). It will be attempted in the present article, to collate the findings of the several groups of workers who have synthesized analogues in order to illustrate some of the salient features of the relationship of structure and activity, rather than to reproduce the biological data for all the known analogues.

How does a hormone molecule exert its biological activity? It must interact with the macromolecule which is the primary receptor and bring about a change in either the chemical or the physico-chemical structure of this molecule, thus initiating a chain of events which results in the observed response. It is the modification of this initial hormone–receptor

TABLE 1. BIOLOGICAL ACTIONS OF THE NEUROHYPOPHYSIAL PEPTIDES

Biological action	Most potent naturally occurring peptide
Contraction of rat uterus	oxytocin
Contraction of myoepithelium of lactating mammary glands of rabbits or guinea pigs (milk ejection)	oxytocin
Lowering of blood-pressure in chickens	oxytocin
Inhibition of diuresis in water-loaded rats (antidiuretic)	arginine vasopressin
Raising blood pressure of rats	arginine vasopressin
Stimulation of the transport of sodium across amphibian bladders (natriferic action)	arginine vasotocin
Increase in the rate of osmotically induced efflux of water from isolated bladders of amphibians	arginine vasotocin
Contraction of the oviducts of birds, reptiles and amphibians	arginine vasotocin

interaction which is being followed in the study of the structure–action relationships of a series of chemical analogues. One may consider the interaction of hormone and receptor as occurring in two stages. First the peptide may be bound at a specific site on the receptor molecule, and then there follows an interaction between the "active center" of the hormone and a sensitive site on the receptor, resulting in a chemical or conformational change in the latter. Alternatively, the binding of the hormone to the receptor may itself induce a change in the conformation of this molecule which brings about the biological response, in which case the concept of an active center is unnecessary. These kinds of interactions are similar to those which occur between an enzyme and its substrate and for which a good deal of the chemical events have been elucidated (see, for example, Hartley, 1964). In analysing the changes in the biological activity of a peptide induced by a single alteration in chemical structure, one must be aware that the change may be due: (a) to an alteration in the overall three-dimensional shape of the molecule so that, for steric reasons, the interaction with the receptor is altered, (b) to an alteration at the specific binding site such that the affinity of the receptor for the peptide is changed, (c) to an alteration of the "active center" if one exists.

Returning now to the neurohypophysial hormones, the structure of oxytocin is shown in Fig. 1 and it can be seen that, (as discussed in Chapter 2) it is a peptide of nine amino acid residues, the first six of which are part of a 20-membered ring formed by disulfide linkage between the hemicystine residues at positions 1 and 6. It is sometimes convenient to regard all the analogues of neurohypophysial hormones, both natural and synthetic, as derivatives of oxytocin, and in this way arginine vasopressin whose structure is shown in Fig. 2 (a) is designated [3-phenylalanine, 8-arginine] oxytocin.

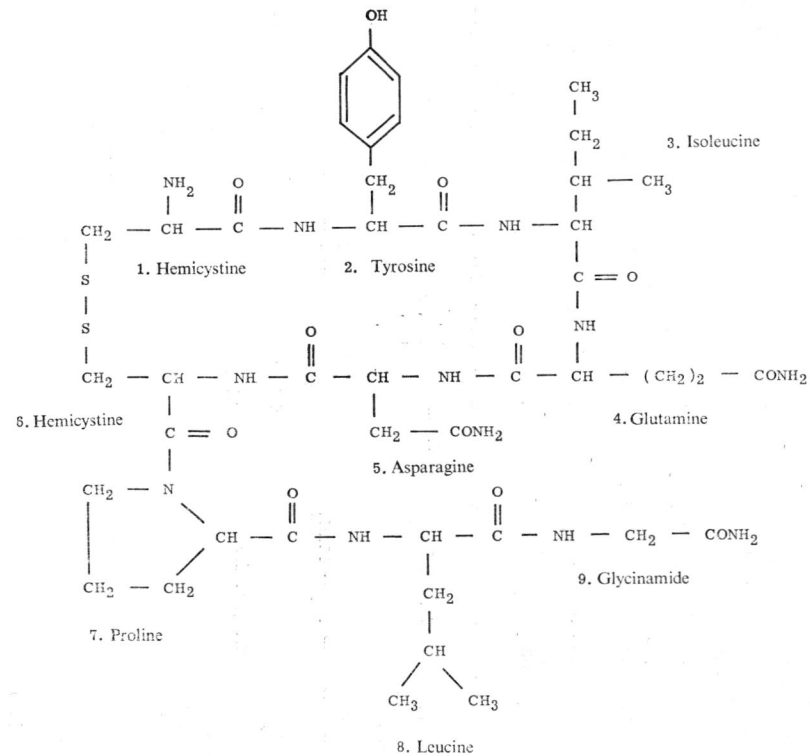

Fig. 1. Oxytocin.

STRUCTURAL AND BIOLOGICAL RELATIONSHIPS OF THE MAMMALIAN NEUROHYPOPHYSIAL HORMONES

It became apparent in the 1920s (see Chapter 1) that the various biological actions which had been ascribed to extracts of the posterior pituitary glands fell into one or other of two groups, and that preparations rich in the activities of one group or the other could be separated by chemical fractionation. The concept grew up of a pressor-antidiuretic

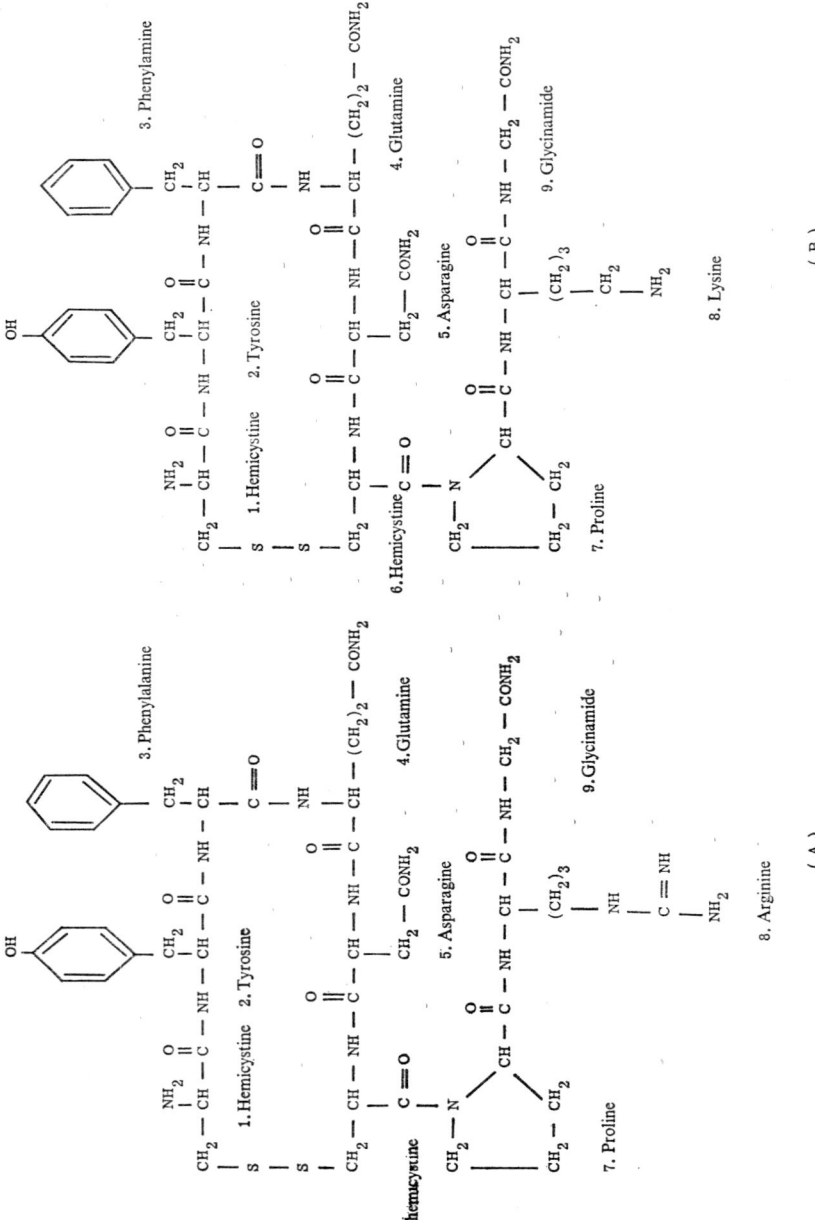

FIG. 2. (a) Arginine vasopressin; (b) Lysine vasopressin

TABLE 2. BIOLOGICAL ACTIVITIES OF THE MAMMALIAN NEUROHYPOPHYSIAL HORMONES

Hormone	Potency (Units/mg)*					
	Uterotonic (isolated rat uterus)		Milk-ejection (rabbit)	Vasodepressor (chicken)	Antidiuretic (rat)	Vasopressor (rat)
	$-Mg^{2+}$	$+Mg^{2+}$				
Oxytocin	450	405	380	450	1.1	2.7
Arginine vasopressin	9	21	51	42	400	400
Lysine vasopressin	5	12	51	28	165	270

* Calculated from Sawyer (1965).

substance (vasopressin) on the one hand and a uterotonic, avian depressor, milk-ejecting hormone (oxytocin) on the other, and overlap of the activities of the two fractions was regarded as the result of mutual contamination. When, however, the hormones were prepared in pure form it was found that they had many biological activities in common, and the situation was rationalized when the chemical structures of the hormones were determined and they were found to be very closely related molecules (Figs. 1 and 2). The vasopressins differ from oxytocin by only two amino acid residues: lysine vasopressin which occurs in the neurohypophyses of pigs and some other pig-like animals (see previous chapter) differs from oxytocin by having a phenylalanine residue in place of isoleucine in position 3 and by having the basic amino acid lysine in place of the neutral amino acid leucine in position 8. Arginine vasopressin, which is the most common mammalian antidiuretic hormone, differs from lysine vasopressin only in the way that its name suggests, namely that the basic amino acid in position 8 is arginine rather than lysine. In view of the apparent close structural similarity of oxytocin and the vasopressins, it is perhaps surprising, on first glance, that their biological activities are as divergent as they are (Table 2), even though the differences are of degree rather than of quality. However, when it is realized that the change at position 8 has meant the introduction of a positive charge into the molecule and that this may markedly alter the conformation of the peptide as well as influence its interaction with charged areas on the receptor molecule, the differences in biological potency are more understandable. Moreover, slight alterations in the structure of the neurohypophysial hormones will, because of the small size of these peptides, have a greater influence on the shape of the whole molecule than similar modifications would have on the gross structure of larger polypeptides or proteins.

STRUCTURAL REQUIREMENTS FOR UTEROTONIC, AVIAN DEPRESSOR AND MILK-EJECTING ACTIVITIES

When oxytocin is compared with arginine vasopressin (Table 2) it is seen that the replacement of phenylalanine by isoleucine at position 3 and of arginine by leucine at position 8 (Figs. 1 and 2) results in a fifty fold increase in the uterotonic activity *in vitro*. Thus it was immediately apparent that the nature of the amino acids in these two positions is an important factor in the determination of the biological activity profile of the peptides. Several synthetic analogues have been prepared with a view to establishing the degree of specificity in each of these positions. Table 3 shows the effect of amino acid substitutions in position 8, on the activity of the oxytocin molecule and, although all the analogues have a significantly lower rat uterus potency than oxytocin, only [8-ornithine]-

TABLE 3. EFFECT OF MODIFYING THE AMINO ACID IN POSITION 8 OF OXYTOCIN ON SOME OF ITS BIOLOGICAL ACTIVITIES

Amino acid in position 8	Potency (Units/mg)				Reference†
	Uterotonic (rat)		Avian depressor (chicken)	Milk ejecting (rabbit)	
	$-Mg^{2+}$	$+Mg^{2+}$*			
Leucine (oxytocin)	450	405	450	380	Sawyer (1965)
Isoleucine	289	363	498	328	Jaquenoud and Boissonnas (1961)
Valine	200		280	310	Jaquenoud and Boissonnas (1961)
Citrulline	202	312	225	238	van Dyke, Sawyer and Overweg (1963)
Ornithine	42	63	90	95	Berde *et al.* (1964)
Lysine	78	148	210	180	Huguenin and Boissonnas (1962)
Arginine	125	238	288	275	Sawyer (1965)

* Wherever uterotonic potencies in the presence of Mg^{2+} are quoted, they have been calculated from Sawyer (1965).

† In this and subsequent tables, a reference is given to the quotation of the biological activity rather than to the synthesis of an analogue. Many analogues have been synthesized and tested in more than one laboratory, but unless there is a discrepancy only one reference has been given.

oxytocin and [8-lysine]-oxytocin have less than 25% of the activity of oxytocin itself. Moreover, in the presence of magnesium ions (which is perhaps a more physiological condition) the differences between the potency of oxytocin and those of the analogues is much smaller, suggesting that, at least under these conditions, the amino acid at position 8 plays a minor role in the hormone–receptor interaction. Similarly, it can be seen from Table 3 that there is also a low specificity for position 8 in the avian depressor and milk-ejecting activities of these peptides. The relationship of chemical structure and milk-ejecting activity is considered in more detail in Chapter 8.

In contrast to the relatively low specificity of position 8, Table 4 shows that substitutions of the amino acid at position 3 markedly alter the activity of oxytocin. Of all the 3-substituted analogues of oxytocin that have been prepared, only those in which there is a methylene group in the same spatial position as the terminal methyl group of isoleucine [3-β-diethylalanine]-oxytocin and [3-L-cyclopentylglycine]-oxytocin, have appreciable uterotonic, avian depressor and milk-ejecting activities (Table 4). [3-Valine]-oxytocin which lacks this methylene group is a partial exception in view of its milk-ejecting and magnesium-dependent uterotonic activity suggesting a lower specific requirement for these actions.

In trying to determine more precisely the contribution that each amino acid in the molecule of oxytocin makes to the biological activity of the hormone, du Vigneaud and his associates have synthesized a number of structural analogues in which the chemical functional groups have been replaced one by one with hydrogen (du Vigneaud, 1964). The six chemical functional groups of oxytocin, which incidentally also occur in the vasopressins, are the disulfide bridge connecting the half-cystine residues at positions 1 and 6, the free amino-terminal group, the phenolic hydroxyl group of tyrosine and the three carboxamide groups of glutamine, asparagine and glycinamide. Table 5 shows the biological activities of the peptides prepared by du Vigneaud and his colleagues and it is at once apparent that all the functional groups except one, contribute in some measure to the potency of the hormone. The exception is the terminal amino group, since the peptide in which this group is replaced by hydrogen, deamino-oxytocin, has a higher potency than the naturally occurring hormone (Hope, Murti and du Vigneaud, 1962). The discovery that deamino-oxytocin is a highly potent analogue provides a salutary lesson in the caution which must be applied when interpreting results from analogues in which functional groups have been blocked. The observation that N-acetyloxytocin has very little uterotonic activity and no avian depressor activity (Boissonnas et al., 1961) led to the suggestion

TABLE 4. EFFECT OF MODIFYING THE AMINO ACID IN POSITION 3 OF OXYTOCIN ON SOME OF ITS BIOLOGICAL ACTIVITIES

Amino acid in position 3	Potency (Units/mg)				Reference
	Uterotonic (rat)		Avian Depressor (chicken)	Milk ejecting (rabbit)	
	$-Mg^{2+}$	$+Mg^{2+}$*			
Isoleucine (oxytocin)	450	405	450	380	Sawyer (1965)
Allo-isoleucine	24		19	125†	Nesvadba, Honzl and Rudinger (1963)
Diethylalanine	305		313	400	Eisler, Rudinger and Šorm (1966)
Cyclopentylglycine	252		226	380	Eisler, Rudinger and Šorm (1966)
Cyclohexylglycine	8.2		8.5	40	Eisler, Rudinger and Šorm (1966)
Valine	59	212	58	207	Berde, Cerletti and Konzett (1961)
Nor-valine	7		14	85†	Nesvadba and Rudinger (1963)
Leucine	6		10	35†	Nesvadba, Honzl and Rudinger (1963)
Nor-leucine	7		20	25†	Nesvadba, Honzl and Rudinger (1963)
Phenylalanine	20	28	68	110	Katsoyannis (1957)
Tyrosine	0.1		0.03	1.5	Boissonnas and Guttmann (1960)
Tryptophan	0.04		0.1	0.1	Guttmann and Boissonnas (1960)

* Calculated from Sawyer (1965).
† Milk ejection in guinea pig.

that a free amino group was necessary for activity but this has been disproved by the properties of deamino-oxytocin. Neither N-acetyl-oxytocin (Boissonnas et al., 1961; Smyth, 1967a) nor N-carbamyloxytocin (Smyth, 1967b), both of which have very low uterotonic activity, act as oxytocin inhibitors, and would therefore appear not to bind very well at the oxytocin receptors. Thus the low activity of these analogues appears to be due not to a masking of the amino group, but to steric hindrance produced by the added blocking group. Indeed, it seems that even the amino group itself may hinder hormone-receptor interaction.

TABLE 5. BIOLOGICAL ACTIVITIES OF ANALOGUES OF OXYTOCIN IN WHICH THE CHEMICAL FUNCTIONAL GROUPS HAVE BEEN REPLACED ONE BY ONE WITH HYDROGEN

Peptide	Biological activity (Units/mg)*		
	Uterotonic ($-Mg^{2+}$)	Avian depressor	Milk ejecting
Oxytocin	485	500	410
1,6-Dethio-oxytocin	0	0	–
1-Deamino-oxytocin †	750	900	500
2-Deoxy-oxytocin ([2-Phenylalanine]-oxytocin)	30	60	60
4-Decarboxamido-oxytocin	70	110	225
5-Decarboxamido-oxytocin	0.2 – 0.3	0.2 – 0.3	1
9-Decarboxamido-oxytocin	7	<0.02	4

* From du Vigneaud (1964).
† These data were obtained with a crystalline preparation.

Among the earlier synthetic analogues of oxytocin which were studied (Bodanszky and du Vigneaud, 1959; Konzett and Berde, 1959) was [2-phenylalanine]-oxytocin, a peptide lacking the tyrosine hydroxyl group present in position 2 in the parent hormone. This analogue, which is also known as deoxy-oxytocin, has about 5% of the uterotonic activity of oxytocin, although its milk-ejecting activity is closer to 20%. No inhibition of oxytocin has been observed with [2-phenylalanine]-oxytocin and this suggests that the low potency is due, at least in part, to an impaired ability to bind to the receptor rather than to a lowered intrinsic activity, although Rudinger and Krejčí (1962) point out that the shape of the dose-response curve of this analogue suggests that the low potency is not due to decreased binding alone. However, analogues in which the hydrogen of the tyrosine hydroxyl has been substituted by a larger group are inhibitors of the parent hormone—at least in its uterotonic activity. For example, when the hydrogen is replaced by a methyl group, the resulting analogue, [2-O-methyltyrosine]-oxytocin, has a very low (less than 1% that of oxytocin) uterotonic potency of its own, and can completely inhibit the activity of oxytocin (Bissett, 1963, 1964). Analysis of the concentration dependence of the inhibition shows (Rudinger and Krejčí,

1962) that the analogue acts as a competitive inhibitor of oxytocin and thus binds at the same site(s) as the hormone. It is interesting to note that although [2-*O*-methyltyrosine]-oxytocin is an inhibitor of the uterotonic action of oxytocin it does not appear to inhibit the milk-ejecting activity of the hormone (Bisset, 1964). Other analogues in which a large group has been attached to the tyrosine oxygen atom [2-*O*-ethyltyrosine]-oxytocin (Rudinger and Jošt, 1964), *N*-acetyl-*O*-acetyloxytocin (Smyth, 1967a) and *N*-carbamyl-*O*-carbamyloxytocin (Smyth, 1967b) are also inhibitors of the uterotonic action of oxytocin. These findings would indicate that the tyrosine hydroxyl is involved in a hormone–receptor interaction other than binding alone or, in other words, that it is part of the "active center" of the molecule. Two analogues in which the tyrosine hydroxyl has been completely replaced, [2-*p*-methylphenylalanine]-oxytocin and [2-*p*-ethylphenylalanine]-oxytocin, are also inhibitors of the parent hormone (Rudinger and Jošt, 1964). This is perhaps a little surprising in view of the absence of inhibitory properties of [2-phenylalanine]-oxytocin and it suggests that a *para* substituent increases the binding capacity of the peptide.

Two more of the chemical functional groups in oxytocin are the carboxamide groups on the glutamine residue at position 4 and the asparagine at position 5. There is a striking difference between the specificity requirements for each of these very similar amino acids, the requirement being much more stringent for the 5-asparagine than for the 4-glutamine. A low specificity for glutamine would be expected since position 4 is one in which changes occur naturally, in hormones where glutamine is replaced by serine in [4-serine, 8-isoleucine]-oxytocin (Acher *et al.*, 1962; Follett and Heller, 1963) which occurs in bony fishes, and in [4-serine, 8-glutamine]-oxytocin which occurs in some cartilaginous fishes (Acher *et al.*, 1965).

Replacement of the glutamine residue by asparagine, [4-asparagine]-oxytocin (Jaquenoud and Boissonnas, 1962a), or removal of its functional group, 4-decarboxamido oxytocin (du Vigneaud *et al.*, 1964), yielded analogues which retained a moderate amount of activity (e.g. see Table 5). However, the introduction of a negative charge at position 4 by the removal of the amide group alone gave the analogue [4-glutamic acid]-oxytocin with very low activities (Photaki and du Vigneaud, 1965). One effect of replacing the 4-glutamine, at least with serine, on the uterotonic action, is the greater sensitivity to the concentration of magnesium ions in the suspension fluid. Thus the ratio of the uterotonic activity of [4-serine, 8-isoleucine]-oxytocin in the presence of 0.5 mM Mg^{2+} to that in the absence of the ion is around 3, a property which was important in the discovery of the hormone (Heller *et al.*, 1961). This change in magnesium potentiation may be interpreted (Rudinger, 1967) as being due to the removal of a magnesium-insensitive binding site so that magnesium-dependent ones are relatively more prominent, or to the replacement of a magnesium-insensitive site by a magnesium-dependent one.

In contrast to the low specificity for glutamine in position 4, there seems to be an almost absolute requirement for asparagine at position 5. Simple removal of the carboxamide group (Guttman and Boissonnas, 1963; du Vigneaud *et al.*, 1964), or even its displacement from the ring by the insertion of one extra methylene group to give [5-glutamine]-oxytocin (Jaquenoud and Boissonnas, 1962a), led to almost complete loss of activity in all the biological tests. This being so it is not surprising that [5-valine]-oxytocin (Walter and Schwartz, 1966) and the analogue in which the asparagine and glutamine residues have been interchanged, [4-asparagine, 5-glutamine]-oxytocin (Jaquenoud and Boissonnas, 1962a) are also almost devoid of activity.

The terminal glycinamide also appears to play an important role in the binding of hormone to the receptor. Removal of the carboxamide functional group to give 9-decarboxamido oxytocin (Branda and du Vigneaud, 1966) or of the amide group alone as in [9-glycine]-oxytocin (Ferrier and du Vigneaud, 1966) results in analogues with very little activity, as does removal of the glycine residue altogether (Jaquenoud and Boissonnas, 1962b). Replacement of glycine with hydrazino acetic acid or addition of this grouping to its carboxyl terminus also yield peptides with very little activity although the latter compound, in which the glycine residue as such is intact, is much more active than the former (Niedrich, Wiegershausen and Göres, 1964). Addition of a methyl group to the nitrogen of the glycine residue to give [9-sarcosine]-oxytocin (Cash *et al.*, 1962) also markedly decreases the activity of the hormone but to a much lesser degree than the other modifications of glycine which have been discussed.

The 1 : 6 disulfide link present in all the neurohypophysial hormones has attracted much attention as a possible active site. Observation of the effects of the sulfhydryl-blocking agent N-ethyl maleimide on the amphibian bladder water-transporting activity of neurohypophysial hormones led to the suggestion (Schwartz *et al.*, 1964) that the disulfide bond in the hormone was reacting with free sulfhydryl groups in the receptor thus initiating a series of thiol-disulfide exchanges which, in the case of the amphibian bladder, resulted in a structural change in a component of a water-permeability barrier. Desulfurization of oxytocin with Raney-nickel leads to complete loss of activity (Turner, Pierce and du Vigneaud,

1951). However, desulfurization completely alters the configuration of oxytocin since the resulting peptide has no stable hexapeptide ring, and it is known that even increasing the size of this 20-membered ring by one carbon atom as in [1-γ-mercaptobutyric acid]-oxytocin results in a very feebly active peptide (Jarvis, Ferrier and du Vigneaud, 1965). This finding was foreshadowed by the earlier (Ressler and du Vigneaud, 1957) observation that the 4-isoglutamine analogue of oxytocin was virtually without activity, and in the light of present knowledge of the low specificity at position 4 this loss of activity must be due to the increase (from 20–22) in size of the ring. Replacement of one or both of the sulfur atoms with selenium has little effect on the potency of oxytocin (Walter and du Vigneaud, 1965; 1966), but this does not argue very strongly against the importance of a disulfide bond for activity, since a diselenide bond might be expected to have similar properties. More pertinent information about the contribution of the disulfide bond to the activity of neurohypophysial hormones is obtained from analogues in which one, or both of the sulfur atoms have been replaced by methylene groups and in which the size of the ring remains virtually the same (Jošt and Rudinger, 1967). Figure 3 shows the structure of these analogues and gives their potencies, and it is at once apparent that the disulfide bridge as such is not essential to activity. However, the lower potency of the 1,6 dicarba-analogue indicates nevertheless that the disulfide bond may play a part in the binding of hormone to receptor, perhaps by the kind of thiol-disulfide interchange envisaged by Schwartz *et al*. (1964), and this suggestion is supported by the observation that glutathione acts as a competitive inhibitor of oxytocin on the isolated rat uterus (Bentley, 1964). In addition, the disulfide bond is important for the correct spatial orientation of other binding sites and the possible "active center".

Munsick (1960) determined the uterotonic potency *in vitro*, relative to the International Standard, of several analogues of oxytocin on isolated rat uteri suspended either in a magnesium-free medium or in one containing 0.5 mM Mg^{2+}. All the analogues which he used, except oxytocin itself, showed an increased potency in the presence of magnesium ions. The ratio
$$\frac{\text{Potency} + Mg^{2+}}{\text{Potency} - Mg^{2+}}$$
is a useful parameter for the pharmacological characterization of neurohypophysial hormones, and has led to the discovery of new hormones in pituitary extracts from lower vertebrates (see previous chapter). The potentiation of uterotonic activity in the presence of magnesium ions provides some pharmacological basis for the earlier observation (Berde,

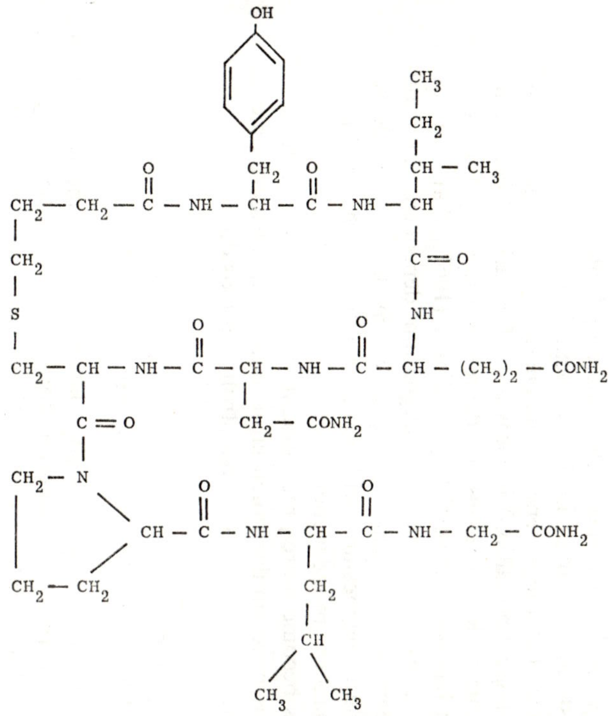

Chemical Structure and Biological Activity

FIG. 3. (a) 1-carba-1-deamino-oxytocin; (b) 1,6-dicarba-1-deamino-oxytocin, analogues in which one or both sulfurs of the disulfide bond have been replaced with methylene groups

Rat uterus, 300 U/mg; Chicken depressor, 125 U/mg; Guinea pig milk ejection 450 U/mg
(A)

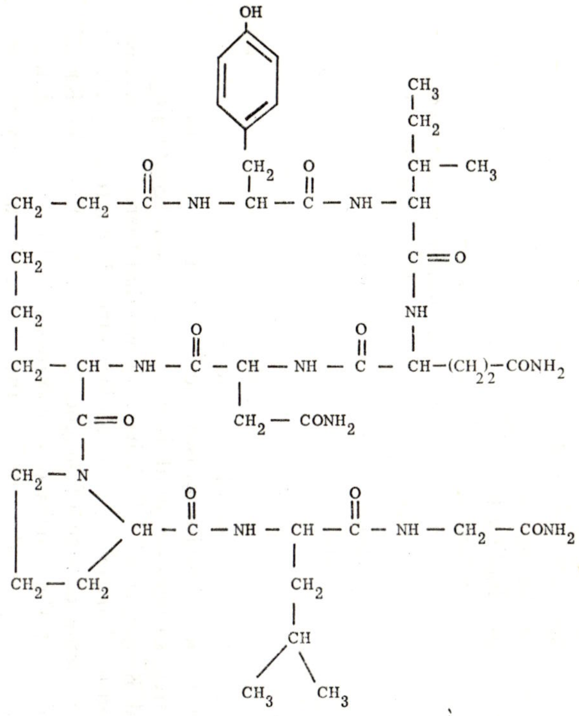

Rat uterus, 9 U/mg; chicken depressor, 2·5 U/mg; Guinea pig milk ejection, 3 U/mg.
(B)

Doepfner and Konzett, 1957) that the potency of several analogues was greater when tested on the uterus *in vivo* than on the isolated organ, and for Fitzpatrick's (1956) finding that the activity of Pitressin on the cow uterus *in vivo* was potentiated by an increase in the serum magnesium concentration, while the activity of Pitocin was not so potentiated. The lack of potentiation of the activity of oxytocin itself by magnesium

i.e. $$\frac{\text{Potency} + \text{Mg}^{2+}}{\text{Potency} - \text{Mg}^{2+}} = 1$$

is a mathematical rather than a pharmacological phenomenon, since oxytocin is the reference substance in both assays. In fact there is an increase in the absolute potency of oxytocin, since there is always a decrease in the threshold dose for an isotonically contracting uterus when a magnesium free suspension fluid is replaced by one containing 0.5 mM Mg^{++}, and Krejčí *et al.* (1964) have shown that there is an increase in the maximum tension developed in an isometrically contracting uterus subjected to the same change of magnesium concentration. As Krejčí *et al.* (1964) point out, the paucity of our knowledge of uterine physiology makes it difficult to suggest the cause of the changes induced by magnesium ions. It is probable that the general excitability of the muscle cells may be altered by changes in ion concentrations perhaps through changes in membrane potential. However, the differential effects of the various peptides suggests an alteration in the oxytocin–receptor interaction, and it seems possible that the absence of magnesium ions (since this is the more unphysiological condition) induces a conformational change in the receptor molecule which increases the degree of specificity for oxytocin. Alternatively it has been suggested by Rudinger (1967), that some of the binding sites in oxytocin may be magnesium-dependent and others magnesium-independent, so that analogues which show a high degree of potentiation with magnesium will have resulted from modifications involving a magnesium-independent site(s) such that the magnesium-dependent ones become more predominant. Bentley (1965) has found that manganous ions have similar potentiating effects on the uterotonic activities of analogues of oxytocin, but that strontium ions do not.

THE INFLUENCE OF STRUCTURAL CHANGES ON PRESSOR-ANTIDIURETIC ACTIVITY

Arginine vasopressin and the closely related peptide lysine vasopressin are the mammalian pressor-antidiuretic hormones, the latter being present in the pituitary glands of certain pig-like animals and the former being widely distributed throughout the mammals. Perhaps the greatest structural difference between the vasopressins and oxytocin (Figs. 1 and 2) is the presence of a basic amino acid at position 8 instead of the neutral leucine, thus resulting in the introduction of an additional chemical functional group into the molecule. This change, together with the substitution of phenylalanine for isoleucine at position 3 transforms a peptide with predominantly uterotonic, milk-ejecting and avian depressor activities into one with very pronounced mammalian vasopressor and antidiuretic potencies (Table 2). In much the same way as has been discussed for the oxytocin series, analogues were prepared to see which of the two amino acid substitutions, the phenylalanine at position 3 or the basic amino acid at position 8, is the more important for the manifestation of pressor-antidiuretic activity. Table 6 shows the effects of combining the ring of oxytocin with the side chain of vasopressin and *vice versa*. It can be seen that although the phenylalanine at position 3 contributes to the antidiuretic, and, to a lesser extent, to the pressor activity—as shown by the fact that [3-phenylalanine]-oxytocin is a better antidiuretic and pressor agent than oxytocin—it would seem that it is the substitution of arginine or lysine for leucine at position 8 which is largely responsible for the high pressor-antidiuretic activity which distinguishes the vasopressins from oxytocin. This is in contrast with the observations discussed above which show that the isoleucine in position 3 of oxytocin is more important for the uterotonic, milk-ejecting and avian depressor activities than the amino acid in position 8. Discussion of the relative influence of individual amino acids on the potency of these peptides is a very useful exercise but must be carried out with caution. Table 6 shows that lysine vasotocin does not entirely fit the hypothesis which has just been expounded, since its antidiuretic potency is no greater than that of [3-phenylalanine]-oxytocin and is only 15% that of lysine vasopressin. It would appear, therefore, that although the replacement of phenylalanine by isoleucine has very little effect on the interaction of the antidiuretic receptor molecule and the basic residue at position 8 when this is arginine, the nature of lysine is such that its interaction is very much reduced under these conditions. This serves to underline the importance of the spatial relationship of the various reactive parts of the molecule for hormonal activity. In other words, although the basicity of residue 8 may be a prime factor in the production of an antidiuretic response, it can only come into play if the shape of the molecule as a whole is such that the basic residue can "react" with the relevant part of the receptor.

Returning to the importance of the basicity of residue 8, it was first suggested by Katsoyannis and du Vigneaud (1958) that it was an essential

TABLE 6. BIOLOGICAL PROPERTIES OF ANALOGUES IN WHICH THE RING OF OXYTOCIN IS JOINED TO THE SIDE CHAIN OF VASOPRESSIN AND *vice versa*

Peptide	Amino acid in position		Potency (Units/mg)					Reference
	3	8	Uterotonic ($-Mg^{2+}$)	Milk ejecting	Avian depressor	Antidiuretic	Vasopressor	
[8-arginine]-vasopressin	Phe	Arg	9	51	42	400	400	Sawyer (1965)
[8-lysine]-vasopressin	Phe	Lys	5	51	28	165	270	Sawyer (1965)
[3-phenylalanine]-oxytocin	Phe	Leu	20	110	68	22	4.2	Katsoyannis (1957)
Oxytocin	Ile	Leu	450	380	450	1.1	2.7	Sawyer (1965)
[8-arginine]-oxytocin	Ile	Arg	125	275	288	195	245	Sawyer (1965)
[8-lysine]-oxytocin	Ile	Lys	78	108	210	24	130	Huguenin and Boissonnas (1962)

factor in determining pressor-antidiuretic activity as a result of observations on the potency of a series of peptides in which the amino acid at position 8 was, in turn, leucine, histidine, lysine and arginine. Since then, many more 8-substituted analogues have been synthesized and the biological properties of a selection of these are given in Table 7. Two points of interest are illustrated by this Table. Firstly, it shows that peptides with a basic amino acid at position 8 (arginine, lysine, ornithine and 2 : 4 diaminobutyric acid) have pronounced pressor and antidiuretic activities, whereas those with neutral residues in this position (histidine is

TABLE 7. EFFECT OF THE AMINO ACID IN POSITION 8 ON THE (RAT) VASOPRESSOR AND (RAT) ANTIDIURETIC ACTIVITIES OF PEPTIDES IN THE VASOPRESSIN SERIES

Amino acid in position 8	Potency (Units/mg)		Reference
	Vaso-pressor	Antidi-uretic	
L-Arginine	400	400	Sawyer (1965)
L-Lysine	270	165	Sawyer (1965)
L-Ornithine	360	88	Berde, Boissonnas, Huguenin and Stürmer (1964)
L-2:4 Diaminobutyric acid	149	120	Zaoral and Šorm (1966a)
L-Citrulline	30	38	van Dyke, Sawyer and Overweg (1963)
L-Leucine	4	22	Katsoyannis (1957)
D-Arginine	4.1	114	Zaoral, Kolc and Šorm (1967a)
D-Lysine	0.75	6–10	Zaoral, Kolc and Šorm (1967a)
D-2:4 Diaminobutyric acid	3.6	120	Zaoral and Šorm (1966b)

neutral at physiological pH) generally have low activities. However, shape also plays a part in determining potency, since the analogue containing citrulline, which is very similar sterically to arginine but has no positive charge, shows a high potency in both pressor and antidiuretic assays. The second interesting feature shown in Table 7 is the dissociation of pressor from antidiuretic activity in analogues in which the basic residue in position 8 is in the D-configuration. Thus, although the biological receptor for the pressor response has a very high degree of specificity for an L-isomer at residue 8, the antidiuretic receptor has a very much lower specificity. Again lysine seems to be an exception and [8-D-lysine]-vasopressin is a poor antidiuretic substance. This seems to suggest that the interaction of the receptor with lysine is much more tenuous than that with arginine, and perhaps is one of the factors responsible for the very narrow natural distribution of lysine vasopressin compared with that of the arginine congener.

The high antidiuretic to pressor ratio for the D-arginine isomer of vasopressin allows an explanation to be advanced for some very early results of Heller (1939). He found that when Pitressin (Parke, Davis and Co.) was heated at alkaline pH the pressor activity was destroyed to a much greater extent than the antidiuretic activity. For example, after heating for 90 min at 99° and pH 10, the ratio of antidiuretic to pressor activity changed from 1 : 1 to 12 : 1. One of the changes that is likely to occur when a polypeptide is heated at alkaline pH is racemization of some of the constituent amino acids and, if one can extrapolate from the action of dilute sodium hydroxide on adrenocorticotropin (ACTH), one of the amino acids most likely to racemize is arginine (Pickering and Li, 1964). Thus it seems possible that Heller had made [8-D-arginine]-vasopressin some 30 years before its chemical synthesis (Zaoral, Kolc and Šorm 1967a). One of the analogues shown in Table 7, [8-ornithine]-vasopressin also shows dissociated pressor and antidiuretic activities but in this case the pressor potency is the greater. By replacing the tyrosine residue at position 2 with a phenylalanine residue (i.e. by producing the deoxy analogue) this dissociation is even more enhanced, since this peptide, [2-phenylalanine, 8-ornithine]-vasopressin has a $\frac{\text{pressor}}{\text{antidiuretic}}$ ratio of about 10—which can be increased to 220 by replacing the 3-phenylalanine with isoleucine to give [2-phenylalanine, 8-ornithine]-oxytocin (Berde et al., 1964). A similar increase of pressor relative to antidiuretic activity is found in deoxy-lysine vasopressin but the reverse is true for deoxy-arginine vasopressin (Berde et al., 1964).

In general, apart from the special cases of residues 3 and 8, modifications of the amino acids of vasopressin produce similar effects on its activity as the same structural changes on the activity of oxytocin. Blocking or removal of the terminal amino group of the vasopressins have much the same effects on the pressor-antidiuretic actions of these hormones as the same modifications have on the uterotonic action of oxytocin. Thus the N-acetylated vasopressins have little or no activity (Studer and Cash, 1963; Cash and Smith, 1963) whereas removal of the amino group generally leads to enhanced antidiuretic activity (Table 8). It is interesting to note that the pressor potencies of the deamino analogues are in general somewhat lower than those of the complete peptides and this may reflect the importance of the positive charge of the molecule as a whole, rather than of residue 8 alone, for full reaction with the pressor

TABLE 8. EFFECTS OF THE ABSENCE OF THE TERMINAL AMINO GROUP ON THE BIOLOGICAL ACTIVITY OF POTENT VASOPRESSOR AND ANTIDIURETIC PEPTIDES IN THE VASOPRESSIN SERIES

Amino acid in position 8	Potency (Units/mg)				Reference
	Vasopressor		Antidiuretic		
	Intact peptide	1-deamino derivative	Intact peptide	1-deamino derivative	
L-Arginine	400	370	400	1300	Huguenin and Boissonnas (1966)
L-Lysine	243	126	203	301	Kimbrough et al., (1963)
L-Ornithine	360	355	88	202	Berde and Boissonnas (1966)
D-Arginine	4.1	11	114	870	Zaoral, Kolc and Šorm (1967b)
D-Lysine	0.75	1.05	6–10	3.8	Zaoral, Kolc and Šorm (1967b)
D-:4 Diamino-2butyric acid	3.6	2.05	120	360	Zaoral, Kolc and Šorm (1967b)

receptor (Kimbrough et al., 1963). However, the properties of the D-isomers of the vasopressins are not in accord with this suggestion.

The tyrosine residue in position 2 seems to play a similar role in the initiation of the pressor response of vasopressin as it does in the uterotonic effect of oxytocin. Thus [2-O-methyltyrosine, 8-lysine]-vasopressin has a low intrinsic pressor activity and acts as an inhibitor in the pressor assay, and the O-ethyl derivative is also an inhibitor (Zaoral and Šorm, 1964).

Another feature in common with the oxytocin series is the low specificity of the glutamine in position 4. For example, [4-asparagine, 8-lysine]-vasopressin is a good pressor-antidiuretic substance (Zaoral et al., 1963), although Zaoral and Šorm (1964) point out that the very high antidiuretic potency originally claimed for this peptide (about three times that of lysine vasopressin) is misleading, since the dose-response lines of the analogue and the natural hormone intersect at a dose of about 10^{-7}mg. Thus the 4-asparagine analogue appears more potent than lysine vasopressin at doses below 10^{-7}mg and less potent at doses above this level. Nevertheless, this analogue is a potent pressor-antidiuretic substance and demonstrates the low specific requirement at position 4.

Finally it might be mentioned that the integrity of the ring is as much a requirement for pressor-antidiuretic activity as it is for oxytocic activity and this has been demonstrated by the synthesis of dethio-derivatives of the vasopressin (Huguenin and Guttmann, 1965) which are compounds with negligible activity.

STRUCTURE-ACTIVITY CONSIDERATIONS OF THE ACTIONS OF NEUROHYPOPHYSIAL HORMONES ON AMPHIBIAN BLADDERS

Neurohypophysial hormones increase the transport across the wall of the bladder of both water, measured by loss in weight (Bentley, 1958; Sawyer, 1960) and sodium, measured by a change in the short-circuit current (Ussing and Zerahn, 1951; Maetz, Morel and Race, 1959). Information on the specific activities of analogues of the neurohypophysial hormones in these systems comes mainly from three sources. Rasmussen *et al.* (1963) have studied the hydro-osmotic effects of 34 analogues on the bladder of the toad *(Bufo marinus)* and Sawyer (1965) lists potencies for this action on the bladder of the bullfrog *(Rana catesbiana)*. Sodium transport-stimulating (natriferic) activity has been studied largely in the laboratory of Morel using the bladder of the edible frog *(Rana esculenta)*, and the natriferic potency of many analogues is listed by Morel and Bastide (1964). Table 9 compares the frog bladder natriferic activity with the water transporting activity of both frog and toad bladders for a selection of analogues, and is compiled from the results of these three groups of workers.

Arginine vasotocin (Fig. 4) is by far the most active peptide in each of these amphibian bioassay procedures which might have been expected from the fact that this peptide is one of the hormones present in amphibian neurohypophyses (Acher *et al.*, 1960; Heller and Pickering, 1961; Sawyer, Munsick and van Dyke, 1961). Any alteration in the structure of arginine vasotocin leads to a diminished potency in each of these tests; although substitution of amino acid residue 8 seems to be the least harmful of the modifications which have been tested. Indeed omission of residue 8 altogether results in an analogue, [des-8-leucine]-oxytocin, with as much, or slightly more natriferic activity than oxytocin (Morel and Bastide, 1964), and even the peptide lacking all the amino acids of the side chain and consisting of the amide of the oxytocin ring has a potency

TABLE 9. EFFECT OF MODIFICATIONS OF THE MOLECULE OF 8-ARGININE OXYTOCIN, (ARGININE VASOTOCIN, AVT), ON ITS ABILITY TO STIMULATE WATER MOVEMENT AND SODIUM TRANSPORT ACROSS AMPHIBIAN BLADDERS

Analogue	Amino acids different from AVT	Frog natriferic activity (U/mg)[1]	Hydro-osmotic activity (U/mg)	
			Frog[2]	Toad[3]
[8-Arginine]-oxytocin	None	1,140	114,000	11,250
[8-Lysine]-oxytocin	$Arg^8 \rightarrow Lys^8$	940	14,850	2,812
[8-Isoleucine]-oxytocin	$Arg^8 \rightarrow Ile^8$	507	1,670	900
[8-Citrulline]-oxytocin	$Arg^8 \rightarrow Cit^8$		800	750
[8-Glycine]-oxytocin	$Arg^8 \rightarrow Gly^8$		380	
Oxytocin	$Arg^8 \rightarrow Leu^8$	450	450	450
Deamino-oxytocin	$Arg^8 \rightarrow Leu^8$ $CyS^1 \rightarrow 1\text{-}\beta\text{-}$mercaptopropionic acid	190		51
[8-Arginine]-vasopressin	$Ile^3 \rightarrow Phe^3$	33	23	146
[8-Lysine]-vasopressin	$Ile^3 \rightarrow Phe^3$ $Arg^8 \rightarrow Lys^8$	5.4	2	45
[deamino-8-Lysine] vasopressin	$Ile^3 \rightarrow Phe^3$ $Arg^8 \rightarrow Lys^8$ $CyS^1 \rightarrow 1\text{-}\beta\text{-}$mercaptopropionic acid			4
[8-Citrulline]-vasopressin	$Ile^3 \rightarrow Phe^3$ $Arg^8 \rightarrow Cit^8$		3.9	18
[3-Phenylalanine]-oxytocin	$Ile^3 \rightarrow Phe^3$ $Arg^8 \rightarrow Leu^8$	1.8	6	1.4
[3-allo-Isoleucine]-oxytocin	$Ile^3 \rightarrow aIle^3$ $Arg^8 \rightarrow Leu^8$	8.9		38
[3-Valine]-oxytocin	$Ile^3 \rightarrow Val^3$ $Arg^8 \rightarrow Leu^8$	49	<12	14
[4-Asparagine]-oxytocin	$Arg^8 \rightarrow Leu^8$ $Gln^4 \rightarrow Asn^4$	18		450
[4-Serine, 8-isoleucine]-oxytocin	$Arg^8 \rightarrow Ile^8$ $Gln^4 \rightarrow Ser^4$	5.3	6	180
[2-Phenylalanine]-oxytocin	$Arg^8 \rightarrow Leu^8$ $Tyr^2 \rightarrow Phe^2$	36	24	11.2

1. Morel and Bastide (1964).
2. Calculated from Sawyer (1965).
3. Rasmussen et al. (1963).

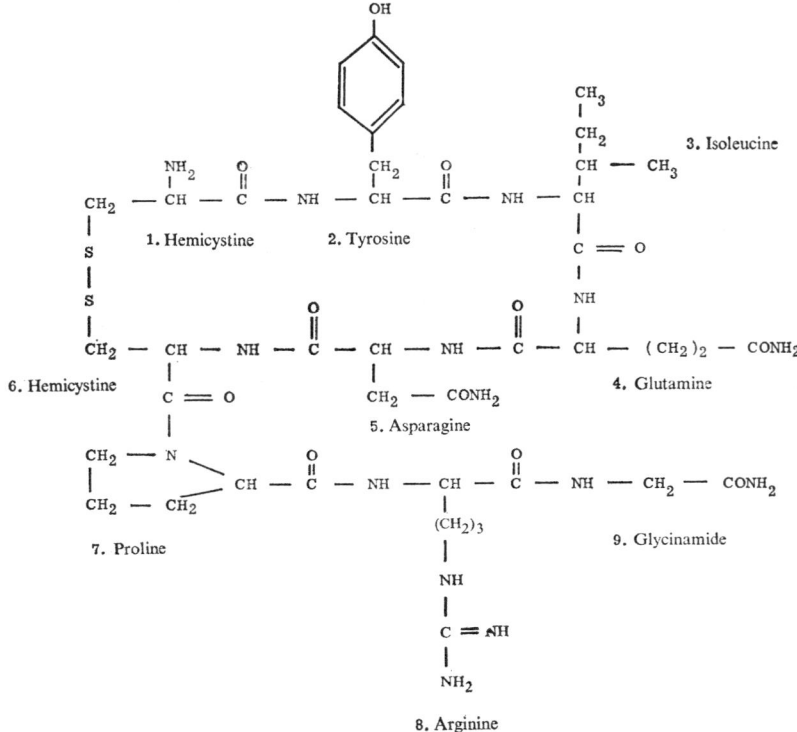

Fig. 4. [8-Arginine]-oxytocin, arginine vasotocin.

of 33 Units/mg when tested on water transport on the toad bladder (Rasmussen et al., 1963).

In contrast with its effect on the uterotonic and antidiuretic activities of these peptides, removal of the terminal amino group decreases the natriferic and water-transfer potencies in both frog and toad bladders. In general there is a high specific requirement for isoleucine at residue 3 but the toad bladder receptors appear to be able to tolerate the substitution of phenylalanine in this position provided that arginine, lysine or isoleucine are present in position 8. There is a similar difference in the requirements of frog and toad receptors for the amino acid in position 4. Any change from the glutamine normally present in this position markedly lowers both sodium and water transport-stimulating activities of the peptides when tested on frog bladders, whereas the potency is much less affected when obtained from the effect on water transport across toad bladders, and [4-asparagine] oxytocin is as potent as oxytocin in this system. It will be recalled that there is a low specific requirement for the 4 glutamine in all the mammalian test systems. The variability experienced in bladder assays makes it dangerous to compare absolute potencies obtained in different laboratories and thus no attempt has been made to distinguish structural requirements for natriferic activity from those of water-movement activity.

Of all the 34 analogues tested by Rasmussen et al. (1963) only one, [2-serine, 8-lysine]-vasopressin, showed no activity at all, and they interpret their results with the other analogues as suggesting that the variation in potency they observed was due to changes in the affinity of the peptides for the toad bladder receptors rather than a change in intrinsic activity. These authors found also that apart from the exception mentioned above, only by destroying (reducing) the disulfide bond, and thus losing the integrity of the ring structure, could the activity be abolished. Increase in the size of the ring by insertion of a methylene group between the two sulfur atoms gave a peptide [1,6-djenkolic acid-8-lysine]-vasopressin with very low potency for the stimulation of water transport across toad bladders (Schwartz, Howard and Guggenheim, 1964). The analogues in which one or both of the sulfur atoms have been replaced with methylene groups (Fig. 3) have respectively 0.4% and 0.03% of the natriferic activity of oxytocin, i.e. 1.8 U/mg and 0.14 U/mg (Jošt and Rudinger, 1967). Thus although a disulfide bond is not absolutely essential for natriferic activity it plays a major role in the production of this effect and is more important for natriferic than for uterotonic activity.

SYNTHETIC PEPTIDES WITH PROTRACTED ACTIVITY—HORMONOGENS

Rudinger, Šorm and their co-workers have synthesized a series of analogues in which additional amino acids or short peptide chains have been attached at the NH_2-terminus of oxytocin and vasopressin. The rationale for the synthesis of these analogues was the prediction that the free hormones would gradually be liberated from them *in vivo* after the stepwise removal of the additional amino acid residues by the action of aminopeptidases. The biological properties of a group of such analogues of oxytocin (Beránková-Ksandrová et al., 1966) are in accord with this hypothesis. There was a prolongation of the antidiuretic effects of these peptides compared with that of oxytocin and, in general, the degree of prolongation (index of persistence) increased with the length of the attached peptide. Moreover, there was an inverse relationship between the index of persistence and the specific activity of the analogues, a finding which is consistent with the view that their activity is due to the gradual release of oxytocin, and which justifies the name *hormonogens* for this group of analogues. The avian depressor and milk ejecting activities of these hormonogens were also studied by Beránková-Ksandravá, *et al.* (1966) and found to be prolonged, although the results were complicated by tachyphylaxis. Nevertheless, the hormonogens did produce protracted responses and these could be matched by continuous infusions of oxytocin which produced similar tachyphylactic effects as the hormonogens. Similar hormonogens related to vasopressin have been synthesized and show protracted pressor and antidiuretic activities (Kasafírek *et al.*, 1966).

SOME GENERAL CONCLUSIONS

In spite of the wealth of information available, it is difficult to make any positive conclusions on the relationship of structure and activity in the series of peptides related to the neurohypophysial hormones, and it is only possible to look for some pointers towards the final solution. An intact hexapeptide ring is essential for activity and the neurohypophysial hormones and analogues with an intact ring are the only peptides which are known to initiate milk-ejecting or amphibian bladder effects. Straight chain peptides of a similar size to oxytocin, like angiotensin and bradykinin, which stimulate the isolated rat uterus have no effect on milk-ejection (Bisset and Lewis, 1962) or water transport across the toad bladder (Rasmussen *et al.*, 1963).

What is the importance of the various amino acids in oxytocin and vasopressin? It is difficult to implicate any given amino acid in an active center rather than a binding site, with the possible exception of the tyrosine at position 2 where the inhibitory properties of the methoxy and ethoxy derivatives suggest that this residue may be involved in the initiation of response, although this conclusion can be reached only with regard to uterotonic and vasopressor responses.

The asparagine in position 5 appears to be an important binding site in all of the test systems. Any modification of the residue, however slight, leads to a drastic reduction in activity. This is in contrast to low specific requirement for glutamine in position 4 in all but the frog bladder receptors.

Uterotonic activity is very sensitive to changes in residue 3 where the isoleucine present in oxytocin seems to be very much involved in the binding to the myometrial receptors presumably by lipophilic interactions of its terminal methyl group (Nesvadba *et al.*, 1963; Rudinger and Jošt, 1964; Chimiak and Rudinger, 1965; Eisler, Rudinger and Šorm, 1966). Similarly, pressor-antidiuretic activity is largely associated with the presence of a basic residue in position 8, although it may be worth while to repeat the warning that the molecule must be considered as a whole rather than as the sum of the individual amino acids. This is shown in Table 6 by the pressor-antidiuretic properties of peptides in which the basic amino acid at residue 8 is lysine.

REFERENCES

BOOKS, REVIEWS, AND MONOGRAPHS

BERDE, B. and BOISSONNAS, R. A. (1966). Synthetic analogues and homologues of the posterior pituitary hormones. *The Pituitary Gland*, vol. 3, pp. 624–661. Harris, G. W. and Donovan, B. T. (eds.). Butterworths, London.

BERDE, B., CERLETTI, A. and KONZETT, H. (1961). The biological activity of a series of peptides related to oxytocin. *Oxytocin*, pp. 247–264. Caldeyro-Barcia, R. and Heller, H. (eds.). Pergamon Press, Oxford.

BISSET, G. W. (1964). The effect on milk-ejecting activity of modifying two functional groups in oxytocin. *Oxytocin, Vasopressin and Their Structural Analogues* vol. 10, pp. 21–29. Proc. 2nd Int. Pharmacol. Meeting, Rudinger, J. (ed.). Pergamon Press, Oxford.

DU VIGNEAUD, V. (1964). An organic chemical approach to the study of the significance of the chemical functional groups of oxytocin to its biological activities. *Proc. Robert A. Welch. Foundation Conf. Chem. Res. VIII. Selected topics in modern biochemistry*, pp. 133–147.

HARTLEY, B. S. (1964). The structure and activity of chymotrypsin. *Structure and Activity of Enzymes*. Goodwin, T. W., Harris, J. I. and Hartley, B. S. (eds.). Academic Press, London.

KREJČÍ, I., POLACEK, I., KUPKOVA, B. and RUDINGER, J. (1964). Dose-response analysis of the action of some oxytocin analogues on the isolated uterus: the effect of ions. *Oxytocin, Vasopressin and Their Structural Analogues* vol. 10, pp. 117–122. Proc. 2nd Int. Pharmacol. Meeting, Rudinger, J. (ed.). Pergamon Press, Oxford.

MOREL, F. and BASTIDE, F. (1964). Relationship between the structure of several analogues of oxytocin and their "natriferic" activity *in vitro*. *Oxytocin, Vasopressin and Their Structural Analogues* vol. 10, pp. 47–55. Proc. 2nd Int. Pharmacol. Meeting, Rudinger, J. (ed.). Pergamon Press, Oxford.

NIEDRICH, H., WIEGERSHAUSEN, B. and GÖRES, E. (1964). Synthesis and activity of oxytocin analogues with carboxyl-terminal hydrazinoacetic acid. *Oxytocin, Vasopressin and Their Structural Analogues* vol. 10, pp. 173–176. Proc. 2nd Int. Pharmacol. Meeting, Rudinger, J. (ed.). Pergamon Press, Oxford.

RUDINGER, J. and JOŠT, K. (1964). Synthetic analogues of oxytocin and vasopressin: structural relations. *Oxytocin, Vasopressin and Their Structural Analogues*, vol. 10, pp. 3–19. Proc. 2nd Int. Pharmacol. Meeting, Rudinger, J. (ed.). Pergamon Press, Oxford.

SCHWARTZ, I. L. and LIVINGSTON, L. M. (1964). Cellular and molecular aspects of the antidiuretic action of vasopressins and related peptides. *Vitamins and Hormones*, 22: 261–358.

SCHWARTZ, I. L., RASMUSSEN, H., MARC-AURELE, J. and CHRISTMAN, D. (1964). Molecular phenomena related to the mechanism of action of vasopressin on membrane permeability. In: *The Biochemical Aspects of Hormone Action.* Eisenstein, A. B. (ed.). J. & A. Churchill, London

ZAORAL, M. and ŠORM, F. (1966). Preparation and biological activity of some new lysine vasopressin analogues. *Oxytocin, Vasopressin and Their Structural Analogues* vol. 10, pp. 167–171. Proc. 2nd Int. Pharmacol. Meeting, Rudinger, J. (ed.). Pergamon Press, Oxford.

ORIGINAL PAPERS

ACHER, R., CHAUVET, J., CHAUVET, M. T. and CREPY, D. (1962). Isolement d'une nouvelle hormone neurohypophysaire, l'isotocin, présente chez les poissons osseux. *Biochim. Biophys. Acta*, **58**: 624–625.

ACHER, R., CHAUVET, J., CHAUVET, M. T. and CREPY, D. (1965). Phylogenie des peptides neurohypophysaires: la glumitocine (Ser_4-Gln_8-ocytocine) présente chez un poisson cartilagineux, la raie *(Raia clavata)*. *Biochim. Biophys. Acta*, **107**: 393–396.

ACHER, R., CHAUVET, J., LENCI, M. T., MAETZ, J. and MOREL, F. (1960). Présence d'une vasotocine dans la neurohypophyse de la grenouille *(Rana esculenta)*. *Biochim. Biophys. Acta*, **42**: 379–380.

BENTLEY, P. J. (1958). The effects of neurohypophysial extracts on water transfer across the wall of the isolated urinary bladder of the toad *Bufo marinus*. *J. Endocrin.*, **17**: 201–209.

BENTLEY, P. J. (1964). The effects of N-ethylmaleimide and glutathione on the isolated rat uterus and frog bladder with special reference to the action of oxytocin. *J. Endocrin.*, **30**: 103–113.

BENTLEY, P. J. (1965). The potentiating action of magnesium and manganese on the oxytocic effect of some oxytocin analogues. *J. Endocrin.*, **32**: 215–222.

BERÁNKOVÁ-KSANDROVÁ, Z., BISSET, G. W., JOŠT, K., KREJČÍ, I., PLIŠKA, V., RUDINGER, J., RYCHLÍK, I. and ŠORM, F. (1966). Synthetic analogues of oxytocin acting as hormonogens. *Brit. J. Pharmacol., Chemother.*, **26**: 615–632.

BERDE, B., BOISSONNAS, R. A., HUGUENIN, R. L. and STÜRMER, E. (1964). Vasopressin analogues with selective pressor activity. *Experientia*, **20**: 42–43.

BERDE, B., DOEPFNER, W. and KONZETT, H. (1957). Some pharmacological actions of four synthetic analogues of oxytocin. *Brit. J. Pharmacol., Chemother.*, **12**: 209–214.

BISSET, G. W. (1963). Synthetic analogues of oxytocin acting as antagonists. *J. Physiol, Lond.*, **165**: 69–70.

BISSET, G. W. and LEWIS, G. P. (1962). A spectrum of pharmacological activity in some biologically active peptides. *Brit. J. Pharmacol., Chemother.*, **19**: 168–182.

BODANSZKY, M. and DU VIGNEAUD, V. (1959). Synthesis of a biologically active analog of oxytocin, with phenylalanine replacing tyrosine. *J. Amer. Chem. Soc.*, **81**: 6072–6075.

BOISSONNAS, R. A. and GUTTMANN, S. (1960). Synthèse d'analogues de l'oxytocine et de la lysine-vasopressin contenant de la phénylalanine ou de la tyrosine en positions 2 et 3. *Helv. Chim. Acta*, **43**: 190–200.

BOISSONNAS, R. A., GUTTMANN, S., BERDE, B. and KONZETT, H. (1961). Relationships between the chemical structures and the biological properties of the posterior pituitary hormones and their synthetic analogues. *Experientia*, **17**: 377–390.

BRANDA, L. A. and DU VIGNEAUD, V. (1966). Synthesis and pharmacological properties of 9-decarboxamido oxytocin. *J. Med. Chem.*, **9**: 169–172.

Cash, W. D., Mahaffey, L. M., Buck, A. S., Nettleton, D. E. Jr., Romas, C. and du Vigneaud, V. (1962). Synthesis and biological properties of 9-sarcosine oxytocin. *J. Med. Chem.*, **5**: 413–423.
Cash, W. D. and Smith, B. L. (1963). Synthesis and biological properties of 1-acetyl-8-lysine-vasopressin. *J. Biol. Chem.*, **238**: 994–997.
Chimiak, A. and Rudinger, J. (1965). Amino acids and peptides LIII. Synthesis and some biological properties of 3-O-methylthreonine oxytocin. *Colln. Czech. Chem. Commun.*, **30**: 2592–2599.
du Vigneaud, V., Denning, G. S. Jr., Draborek, S. and Chan, W. Y. (1964). The synthesis and pharmacological study of 4-decarboxamido-oxytocin (4-α-aminobutyric acid-oxytocin) and 5-decarboxamido-oxytocin (5-alanine-oxytocin). *J. Biol. Chem.*, **239**: 472–478.
van Dyke, H. B., Sawyer, W. H. and Overweg, N. I. A. (1963). Pharmacologic activities of the 8-citrulline analogues of oxytocin and vasopressin. *Endocrinology*, **73**: 637–639.
Eisler, K., Rudinger, J. and Šorm, F. (1966). Amino acids and peptides. LXV. Analogues of oxytocin with isoleucine replaced by L-diethylalanine, L-cyclopentylglycine and L- and D-cyclohexylglycine. *Colln. Czech. Chem. Commun.*, **31**: 4563–4580.
Ferrier, B. M. and du Vigneaud, V. (1966). 9-Deamidooxytocin, an analog of the hormone containing a glycine residue in place of the glycinamide residue. *J. Med. Chem.*, **9**: 55–57.
Fitzpatrick, R. J. (1956). The *in vivo* potentiation by magnesium salts of the uterine response to posterior pituitary extracts in the bovine. *J. Pharm. Pharmacol.*, **8**: 403–409.
Follett, B. K. and Heller, H. (1963). Pharmacological comparison between the teleost hormone, ichthyotocin, and synthetic 4-ser, 8-ileu oxytocin. *Biochem. Pharmacol.*, **12**, Suppl. p. 183.
Guttmann, S. and Boissonnas, R. A. (1960). Synthèse de dix analogues de l'oxytocine et de la lysine-vasopressine, contenant de la sérine et de l'histidine ou du tryptophane en position 2 ou 3. *Helv. Chim. Acta*, **43**: 200–216.
Guttmann, S. and Boissonnas, R. A. (1963). Synthèse de la Sér⁴-oxytocine, de l'Ala⁴-oxytocine, de la Sér⁵-oxytocine et de l'Ala⁵-oxytocine. *Helv. Chim. Acta*, **46**: 1626–1636.
Heller, H. (1939). The effect of the hydrogen-ion concentration on the stability of the antidiuretic and vasopressor activities of posterior pituitary extracts. *J. Physiol., Lond.*, **96**: 337–347.
Heller, H. and Pickering, B. T. (1961). Neurohypophysial hormones of non-mammalian vertebrates. *J. Physiol., Lond.*, **155**: 98–114.
Heller, H., Pickering, B. T., Maetz, J. and Morel, F. (1961). Pharmacological characterisation of the oxytocic peptides in the pituitary of a marine teleost fish *(Pollachius virens)*. *Nature, Lond.*, **191**: 670–671.
Hope, D. B., Murti, V. and du Vigneaud, V. (1962). A highly potent analogue of oxytocin, desamino-oxytocin. *J. Biol. Chem.*, **237**: 1563–1566.
Huguenin, R. L. and Boissonnas, R. A. (1962). Synthèses de la Phé²-arginine vasopressine et de la Phé²-arginine vasotocine et nouvelles synthèses de l'arginine vasopressine et de l'arginine vasotocine. *Helv. Chim. Acta*, **45**: 1629–1643.
Huguenin, R. L. and Boissonnas, R. A. (1966). Synthése de la desamino¹-Arg⁸-vasopressine et de la desamino¹-Phé²-Arg⁸-vasopressine, deux analogues possedant une activité antidiurétique plus elevée et plus selective que celle des vasopressines naturelles. *Helv. Chim. Acta*, **49**: 695–705.

HUGUENIN, R. L. and GUTTMANN, S. (1965). Synthese de l'Ala^1-Ala^6-Arg^8-vasopressine et de l'Ala^1-Ala^6-Lys^8-vasopressine, ainsi que de la (désamino-Ala)^1-Arg^8-vasopressine et de la (désamino-Ala)^1-Ala^6-Lys^8-vasopressine. *Helv. Chim. Acta*, **48**: 1885–1898.

JAQUENOUD, P. A. and BOISSONNAS, R. A. (1961). Synthèse de la Ileu^8-oxytocine et de la Val^8-oxytocine, deux analogues de l'oxytocine modifiés dans la chaîne latérale. *Helv. Chim. Acta*, **44**: 113–122.

JAQUENOUD, P. A. and BOISSONNAS, R. A. (1962a). Synthèse de l'Asp(NH$_2$)^4-oxytocine, de la Glu(NH$_2$)^5-oxytocine et de l'Asp(NH$_2$)^4-Glu(NH$_2$)^5-oxytocine. *Helv. Chim. Acta*, **45**: 1601–1607.

JAQUENOUD, P. A. and BOISSONNAS, R. A. (1962b). Synthèse de la dé-pro^7-oxytocine, de la dé-leu^8-oxytocine et de la dé-gly^9-oxytocine. *Helv. Chim. Acta*, **45**: 1462–1472.

JARVIS, D., FERRIER, B. M. and DU VIGNEAUD, V. (1965). The effect of increasing the size of the ring present in deamino oxytocin by one methylene group on its biological properties. The synthesis of 1-β-mercaptobutyric acid-oxytocin. *J. Biol.Chem.*, **240**: 3553–3557.

JOŠT, K. and RUDINGER, J. (1967). Amino acids and peptides. LXIX. Synthesis of two biologically active analogues of deamino-oxytocin not containing a disulphide bond. *Colln. Czech. Chem. Commun.*, **32**: 1229–1241.

KASAFÍREK, E., RABEK, V., RUDINGER, J. and ŠORM, F. (1966). Amino acids and peptides. LXVI. Synthesis of ten extended-chain analogues of lysine vasopressin. *Colln. Czech. Chem. Commun.*, **31**: 4581–4591.

KATSOYANNIS, P. G. (1957). Oxypressin, a synthetic octapeptide amide with hormonal properties. *J. Amer. Chem. Soc.*, **79**: 109–111.

KATSOYANNIS P. G. and DU VIGNEAUD, V. (1958). The synthesis of the histidine analog of the vasopressins. *Arch. Biochem. Biophys.*, **78**: 555–562.

KIMBROUGH, R. D. JR., CASH, W. D., BRANDA, L. A., CHAN, W. Y. and DU VIGNEAUD, V. (1963). Synthesis and biological properties of 1-desamino-8-lysine vasopressin. *J. Biol. Chem.*, **238**: 1411–1414.

KONZETT, H. and BERDE, B. (1959). The biological activity of a new analogue of oxytocin in which the tyrosyl group is replaced by phenylalanyl. *Brit. J. Pharmacol., Chemother.*, **14**: 133–136.

MAETZ, J., MOREL, F. and RACE, B. (1959). Mise en evidence dans la neurohypophyse de *Rana esculenta* L. d'un facteur hormonal nouveau stimulant le transport actif de sodium à travers la peau. *Biochim. Biophys. Acta*, **36**: 317–326.

MUNSICK, R. A. (1960). Effect of magnesium ion on the response of the rat uterus to neurohypophysial hormones and analogues. *Endocrinology*, **66**: 451–457.

NESVADBA, H., HONZL, J. and RUDINGER, J. (1963). Amino acids and peptides. XXXVII. Some structural analogues of oxytocin modified in position 3 of the peptide chain: synthesis and some chemical and biological properties. *Colln. Czech. Chem. Commun.*, **28**: 1691–1705.

PHOTAKI, I. and DU VIGNEAUD, V. (1965). 4-Deamidooxytocin, an onolog of the hormone containing glutamic acid in place of glutamine. *J. Amer. Chem. Soc.*, **87**: 908–913.

PICKERING, B. T. and LI, C. H. (1964). Adrenocorticotropins. XXIX. The action of sodium hydroxide on adrenocorticotropin. *Arch. Biochem. Biophys.*, **104**: 119–127.

RASMUSSEN, H., SCHWARTZ, I. L., YOUNG, R. and MARC-AURELE, J. (1963). Structural requirements for the action of neurohypophysial hormones upon the isolated amphibian urinary bladder. *J. Gen. Physiol.*, **46**: 1171–1189.

Ressler, C. and du Vigneaud, V. (1957). The isoglutamine isomer of oxytocin: its synthesis and comparison with oxytocin. *J. Amer. Chem. Soc.*, **79**: 4511–4515.

Rudinger, J. (1967). Synthetic analogues of oxytocin: an approach to problems of hormone action. *Proc. R. Soc.*, **B170**, 17–26.

Rudinger, J. and Krejčí, I. (1962). Dose-response relations for some synthetic analogues of oxytocin, and the mode of action of oxytocin on the isolated uterus. *Experientia*, **18**: 585–588.

Sawyer, W. H. (1960). Increased permeability of the bullfrog *(Rana catesbiana)* bladder *in vitro* in response to synthetic oxytocin and arginine vasotocin and to neurohypophysial extracts from non-mammalian vertebrates. *Endocrinology*, **66**: 112–120.

Sawyer, W. H. (1961). Neurohypophysial hormones. *Pharmacol. Rev.*, **13**: 225–277.

Sawyer, W. H., (1965). Active principles from a cyclostome *(Petromyzon marinus)* and two cartilaginous fishes *(Squalus acanthias and Hydrolagus collei)*. *Gen. Comp. Endocrin.*, **5**: 427–439.

Sawyer, W. H., Munsick, R. A. and van Dyke, H. B. (1961). Evidence for the presence of arginine vasotocin (8-arginine oxytocin) and oxytocin in neurohypophyseal extracts from amphibians and reptiles. *Gen. Comp. Endocrin.*, **1**: 30–36.

Schwartz, I. L., Howard, J. D. and Guggenheim, M. A. (1964). Unpublished observations cited by Schwartz and Livingston (1964) (*q.v.* p. 293).

Smyth, D. G. (1967a). Acetylation of amino and tyrosine hydroxyl groups. Preparation of inhibitors of oxytocin with no intrinsic activity on the isolated uterus. *J. Biol. Chem.*, **242**: 1592–1598.

Smyth, D. G. (1967b). Carbamylation of amino and tyrosine hydroxyl groups. Preparation of an inhibitor of oxytocin with no intrinsic activity on the isolated uterus. *J. Biol. Chem.*, **242**: 1579–1591.

Studer, R. O. and Cash, W. D. (1963). Synthesis of 1-acetyl-8-arginine-vasopressin and a study of its effects in the rat pressor assay. *J. Biol. Chem.*, **238**: 657–659.

Turner, R. A., Pierce, J. G. and du Vigneaud, V. (1951). The desulfurisation of oxytocin. *J. Biol. Chem.*, **193**: 359–361.

Ussing, H. H. and Zerahn, K. (1951). Active transport of sodium as the source o electric current in short-circuited isolated frog skin. *Acta Physiol. Scand.*, **23** 110–127.

Walter, R. and Schwartz, I. L. (1966). 5-Valine-oxytocin and 1-deamino-5-valine-oxytocin. Synthesis and some pharmacological properties. *J. Biol. Chem.*, **241**: 5500–5503.

Walter, R. and du Vigneaud, V. (1965). 6-Hemi-L-selenocystine oxytocin and 1-deamino-6-hemi-L-selenocystine oxytocin, highly potent isologs of oxytocin and 1-deamino-oxytocin. *J. Amer. Chem. Soc.*, **87**: 4192–4193.

Walter, R. and du Vigneaud, V. (1966). 1-Deamino-1,6-L-selenocystine oxytocin, a highly potent isolog of 1-deamino-oxytocin. *J. Amer. Chem. Soc.*, **88**: 1331–1332.

Zaoral, M., Kolc, J. and Šorm, F. (1967a). Amino acids and peptides. LXX. Synthesis of D-Arg^8- and D-Lys^8-vasopressin. *Colln. Czech. Chem. Commun.*, **32**: 1242–1249.

Zaoral, M., Kolc, J. and Šorm, F. (1967b). Amino acids and peptides. LXXI. Synthesis of 1-deamino-8-D-aminobutyrine vasopressin, 1-deamino-8-D-lysine vasopressin and 1-deamino-8-D-arginine vasopressin. *Colln. Czech. Chem. Commun.*, **32**: 1250–1257.

ZAORAL, M., PLÍSKA, V., RAZABECK, K. and ŠORM, F. (1963). Synthesis of a highly effective analogue of lysine vasopressin. *Colln. Czech. Chem. Commun.*, **28**: 746–747.

ZAORAL, M. and ŠORM, F. (1966a). Amino acids and peptides. LIX. Synthesis and some biological properties of L-DAB^8-vasopressin. *Colln. Czech. Chem. Commun.*, **31**: 90–97.

ZAORAL, M. and ŠORM, F. (1966b). Amino acids and peptides. LX. Synthesis of D-DAB^8-vasopressin. *Colln. Czech. Chem. Commun.*, **31**: 310–314.

CHAPTER 5

STORAGE OF NEUROHYPOPHYSIAL HORMONES AND THE MECHANISM FOR THEIR RELEASE

K. Lederis and K. Jayasena*

*Department of Pharmacology,
University of Bristol, Bristol, England*

INTRODUCTION

For a long time the production of the neurohypophysial hormones was thought to occur in the posterior pituitary and the hormone storing and releasing functions were held to represent only the secondary functions of the organ until Bargmann (1949) confirmed the concept of neurosecretion already postulated by Speidel (1919, 1922) and repeatedly advocated by E. and B. Scharrer since 1928. Experimental evidence obtained in 1942 was interpreted as indicating that the posterior pituitary elaborates and stores the active principles in the form of a parent protein molecule from which active side chains are split off differentially and secreted (released) separately into the blood stream according to requirements (van Dyke *et al.*, 1942).

During recent years the neurohypophysis has been widely accepted as having probably no other functions than those of storing, and releasing, vasopressin and oxytocin (for recent reviews see Heller, 1963; Heller and Ginsburg, 1966; Sawyer, 1966; Lederis, 1967). The production of hormones is now usually ascribed to the neurosecretory cells of the anterior hypothalamus (see Bargmann and Scharrer, 1951; Hild and Zetler, 1953: Bern and Knowles, 1966). However, as an alternative, the elaboration of the hormones in the neurohypophysis is still being considered. Production of oxytocin by mitochondria in the neurohypophysis was suggested by Green and Maxwell (1959). Other evidence suggests

---

* Present address: Department of Pharmacology, Faculty of Medicine, University of Ceylon, Ceylon.

the elaboration of the stainable neurosecretory material (being held to be analogous with posterior pituitary hormones) in the neural lobe (Christ, Engelhardt and Diepen, 1958; Diepen, Engelhardt and Smith-Agreda, 1954; Christ, 1960, 1962; Dellmann, 1960, 1962). Sachs and Takabatake (1964) in investigations of the biosynthesis of vasopressin have come to the conclusion that a precursor of neurohypophysial hormones may be formed in the perikarya of the hypothalamic neurosecretory cells and that the "activation" of the peptides occurs later in the neural lobe (see Chapter 6). Estimations of hormones in the anterior hypothalamus (Vogt, 1953) or in the supraoptic and paraventricular nuclei separately (van Dyke, Adamsons and Engel, 1957; Lederis, 1961, 1962a) also favor the view that a final elaboration ("activation") of the active peptides, or at least of oxytocin (possibly from the precursor postulated by Sachs and Takabatake), may continue in the infundibular process. Such findings necessitate a modification of views on the mode and site of production of the neurohypophysial hormones and on the function of the infundibular process, since otherwise the striking differences in the vasopressin : oxytocin (V/O) ratios between the hypothalamus and the neural lobe of the dog (suggesting the appearance *de novo* of oxytocin in the latter) would be difficult to explain (Vogt, 1953; van Dyke *et al.*, 1957; Lederis, 1962a). Until more detailed evidence on the biosynthesis of the neurohypophysial hormones becomes available it should be borne in mind that the neural lobe may have a multiple function, i.e. not only that of storage and release but also that of performing the final steps in the elaboration of the neurohypophysial hormones.

STORAGE OF VASOPRESSIN AND OXYTOCIN

THE NEURAL LOBE AS A HORMONE DEPOT

A role of the neural lobe as a storage depot is indicated by the fact that it contains hormones in quantities many times greater than those required for the daily control of body water and electrolytes or for the immediate supply of these hormones under conditions such as parturition or lactation. Compared with the anterior hypothalamus, where the main hormone synthesis seems to occur, the neural lobe contains up to several hundred times more hormones (Table 1). This relationship between the hypothalamic and the neurohypophysial hormone contents speaks against the suggestion of Jasinski, Gorbman and Hara (1966) that the entire neuron can be considered as a storage area. The alternative explanation offered by the same workers seems more likely: Jasinski *et al.* (1966) suggest that a varia-

TABLE 1. HORMONE CONTENT OF MAMMALIAN HYPOTHALAMUS (from Heller, 1966) Data from von Schlichtegroll (1954), van Dyke, Adamsons and Engel (1957) and Lederis (1961, 1962a).

Species	Vasopressin (V) (Percentage of neural lobe content)	Oxytocin (O) (Percentage of neural lobe content)	V:O ratio Hypothalamus	V:O ratio Neural lobe
Man	4.6	5.9	1.9	1.6
Macaque	0.4	—	—	—
Ox	0.6	0.5	1.7	1.4
Sheep	0.5	0.6	1.9	1.8
Camel	0.4	1.2	1.1	3.3
Pig	0.7	0.6	2.1	1.6
Elephant	1.6	0.2	7.0	1.0
Dog	2.5	0.2	15.1	1.2
Cat	—	—	1.0	1.3
Rabbit	1.9	1.4	4.0	2.9
Rat	1.4	1.0	2.3	1.6

tion in the amount of cytoplasmic accumulation of the neurosecretory material in the "somal and axonal *storage* area may subserve the function of initiation or arrest for the process of new synthesis of the neurosecretory material". It has been estimated that in the dog, whose posterior lobe contains 6–20 units of vasopressin, a maximum antidiuresis is obtained by the discharge into the blood stream of about 300 μU of vasopressin/min (Noble, 1957); this is equivalent to the release of only about 430 mU/24 hr — i.e. only 2–7% of the total hormone stored. Even without any repletion from the synthetic area, the storage depot—the neural lobe—in the dog would therefore suffice to effect the maintenance of water balance under conditions necessitating continuous antidiuresis for 30–50 days.

Several other reasons for the biological necessity of a storage depot for the neurohypophysial hormones can be envisaged: (1) A minimal rate of hormone production and immediate release, without storage would be sufficient for maintenance of water balance under normal conditions. However a depot is necessary to meet the sustained demand for large quantities of hormones under certain physiological (e.g. parturition, lactation) or emergency (e.g. dehydration, hemorrhage) conditions, so that sufficient quantities of the stored hormones can be mobilized and utilized for prolonged periods of time with or without simultaneous hormone production to replenish the depleted depot. (2) An equally, or more important necessity for a storage organ is the existence of a blood–brain barrier in the upper region of the system—in the hypothalamus (Wislocki and King, 1936; Harris, 1960). The neurohypophysial blood supply, on the other hand, has been shown to lie outside the barrier (Ortmann, 1957). Irrespective of the hormone content in the hypothalamus, from where release into the blood stream is limited or does not occur at all (Harris, 1960), a storage depot is necessary outside the barrier so that the neurohypophysial hormones can easily move into the blood stream from the neural lobe, and also possibly in the reverse direction (Palay, 1955).

HORMONE CONTENT IN THE MAMMALIAN NEUROHYPOPHYSIS

The hormone content and even more so the ratio vasopressin to oxytocin appears to be genetically controlled. When the V/O ratios in different classes of vertebrates are considered on the molar basis (Follett, 1963) it is evident that they are characteristic, e.g. for taxonomic groups (Ferguson and Heller, 1965; Heller, 1966; Heller and Spickett, 1967) agreeing well with morphological classification of mammals. Different mole ratios of vasopressin and oxytocin are found in mammals between, and within, the various orders (see Chapter 3).

The hormone ratios seem to remain substantially constant from infancy through adult life to senility, if the findings on rats can be applied to other mammals. In the adult rat the V/O ratio is near unity. The same applies to infant animals (Heller and Lederis, 1959)—provided that treatment with acetone is avoided prior to extraction of pituitaries—and to old—senile—rats (Heller, Lederis and Rodeck, 1960). During the estrus cycle, and in pregnancy (Acher, Chauvet and Olivry, 1956; Heller, 1959) the V/O ratio does not change, although the absolute hormone amounts may change significantly. During lactation an increase in the V/O ratio above unity has been found by some workers (Dicker and Tyler, 1953a, 1953b; Acher and Fromageot, 1957), but not by others (Heller, 1959; Denamur and Martinet, 1953; Cowie and Folley, 1957).

However, the importance of a repletion—increased synthetic activity—is often neglected under conditions when sustained release at a high rate of either vasopressin (e.g. dehydration) or oxytocin (e.g. lactation) is required. Only circumstantial evidence for the constancy of the hormone content has been available until recently. Thus during chronic dehydration the hormone content in the infundibular process of the rat may increase during the first 48–72 hr (Ames and van Dyke, 1950; Dicker and Nunn, 1957). Only after 4 days of continued withdrawal of water (or administration of hypertonic saline) does the hormone content begin to fall (Simon and Kardos, 1934; Dicker and Nunn, 1957). Such findings suggest that the stimulus of dehydration initiates not only the release of vasopressin at a higher rate but also increases the synthetic activity of the hypothalamo-neurohypophysial system in order to maintain the, perhaps genetically, predetermined storage levels. The synthetic capability of the system is limited as shown by the progressive fall of the stored reserves at an advanced state of dehydration (4th–14th day of chronic dehydration (Lederis, 1962a). Direct evidence to substantiate a dependence between release (depletion) and an attempted repletion of the stored hormone levels has been provided by Sachs and Takabatake (1964). They found in experiments *in vitro* that synthesis *de novo* of vasopressin by the hypothalamus of the dehydrated guinea pig was more than 300% higher than that by controls which, before the experiment, had free access to drinking water.

The absolute amounts of hormones in the neural lobe seem to be reasonably constant for any species subject to experimental or environmental influences, but may vary considerably between species. Thus it appears that, related to body weight, the neural lobe of a large animal contains less hormones than that of the smaller species (see Table 2). The vasopressin content calculated/kg body weight, may be up to 200 times higher in the rat and the guinea pig than man, ox, elephant or the domestic pig, with the dog, sheep and rabbit falling between the two extremes.

TABLE 2. VASOPRESSIN CONTENT, CALCULATED IN RELATION TO BODY WEIGHT, IN NEURAL LOBES OF SOME MAMMALS

Species	Average body weight (kg)	Vasopressin content	
		mU/gland	mU/kg b.wt.
Indian elephant (1)	5000	100,500	20
Hippopotamus*	3000	24,300	8
Algerian camel (3)	650	130,000	200
Ox (1)	500	96,400	192
Pig (1)	80	17,300	215
Man (1)	70	15,200	220
Sheep (1)	35	20,300	570
Dog (1, 3)	15	17,000	1130
Rabbit (1)	2.5	3430	1550
Guinea-pig (2)	0.5	2325	4650
Rat (2)	0.2	850	4250

(1) From Lederis, 1962a; (2) Heller and Lederis, 1959; (3) van Dyke *et al.*, 1957.
* Heller and Lederis, unpublished observations.

VASOPRESSIN AND OXYTOCIN IN SUBCELLULAR PARTICLES

The first attempts to isolate cell particles, with which the neurohypophysial hormones are associated or in which they are lodged, appear to have been made by Schiebler (1952). Homogenates of bovine neurohypophyses were centrifuged at 12,000 g—60,000 g, and a particle fraction was obtained which showed appreciable amounts of succinic dehydrogenase activity and also quantities of Gomori-positive material. It was concluded that the neurohypophysial hormones were associated with mitochondria, although some smaller particles (elementary granules), ranging from 50–250 nm, were also observed with the electron microscope in the "Gomori-positive, mitochondrial" fraction.

Similar conclusions were reached by Pardoe and Weatherall (1955) who prepared subcellular particles by differential centrifugation of rat posterior pituitary homogenates. The distribution of hormones was measured by estimating the pressor, oxytocic and antidiuretic activities in the fractions. Two main conclusions were reached: (1) that the neurohypophysial hormones occur in the "mitochondrial" fraction and (2) that vasopressin and oxytocin may be lodged in separate particles, owing to different yields of the two hormones when using centrifugation media of differing molarities (0.25 M and 0.8 M sucrose). It is now known that the interpretation of the findings was erroneous and that this was due to the, at that time, limited knowledge of particulate composition of cell fractions. Differential centrifugation techniques were in their infancy and were usually applied to liver homogenates. It was subsequently shown in numerous laboratories that the term "mitochondrial" could be applied to fractions obtained at centrifugal forces ranging from 2700 g (Harman and Feigelson, 1952) to as high as 34,000 g (La Bella and Brown, 1959) or even 250,000 g (Appelmans, Wattiaux and De Duve, 1955). De Duve and his co-workers (De Duve et al. 1955) established that (a) the conventional differential centrifugation procedures (in use at that time) did not permit the isolation of homogenous cell fractions and (b) that "mitochondria are cellular particles of a great variety of sizes and shapes having but one feature in common—the localization of oxidizing enzymes of the cell".

Further attempts were made to investigate the subcellular localization of neurohypophysial hormones in the light of improved differential and density gradient centrifugation techniques. Lederis and Heller (1960) obtained fractions from rabbit neurohypophyses and found that the bulk of the sedimentable vasopressin and oxytocin occurred in a fraction (obtained at 30,000 g for 60 min in 0.44 M sucrose) which consisted mainly

of elementary granules, as seen with the electron microscope. The observation of Pardoe and Weatherall (1955) that vasopressin and oxytocin may be associated with different particles was confirmed by density-gradient centrifugation experiments (Heller and Lederis, 1961). After differential and density gradient centrifugation experiments, combined with hormone estimations in, and electron microscopical examination of, the fractions, the isolation, identification and properties of the hormone-containing particles of the rabbit neurohypophysis were described by Heller and Lederis (1962) and Barer, Heller and Lederis (1963). Confirmation of the subcellular localization of neurohypophysial hormones in the elementary granules was provided by independent, and, in several cases simultaneous, observations in other laboratories (Weinstein, Malamed and Sachs, 1961; La Bella, Beaulier and Reiffenstein, 1962, 1963; La Bella and Sanwal, 1965; Ishii *et al.*, 1962; Gessner *et al.*, 1965). Using similar centrifugation procedures it was shown that neurohypophysial hormones occur in the elementary granules also in the human posterior pituitary (Daniel and Lederis, unpubl.) and in a teleost fish (Lederis, 1962b). Density gradient centrifugation experiments (Heller and Lederis, 1961; La Bella *et al.*, 1962; Lederis and Kauz, 1965) in conjunction with hormone estimations in various parts of the hypothalamo-neurohypophysial system (Vogt, 1953; Adamsons *et al.*, 1956; Lederis, 1961, 1962a) favor the postulated existence of separate neurones responsible for the synthesis, storage and release of one hormone only, the "vasopressinergic" or "oxytocinergic" neurons and their fibers suggested by Heller (1961). Recent interesting and extensive investigations by Valtin and his co-workers (see Valtin, 1967; Sokol and Valtin, 1967) of the hypothalamo-neurohypophysial system in the Brattleboro strain of rats with hereditary hypothalamic diabetes insipidus have provided direct evidence in support of the existence of the "vasopressinergic and oxytocinergic" neurones.

"NEUROSECRETORY MATERIAL" AND THE
NEUROHYPOPHYSIAL HORMONES

Pronouncements on the hormone content of the neural lobe have frequently been based on morphological (light- or electron microscopical) observations. It is now apparent that such pronouncements do not always agree with the measurements of hormone content. An attempt will be made to provide some examples of pitfalls when conclusions on hormone content are drawn from observation of morphological appearances. For example, dehydration, either by water withdrawal or by administration of a hypertonic NaCl solution in rats (Ortmann, 1951; Leveque and Scharrer, 1953;

Duchen, 1962) produces a demonstrable decrease of the light-microscopically demonstrable neurosecretory material. A simultaneous and parallel depletion of hormones is usually assumed because "increased hormone release" is known to occur after such experimental procedures (Gilman and Goodman, 1937; Verney, 1947). It is generally agreed that the above statement is true in principle. However, it has been shown equally clearly in the same species that during the initial period (1–3 days) of dehydration, by which time the depletion of the (Gomori) stainable material has occurred, the hormone content in the neural lobe does not alter much (Ames and van Dyke, 1950; Dicker and Nunn, 1957; Heller and Lederis, 1959). A fall in the amount of stored hormones occurs only after prolonged dehydration.

Changes in the electron microscopical appearance can also lead to conclusions which may result in erroneous assessments of hormone content. Ether anesthesia is one of the well documented stimuli for "massive release" of neurohypophysial hormones (Ginsburg and Heller, 1952; Ames and van Dyke, 1952; Dicker, 1953; Thorn and Silver, 1957; Chaudhury and Walker, 1958). Loss of the electron-dense material from the elementary granules of the infundibular process can occur as soon as 10 min after exposure of the animal to ether as shown by Gerschenfeld, Tramezzani and De Robertis (1960) in toads, after 30 min in rabbits (Barer and Lederis, 1966) and after 60 min in rats (Daniel and Lederis, 1966b). In the latter two instances it was shown, by combining electron microscopical observations with hormone estimations in the same experiment, that the stored hormone content had not changed at the time at which the electron microscopically observed "depletion" had occurred (Plates 1–6). The attention of the reader is drawn to the fact that a "massive release" in physiological terms may amount to a 100-fold or even 1000-fold increase in the blood concentration of vasopressin (Ginsburg and Brown, 1957) as compared with the "basal release", which is not measurable with the conventional assay procedures. Since such an increase in vasopressin content in the blood can be achieved by secreting less than 1% of the total hormone content of the storage depot—the neural lobe—it can be concluded that a period of time of stimulation by ether in excess of 1 hr would be necessary before a reliably measurable decrease of the stored hormones could be shown (Daniel and Lederis, 1966b).

The morphological demonstration of the depletion of the stainable or of the electron-dense material cannot, therefore, be used as a measure of hormone content of neural lobe. Such morphological changes may demonstrate, at best, some as yet undefined alterations in the hormone storage mechanism. It could be argued that stimuli which initiate hormone release

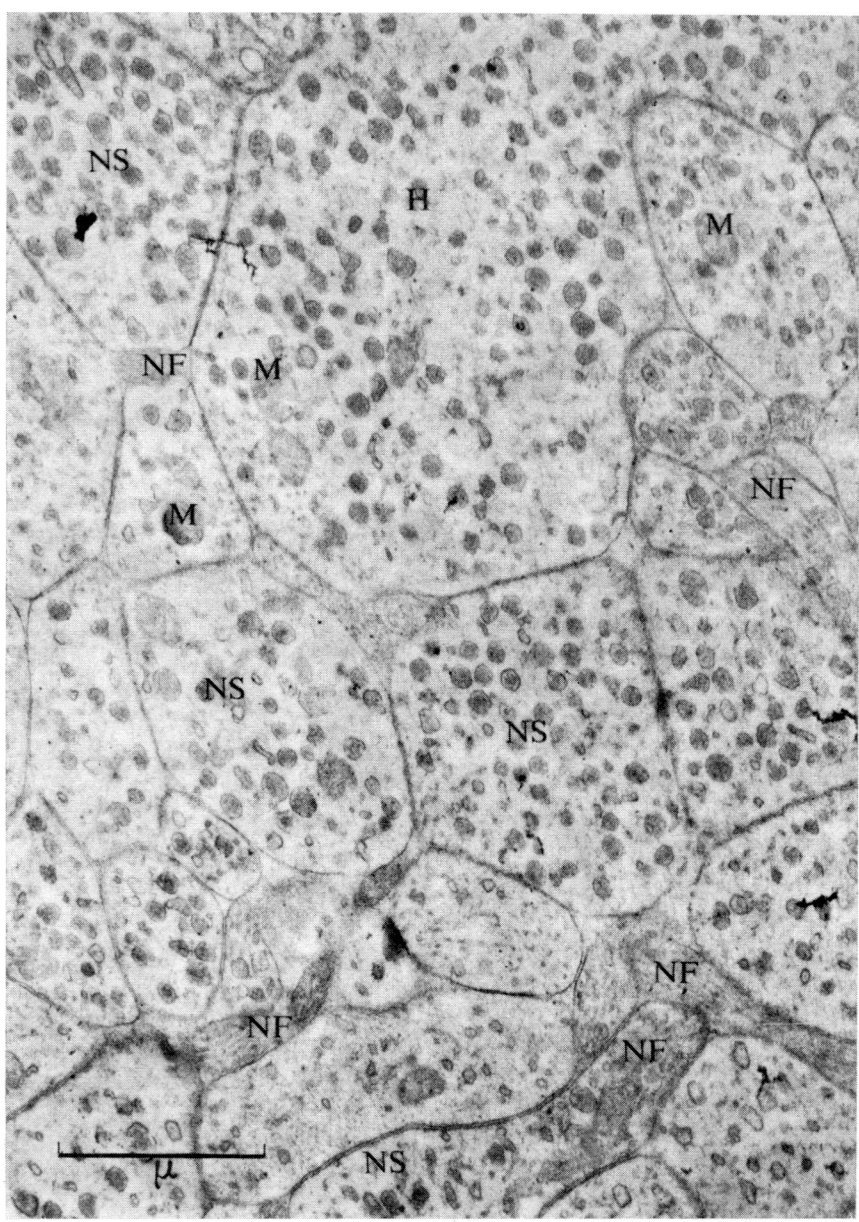

PLATE 1. Electron-micrograph of a neural lobe of a control rat (see Fig. 2). Nerve swellings (or terminals) (NS) and a "Herring-body" (H) containing numerous elementary granules with electron-dense cores. M, mitochondria; NF, non-dilated nerve fibers in which microtubules can be seen, the latter are not usually visible in the nerve swellings (or terminals). (From Daniel and Lederis, 1966b).

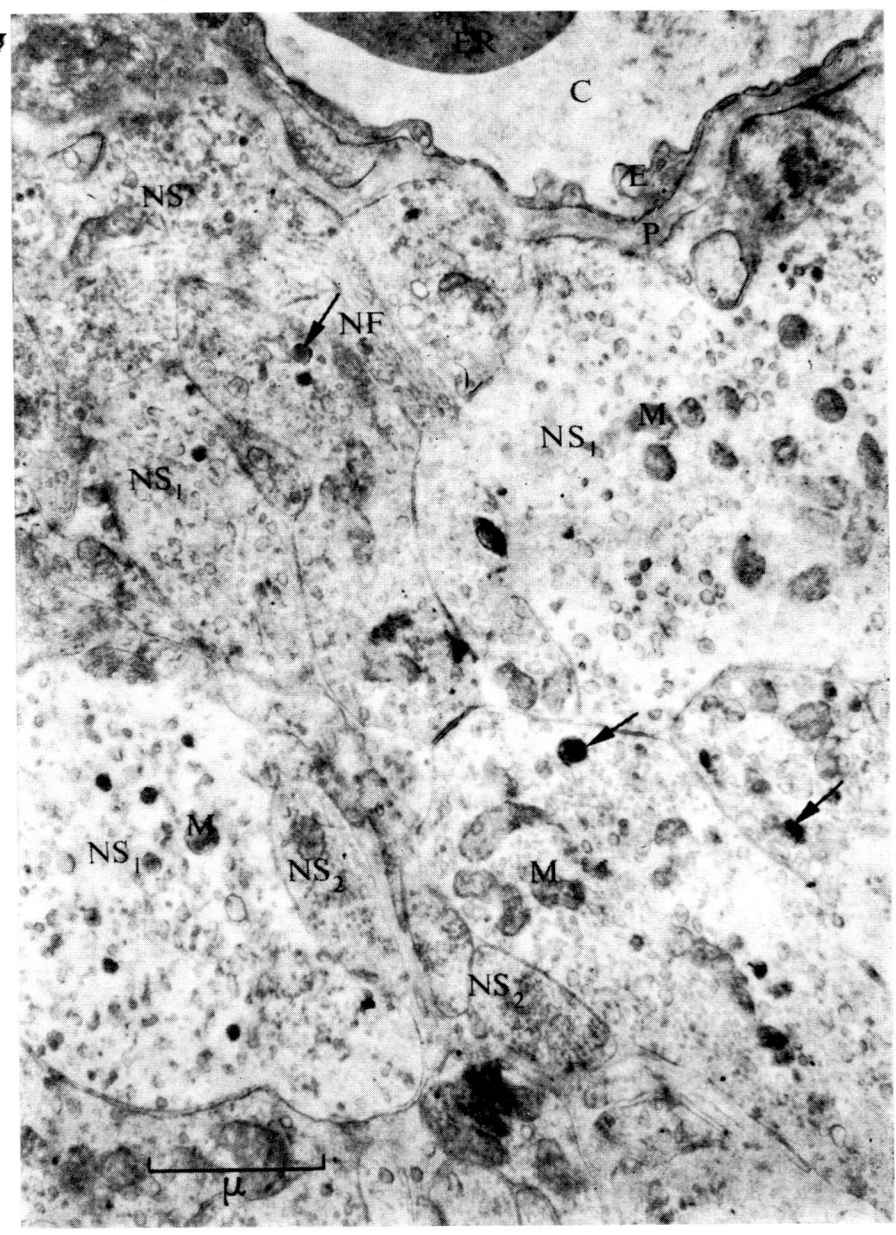

PLATE 2. Neural lobe of a rat which had been kept under ether anesthesia for 60 min (see Fig. 2). Lack of electron-dense contents apparent in most elementary granules in nerve swellings (NS_1). NF, nerve fiber dilating into a swelling (NS), microtubules visible in the former. M, mitochondria; C, capillary lumen; ER, erythrocyte; E, capillary endothelium; P, perivascular space; arrows, dense bodies frequently seen in nerve swellings of stimulated neural lobes. (From Daniel and Lederis, 1966b).

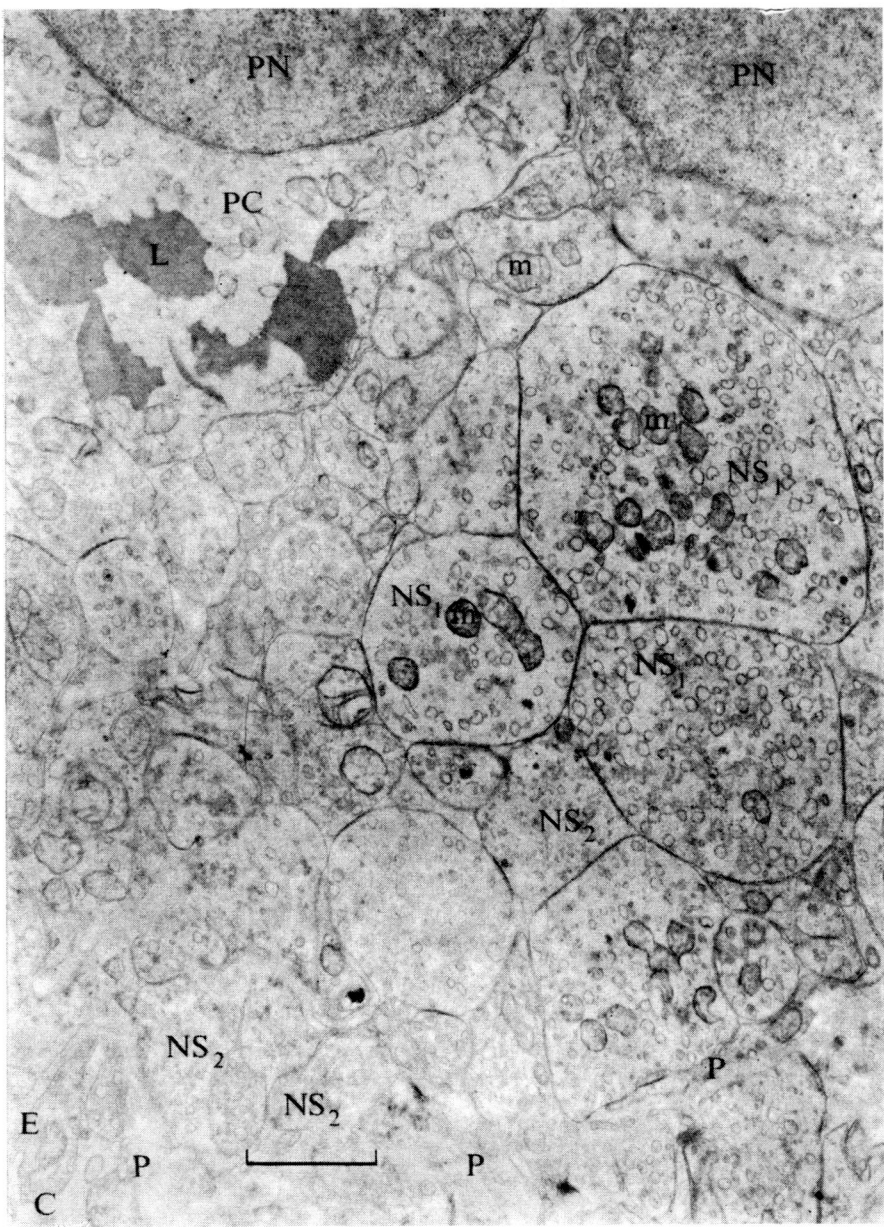

PLATE 3. Neural lobe of a rat after ether anesthesia and hemorrhage (see Fig. 2). Note complete lack of the electron-dense content in the elementary granules. NS_1, nerve swellings (or terminals) with electron-optically "empty" elementary granules; NS_2, nerve swellings (or terminals) containing only small "synaptic" vesicles; PN, nuclei of pituicytes; PC, pituicyte cytoplasm in which dense lipid droplets (L) are seen; C, capillary lumen; E, capillary endothelium; P, perivascular spaces; M, mitochondria. (From Daniel and Lederis, 1966b).

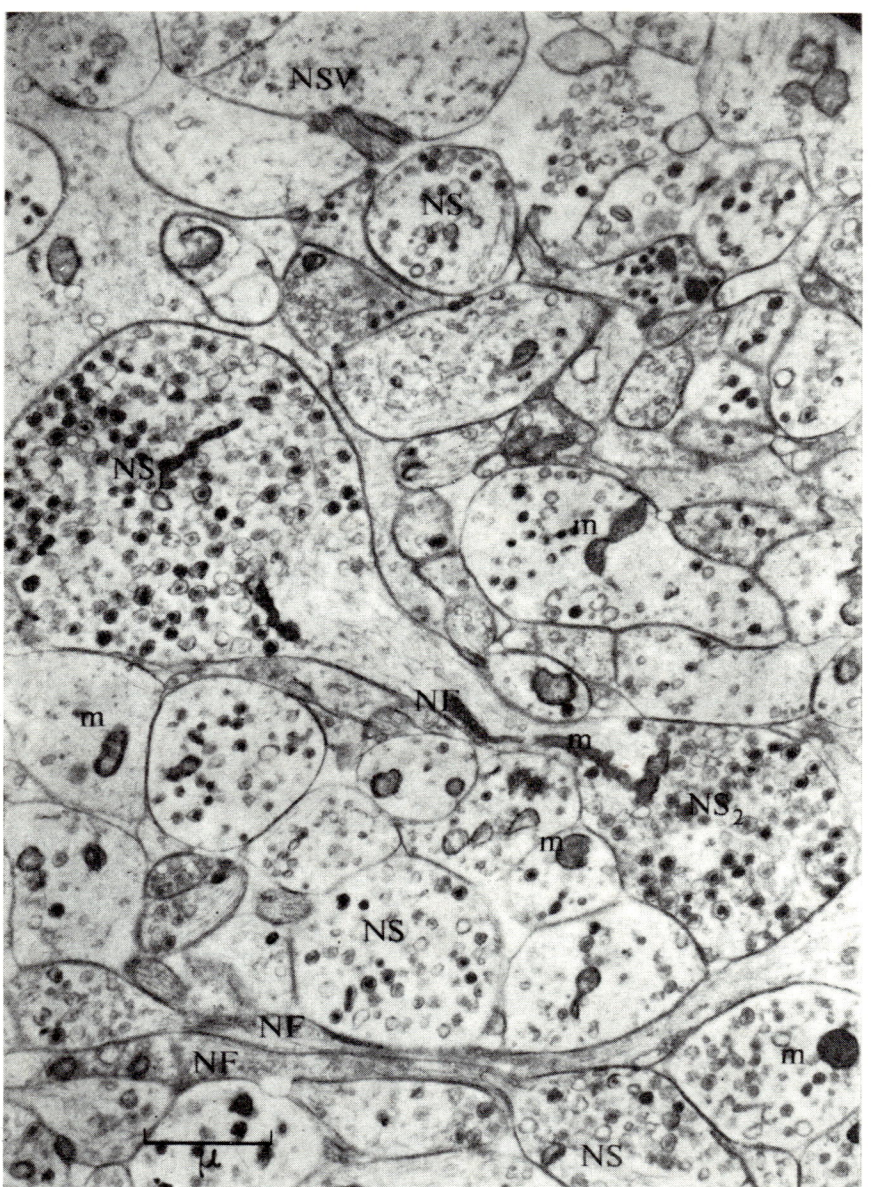

PLATE 4. Neural lobe of an adult male rabbit. NF, nerve fibers continuous with one or more swellings (NS_1, NS_2); NSV, nerve swelling containing small vesicles; M, mitochondria. (From Barer and Lederis, 1966).

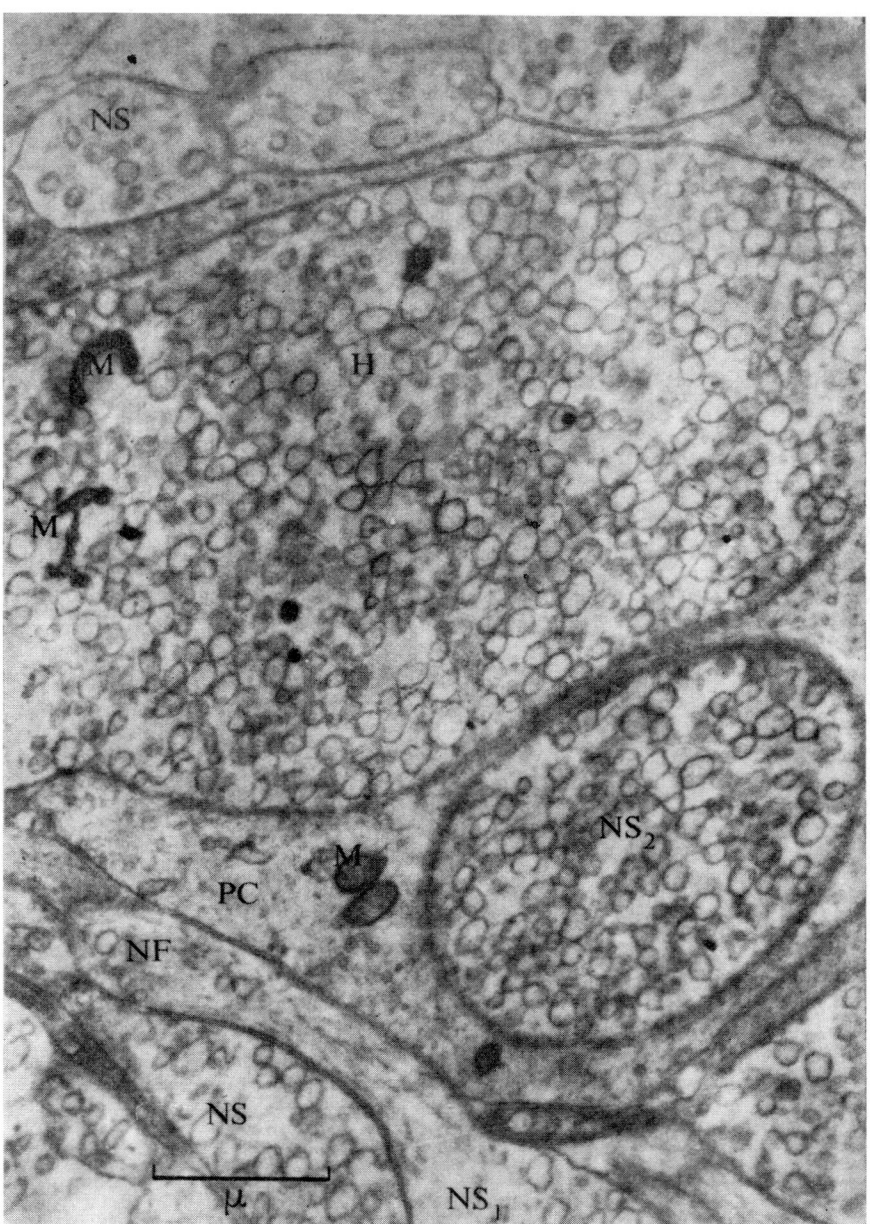

PLATE 5. Section of a neural lobe of a rabbit which had been kept under ether anesthesia for 30 min. Note lack of electron-dense cores in the elementary granules. Large nerve swelling or terminal (Herring body) in upper middle of micrograph (H); other nerve swellings (NS), one of which (NS$_1$) is continuous with a non-dilated nerve fiber (NF); M, mitochondria; PC, a pituicyte process in which a nerve swelling (NS$_2$) is embedded. (From Barer and Lederis, 1966).

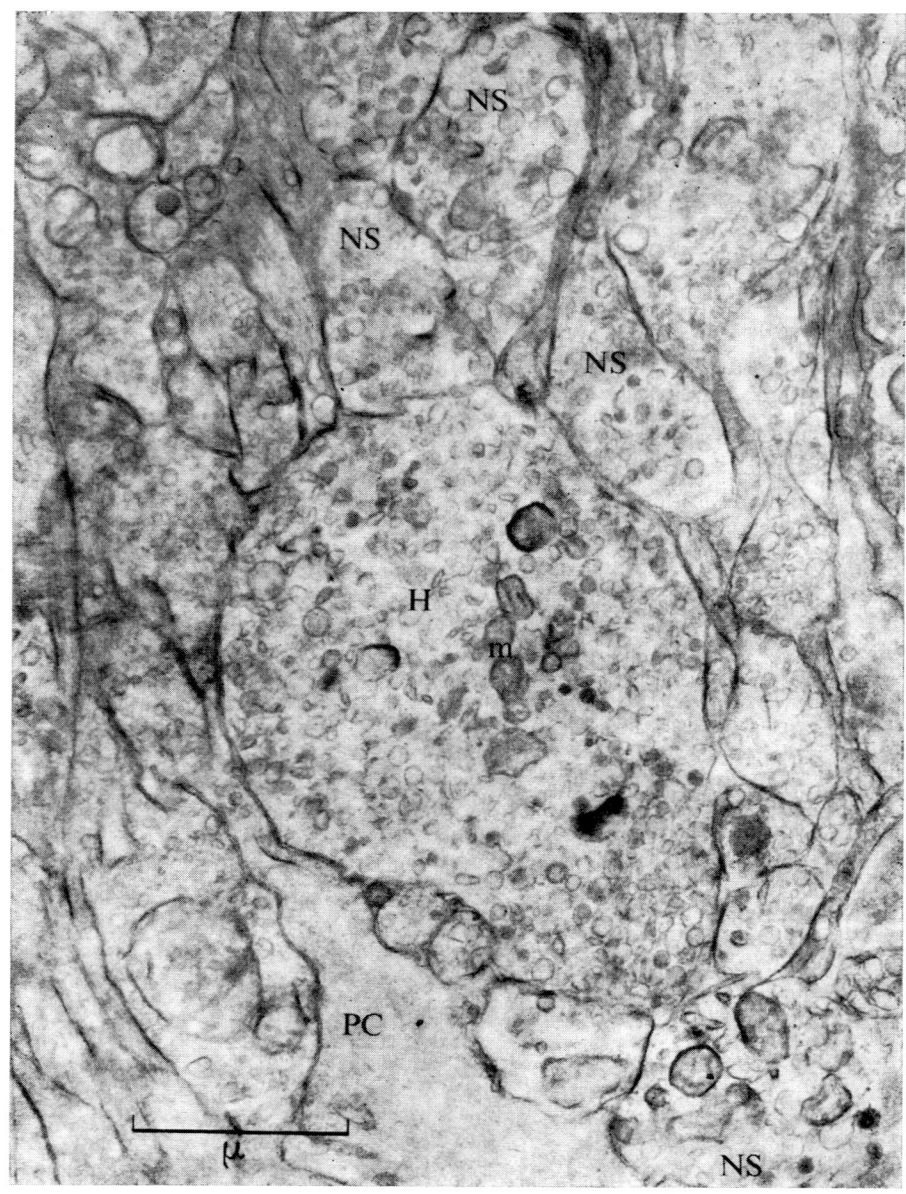

PLATE 6. Neural lobe of a rabbit kept on dry diet for 14 days. A pronounced loss of the electron-dense cores is apparent in the elementary granules of all nerve swellings (NS); H, "Herring-body"; M, mitochondria; PC, process of a pituicyte. (From Barer and Lederis, 1966).

at an increased rate produce changes in the nature of the so called neurosecretory (the stainable or the electron-dense) material. There are several possibilities: (1) the usual "neurosecretory stains" (in light-microscopy) may no longer react with, or osmium (in electron microscopy) may no longer be taken up by, the neurosecretory material. (2) a redistribution of the neurosecretory material (hormones and/or carrier protein–neurophysin) may occur in one of two ways: (a) intraneuronal movements of the hormone–neurophysin complex: some hormone (with or without neurophysin) may leave the elementary granules but may remain within the nerve swellings (or terminals), or (b) the peptide hormones themselves (with or without neurophysin) may move out of the granules, leave the nerve swellings and be then distributed through the extensive perivascular channels of the neural lobe by passive diffusion or by an "active" process (Barer and Lederis, 1966). The latter view is supported by experimental evidence showing that the proportions of free (diffusible) and bound (intragranular?) hormones change in favor of the former when the posterior pituitary is subjected to hormone-releasing stimuli (see: Release of neurohypophysial hormones).

RELEASE OF NEUROHYPOPHYSIAL HORMONES

RELEASE MECHANISMS

The physiological mechanism by which vasopressin is released was defined by Verney (1947). According to this view, osmotically sensitive cells in the anterior hypothalamus constitute the direct link between the demand for ADH and its release; small changes in the osmotic pressure of the blood stimulate the osmoreceptors and ADH is released (Jewell, 1953; Ames, Moore and van Dyke, 1950; Abrahams and Pickford, 1954). Recent evidence from experiments *in vitro* (Douglas 1963) outlines cellular events which may explain the finer mechanisms concerned with the release of vasopressin and oxytocin. According to this concept, which has been formulated as "stimulus-secretion coupling" (Douglas and Rubin, 1965; Douglas and Poisner, 1964a, 1964b), depolarization of the neuronal membrane (by potassium) followed by an influx of calcium ions results in an increase of free vasopressin. Further work *in vitro* showed (Daniel and Lederis, 1963, 1966a, 1966b, 1967; Dicker, 1966) that the same procedure releases also oxytocin. Daniel and Lederis (1967) investigated the kinetics of hormone release *in vitro* and measured the rate at which vasopressin and oxytocin are released during prolonged stimulation by K^+/Ca^{++} *in vitro*. The highest rate of release was shown to occur during the first 10–20 min of incubation. During the subsequent 60–70 min even the depolarized neural lobes released only small quantities of vasopressin and oxytocin (Fig. 1).

These results indicate that the physiological release of neurohypophysial hormones can occur without the involvement of "transmitter substances". The following events seem likely to precede hormone release: an appropriate stimulus activates the reflex arc for the release of vasopressin or oxy-

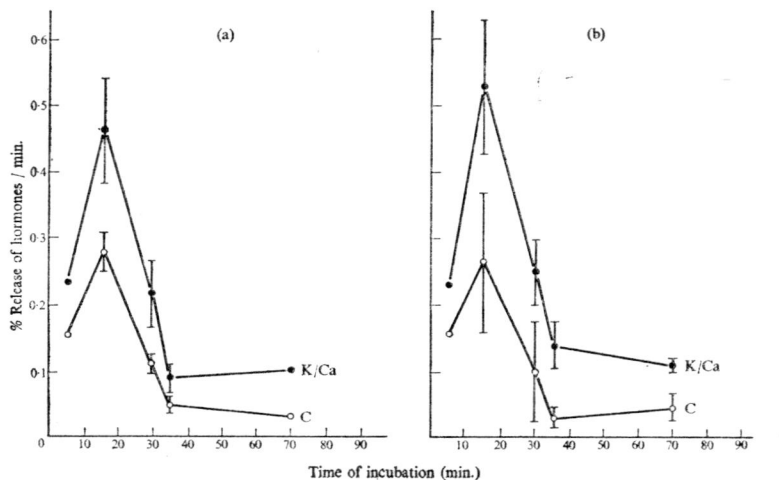

FIG. 1. Average rate of hormone release (Fig. 1a, vasopressin; Fig. 1b, oxytocin) from halved neural lobes of rats *in vitro* in relation to duration of incubation. C, controls in phosphate buffer; K/Ca, in buffer containing 56 mM K^+ and 4 mM Ca^{2+}. Means and S. E. from six experiments. (From Daniel and Lederis, 1967.)

tocin or both. Part of this reflex arc may involve the activation of cholinergic neurones (see below) acting on the cell bodies of the supraoptic and paraventricular nuclei of the hypothalamus thus setting up action potentials and propagating impulses along the hypothalamo-neurohypophysial nerve fibers. On arrival of the impulses at the nerve terminals in the neural lobe (or at any other swelling along the neurohypophysial section of the nerve fibers as suggested by Barer and Lederis, 1966), depolarization of the neuronal membrane promotes influx of Ca^{++} into the fiber. It is not known how the subsequent reaction—after Ca^{++} has entered the nerve terminal (or swelling)—proceeds. It cannot be excluded that calcium is only an intermediate link in the release of neurohypophysial hormones and that further, as yet unknown, neuronal events resulting in the freeing of hormones, occur. On the other hand, the site and mode of action of calcium is indicated by the finding that the presence of Ca^{++} inhibits, or at least diminishes, the binding of vasopressin and oxytocin to the carrier protein, neurophysin, *in vivo* and *in vitro* (Smith and Thorn, 1965; Ginsburg, Jayasena and Thomas, 1966a; see also below, p. 137). Following the freeing of hormones from the carrier protein no further mechanism, involving other mediator or transmitter substances, for hormone release need be postulated—passive gradient diffusion of the free peptides out of the neurone, through the interneuronal spaces, and into the blood vessels, would suffice (Barer and Lederis, 1966).

If the change of the stored hormone-carrier complex, resulting in the setting free of vasopressin and oxytocin, is accepted as the decisive part of the releasing process, the actual movement of the freed hormones would depend only on the quantities of the hormones in the intra- and extra-neuronal "compartments" (Thorn, 1965, 1966). No further active release process would be necessary, and it could be expected that after appropriate stimulation a greater proportion of the total hormone content in the neural lobe would be changed to the free, diffusible, form, i.e. increase in the free hormone pool (Thorn, 1966). Recent experiments *in vitro* have shown that

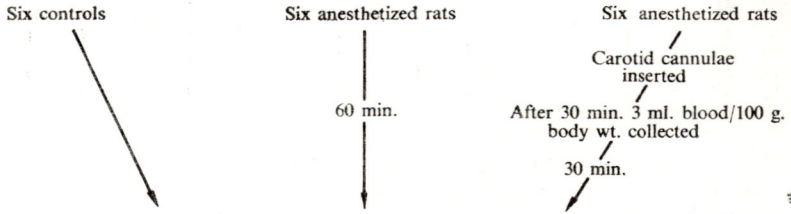

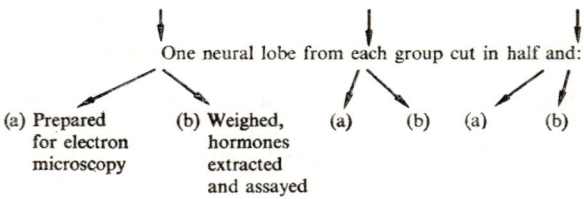

FIG. 2. Experimental procedure to investigate ultrastructural changes and the effects on hormone release of ether anesthesia, and ether-and-hemorrhage, on rat neural lobes *in vivo* and *in vitro*. (From Daniel and Lederis, 1966b.)

such a mechanism, for increasing the free hormone pool, exists. Daniel and Lederis (1966b) stimulated hormone release in rats *in vivo* by ether anesthesia and severe hemorrhage (Fig. 2). When the stimulated neural lobes were subsequently incubated *in vitro* in physiological buffer solutions, significantly higher quantities ($P < 0.01$) of vasopressin were released into the incubation medium from these neural lobes as compared with controls from non-stimulated animals (Fig. 3).

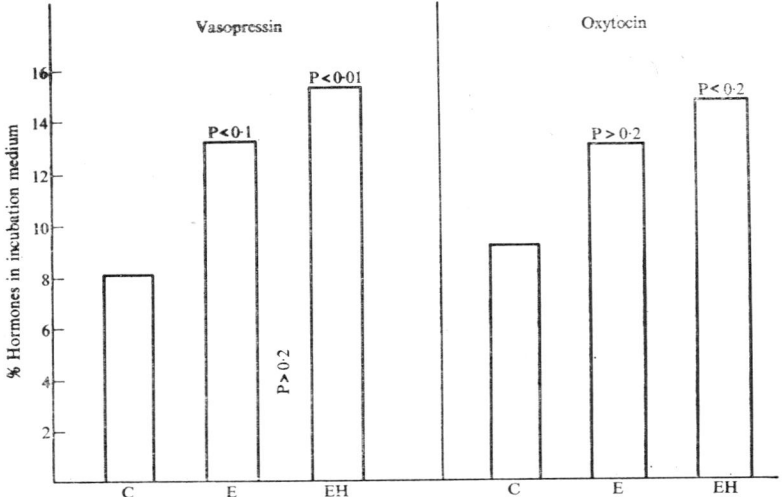

FIG. 3. Incubation of halved neural lobes of rats in phosphate buffer for 40 min at 37°. Vasopressin and oxytocin (as percentage of the total gland content) released into the incubation medium. C, controls; E, ether anesthesia; EH, ether anesthesia and hemorrhage. P = difference between controls and the experimental groups (From Daniel and Lederis, 1966b).

SEPARATE RELEASE OF VASOPRESSIN AND OXYTOCIN

Early electrical stimulation experiments tended to show that both neurohypophysial hormones are released simultaneously (Harris, 1948). This was concluded from observations that electrical stimulation of the neural lobe or of the infundibular stem caused antidiuresis (Harris, 1947) and increased uterine activity (Harris, 1948). Electrical stimulation of the hypothalamus (supraoptic or paraventricular nuclei or hypothalamo-hypophysial tract) in lactating goats and sheep was also shown to inhibit water diuresis and to stimulate milk ejection (Andersson, 1951a,b, 1957; Andersson and McCann, 1955). Similarly, intracarotid administration of acetylcholine or of hypertonic saline, or emotional stress, in the dog, indicated the release of both hormones (Abrahams and Pickford, 1954).

Such evidence has sometimes lead to conclusions that "...any stimulus that releases one hormone, releases the other simultaneously" (Dicker, 1961).

In contrast to the evidence favoring simultaneous release of both hormones, a large volume of work has now shown that specific stimuli cause the preferential or exclusive release of only one hormone. Thus, suckling in lactating women, cows and rabbits was shown to stimulate mainly milk ejection (Peeters and Coussens, 1950; Kalliala and Karvonen, 1951; Cross, 1951; Theobald, 1959; Gaitan, Coba and Mizrachi, 1964). Chronic dehydration in rabbits produces a more pronounced depletion of the vasopressin stores although some depletion of the stored oxytocin also occurs (Lederis, 1962a). Other evidence employing up-to-date methods of hormone estimation in blood (Beleslin *et al.*, 1967) has (see Fig. 4) confirmed conclusively the findings of Chaudhury and Walker (1958) and Ginsburg and Smith (1959) that hemorrhage causes a pronounced release of vasopressin but not of oxytocin. However, Dyball (1968) could detect oxytocin as well as vasopressin in jugular blood of rats after severe hemorrhage. His findings differ from those of Beleslin *et al.* (1967) who could only detect vasopressin but not oxytocin in the blood of cats after a severe hemorrhage. It cannot be excluded that species differences may account for these different findings. On the other hand it could be postulated that the stimulus used by Dyball who withdrew 40 ml blood/kg b.w. was more severe and may have reflexly stimulated an "unspecific" release of oxytocin.

The evidence quoted above favors the view that separate physiological reflex arcs are available for the release of one hormone following a specific stimulus. However, it seems that under many experimental conditions excessively severe or prolonged specific stimuli may become "unspecific", i.e. may reflexly stimulate the release of both hormones. Thus, prolonged dehydration in dogs or in rabbits results in a pronounced depletion of vasopressin in the neurohypophysis accompanied by a less pronounced loss of oxytocin (Hild and Zetler, 1953; Lederis, 1962a). Experiments of Daniel and Lederis (1966b) on the rat neurohypophysis *in vitro*, after stimulation of hormone release *in vivo* (Table 3, also see Fig. 3) by ether anesthesia and hemorrhage showed a significant decrease in the vasopressin content of the neural lobe. The release of vasopressin *in vitro*, from the neural lobes which had been stimulated *in vivo*, was significantly higher as compared with controls. An increased release of oxytocin was indicated but was not significantly different from controls.

Ultracentrifugation experiments in lactating rabbits, in which considerably larger quantities of free oxytocin than vasopressin were found, indicate a change in the neural lobe for a preferential release of oxytocin

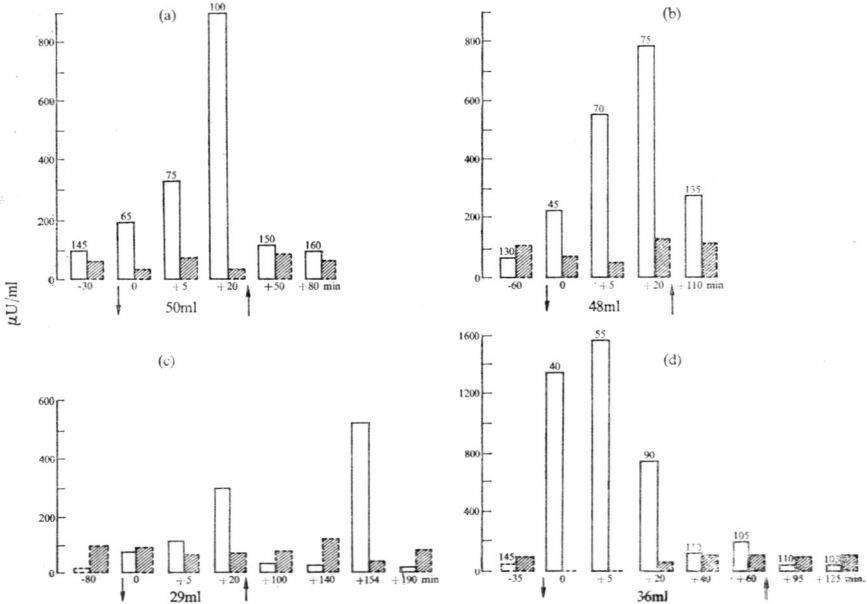

FIG. 4. Concentrations in $\mu U/ml$ of vasopressin (open columns) and oxytocin (hatched columns) in blood samples collected from external jugular vein of dogs before and after hemorrhage. Dotted line gives minimum concentrations detectable in the assays for those samples in which no activity was found. Arrows indicate withdrawal (↓) of blood during hemorrhage and its replacement (↑). Figures below base-line indicate times (in min) at which samples (4 ml) were collected before (−) or after (+) blood withdrawal. All samples collected over 2 min. Figures above columns give blood pressure in mmHg.

Expt. a. 50 ml of blood withdrawn. 4 ml dextran injected intravenously simultaneously with collection of each blood sample.

Expt. b. 48 ml of blood withdrawn. 4 ml of this blood injected simultaneously with the collection of each of the two samples at +5 and +20 min and only 40 ml of blood replaced followed by 12 ml dextran intravenously.

Expt. c. 29 ml of blood withdrawn at 0 min and 46 ml at +140 min. Replacement of blood followed by intravenous injection of dextran, 12 ml first time and 8 ml second time.

Expt. d. 36 ml of blood withdrawn. 4 ml dextran injected intravenously simultaneously with collection of each blood sample (From Beleslin *et al.*, 1967).

TABLE 3. CHANGES IN HORMONE CONTENT IN THE POSTERIOR PITUITARY OF THE RAT DUE TO HORMONE RELEASE *in vivo* AFTER ETHER ANESTHESIA (E) AND ETHER AND HEMORRHAGE (EH).

Series	Hormone content	Vasopressin			Oxytocin		
		C	E	EH	C	E	EH
1	mU/gland	1012	890	696*	840	882	711
1	mU/100 g body weight	369	309	264*	325	310	250
2	mU/mg wet gland	945	833	542***	832	954	682**

* $P > 0.1$.   ** $P > 0.05$.   *** $P > 0.01$.

Series 1: Hormone content in incubated glands (amount in incubation medium plus amount in gland extract).
Series 2: Hormone content in fresh weighed portions of neural lobes.
P, difference between C (controls) and EH.
(Daniel and Lederis, 1966b).

(Lederis, 1967b). On the other hand, experiments with dehydrated rabbit neural lobes have shown an increase in the free vasopressin content (Barer *et al.*, 1963). Whereas only about 20% of both hormones remain in the final supernatant ("free hormones") when differential centrifugation is carried out with homogenates of adult male rabbit neural lobes (Lederis and Heller, 1960; Heller and Lederis, 1962; Barer *et al.*, 1963) more than 80% of the total oxytocin content of the lactating rabbit neural lobe remains in the final supernatant (Lederis, 1967b). The same experiments showed a less pronounced increase in free vasopressin (Table 4).

Such experimental evidence indicates that (a) releasing stimuli affect the storage mechanism by altering the proportions of free and bound hor-

TABLE 4. DIFFERENTIAL CENTRIFUGATION OF RABBIT POSTERIOR PITUITARY HOMOGENATES ACCORDING TO THE PROCEDURE OF BARER, HELLER AND LEDERIS (1963) % OF SEDIMENTABLE (INTRAGRANULAR) AND FREE (EXTRAGRANULAR) HORMONES.

Animals	Vasopressin (%)		Oxytocin (%)	
	Sedimentable	Free	Sedimentable	Free
Male controls	78.4	21.6	77.8	22.2
Lactating (21 days)	41.5	58.5	16.9	83.1
Infant (21 days)	47.8	52.2	39.1	60.9
Dehydrated (7 days)	52.8	47.2	49.2	50.8

TABLE 5. EXPERIMENTAL RELEASE OF NEUROHYPOPHYSIAL HORMONES

Releasing stimulus	Vaso-pressin	Oxytocin	Author
Drugs			
Yohimbine	+		Fugo (1944).
Morphine	+		de Bodo (1944), Giere and Eversole (1954), Giarman, Mattie and Stephenson (1953), Schnieden and Blackmore (1955).
Nicotine	+		Motzfeldt (1917), Burn, Truelove and Burn (1945), Taylor and Walker (1951) de Wied and Jinks (1958).
	+	+	Bisset and Walker (1957).
Acetylcholine	+		Pickford (1939, 1947), Pickford and Watt (1951).
	+	+	Abrahams and Pickford (1954).
		+	Pickford (1959, 1960).
Anticholinesterases	+		Pickford (1947), Duke, Pickford and Watt (1950).
	+	+	Abrahams and Pickford (1956).
Ferritin	+		Baez, Mazur and Shorr (1952).
Adenosine triphosphate	+		Dexter, Stoner and Green (1954).
Histamine	+		de Wied and Jinks (1958).
Reserpine	+		Chaudhury, Chaudhury and Lu (1962).
Bradykinin	+		Rocha e Silva and Malnic (1964).
Electrical stimulation of the central nervous system and supraopticohypophysial tract		+	Haterius and Ferguson (1938), Cross and Harris (1952), Cross (1953, 1955a), Tindal, Knaggs and Turvey (1967).
	+		Harris (1948), Fang, Liu and Wang (1962), Mills and Wang (1964a, 1964b).
	+	+	Andersson and McCann (1955), Harris (1947), Bisset, Hilton and Poisner (1967).
Stressful stimuli and anesthetics	+		Rydin and Verney (1938), Verney (1947), Heller and Smirk (1932), de Bodo and Prescott (1945), Kelsall

TABLE 5 (cont.)

Releasing stimulus	Vaso-pressin	Oxytocin	Author
Hemorrhage	+	+	(1949), Ames and van Dyke (1952), Ginsburg and Heller (1953), Dicker (1953), Giere and Eversole (1954), Ginsburg and Brown (1956), Thorn and Silver (1957). Chaudhury and Walker (1958). Rydin and Verney (1938), Ginsburg and Heller (1953), Ginsburg and Brown (1956, 1957), Ginsburg and Smith (1959), Baratz and Ingraham (1959), Weinstein, Berne and Sachs (1960), de Wied (1960), Dyball (1966), Beleslin et al. (1967).
Osmotic stimulation (Injection of hypertonic solutions, water deprivation etc.)	+		Gilman and Goodman (1937), Kuschinsky and Liebert (1939), Verney (1947), Heller (1949), Ames, Moore and van Dyke (1950), Morel (1955), Friedman, Hinke and Friedman (1956), Zuidema and Clark (1957), Dicker and Nunn (1958), Siddiqi and Walker (1960), de Wied (1960), Moses (1963, 1964), Little and Radford (1964), Kastin (1967), de Wied and László (1967), Share (1961, 1962).
		+	Andersson (1951a), Holland, Cross and Sawyer (1959).
	+	+	Pickford (1960), Abrahams and Pickford (1954).
Vagotomy and carotid occlusion	+		Share and Levy (1962), Usami, Peric and Chien (1963), Chien, Peric and Usami (1963), Clark and Rocha e Silva (1966).
Carotid sinus receptor stimulation	+		Share and Levy (1966), Share (1967).
Vagal stimulation (central)	+		Chang et al. (1937, 1939), Mills and Wang (1964a, 1964b), Dyball (1966).
		+	Chang et al. (1938), Andersson (1951b), Siddiqi and Walker (1960).

TABLE 5 (cont.)

Releasing stimulus	Hormone released		Author
	Vasopressin	Oxytocin	
Vagal stimulation (peripheral)	+		Beleslin *et al.* (1967).
Calcium chloride injection	+		Thorn, Smith and Skadhauge (1965), Dyball (1968).
Suckling or mammary stimulation		+	Waller (1938), Cross (1955b), Grosvenor and Turner (1956, 1957a, 1957b), Martinet and Denamur (1960), Chaudhury (1961), Fitzpatrick (1961), Fuchs and Wagner (1963), Folley, and Knaggs (1965a), Ishikawa, Koizumi and Brooks (1966).
	+	+	Peeters *et al.* (1949), Peeters and Coussens (1950), Peeters, Stormorken and Vanschoubroek (1960), Cross (1950, 1951), Theobald (1959), Kalliala and Karvonnen (1951), Kalliala, Karvonen and Leppänen (1952).
Parturition, dilatation of the birth canal and cervical stimulation.		+	Ferguson (1941), Andersson (1951a), Cross (1959), Fitzpatrick (1961), Fitzpatrick and Warmsley (1962), Folley and Knaggs (1965b), Fuchs (1966).
	+	+	Debackere and Peeters (1960b), Debackere and Peeters (1960a).
Coitus and ejaculation	+		Friberg (1953).
	−	+	Fitzpatrick (1957), Cross (1961), Debackere and Peeters (1961).

mones in favor of the former, (b) that *specific* stimuli, e.g. dehydration or hemorrhage increase the free vasopressin pool, whereas lactation lowers the pool of bound oxytocin.

It can, therefore, be concluded that separate mechanisms exist for the release of each of the two neurohypophysial hormones independently, upon specific stimulation, but that a strong or prolonged specific stimulus may result in the release of both hormones, this being analogous with the general properties of the central nervous system, i.e. spread of stimuli.

Table 5 gives a summary of a number of experimental stimuli which cause the release of neurohypophysial hormones and indicates whether the release of one, the other, or both hormones was observed.

A comprehensive account of a variety of physiological, experimental, and pathological stimuli for the release of neurohypophysial hormones has recently been given by Heller and Ginsburg (1966) and by Ginsburg (1968a).

ACETYLCHOLINE AND THE RELEASE OF NEUROHYPOPHYSIAL HORMONES

Acetylcholine, acting centrally, has been shown to be implicated in the release of vasopressin and oxytocin. Chang *et al.* (1937, 1938) found that the stimulation of the central end of the cut vagus in dogs produced vasopressor and oxytocic effects and that these effects did not occur after section of the infundibular stalk or after hypophysectomy. Pickford and her co-workers (Pickford, 1939, 1947; Duke, Pickford and Watt, 1950; Pickford and Watt, 1951; Abrahams and Pickford, 1954) in a variety of experiments involving the administration of acetylcholine into the venous or arterial circulation, or near the supraoptic nuclei, consistently observed antidiuresis, and also effects on the uterus or milk ejection in dogs, and showed that these effects were due to the release of vasopressin and oxytocin.

The hypothesis that acetylcholine is involved in the release of hormones by a direct local action on the nerve endings in the neural lobe, has been repeatedly advocated on circumstantial evidence. The histochemical demonstration of cholinesterases in the pars nervosa of some mammalian species (Bloom, 1960, in the hedgehog; Koelle and Geesey, 1961, in the cat; Holmes, 1961, in the macaque monkey; Holmes, 1964, in the hedgehog) and the definition of electron microscopically visible small vesicles in the neurohypophysis as "synaptic" (Palay, 1957; Green and Maxwell, 1959; Gerschenfeld, Tramezzani and de Robertis, 1960) have been interpreted by Koelle (1961) and de Robertis (1962) as indicating that the neurohypophysis is a cholinergic organ. According to Koelle (1961) acetylcholine is involved in the release of neurohypophysial hormones by its action on the hypothalamic cell bodies and also by local action on the nerve terminals. Koelle suggests that acetylcholine, as well as the hormones vasopressin and oxytocin, occurs in the terminals of the neurohypophysial nerve endings, that it can be released from these endings to act back on them and thus be concerned in the release of the hormones from the same endings.

Low concentrations of choline acetylase in the neural lobe were found by Feldberg and Vogt (1948). Occurrence of a "cholinergic substance" in the pars nervosa of domestic cattle was reported by Uemura, Kobayashi and Ishii (1963). More detailed examination of the rabbit neurohypophysis for its content of acetylcholine and related enzymes (Lederis and Livingston, 1966, 1968a; Lederis, 1966; Livingston, 1966; Livingston and Lederis, 1967) has shown that acetylcholine, acetylcholinesterase (together with other cholinesterases) and choline acetylase occur in the posterior pituitary in varying quantities (Table 6). Acetylcholine has also been demonstrated in neural lobes of other mammalian species, including man, ox, rat and hedgehog (Lederis, 1967a).

TABLE 6. ACETYLCHOLINE, ACETYLCHOLINESTERASE AND CHOLINE ACETYLASE IN THE NEURAL LOBE AND ANTERIOR HYPOTHALAMUS OF THE RABBIT (FROM LEDERIS AND LIVINGSTON, 1968a)

Activity	Neural lobe (Means ± S.E.)	Hypothalamus (Means ± S.E.)
Acetylcholine (μg/g fresh tissue)	4.38 ± 0.98 (11 expts.)	4.87 ± 1.53 (7 expts.)
Acetylcholinesterase (μM substrate hydrolyzed/min/g fresh tissue)	1.74 ± 0.11 (14 expts.)	3.78 ± 0.60 (18 expts.)
Choline acetylase (μg acetylcholine produced/ hour/g fresh tissue)	87 ± 22 (12 expts.)	378 ± 149 (16 expts.)

Attempts have also been made at determining with which subcellular organelles of the neural lobe acetylcholine is associated and whether it occurs in the "neurosecretory" (hormone-containing) or separate "non-neurosecretory" nerve endings (for definition of these terms and for description of granules and vesicles in the neural lobe see a recent review by Bern and Knowles, 1966; also Oota, 1963; Oota and Kobayashi, 1962; Lederis, 1964a, 1964b). Evidence was obtained from experiments with rabbit neural lobe homogenates combining density gradient centrifugation with simultaneous hormone and acetylcholine estimation in, and electron microscopical examination of, the gradient fractions (see Fig. 5) that, (a) acetylcholine occurs in the small ("synaptic") vesicle fraction (Whittaker, 1959) and (b) that at least some acetylcholine probably occurs in nerve endings other than those in which the neurohypophysial hormones are found (Lederis, 1967a; Lederis and Livingston, 1968b). According to the findings of Feldberg and Vogt, (1948) the neurohypophysis cannot be

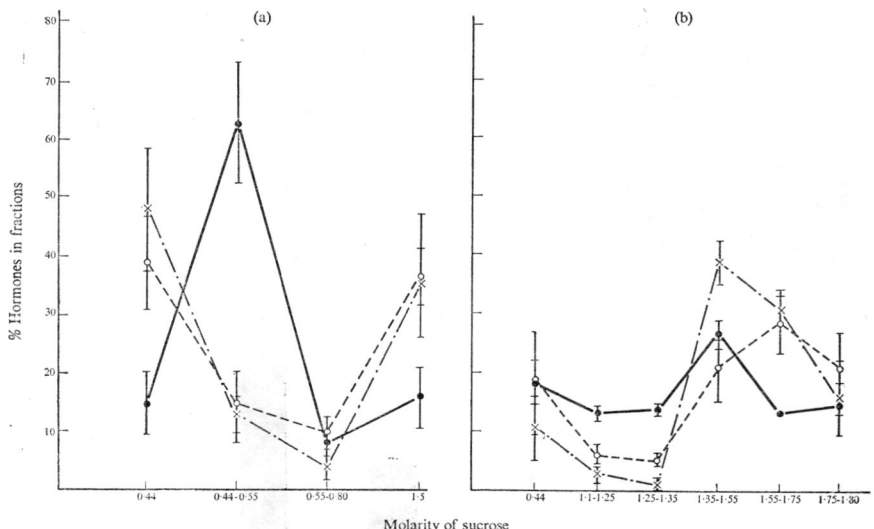

Fig. 5. Distribution (%) of acetylcholine •—•, vasopressin o———o and oxytocin ×—·—× after density gradient centrifugation of rabbit neural lobe homogenates.

a. Distribution of the three activities in subcellular particles after centrifugation of disrupted nerve endings in a continuous sucrose gradient 0.44—0.8 M layered over 1.5 M sucrose (means and S. E. from 5 experiments).

b. Distribution of activities in fractions after centrifugation of undisrupted nerve endings in a continuous gradient of 1.1—1.8 M sucrose (means and S. E. from 4 experiments). (From Lederis and Livingston, 1968b).

considered as a cholinergic organ despite the occurrence there of acetylcholine and related enzymes, e.g. the choline acetylase concentration in cholinergic systems is much higher. Moreover, these workers found that most tissues of the body are able to synthesize small quantities of acetylcholine. Investigations *in vitro* under suitable experimental conditions under which the release of vasopressin and oxytocin can be easily stimulated (Douglas, 1963; Daniel and Lederis, 1963, 1966b), have shown that acetylcholine does not promote hormone release when acting directly on the neural lobe (Douglas and Poisner, 1964a; Daniel and Lederis, 1966a, 1967; Dicker, 1966). When, however, the isolated hypothalamus with the neural lobe attached ("intact hypothalamo-neurohypophysial system", Daniel and Lederis, 1967) was incubated under the same experimental conditions in a buffer containing acetylcholine, 10^{-7} mg/ml, with or without eserine, a significant increase in the release of vasopressin ($P < 0.05$) and a highly significant increase ($P < 0.01$) in the release of oxytocin occurred (Fig. 6).

In the light of this evidence it seems unlikely that acetylcholine has a dual role in the release of neurohypophysial hormones as postulated by Koelle (1961) and de Robertis (1962). There are indications that acetylcholine may have a vasomotor function in the neurohypophysis. Prelimin-

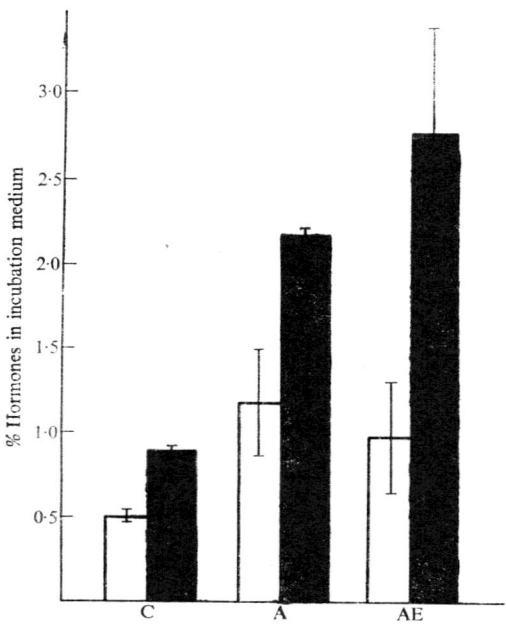

FIG. 6. Percentage of vasopressin (□) and oxytocin (■) released into incubation medium from isolated intact hypothalamo-neurohypophysial systems. Means and S. E. from eight experiments. C, controls in phosphate buffer, A, in buffer containing 10-7 mg/ml acetylcholine, AE, in buffer containing acetylcholine and eserine 10^{-7} mg/ml. (From Daniel and Lederis, 1967).

ary observations in histochemical experiments with the electron microscope suggest that acetylcholinesterase and other esterases are distributed mainly in and around the blood vessels of the rabbit neurohypophysis (Lederis and Livingston, unpublished observations). The histochemical demonstration of sympathetic nerve fibers around the blood vessels (Dahlström and Fuxe, 1966) and the electron microscopical observations of nerve endings with the characteristic appearance of noradrenaline-containing nerve terminals in close proximity to blood vessels of mammalian neurohypophyses (Lederis, 1967c), or those of teleost fishes (Follenius, 1967), together with the distribution of acetylcholinesterase in similar areas, suggest that both components of the autonomic nervous system occur in the neurohypophysis and that these components may have a vasomotor role in the posterior pituitary. Observations, showing an increase in volume of the neurohypophysis during dehydration and suggesting increased blood supply (Legait, 1964; Streefkerk, 1967; Friesen and Astwood, 1967) support the above assumption.

THE NEUROPHYSIN–HORMONE COMPLEX

THE NATURE AND THE HORMONE-BINDING PROPERTIES OF NEUROPHYSIN

Until the chemical structure of the neurohypophysial hormonal peptides was established by du Vigneaud and his colleagues, differing views were held on the nature of the hormones. Biological evidence suggested the existence of up to three active substances (Hild and Zetler, 1951; Bargmann, 1957), but other evidence supported the "unitary posterior pituitary hormone theory" (Abel, 1930). The latter view was favored on the grounds of findings by McArthur (1931), Rosenfeld (1940) and van Dyke and his colleagues (van Dyke *et al.*, 1942) who showed that a protein of the molecular weight of about 30,000 could be isolated either by ultracentrifugation (Rosenfeld) or by salt-precipitation (McArthur, van Dyke *et al.*). The "van Dyke protein" was later investigated by Acher and his co-workers (Acher, Chauvet and Olivry, 1956; Acher and Fromageot, 1957) who concluded that "further investigations are necessary to determine whether the complex formed by vasopressin, oxytocin and inert protein is an artefact of extraction or whether it has biological significance" (Acher and Fromageot, 1957). However, Chauvet, Lenci and Acher (1960) later obtained a protein fraction from sheep neurohypophyses and showed that it had no hormonal activity but could form non-dialysable complexes with vasopressin and oxytocin; the name "neurophysin" was given to this protein.

During the last few years the nature, properties and hormone-binding capacity of neurophysin have been studied in greater detail in several laboratories (Ginsburg and Ireland, 1963, 1964, 1965, 1966; Ginsburg, Jayasena and Thomas, 1966a, 1966b; Stouffer, Hope and du Vigneaud, 1963; Hope, Schachter and Frankland, 1964; Hollenberg and Hope, 1967;

Smith and Thorn, 1965; Thorn, 1966; for recent reviews, see Ginsburg 1968a, 1968b). A relatively pure preparation of neurophysin with a molecular weight of about 25,000 was obtained from beef neural lobes and the maximum hormone-binding capacity of 7 molecules of oxytocin and 4 molecules of arginine vasopressin (AVP) per molecule neurophysin was calculated (Ginsburg and Ireland, 1965). When the hormone-binding capacity of porcine neurophysin was investigated (Ginsburg, Jayasena and Thomas, 1966a) it was again found that more oxytocin than lysine vasopressin (LVP) was bound by each molecule of porcine neurophysin (14 molecules and 4 molecules respectively). The binding maxima arrived at from experiments with highly purified neurophysin under optimal conditions, such as optimum pH and concentration of protein (Ginsburg and Ireland, 1965) are not thought to apply *in situ*, i.e. in the elementary granules. Ginsburg and Ireland (1966) calculated the neurophysin and hormone content in the isolated granules and concluded that, firstly, about 50% of the acid-soluble protein in the granules is represented by neurophysin and secondly, that the average hormone content (oxytocin plus vasopressin) of a single granule was $0.5-1.0 \times 10^{-13}$ units. Calculated for each molecule of neurophysin this would result in 1.0–1.6 molecules of peptide hormone. This is considerably below the maximum binding capacity *in vitro* and may be accounted for by the intracellular pH being considerably above the optimum hormone-binding pH 5.8 (Ginsburg and Ireland, 1964).

The bovine neurophysin obtained by Ginsburg and Ireland (for a diagrammatic summary of the method of preparing neurophysin see Fig. 7) was resolved into two components. The fast-moving fraction, of an estimated molecular weight of 90,000, did not bind the neurohypophysial hormones as shown by dialysis experiments, but the other component (mol. wt. about 20,000) did. Homogeneity tests on the porcine neurophysin by Ginsburg *et al*. (1966a), while indicating only one component by Sephadex G-25 gel filtration and by ultracentrifugation, yielded two major components by the variable solubility (Smithies, 1954) test. Further analysis of the porcine neurophysin was attempted, (Ginsburg, Jayasena and Thomas, 1966b) and a chromatographic separation on DEAE-Sephadex into two subfractions was achieved. Dialysis experiments with the two neurophysin fractions according to the method of Ginsburg and Ireland (1964), showed that one fraction formed non-dialyzable complexes with oxytocin only while the other bound both oxytocin and LVP.

A greater degree of heterogeneity of neurophysin than that observed by Ginsburg and his co-workers was recently reported (Frankland *et al*., 1966; Hope and Hollenberg, 1966). Separation of neurophysin into six distinct protein fractions was achieved by Hollenberg and Hope (1967). One component, containing relatively little cystine, lacked the ability to form complexes with the hormones and was suggested to be of a molecular weight of above 50,000. This component may be the same as that isolated

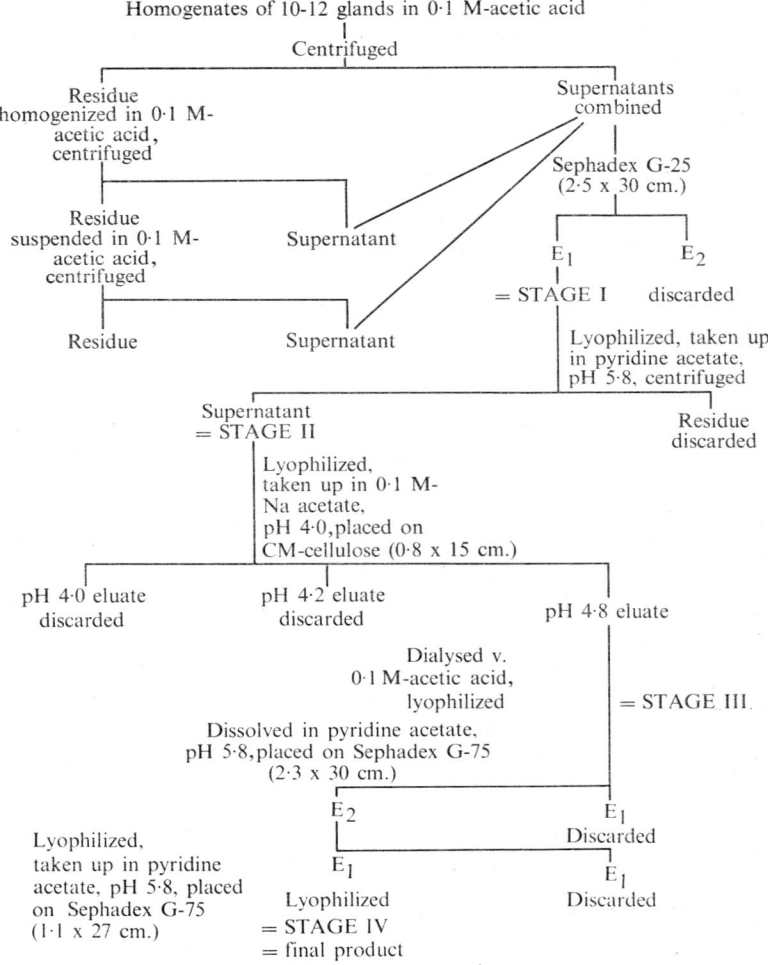

FIG. 7. Preparation of bovine neurophysin. E_1 and E_2 refer to fractions eluted from Sephadex columns. E_1, eluted in the void volume (V_0). E_2, eluted at volumes greater than the V_0 (From Ginsburg and Ireland, 1965).

by Ginsburg and Ireland (1965) of an estimated molecular weight of 90,000. Two of the remaining five neurophysin fractions of Hollenberg and Hope were found to bind oxytocin and vasopressin: one fraction binding about 10 units of each hormone/mg protein, the other only about 2 U/mg; the workers assume that the other three fractions also bind the hormones although no experimental evidence in support of this assumption was presented. In a later publication from the same laboratory (Dean and Hope, 1967) only two neurophysin components were found. These were obtained from isolated elementary granules, and the authors conclude that several constituents of neurophysin, described in the earlier publication (Hollenberg and Hope, 1967), may have arisen as a result of "minor changes in the granular protein during the isolation of the protein". The hormone-binding properties of the two neurophysins were, however, not investigated. It would be of interest to know whether both or only one of these proteins can bind the hormones and also whether a hormone-binding specificity similar to that shown for the porcine neurophysins by Ginsburg et al. (1966b) could be demonstrated in another species.

The isolation of two neurophysins, with different hormone-binding characteristics, from the pig neurohypophysis by Ginsburg et al. (1966b), while allowing for the possibility of denaturation of protein during the preparative procedures, suggests the existence of specific neurophysins for each of the two hormones. The results with porcine neurophysin may be interpreted as showing that oxytocin and vasopressin are stored in association with two separate neurophysins—the "oxytocin neurophysin" may have been separated in a pure form; the other fraction which binds both hormones may be a mixture of "oxytocin neurophysin" and "vasopressin neurophysin". Furthermore, the higher capacity of both the porcine and bovine neurophysins for oxytocin binding may be taken to show that the "oxytocin neurophysin" is present in larger quantities or, alternatively, that it is extracted more efficiently, under the experimental conditions employed, than the "vasopressin neurophysin".

NEUROPHYSIN AND THE STORAGE AND RELEASE
OF THE ACTIVE PEPTIDES

The mechanism of neurophysin–hormone binding is thought to involve an electrostatic interaction (Hasselbach and Piguet, 1952; Acher and Fromageot, 1957; Stouffer, Hope and du Vigneaud, 1963; Ginsburg and Ireland, 1964), the binding sites being between the free α-amino group of a hemicystine residue in the peptide and carboxyl groups in the protein. This view is supported by the findings that (a) an analogue of oxytocin lacking the free amino group (desamino oxytocin) is not bound by bovine neurophysin (Stouffer et al., 1963) and (b) that the pH dependence of hormone binding by neurophysin (optimum pH 5.2–5.8) was compatible only with the involvement of the free amino group of the peptides in complex formations with carboxyl groups in neurophysin (Ginsburg and Ireland, 1963, 1964). The amino acid composition of bovine and porcine neurophysin (Block and van Dyke, 1952; Frankland et al., 1966; Ginsburg et al., unpublished results, 1966), shows a high content of cystine and, perhaps significantly, also a high content of dicarboxylic acids.

The finding of two separate components in bovine and porcine neurophysin by Ginsburg, Jayasena and Thomas (1966a), has been interpreted (Ginsburg, 1968b) as suggesting that ionic association alone does not explain the high degree of specificity; it could be that only a primary link may be established by ionic association and the binding specificity of one hormone to one of the two neurophysins may be conferred by other forces, possibly a secondary disulfide interchange or lipophilic interaction between other sites (Ginsburg and Ireland, 1965; Ginsburg, 1968a).

Effects of calcium ions on hormone binding by neurophysin, and molecular aspects of hormone release

The elucidation of the stimulus-secretion coupling phenomenon (see p. 119) has advanced the understanding of the likely processes involved in the release of vasopressin and oxytocin. It is still not known what role neurophysin plays in the discharge of hormones. It seems unlikely that the hydrogen ion concentration could change drastically upon arrival of hormone-releasing impulses; it is even less likely that the maintenance of the intact hormone–neurophysin complex at the optimal binding pH (5.2–5.8) can occur within the nerve endings (or swellings) under physiological conditions.

Several investigations *in vivo* (Thorn, Smith and Skadhauge, 1965) and *in vitro* (Smith and Thorn, 1965; Thorn, 1966) have shown that calcium can prevent the binding of arginine vasopressin to bovine neurophysin. Ginsburg, Jayasena and Thomas (1966a) confirmed these findings and showed that binding of lysine vasopressin and oxytocin by porcine neurophysin was inhibited in the presence of Ca^{++}. These workers found in dialysis experiments that the calcium concentration for inhibition of binding was critical at varying concentrations of hormones and of neurophysin, i.e. no significant inhibition was found when the Ca^{++} concentration was 0.25×10^{-6} M, while at 1.0×10^{-6} M the inhibition was complete (Table 7). Attempts at elucidation of the mode of action of Ca^{++} on the

TABLE 7. EFFECT OF VARYING CONCENTRATIONS OF CALCIUM ON THE BINDING OF LVP AND OXYTOCIN BY 32 μG OF NEUROPHYSIN. (THE RESULTS ARE EXPRESSED AS PERCENTAGE INHIBITION OF BINDING GIVEN BY 100 $(B_{-Ca} - B_{+Ca})/B_{-Ca}$ WHERE B_{+Ca} = UNITS BOUND IN PRESENCE OF CALCIUM; B_{-Ca} = UNITS BOUND IN ABSENCE OF CALCIUM.)

	Units	n moles	10^6[Ca]moles/l.							
			0	0.125	0.25	0.3	0.4	0.5	1.0	2.5
Oxytocin	1.63	3.9	0	0	14	–	–	36	100	100
	0.98	2.3	0	–	–	–	–	29	–	–
	0.65	1.5	0	–	–	–	–	20	–	–
LVP	3.06	10.4	0	–	0	25	35	–	–	–
	1.53	5.6	0	18	11	36	55	100	100	100
	0.76	2.75	0	–	0	25	35	–	–	–

0 = no inhibition of binding. 100 = complete inhibition of binding.
(From Ginsburg, Jayasena and Thomas, 1966b).

hormone–protein complex (by using $^{45}Ca^{++}$ in similar dialysis experiments) have not produced any clear evidence, other than that showing a lack of pronounced binding of Ca^{++} by either neurophysin or the hormone peptides. The findings were interpreted as suggesting that Ca^{++} may interact with a site on neurophysin different from that for the hormones. Thomas and Ginsburg (1966), who studied the kinetics of the inhibition by cystine of vasopressin binding by neurophysin, suggest that an allosteric transformation of the protein occurs during the binding of the peptide. On this evidence it cannot be excluded that Ca^{++} may cause an allosteric change in reverse thus occluding the sites at which hormones may be bound to neurophysin. Such a hypothesis would seem attractive in explaining the drastic changes in the light- or electron-microscopical appearance of the stimulated posterior pituitary. It could be envisaged that an allosteric transformation of neurophysin, possibly initiated by Ca^{++}, does not only break the protein–peptide hormone bonds, but that it also makes inaccessible the sites for binding of heavy metals (as in electron microscopy) or the disulfide bridges for the oxidative staining reactions (as in light microscopy). The earlier suggestion (Lederis, 1964b, 1965a, 1965b; Daniel and Lederis, 1966b) that lack of stainability of the "neurosecretory material", or of electron density in the elementary granules, "occurs as a result of physicochemical changes in the hormone–neurophysin complex" could thus be substantiated. Conformational changes of the neurophysin–hormone complex as a likely reason for loss of stainability or of electron density have been suggested by Barer and Lederis (1966).

The action of Ca^{++} on the inhibition of neurophysin–hormone binding *in vivo* and *in vitro* was shown to be effective when using the intact neural lobe (fiber swellings or terminals) and also when acting on neural lobe slices. When isolated elementary granules are exposed to calcium ions, in a concentration sufficient to produce hormone release from the intact or sliced neural lobe, no loss of hormones occurs (Daniel and Lederis, 1963; Ginsburg and Ireland, 1966). This may be due to the relatively higher concentration of neurophysin in the granules as compared with experiments *in vivo*, or experiments on the posterior pituitary *in vitro* in which the intragranular and extragranular, and possibly extraneuronal, concentrations of neurophysin may be in equilibrium. Ginsburg (1968b) suggests that free hormones as well as neurophysin-hormone complexes occur, in addition to their location in the elementary granules, also "in one or more of the extragranular compartments, but almost certainly at much lower concentrations than in the neurosecretory particles".

In view of the conclusions reached by Thorn (1966) and by Ginsburg and his co-workers (Ginsburg and Ireland, 1966; Ginsburg, 1968a, 1968b) it would seem likely that Ca^{++} may act on the neurophysin–hormone complexes of the "extragranular pool" rather than those of the intragranular one. Ginsburg (1968b) proposed a "model for the complex dissociation theory of hormone release" (see Fig. 8). This model proposes that in the "resting" condition (*A*) free and bound hormones occur in granules and in an extragranular compartment, neurophysin and neurophysin-bound hormones being highly concentrated in the former and there being no concentration gradient for free hormones (assuming that the granular membrane does not impede diffusion of free hormones). Influx of Ca^{++} coincident with the arrival of a wave of depolarization (*B*) causes dissociation of the extragranular hormone–neurophysin complex and the free hormones diffuse out of the nerve swelling. With recovery toward the resting state, hormone–neurophysin complexes reform in the extragranular compartment (*C*) followed, as equilibrium is reestablished, by a net flux of free hormones from the granules and the dissociation of some intragranular complexes (*D*). Such a model seems feasible and is supported by the observed alteration in the subcellular distribution of hormones in infant, lactating and dehydrated rabbits (Barer *et al.*, 1963; Lederis, 1967b). The increase in the free hormone pool in stimulated (hypersecreting) posterior pituitaries of rats after ether anesthesia and hemorrhage (Daniel and Lederis, 1966b), could also be held to support the sequence of events: depolarization → influx of Ca^{++} → dissociation of neurophysin–hormone complexes → diffusion (or active transport?) of hormones into the blood.

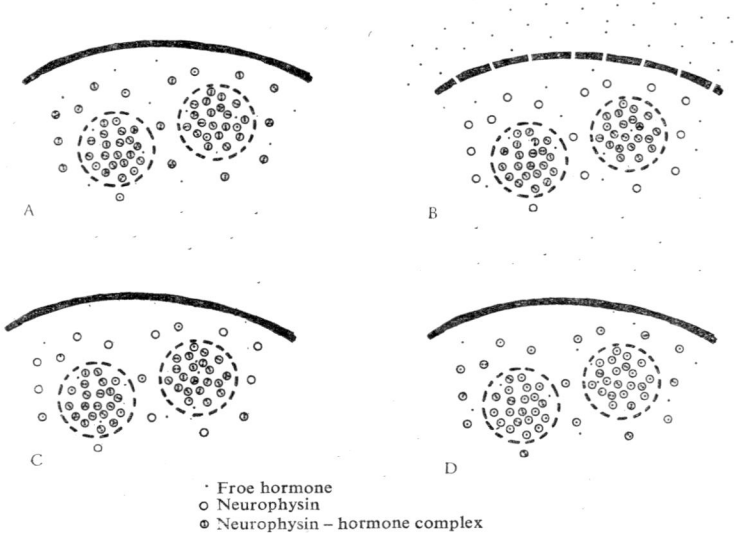

· Free hormone
o Neurophysin
⊙ Neurophysin – hormone complex

FIG. 8. Simplified model for the "enhanced diffusibility" theory of hormone release. The diagrams represent a neuronal membrane enclosing two neurosecretory granules and extragranular space. A, resting state; B, depolarization and Ca^{2+} influx; C, repolarization; D, intracellular repolarization (From Ginsburg, 1968b).

Are the hormone–neurophysin complexes or free peptides released?

A preliminary report has recently appeared (Sachs, Fawcett and Haller, 1967) of findings which seem to contradict the view that neurophysin–hormone complexes are dissociated by Ca^{++} and that the free peptide hormones are released. Sachs and his co-workers infused ^{35}S-cystine into the third ventricle of dehydrated dogs and found ^{35}S-labeled vasopressin and neurophysin in the neural lobe of these dogs killed 10 days after administration of the labeled cystine. After incubation of the neural lobes of such dogs *in vitro* in a medium containing 56 mM K^+, radioactive vasopressin and proteins were found in the incubation medium. From this observation Sachs *et al.* concluded that "vasopressin (ADH) and its carrier proteins (neurophysins) are released simultaneously since more than half of the ^{35}S-protein released into the medium had gel-filtration and electrophoretic properties almost identical with those of beef neurophysin". Moreover, they express the view that "this finding is inconsistent with the postulate that cytoplasmic neurophysin-vasopressin complexes are dissociated by Ca^{++}, resulting in the secretion of ADH alone (Ginsburg and Ireland, 1964). Our results are also at variance with the previous failure to demonstrate neurophysin secretion by indirect methods (Thorn, 1966)".

The issue arises now which of the two differing findings corresponds with, or comes nearer to, the physiological mode of release of neurohypophysial hormones. The finding of neurophysin (or at least of a neurophysin-like protein) in the incubation medium may indicate, in addition to the possible release of intact protein–hormone complexes, several possibilities: (1) the finding of neurophysin (or neurophysin-like protein?) in the medium does not necessarily indicate the release of hormone–protein complexes—"leaking" of neurophysin due to mechanical damage or to partial simulation only of physiological conditions in the experiments *in vivo*, cannot be excluded; (2) similar "leaking" of hormone–neurophysin complexes may occur under *in vitro* conditions. Thorn's (1966) experiments were done on rats, and failure to detect neurophysin may have been due to insufficient amount of the protein in the medium; (3) no calcium ions were present in the incubation medium used. It would be of considerable interest to know how the release of hormones and of neurophysin would be affected if Ca^{++} at the concentration usually employed in the Douglas (1963) type of experiment were included in the medium.

Ginsburg and Jayasena (unpublished observations, cited by Ginsburg, 1968b) found in recent experiments that a protein with immunological and hormone-binding properties of neurophysin can be isolated from serum and certain target organs (uterus, mammary gland, kidney, liver, spleen, brain). It could be postulated that a similar protein is present in the "extracellular" (extraneuronal) compartments of the neural lobe. It could be further speculated that the hormonal peptides, once they leave the nerve endings may be continually attached to neurophysin-like proteins; such similar, though not necessarily identical, proteins may be present in the extracellular space of the neural lobe and in the blood for transport purposes and, finally, in the target organs in a role of receptors or "inactivators".

REFERENCES

BOOKS, REVIEWS, AND MONOGRAPHS

ACHER, R. and FROMAGEOT, C. (1957). The relationship of oxytocin and vasopressin to active proteins of posterior pituitary origin. *The Neurohypophysis*, pp. 39–50. Heller, H. (ed.). Butterworths, London.

ANDERSSON, B. (1957). Polydipsia, antidiuresis and milk ejection caused by hypothalamic stimulation. *The Neurohypophysis*, pp. 131–138. Heller, H. (ed.). Butterworths, London.

BARGMANN, W. (1957). Relationship between neurohypophysial structure and function. *The Neurohypophysis*, pp. 11–22. Heller, H. (ed.). Butterworths, London.

BERN, H. and KNOWLES, F. G. W. (1966). Neurosecretion. *Neuroendocrinology*. Martini, L. and Ganong, W. F. (eds.). Academic Press, London and New York.

CHRIST, J. F. (1960). Hypothalamic-hypophysial neurosecretion (Histological changes in the neurosecretory system of the rabbit after electrical stimulation). *Mem. Soc. Endocr.*, 9: 19–26.

CHRIST, J. F. (1962). The early changes in the hypophysial neurosecretory fibres after coagulation. *Neurosecretion. Mem. Soc. Endocr.*, 12: 125–147.

CHRIST, J. F., ENGELHARDT, F. and DIEPEN, R. (1958). Über Begleiterscheinungen der Neurosekretion im Silberbild. *II Int. Symp. Neurosekretion*, pp. 30–41. Bargmann, W., Hanström, B., Scharrer, B. and Scharrer, E. (eds.). Springer, Heidelberg.

COWIE, A. T. and FOLLEY, S. J. (1957). Neurohypophysial hormones and the mammary gland. *The Neurohypophysis*, pp. 183–202. Heller, H. (ed.). Butterworths, London.

CROSS, B. A. (1959). Neurohypophysial control of parturition. *Recent Prog. Endocr. Reprod.* pp. 414–455. Lloyd, C. W. (ed.). Academic Press, New York.

CROSS, B. A. (1961). Neural control of oxytocin secretion. *Oxytocin*, pp. 24–46. Caldeyro-Barcia, R. and Heller, H. (eds.). Pergamon Press, London.

VAN DYKE, H. B., ADAMSON, K. JR., and ENGEL, S. L. (1957). The storage and liberation of neurohypophysial hormones, *The Neurohypophysis*, pp. 65–76. Heller, H. (ed.). Butterworths, London.

FITZPATRICK, R. J. (1957). On oxytocin and uterine functions. *The Neurohypophysis*, pp. 203–217. Heller, H. (ed.). Butterworths, London.

FITZPATRICK, R. J. (1961). The estimation of small amounts of oxytocin in blood. *Oxytocin* pp. 358–379. Caldeyro-Barcia, R. and Heller, H. (eds.). Pergamon Press, Oxford.

FOLLENIUS, E. (1968). Cytologie des systèmes neurosécréteurs hypothalamo-hypophysaires des poissons téléosteens. *Neurosecretion*, pp. 42–55 Stutinsky, F. (ed.). Springer, Heidelberg.

FOLLEY, S. J. and KNAGGS, G. S. (1965a). Oxytocin levels in the blood of ruminants with special reference to the milking stimulus. *Advances in Oxytocin Research*, pp. 37–49. Pinkerton, J. H. M. (ed.). Pergamon Press, Oxford.

GINSBURG, M. (1968a). Production, release, transportation and elimination of the neurohypophysial hormones. *Handbuch der Pharmakologie* vol. 23, pp 286–371. Springer, Heidelberg.

GINSBURG, M. (1968b). Molecular aspects of neurohypophysial hormone release. *Proc. R. Soc. B*, **170**: 27–36.

GINSBURG, M. and HELLER, H. (1952). Unpublished observations cited by Heller, H. *The Suprarenal Cortex*, pp. 187–195. Yoffey, J. M. (ed.). Butterworths, London,

GINSBURG, M. and BROWN, L. M. (1957). The effects of haemorrhage and plasma. hypertonicity on the neurohypophysis. *The Neurohypophysis*, pp. 109–130. Heller, H. (ed.). Butterworths, London.

GREEN, J. D. and MAXWELL, D. J. (1959). The comparative anatomy of the hypophysis and observations on the mechanism of neurosecretion. *Comparative Endocrinology* pp. 368–392. Gorbman, A. (ed.). Wiley, New York.

HARRIS, G. W. (1960). Central control of pituitary secretion. *Handbook of Physiology*, section 1, vol. 2, pp. 1007–1038. Field, J. (ed.). Amer. Physiol. Soc., Washington.

HELLER, H. (1959). The neurohypophysis during the estrous cycle, pregnancy and lacta-

tion. *Recent Progress in the Endocrinology of Reproduction*, pp. 365–378. Lloyd, C. W. (ed.). Academic Press, London and New York.
HELLER, H. (1961). Occurrence, storage and metabolism of oxytocin. *Oxytocin*, pp. 3–23. Caldeyro-Barcia, R. and Heller, H. (eds.). Pergamon Press, London.
HELLER, H. (1963). Neurohypophyseal hormones. *Comparative Endocrinology*, pp. 26–72. von Euler, U. S. and Heller, H. (eds.). Academic Press, London and New York.
HELLER, H. (1966). The hormone content of the vertebrate hypothalamo-neurohypophysial system. *Brit. Med. Bull.*, 22: 227–231.
HELLER, H. and GINSBURG, M. (1966). Secretion, metabolism and fate of the posterior pituitary hormones. *The Pituitary Gland*, vol. 3, pp. 330–373. Harris, G. W. and Donovan, B. T. (eds.). Butterworths, London.
HELLER, H. and LEDERIS, K. (1962). Characteristics of isolated neurosecretory vesicles from mammalian neural lobes. *Mem. Soc. Endocr.*, 12: 35–50.
HELLER, H. and SPICKETT, S. G. (1967). The polymorphism of the neurohypophysial hormones. *Mem. Soc. Endocr.*, 15: 89–106.
LEDERIS, K. (1962a). The distribution of vasopressin and oxytocin in hypothalamic nuclei. *Mem. Soc. Endocr.* 12, 227–236.
LEDERIS, K. (1967). Storage and release of neurohypophysial hormones with special reference to the fine structure of the vertebrate posterior pituitary. *Physiology and Pathology of Adaptation Mechanisms*. Bajusz, E. (ed.). Pergamon Press, Oxford.
LEDERIS, K. (1967b). Storage and release of neurohypophysial hormones; ultrastructural and subcellular studies. *Proc. Symposium on Advances in Endocrinology*. Schering-Berlin, in press.
LEDERIS, K. (1967c). Ultrastructural and biological evidence for the presence and likely function of acetylcholine in the hypothalamo-neurophysial system. *Neurosection* pp. 155–164. Stutinsky, F. (ed.). Springer, Heidelberg.
NOBLE, R. L. (1957). The excretion of posterior pituitary principles in the urine. *The Neurohypophysis*, pp. 97–108. Heller, H. (ed.). Butterworths, London.
PALAY, S. L. (1957). The fine structure of the neurohypophysis, *Progress in Neurobiology II, Ultrastructure and Cellular Chemistry of Neural Tissue*, pp. 310–49. Korey, S. and Nurnberger, J. (eds.), Hoeber, New York.
DE ROBERTIS, E. (1962). Ultrastructure and function in some neurosecretory systems. *Mem. Soc. Endocr.* 12, 3–20.
SAWYER, W. H. (1966). Neurohypophysial principles of vertebrates. *The Pituitary Gland*, vol. 3, pp. 307–319. Harris, G. W. and Donovan, B. T. (eds.). Butterworths, London.
STOUFFER, J. E., HOPE, A. B., and DU VIGNEAUD, V. (1963). Neurophysin, oxytocin and desamino-oxytocin. *Perspectives in Biology*, pp. 65–80. Cori, C. E., Foglia, V. G., Lelair, L. F, and Ochoa, S. (eds.). Elsevier Publ. Co., Amsterdam.
STREEFKERK, J. G. (1967). Functional changes in the morphological appearance of the hypothalamo-hypophysial neurosecretory and catecholaminergic neural system, and in the adenohypophysis of the rat. Thesis, University of Amsterdam, Van Soest, Amsterdam.

ORIGINAL PAPERS

ABEL, J. J. (1930). On the unitary versus the multiple hormone theory of posterior pituitary principle. *J. Pharmac., Exp. Therm.* **40**: 139–169.

ABRAHAMS, V. C. and PICKFORD, M. (1954). Simultaneous observations on the rate of urine flow and spontaneous uterine movements in the dog and their relationship to posterior pituitary lobe activity. *J. Physiol., Lond.*, **126**: 320–346.

ABRAHAMS, V. C. and PICKFORD, M. (1956). The effect of anti-cholinesterases injected into the supraoptic nuclei of chloralosed dogs on the release of the oxytocic factor of the posterior pituitary. *J. Physiol., Lond.*, **133**: 330–333.

ACHER, R., CHAUVET, J. and OLIVRY, G. (1956). Sur l'existence eventuelle d'une hormone unique neurohypophysaire. Relation entre l'ocytocine, la vasopressine et la protéine de van Dyke extraites de la neurohypophyse du boeuf. *Biochim. Biophys. Acta*, **22**: 421–427.

ADAMSONS, K., ENGEL, S., L., VAN DYKE, H. B., SCHMIDT-NIELSEN, B. and SCHMIDT-NIELSEN, K. (1956). The distribution of oxytocin and vasopressin (antidiuretic hormone) in the neurohypophysis of the camel. *Endocrinology*, **58**: 272–278.

AMES, R. G. and VAN DYKE, H. B. (1950). Antidiuretic hormone in the urine and pituitary of the kangaroo rat. *Proc. Soc. Exp. Biol.* **75**: 417–420.

AMES, R. G. and VAN DYKE, H. B. (1952). Antidiuretic hormone in serum or plasma of rats. *Endocrinology*, **50**: 350–360.

AMES, R. G., MOORE, D. H. and VAN DYKE, H. B. (1950). The excretion of posterior pituitary antidiuretic hormone in the urine and its detection in the blood. *Endocrinology*, **46**: 215–227.

ANDERSSON, B. (1951a). Some observations on the neuro-hormonal regulation of milk-ejection. *Acta Physiol. Scand.*, **23**: 1–7.

ANDERSSON, B. (1951b). The effect and localization of electrical stimulation of certain parts of the brain stem in sheep and goats. *Acta Physiol. Scand.*, **23**: 8–23.

ANDERSSON, B. (1951c). Further studies on the milk ejection mechanism in sheep and goats. *Acta Physiol. Scand.*, **23**: 24–30.

ANDERSSON, B. and MCCANN, S. M. (1955). Drinking, antidiuresis and milk ejection from electrical stimulation within the hypothalamus of the goat. *Acta Physiol. Scand.*, **35**: 191–201.

APPELMANS, F., WATTIAUX, R. and DE DUVE, C. (1955). Tissue fractionation studies. 5. The association of acid phosphatase with a special class of cytoplasmic granules in rat liver. *Biochem. J.*, **59**: 438–445.

BAEZ, S., MAZUR, A., and SHORR, E. (1952). Role of the neurohypophysis in ferritin-induced antidiuresis. *Amer. J. Physiol.*, **169**: 123–133.

BARATZ, R. A. and INGRAHAM, R. C. (1959). Sensitive bioassay method for measuring antidiuretic hormone in mammalian plasma. *Proc. Soc. Exp. Biol. Med.*, **100**: 296–299.

BARER, R. and LEDERIS, K. (1966). Ultrastructure of the rabbit neurohypophysis with special reference to the release of the hormones. *Z. Zellforsch. mikrosk. Anat.*, **75**: 201–239.

BARER, R., HELLER, H. and LEDERIS, K. (1963). The isolation, identification and properties of the hormonal granules of the neurohypophysis. *Proc. Roy. Soc. B*, **158**: 388–416.

BARGMANN, W. (1949). Über die neurosekretorische Verknüpfung von Hypothalamus und Neurohypophyse. *Z. Zellforsch. mikrosk. Anat.* **34**: 610–634.

BARGMANN, W. and SCHARRER, E. (1951). The site of origin of hormones of the posterior pituitary. *Amer. Sci.*, **39**: 255–259.
BELESLIN, D., BISSET, G. W., HALDAR, J. and POLAK, R. L. (1967). The release of vasopressin without oxytocin in response to haemorrhage. *Proc. Roy. Soc. B*, **166**: 443–458.
LABELLA, F. S., BEAULIER, G. and REIFFENSTEIN, R. J. (1962). Evidence for the existence of separate vasopressin and oxytocin-containing granules in the neurohypophysis. *Nature, Lond.*, **193**: 173–174.
LABELLA, F. S. and BROWN, J. H. U. (1959). Cell fractionation of anterior pituitary glands from beef and pig. *J. Biophys. Biochem. Cytol.*, **5**: 17–24.
LABELLA, F. S., REIFFENSTEIN, R. J. and BEAULIER, G. (1963). Subcellular fractionation of bovine posterior pituitary glands by centrifugation. *Arch. Biochem.*, **100**: 399–408.
LABELLA, F. S. and SANWAL, M. (1965). Isolation of nerve endings from the posterior pituitary gland. *J. Cell. Biol.*, **25**: 179–193.
BLOCK, R. J. and VAN DYKE, H. B. (1952). Amino acids in posterior pituitary protein. *Arch. Biochem.*, **36**: 1–4.
BLOOM, R. S. (1960). Thesis, University of Birmingham, cited by R. L. Homes, 1961.
BISSET, G. W., HILTON, S. M. and POISNER, A. M. (1967). Hypothalamic pathways for independent release of vasopressin and oxytocin. *Proc. Roy. Soc. B*, **166**: 422–442.
BISSET, G. W. and WALKER, J. M. (1957). The effects of nicotine, hexamethonium and ethanol on the secretion of the antidiuretic and oxytocic hormones of the rat. *Brit. J. Pharmac. Chemother.*, **12**: 461–467.
DE BODO, R. C. (1944). The antidiuretic action of morphine and its mechanism. *J. Pharmac. Exp. Ther.*, **82**: 74–85.
DE BODO, R. C. and PRESTCOTT, K. F. (1945). The antidiuretic action of barbiturates (phenobarbital, amytal, pentobarbital) and the mechanism involved in this action. *J. Pharmac. Exp. Ther.*, **85**: 222–233.
BURN, J. H., TRUELOVE, L. H. and BURN, I. (1945). The antidiuretic effects of nicotine and smoking. *Brit. Med J.*, **i**: 403–406.
CHANG, H. C., CHIA, K. F., HSÜ, C. M. and LIM, R. K. S. (1937). A vago-postpituitary reflex. I. Pressor component. *Chin. J. Physiol.*, **12**: 309–326.
CHANG, H. C., LIM, R. K. S., LÜ, V. M., WANG, C. C. and WANG, K. L. (1938). A vago-postpituitary reflex. III. Oxytocic component. *Chin. J. Physiol.*, **13**: 269–284.
CHANG, H. C., CHIA, K. F., HUANG, J. J. and LIM, R. K. S. (1939). Vago-postpituitary reflex; antidiuretic effect. *Chin. J. Physiol.*, **14**: 161–172.
CHAUDHURY, R. R. and WALKER, J. M. (1958). The release of neurohypophysial hormones in the rabbit by anaesthetics and by haemorrhage. *J. Physiol., Lond.*, **143**: 16p.
CHAUDHURY, R. R. (1961). Release of oxytocin in unanaesthetised lactating rats. *Brit. J. Pharmac. Chemother.*, **17**: 297–304.
CHAUDHURY, R. R., CHAUDHURY, M. R. and LU, F. C. (1962). The mechanism of reserpine-induced antidiuresis in the rat. *Canad. J. Biochem. Physiol.*, **40**: 1465–1472.
CHAUVET, J., LENCI, M. T. and ACHER, R. (1960). L'ocytocine et la vasopressine du mouton. Reconstitution d'un complex hormonal actif. *Biochim. Biophys. Acta*, **38**: 266–272.
CHIEN, S., PERIC, B. and USAMI, S. (1963). The reflex nature of release of antidiuretic hormone upon common carotid occlusion in vagotomised dogs. *Proc. Soc. Exp. Biol. Med.*, **111**: 193–196.

CLARK, B. J. and ROCHA E SILVA, M. (1966). Independent release of vasopressin by carotid occlusion. *J. Physiol., Lond.*, **186**: 142–143.

CROSS, B. A. (1950). Suckling antidiuresis in rabbits. *Nature, Lond.*, **166**: 612–613.

CROSS, B. A. (1951). Suckling antidiuresis in rabbits. *J. Physiol., Lond.*, **114**: 447–453.

CROSS, B. A. (1953). Sympathetic-adrenal inhibition of the neurohypophysial milk-ejection mechanism. *J. Endocr.*, **9**: 7–18.

CROSS, B. A. (1955a). The hypothalamus and the mechanism of sympathetic adrenal inhibition of milk ejection. *J. Endocr.*, **12**: 15–28.

CROSS, B. A. (1955b). Neurohormonal mechanisms in emotional inhibition of milk ejection. *J. Endocr.*, **12**: 29–37.

CROSS, B. A. and HARRIS, G. W. (1952). The role of the neurohypophysis in the milk ejection reflex. *J. Endocr.*, **8**: 148–161.

DAHLSTROM, A. and FUXE, K. (1966). Monoamines and the pituitary gland. *Acta Endocrinologica Copnh.*, **51**: 301–314.

DANIEL, A. R. and LEDERIS, K. (1963). Hormone release from the neurohypophysis *in vitro*. *Gen. Comp. Endocrinol.*, **3**: 693–694.

DANIEL, A. R. and LEDERIS, K. (1966a). Effects of acetylcholine on the release of neurohypophysial hormones *in vitro*. *J. Endocr.*, **34**: x–xi.

DANIEL, A. R. and LEDERIS, K. (1966b). Effect of ether anaesthesia and haemorrhage on hormone storage and ultrastructure of the rat neurohypophysis. *J. Endocr.*, **34**: 91–104.

DANIEL, A. R. and LEDERIS, K. (1967). Release of neurohypophysial hormones *in vitro*. *J. Physiol. Lond.*, **190**: 171–187.

DEAN, R. C. and HOPE, D. B. (1967). The isolation of purified neurosecretory granules from bovine pituitary posterior lobes. Comparison of granule protein constituents with those of neurophysin. *Biochem. J.*, **104**: 1082–1088.

DEBACKERE, M. and PEETERS, G. (1960a). The influence of vaginal distension on milk ejection and diuresis in the lactating cow. *Archs Int. Pharmacodyn. Thér.*, **123**: 462–471.

DEBACKERE, M. and PEETERS, G. (1960b). Le mechanisme de l'ejection du lait par distension vaginal chez le mouton. *Archs Int. Pharmacodyn. Thér.*, **126**: 486–491.

DEBACKERE, M. and PEETERS, G. (1961). La liberation d'une hormone lors de la stimulation des vesicules seminales et des ampoules chez le bouc. *Archs. Int. Pharmacodyn. Thér.*, **130**: 467–469.

DELLMANN, H. D. (1960). Untersuchungen über Morphologie und Entstehung besonderer nervöser Strukturen in der Neurohypophyse des Rindes, und ihre Bedeutung als Bildungstätte des Neurosekrets. *Dtsch. Z. Nervenheilk.*, **180**: 509–529.

DELLMANN, H. D. (1962). Neurohistologische Untersuchungen über die Verknüpfung von Hypothalamus and Hypophyse (unter besonderer Berücksichtigung der Verhältnisse beim Rind). Ein Beitrag zum Problem der Neurosekretion und der hypothalamischen Beeinflussung der Adenohypophyse. *J. Hirnforsch.*, **5**: 249–344.

DENAMUR, R. and MARTINET, J. (1953). Sensibilité de la glande mammaire de la chevre aux hormones posthypophysaires. *C. R. Séanc. Soc. Biol. Paris*, **147**: 1217–1220.

DEXTER, D., STONER, H. B. and GREEN, H. N. (1954). The release of posterior pituitary antidiuretic hormone by adenosine triphosphate. *J. Endocr.*, **11**: 142–159.

DICKER, S. E. (1953). A method for assay of very small amounts of antidiuretic activity with a note on the antidiuretic titre of rat's blood. *J. Physiol., Lond.*, **122**: 149–157.

DICKER, S. E. (1961). Release and metabolism of the neurohypophysial hormones. *J. Pharm. Pharmacol.*, **13**: 449–469.

DICKER, S. E. (1966). Release of vasopressin and oxytocin from isolated pituitary glands of adult and newborn rats. *J. Physiol. Lond.*, **85**: 429–444.
DICKER, S. E. and NUNN, J. (1957). The role of antidiuretic hormone during water deprivation in rats. *J. Physiol., Lond.*, **136**: 235–248.
DICKER, S. E. and NUNN, J. (1958). Antidiuresis in adult and old rats. *J. Physiol., Lond.* **141**: 332–336.
DICKER, S. E. and TYLER, C. (1953a). Estimation of antidiuretic vasopressor and oxytocic hormones in the pituitary glands of dogs and puppies. *J. Physiol., Lond*, **120**: 141–145.
DICKER, S. E. and TYLER, C. (1953b). Vasopressor and oxytocic activities of the pituitary glands of rats, guinea pigs and cats and of human foetuses. *J. Physiol., Lond.*, **121**: 206–214.
DIEPEN, R., ENGELHARDT, F. and SMITH AGREDA, V. (1954). Über Ort und Art der Entstehung des Neurosekrets im supraoptico-hypophysären System hei Hund und Katze. *Anat. Anz.*, Suppl. **101**: 276–288.
DOUGLAS, W. W. (1963). A possible mechanism of neurosecretion. Release of vasopressin by depolarization and its dependence to calcium. *Nature, Lond.*, **197**: 81–82.
DOUGLAS, W. W. and POISNER, A. M. (1964a). Stimulus–secretion coupling in a neurosecretory organ. The role of calcium in the release of vasopressin from the neurohypophysis. *J. Physiol., Lond.*, **172**: 1–18.
DOUGLAS, W. W. and POISNER, A. M. (1964b). Calcium movement in the neurohypophysis of the rat and its relation to the release of vasopressin. *J. Physiol., Lond.*, **171**: 19–30.
DOUGLAS, W. W. and RUBIN, R. P. (1965). Efflux of adenine nucleotides from perfused adrenal glands exposed to nicotine and other chromaffin cell stimulants. *J. Physiol., Lond.*, **179**: 130–137.
DUCHEN, L. W. (1962). The effects of ingestion of hypertonic saline on the pituitary gland in the rat; a morphological study of the pars intermedia and posterior lobe. *J. Endocr.*, **25**: 161–168.
DUKE, H. N., PICKFORD, M. and WATT, J. A. (1950). The immediate and delayed effects of di-isopropyl fluorophosphate injected into the supraoptic nuclei of dogs. *J. Physiol., Lond.*, **111**: 81–88.
DE DUVE, C., PRESSMAN, B. C., GIANETTO, R., WATTIAUX, R. and APPELMANS, F. (1955). Tissue fractionation studies. 6. Intracellular distribution patterns of enzymes in rat liver tissue. *Biochem. J.*, **60**: 604–617.
DYBALL, R. E. J. (1966). Stimuli for the release of antidiuretic hormone. *J. Physiol., Lond.* **186**: 99–100.
DYBALL, R. (1968). Stimuli for the release of neurohypophysial hormones. *Br. J. Pharmac. Chemother* **33**: 319–328.
VAN DYKE, H. B., CHOW, B. F., GREEP, H. O. and ROTHEN, A. (1942). The isolation of a protein from the pars neuralis of the ox pituitary with constant oxytocic, pressor and diuresis-inhibiting effects. *J. Pharmacol. exp. Therm.*, **74**: 190–209.
FANG, H. S., LIU, H. M. and WANG, S. C. (1962). Liberation of antidiuretic hormone following hypothalamic stimulation in the dog. *Amer. J. Physiol.*, **202**: 212–216.
FELDBERG, W. and VOGT, M. (1948). Acetylcholine synthesis in different regions of the central nervous system. *J. Physiol., Lond.*, **107**: 372–381.
FERGUSON, J. K. W. (1941). A study of the motility of the intact uterus at term. *Surgery Gynec. Obstet.*, **73**: 359–366.
FERGUSON, D. R. and HELLER, H. (1965). Distribution of neurohypophysial hormones in mammals. *J. Physiol., Lond.*, **180**: 846–863.

FITZPATRICK, R. J. and WALMSLEY, C. F. (1962). The concentration of oxytocin in bovine blood during parturition. *J. Physiol., Lond.*, **163**: 13-14.
FOLLETT, B. K. (1963). Mole ratios of the neurohypophysial hormones in the vertebrate neural lobe. *Nature, Lond.*, **198**: 693-694.
FOLLEY, S. J. and KNAGGS, G. S. (1965b). Levels of oxytocin in the jugular vein blood of goats during parturition. *J. Endocr.*, **36**: 301-305.
FRANKLAND, B. T.B., HOLLENBERG, M. D., HOPE, D. B. and SCHACHTER, B. A. (1966). Dissociation of oxytocin and vasopressin from their carrier protein by chromatography on Sephadex G-25. *Brit. J. Pharmacol. Chemother.*, **26**: 502-510.
FRIBERG, O. (1953). Antidiuretic effect of coitus in human subjects. *Acta Endocr., Copnh.*, **12**: 193-196.
FRIEDMAN, S. M., HINKE, J. A. M. and FRIEDMAN, C. L. (1956). Neurohypophyseal responsiveness in the normal and senescent rat. *J. Geront.*, **11**: 286-291.
FRIESEN, H. G. and ASTWOOD, E. B. (1967). Changes in neurohypophysial proteins induced by dehydration and ingestion of saline. *Endocrinology*, **80**: 278-287.
FUCHS, A-R. and WAGNER, G. (1963). Quantitative aspects of release of oxytocin by suckling in unanaesthetised rabbits. *Acta Endocr., Copnh.*, **44**: 581-592.
FUGO, N. W. (1944). The antidiuretic action of yohimbine. *Endocrinology*, **34**: 143-148.
GAITAN, E., COBA, E. and MIZRACHI, M. (1964). Evidence for the differential secretion of oxytocin and vasopressin in man. *J. Clin. Invest.*, **43**: 2310-2322.
GERSCHENFELD, H. M., TRAMEZZANI, J. H. and De ROBERTIS, E. (1960). Ultrastructure and function in neurohypophysis of the toad. *Endocrinology*, **66**: 741-762.
GESSNER, H., STERBA, G., BIESOLD, B. and MÜLLER, H. (1965). Verteilung oxytocinhaltiger Partikel in den subcellulären Fraktionen des Rindes. *Biol. Zbl.*, **84**: 205-232.
GIARMAN, N. J., MATTIE, L. R. and STEPHENSON, W. F. (1953). Studies on the antidiuretic action of morphine. *Science, N. Y.*, **117**: 225-226.
GIERE, F. A. and EVERSOLE, W. J. (1954). Effects of adrenal medullary hormones on antidiuretic substance in blood serum. *Science, N. Y.*, **120**: 395-396.
GILMAN, A. and GOODMAN, L. (1937). The secretory response of the posterior pituitary to the need for water conservation. *J. Physiol.*, **90**: 113-124.
GINSBURG, M. and BROWN, L. M. (1956). Effect of anaesthetic and haemorrhage on the release of neurohypophysial antidiuretic hormone. *Brit. J. Pharmac. Chemother.*, **11**: 236-244.
GINSBURG, M. and HELLER, H. (1953). Antidiuretic activity in blood obtained from various parts of the cardiovascular system. *J. Endocr.*, **9**: 274-282.
GINSBURG, M. and IRELAND, M. (1963). The hormone binding protein of the neurohypophysis. *J. Physiol., Lond.*, **169**: 15P.
GINSBURG, M. and IRELAND, M. (1964). Binding of vasopressin and oxytocin to protein in extracts of bovine and rabbit neurohypophyses. *J. Endocr.*, **30**: 131-145.
GINSBURG, M. and IRELAND, M. (1965). The preparation of bovine neurophysin and the estimation of its maximum capacity to bind oxytocin and arginine vasopressin. *J. Endocr.*, **32**: 187-198.
GINSBURG, M. and IRELAND, M. (1966). The role of neurophysin in the transport and release of neurohypophysial hormones. *J. Endocr.*, **35**: 289-298.
GINSBURG, M., JAYASENA, K. and THOMAS P. J. (1966a). Preparation and properties of porcine neurophysin and the influence of calcium on the hormone-neurophysin complex. *J. Physiol., Lond.*, **184**: 387-401.
GINSBURG, M., JAYASENA, K. and THOMAS, P. J. (1966b). Subfractions from porcine

neurophysin with different hormone binding properties. *J. Physiol., Lond.*, **183**: 45–46.
GINSBURG, M. and SMITH, M. W. (1959). The fate of oxytocin in male and female rats. *Brit. J. Pharmacol. Chemother.*, **14**: 327–333.
GROSVENOR, C. E. and TURNER, C. W. (1956). Ergotamine, oxytocin and milk letdown in lactating rat. *Proc. Soc. Exp. Biol. Med.*, **93**: 466–468.
GROSVENOR, C. E. and TURNER, C. W. (1957a). A method of evaluation of milk letdown in lactating rat. *Proc. Soc. Exp. Biol. Med.*, **94**: 816–817.
GROSVENOR, C. E. and TURNER, C. W. (1957b). Evidence for adrenergic and cholinergic components in milk let-down reflex in lactating rat. *Proc. Soc. Exp. Biol. Med.*, **95**: 719–722.
HARMAN, J. W. and FEIGELSON, L. (1952). Studies on mitochondria. The relationship of structure and function of mitochondria from heart muscle. *Expl. Cell Res.*, **3**: 47–58.
HARRIS, G. W. (1947). The innervation and action of the neurohypophysis; an investigation using the method of remote control stimulation. *Phil. Trans. Roy. Soc., Ser B*, **232**: 385–441.
HARRIS, G. W. (1948). The excretion of an antidiuretic substance by the kidney, after electrical stimulation of the neurohypophysis in the unanaesthetised rabbit. *J. Physiol., Lond.*, **107**: 430–435.
HASSELBACH, C. H. and PIGUET, A. R. (1952). Nature et purification partielle de l'ocytocine sur les hormones hypophysaires. *Helv. Clin. Acta*, **35**: 2131.
HATERIUS, H. O. and FERGUSON, J. K. W. (1938). Evidence for the hormonal nature of the oxytocic principle of the hypophysis. *Amer. J. Physiol.*, **124**: 314–321.
HELLER, H. (1949). Effects of dehydration on adult and newborn rats. *J. Physiol., Lond.*, **108**: 303–314.
HELLER, H. and LEDERIS, K. (1959). Maturation of the hypothalamo-neurohypophysial system. *J. Physiol. Lond.*, **147**: 299–314.
HELLER, H. and LEDERIS, K. (1961). Density gradient centrifugation of hormone-containing subcellular granules from rabbit neurohypophysis. *J. Physiol., Lond.*, **158**: 27–28p.
HELLER, H., LEDERIS, K. and RODECK, H. (1960). The hypothalamo-neurohypophysial system in old rats. *J. Endocr.*, **21**: 225–228.
HELLER, H. and SMIRK, F. H. (1932). Studies concerning the alimentary absorption of water and tissue hydration in relation to diuresis. Part IV. The influence of anaesthetics and hypnotics on the absorption and excretion of water. *J. Physiol., Lond.*, **76**: 292–302.
HILD, W. and ZETLER, G. (1951). Über das Vorkommen der Hypophysenhinterlappenhormone im Zwischenhirn. *Arch. exp. Path. Pharmak.* **213**: 139–153.
HILD, W. and ZETLER, G. (1953). Experimenteller Beweis für die Entstehung der sog. Hypophysenhinterlappenwirkstoffe im Hypothalamus. *Pflügers Arch. ges. Physiol.*, **257**: 169–201.
HOLLAND, R. C., CROSS, B. A. and SAWYER, C. H. (1959). E. E. G. correlates of osmotic activation of the neurohypophysial milk-ejection mechanism. *Amer. J. Physiol.*, **196**: 796–802.
HOLLENBERG, M. D. and HOPE, D. B. (1967). Fractionation of neurophysin by molecular-sieve and ion-exchange chromatography. *Biochem. J.*, **104**: 122–127.
HOLMES, R. L. (1961). Phosphatase and cholinesterase in the hypothalamo-hypophysial system in the monkey. *J. Endocr.*, **23**: 63–67.
HOLMES, R. L. (1964). Experimental, histochemical, and ultrastructural contributions

to our understanding of mammalian pituitary function. *Int. Rev. Gen. Exp. Zool.* **1**: 187–241.

HOPE, D. B. and HOLLENBERG, M. D. (1966). Isolation of a new hormone-binding protein from the posterior lobes of bovine pituitary glands. *Biochem. J.*, **99**: 5–6P.

HOPE, D. B., SCHACHTER, B. A. and FRANKLAND, B. T. B. (1964). Dissociation of oxytocin, vasopressin and neurophysin by gel filtration. *Biochem. J.*, **93**:7P.

ISHII, S., YASAMASU, I., KABAYASHI, H., OOTA, Y., HIRANO, T. and TANAKA, A. (1962). Isolation of neurosecretory granules and nerve endings from bovine posterior lobe. *Annot. Zool. Japan.*, **35**: 121–127.

ISHIKAWA, T., KOIZUMI, K. and BROOKS, C. McC. (1966). Electrical activity recorded from the pituitary stalk of the cat. *Amer. J. Physiol.*, **201**: 427–431.

JASINSKI, A., GORBMAN, A. and HARA, T. J. (1966). Rate of movement and redistribution of stainable neurosecretory granules in hypothalamic neurons. *Science, N.Y.* **154**: 776–778.

JEWELL, P. A. (1953). The occurrence of vesiculated neurones in the hypothalamus of the dog. *J. Physiol., Lond.*, **121**: 167–181.

KALLIALA, H. and KARVONEN, M. J. (1951). Antidiuresis during suckling in lactating women. *Amer. Med. Exp. Biol. Fenn.*, **29**: 233–241.

KALLIALA, H., KARVONEN, M. J. and LEPPÄNEN, V. (1952). Release of antidiuretic hormone during nursing in dog. *Annls. Med. Exp. Biol. Fenn.*, **30**: 96–107.

KASTIN, A. J. (1967). MSH and vasopressin activities in pituitaries of rats treated with hypertonic saline. *Fedn. Proc. Fedn. Amer. Socs. Exp. Biol.*, **29**: 255.

KELSALL, A. R. (1949). The inhibition of water diuresis in man by ischaemic muscle pain. *J. Physiol., Lond.*, **109**: 150–161.

KOELLE, G. B. (1961). A proposed dual neurohumoral role of acetylcholine: its function at the pre- and post-synaptic sites. *Nature, Lond.*, **190**: 208–211.

KOELLE, G. B. and GEESEY, C. (1961). Localization of acetylcholinesterase in the neurohypophysis and its functional implications. *Proc. Soc. Exp. Biol. N.Y.*, **106**: 625–628.

KUSCHINSKY, C. and LIEBERT, P. (1939). Untersuchungen über den Hormongehalt des Hypophysenhinterlappens der Ratte unter dem Einfluss von Wasser, Kochsalz und Novasurol. *Klin. Wschr.*, **18**: 823.

LEDERIS, K. (1961). Vasopressin and oxytocin in the mammalian hypothalamus. *Gen. Comp. Endocr.* **1**: 80–89.

LEDERIS K. (1962b). Ultrastructure of the hypothalamo-neurohypophysial system in teleost fishes and isolation of hormone-containing granules from the neurohypophysis of the cod *(Gadus morrhua)*. *Z. Zellforsch., mikrosk. Anat.* **58**: 192–213.

LEDERIS, K. (1964). Fine structure and hormone content of the hypothalamo-neurohypophysial system of the rainbow trout *(Salmo irideus)* exposed to sea water. *Gen. Comp. Endocr.*, **4**: 638–661.

LEDERIS, K. (1965a). An electron-microscopic study of the human neurohypophysis. *Z. Zellforsch., mikrosk. Anat.* **65**: 847–868.

LEDERIS, K. (1965b). Relationships between ultrastructure and function of the vertebrate hypothalamo-neurohypophysial system. Symposium on Neurosecretion, *Proc. 2nd Internat. Congr. Endocrinology, Part II*, pp. 563–569.

LEDERIS, K. (1966). Acetylcholine in the mammalian neurohypophysis. *J. Endocr.*, **37**: xxiv–xxv.

LEDERIS, K. (1967a). Beziehung zwischen der Ultrastruktur der Neurohypophyse und der subcellulären Verteilung von biologisch aktiven Substanzen. *Arch. Pharmak. Exp. Path.*, **257**: 53–93.

LEDERIS, K. and HELLER, H. (1960). Intracellular storage of vasopressin and oxytocin in the posterior pituitary lobe. *Acta Endocr., Copnh.*, Suppl. **51**: 115–116.
LEDERIS, K. and KAUZ, G. (1965). Separation by density gradient centrifugation of different hormone granules from the trout neurohypophysial tissue. *Gen. Comp. Endocr.*, **5**, Comm. No. 56.
LEDERIS, K. and LIVINGSTON, A. (1966). Acetylcholine content in the rabbit neurohypophysis. *J. Physiol., Lond.* **185**: 37–38P.
LEDERIS, K. and LIVINGSTON, A. (1968a). Acetylcholine, acetylcholinesterase and choline acetylase in the anterior hypothalamus and neural lobe of the rabbit. *J. Physiol., Lond.*, in press.
LEDERIS, K. and LIVINGSTON, A. (1967b). Subcellular localisation of acetylcholine in the posterior pituitary of the rabbit. *J. Physiol., Lond.*, **196**: 34–36P.
LEGAIT, H. (1964). Volume réel et volume relatif des lobes hypophysaires du rat dans diverses conditions physiologiques et expérimentales. *C. R. Séanc. Soc. Biol. Paris*, **158**: 619–621.
LEVEQUE, T. F. and SCHARRER, E. (1953). Pituicytes and the origin of the antidiuretic hormone. *Endocrinology*, **65**: 909–919.
LITTLE, J. B. and RADFORD, E. P. (1964). Bio-assay for antidiuretic activity in blood of undisturbed rats. *J. Appl. Physiol.*, **19**: 179–186.
LIVINGSTON, A. (1966). Acetylcholinesterase content of the rabbit neurohypophysis. *J. Physiol., Lond.*, **187**: 37–38P.
LIVINGSTON, A. and LEDERIS, K. (1967). Acetylcholine and related enzyme systems in the rabbit neurohypophysis. *Acta Endocr., Copnh.*, Suppl. **119**: 99.
MARTINET, J. and DENAMUR, R. (1960). Etude preliminaire des mechanismes de l'evacuation du lait de la glande mammaire chez la chevre et la brebis. *Archs Sci. Physiol.*, **14**: 35–96.
MCARTHUR, C. G. (1931). A new posterior pituitary preparation. *Science, N.Y.* **73**: 448.
MILLS, E. and WANG, S. C. (1964a). Liberation of antidiuretic hormone: location of ascending pathways. *Amer. J. Physiol.*, **207**: 1399–1404.
MILLS, E. and WANG, S. C. (1964b). Liberation of antidiuretic hormone: pharmacologic blockade of ascending pathways. *Amer. J. Physiol.*, **207**: 1405–1410.
MOREL, F. (1955). Quelques aspects de la regulation endocrinienne de l'equilibre hydromineral enregistres chez le rat a l'aide du radio-sodium Na^{24}. *Bull. Biol. France. Belg.* Suppl. **39**: 1–110.
MOSES, A. M. (1963). Adrenal-neurohypophysial relationships in the dehydrated rat. *Endocrinology*, **73**: 230–236.
MOSES, A. M. (1964). Inhibition of vasopressin release in rats by chlorpromazine and reserpine. *Endocrinology*, **74**: 889–893.
MOTZFELDT, K. (1917). Experimental studies on the relation of the pituitary body to renal function. *J. Exp. Med.*, **25**: 153–188.
OOTA, Y. (1963). On the synaptic vesicles in the neurosecretory organs of the carp, bullfrog, pigeon and mouse. *Annot. zool. Japon.* **36**: 167–172.
OOTA, Y. and KOBAYASHI, H. (1962). Fine structures of the median eminence and pars nervosa of the pigeon. *Annot. zool. Japon.*, **35**: 128–138.
ORTMANN, R. (1951). Über experimentelle Veränderungen der Morphologie des Hypophysen-Zwischenhirnsystems und die Beziehung der sog. "Gomori Substanz" zum Adiuretin. *Z. Zellforsch. mikrosk. Anat.*, **36**: 92–140.
PALAY, S. L. (1955). An electron microscopic study of the neurohypophysis in normal, hydrated and dehydrated rats. *Anat. Rec.*, **121**: 348.

PARDOE, A. V. and WEATHERALL, M. (1955). Intracellular localization of oxytocic and vasopressor substances in pituitary glands of rats. *J. Physiol., Lond.*, **127**: 201–212.
PEETERS, G. and COUSSENS, R. (1950). The influences of the milking act on the diuresis of the lactating cow. *Archs Int. Pharmacodyn. Thér.*, **84**: 209–220.
PEETERS, G., COUSSENS, R., BOUCKAERT, J. H. and OYAERT, W. (1949). L'influence de la traite sur la diurese de la vache gravide. *Archs Int. Pharmacodyn. Thér.*, **80**: 355–358.
PEETERS, G., STORMORKEN, H. and VANSCHOUBROEK, F. (1960). The effect of different stimuli on milk ejection and diuresis in the lactating cow. *J. Endocr.*, **20**: 163–172.
PICKFORD, M. (1939). The inhibitory effect of acetylcholine on water-diuresis in the dog, and its pituitary transmission. *J. Physiol., Lond.*, **95**: 226–238.
PICKFORD, M. (1947). The action of acetylcholine on the supraoptic nucleus of the chloralosed dog. *J. Physiol., Lond.*, **106**: 264–270.
PICKFORD, M. (1959). Milk ejection in the anaesthetised dog. *J. Physiol., Lond.*, **149**: 41–42.
PICKFORD, M. (1960). Factors affecting milk release in the dog and the quantity of milk released by suckling. *J. Physiol., Lond.*, **152**: 515–526.
PICKFORD, M. and WATT, J. A. (1951). A comparison of the effect of intravenous and intracarotid injections of acetylcholine in the dog. *J. Physiol., Lond.*, **114**: 333–335.
ROCHA E SILVA, M. and MALNIC, G. (1964). Release of antidiuretic hormone by bradykinin. *J. Pharmac. Exp. Ther.*, **146**: 24–32.
ROSENFELD, M. (1940). The native hormones of the posterior pituitary gland. *Bull. Johns Hopkins Hosp.*, **66**: 398–403.
RYDIN, H. and VERNEY, E. B. (1938). The inhibition of water diuresis by emotional stress and by muscular exercise. *Quart. J. Exp. Physiol.*, **27**: 343–374.
SACHS, H. and TAKABATAKE, Y. (1964). Evidence for a precursor in vasopressin biosynthesis. *Endocrinology*, **75**: 943–948.
SACHS, H., FAWCETT, C. P. and HALLER, E. W. (1967). Biosynthesis and release of neurophysin and hormonal peptides. *Proc. 49th Meeting of Endocrine Society, 1967*, Abst. No. 98, p. 77.
SCHIEBLER, T. H. (1952). Cytochemische und elektronenmikroskopische Untersuchungen an granulären Fraktionen der Neurohypophyse des Rindes. *Z. Zellforsch., mikrosk. Anat.* **36**: 563–576.
VON SCHLICHTERGROLL, A. (1954). Vasopressorische und oxytocische Wirkung in Hypothalamus- und Hypophysen hinterlappenextrachen. *Naturwissenschaften*, **4**: 188–189.
SCHNIEDEN, H. and BLACKMORE, E. K. (1955). The effect of nalorphine on the antidiuretic action of morphine in rats and men. *Brit. J. Pharmac. Chemother.*, **10**: 45–50.
SHARE, L. (1961). Acute reduction in extracellular fluid volume and the concentration of antidiuretic hormone in blood. *Endocrinology*, **69**: 925–933.
SHARE, L. (1962). Vascular volume and blood level of antidiuretic hormone. *Amer. J. Physiol.*, **202**: 791–794.
SHARE, L. and LEVY, M. N. (1962). Cardiovascular receptors and blood titre of antidiuretic hormone. *Amer. J. Physiol.*, **203**: 425–428.
SIDDIQI, S. and WALKER, J. M. (1960). Oxytocic activity of rabbits' blood applied directly to superfused rat uterus. *J. Physiol., Lond.*, **152**: 381–390.
SIMON, A. and KARDOS, Z. (1934). Über den Gehalt der Hypophysenhinterlappen normaler und durstender Tiere an Blutdruck- und Uterus wirksamen Stoffen. *Arch. Exp. Path. Pharmak.*, **176**: 238–242.

SMITH, M. W. and THORN, N. A. (1965). The effects of calcium on protein binding and metabolism of arginine vasopressin in rats. *J. Endocr.*, **32**: 141-151.
SMITHIES, O. (1954). The application of four methods for assessing protein homogeneity to crystalline β-lactoglobulin: an anomaly in phase rule solubility tests. *Biochem. J.*, **58**: 31-38.
SOKOL, H. W. and VALTIN, H. (1967). Evidence for the synthesis of oxytocin and vasopressin in separate neurons. *Nature, Lond.*, **214**: 314-316.
SPEIDEL, C. C. (1919). Gland cells of internal secretion in the spinal cord of the skates. *Carnegie Inst., Washington, Publ.* **13**: 1-31.
SPEIDEL, C. C. (1922). Further comparative studies in other fishes of cells that are homologous to the large irregular glandular cells in the spinal cord of skates. *J. Comp. Neur.*, **34**: 303-317.
TAYLOR, N. B. G. and WALKER, J. M. (1951). Antidiuretic substance in human urine after smoking. *J. Physiol., Lond.*, **113**: 412-418.
THEOBALD, G. W. (1959). The separate release of oxytocin and ADH. *J. Physiol., Lond.*, **149**: 443-461.
THOMAS, P. J. and GINSBURG, M. (1966). Inhibition by L-cystine of the binding of lysine 8-vasopressin by porcine neurophysin. *Biochem. J.*, **100**: 9c.
THORN, N. A. (1965). Role of calcium in the release of vasopressin and oxytocin from posterior pituitary protein. *Acta Endocr., Copnh.*, **50**: 357-364.
THORN, N. A. (1966). *In vitro* studies of the release mechanism for vasopressin in rats. *Acta Endocr. Copnh.*, **53**: 644-654.
THORN, N. A. and SILVER, L. (1957). Chemical form of circulating antidiuretic hormone in rats. *J. Exp. Med.*, **105**: 575-583.
THORN, N. A., SMITH, M. W. and SKADHAUGE, E. (1965). The antidiuretic effect of intravenous and intracarotid infusion of calcium chloride in hydrated rats. *J. Endocr.*, **32**: 161-165.
TINDAL, J. S., KNAGGS, G. S. and TURVEY, A. (1967). Studies on the ascending path of the milk-ejection reflex in the brain of the guinea pig. *J. Endocr.*, **37**: XLI.
UEMURA, H., KOBAYSHI, H. and ISHII, S. (1963). Cholinergic substance in the neurosecretory storage-release organs. *Zool. Mag. Tokyo*, **72**: 204-212.
USAMI, S., PERIC, B. and CHIEN, S. (1963). Release of antidiuretic hormone due to common carotid occlusion and its relation with vagus nerve. *Proc. Soc. Exp. Biol. Med.*, **111**: 189-193.
VALTIN, H. (1967). Hereditary hypothalamic diabetes insipidus in rats (Brattleboro strain) *Amer. J. Med.* **42**: 814-827.
VERNEY, E. B. (1947). The antidiuretic hormone and the factors which determine its release. *Proc. Roy. Soc. B*, **135**: 25-106.
VOGT, M. (1953). Vasopressor, antidiuretic and oxytocic activities of extracts of the dog's hypothalamus. *Brit. J. Pharmacol., Chemother.* **8**: 193-196.
WALLER, H. (1938). *Clinical Studies in Lactation.* Heineman, London.
WEINSTEIN, H., BERNE, R. M. and SACHS, H. (1960). Vasopressin in blood; effect of haemorrhage. *Endocrinology*, **66**: 712-718.
WEINSTEIN, H., MALAMED, A. and SACHS, H. (1961). Isolation of vasopressin-containing granules from the neurohypophysis of the dog. *Biochim. Biophys. Acta*, **50**: 386-389.
WHITTAKER, V. P. (1959). The isolation and characterization of acetylcholine-containing particles. *Biochem. J.*, **72**: 694-706.
DE WIED, D. (1960). A simple automatic and sensitive method for the assay of anti-

diuretic hormone with notes on the antidiuretic potency of plasma under different experimental conditions. *Acta Physiol. Pharmac. Néerland.*, **9**: 69–81.
DE WIED, D. and JINKS, R. (1958). Effect of chlorpromazine on antidiuretic response to noxious stimuli. *Proc. Soc. Exp. Biol. Med.*, **99**: 44–45.
DE WIED, D. and LÁSZLO, F. A. (1967). The effect of autonomic blocking agents on ADH-release induced by hyperosmoticity. *J. Endocr.*, **37**: xvi.
WISLOCKI, G. B. and KING, L. S. (1936). The permeability of the hypophysis and hypothalamus to vital dyes with a study of the hypophysial vascular supply. *Amer. J. Anat.*, **58**: 421–477.
ZUIDEMA, G. D. and CLARK, N. P. (1957). Central localisation of the osmotic control centre. *Amer. J. Physiol.*, **188**: 616–618.

CHAPTER 6

BIOSYNTHESIS OF THE NEUROHYPOPHYSIAL HORMONES*

Howard Sachs[†]

Department of Physiology, Western Reserve University School of Medicine, Cleveland, Ohio, 44106.

INTRODUCTION

It is well established that the polypeptide hormones vasopressin and oxytocin are elaborated by a specialized group of neurons whose cell bodies lie in the anterior hypothalamus and whose axons terminate in the neurohypophysis. These neurons fall within the category of what have been termed "neurosecretory cells." They exhibit morphological and functional characteristics of both nerve and glandular cells and are directly concerned with the translation of neural inputs into endocrine function. While no attempt will be made here to examine the varied facets of the activities of these neuroendocrine cells, it is apparent that questions pertaining to the biosynthesis of the neurohypophysial hormones embody a number of fundamental problems in neuroendocrinology and neurochemistry. In the discussion which follows, the biosynthesis of vasopressin and oxytocin is considered not merely with regard to the steps involved in the formation of the polypeptide chains but also with regard to the manner in which the biosynthetic pathway subserves the unique function of these hypothalamic neurons. Their primary function, obviously, is to secrete vasopressin and oxytocin according to the needs of the body and in response to a variety of physiological stimuli. In a number of endocrine organs (e.g. adrenal cortex, gonads, etc.), gland stimulation and hormone secretion are intimately linked with *de novo* hormone biosynthesis; acute secretory stimuli bring about the rapid release of hormone in amounts far greater than that initially present in the gland. In the case of the

---

* The studies of the author were supported in part by grants from the National Institutes of Health (U. S. Public Health Service AM—2650), and the National Science Foundation (GB-5630).
[†] Supported by Research Career Development Award No. 2 K3 AM-14827.

neurohypophysis, however, the biosynthetic and secretory events often appear both spatially and temporally unrelated. In this regard, it is noteworthy that these hypothalamic neurosecretory cells are not only a factory for the synthesis of vasopressin and oxytocin, but they are also a commodious storehouse. Indeed, it is apparent from the available estimates of "basal" ADH secretion, that the neurohypophysis contains enough hormone to maintain a "steady state" rate of secretion of ADH for several weeks.

The early morphological investigations (for recent reviews see Bargmann, 1966, or Bern and Knowles, 1966) indicated that the major storage form of the neurohypophysial hormones were dense granules (called neurosecretory granules or NSG) of about 0.1 to 0.3μ in diameter (Palay, 1957). This concept received direct verification when NSG from the neural lobes of a number of species were isolated in relatively pure form and shown to contain both the polypeptide hormones, oxytocin and vasopressin (Weinstein et al., 1961; LaBella et al., 1962; Barer et al., 1963). Furthermore, recent studies suggest that these hormones are stored (Ginsburg and Ireland, 1966) and released (Sachs et al., 1967a; Sachs, 1967) in association with a group of specific proteins (termed neurophysin) capable of binding oxytocin and vasopressin (van Dyke et al., 1942; Acher and Fromageot, 1957; Ginsburg et al., 1965; Hope and Hollenberg 1966; Breslow and Abrash, 1966). While the NSG are predominantly concentrated in the axon terminals, morphological and biochemical investigations have demonstrated their presence in the cell bodies and along the entire length of the axon (Palay, 1957; Sloper, 1966; Sachs, 1963a).

With this brief introduction, the biosynthesis of oxytocin and ADH may be examined within the context of several pertinent and related questions; these are:

1. Are the NSG self-contained units in that they possess the enzymic machinery for *de novo* hormone biosynthesis; or, are hormone molecules assembled at other intracellular loci and subsequently stored within the NSG?

2. What is the nature of the enzymic pathways involved in the biosynthesis of these octapeptide hormones?

3. Are separate neurons or NSG involved in the formation of each hormone?

4. Which anatomical portions of the neuron engage in hormone biosynthesis?

5. What factors regulate the rate at which hormone biosynthesis occurs?

To what extent are the biosynthetic events responsive to neural inputs? How do neural inputs modulate the cellular biosynthetic processes?

6. Is the biosynthesis of oxytocin and vasopressin related to the biosynthesis of their respective carrier proteins (i.e., is there a functional genetic unit)?

HORMONE BIOSYNTHESIS AND NEUROSECRETION

A number of physiological and anatomical correlates formed the basis for the concept of the "neurosecretory process." This process as formulated by E. and B. Scharrer (1954) and others (see Bargmann, 1966) ascribed an anatomical division of labor to the neurosecretory cell. The cell body in the hypothalamus synthesizes and packages its hormones within NSG which then move as aggregates (neurosecretory material or NSM) in a protoplasmic flow along the axon to the region of the nerve terminals where the release of the hormones occurs. Support for this concept derives from several independent and overlapping observations. These are: (a) There appears to be a good correlation between the intensity of staining (or amount) of NSM and the state of hydration of the animal (Hild, 1951) or in some instances, the hormone content of the pituitary; (b) After section of the nerve fibers, the NSG as well as the hormones disappear distal to the lesion and accumulate in large masses in the swollen stumps of the fibers proximal to the lesion (Hild, 1951; Hild and Zetler, 1953; Sloper and Adams, 1956); (c) Radio-autographic experiments (Sloper et al., 1960) are consistent with "axoplasmic flow," a doctrine, developed and studied most extensively in peripheral nerve (Weiss, 1961).

By and large, the biosynthesis of oxytocin and vasopressin has been studied within the context of this "theory of neurosecretion", and to date no convincing evidence has been brought forward which conflicts with the essential features of the theory (i.e. the absolute requirement of the perikaryon for the synthesis of NSG and/or the hormones, axonal transport, and release of hormones from the neurohypophysis). Nevertheless, a number of studies have indicated that the above formulation of "neurosecretion" might require some modification, and investigations in our own and other laboratories have been directed toward providing more precise descriptions of the intermediate stages of hormone biosynthesis and of the "neurosecretory process."

ANATOMICAL AND INTRACELLULAR LOCI OF HORMONE BIOSYNTHESIS

While the lesion experiments described above demonstrate that the integrity of the hypothalamic neurons is required for the sustained activity of their axonal elements, they do not preclude the possibility that these latter segments can carry out the biosynthesis of oxytocin and vasopressin. For example, it is conceivable that the cell body merely furnishes a necessary and continuous supply of substrates, or cofactors, or that it has to replenish essential but short-lived components of the biosynthetic apparatus. Recent studies on peripheral nerve have indicated that the axon possesses a limited capacity to carry on both protein and RNA synthesis (Koenig, 1967). Furthermore, the results of Vogt (1953), De Robertis (1962) and Christ (1962) suggested that the distal portions of the hypothalamo-neurohypophysial complex (i.e. the neurohypophysis) may play a significant role in the synthesis of one or both of the neurohypophysial hormones. For example, De Robertis (1962) has reported that in at least two species, toad and rat, the size of NSG increases along the hypothalamo-hypophysial tract (contrary to findings of Sloper and Bateson, 1965). Christ (1962) and co-workers, on the basis of histological studies, have also suggested that neurosecretory material may be formed not only in the cell bodies but by all parts of the neurons of the supraoptic and paraventricular nuclei. Vogt (1953), on the basis of the marked differences between hypothalamic and posterior pituitary oxytocin/ADH ratios, postulated that either the posterior lobe must have an important modifying influence on whatever has been formed in the hypothalamus or that the distal portion of the neuron is responsible for oxytocin biosynthesis. While the results of De Robertis, Christ and Vogt may be marshalled in favor of the idea that the axonal elements play a significant role in hormone biosynthesis, the nature of the evidence is at best indirect and is subject to a number of alternative interpretations.

Over the past several years, it has become feasible to study the biosynthesis of vasopressin directly by means of isotope techniques (see Sachs, 1966). Thus, by the introduction of this approach it was possible to pose such questions as: (a) Where in the cell does labeled vasopressin first arise after the intravenous or intraventricular infusion of ^{35}S-cysteine? (b) Which segments of the neuron carry out the biosynthesis of vasopressin independently *(in vivo* and *in vitro)*? (c) Could the isotope results furnish a clue to the nature of the enzymic processes involved in hormone biosynthesis?

The results of our isotope experiments on the incorporation of radioactive amino acids into vasopressin are in accord with the concept that the hypothalamus is the major if not obligatory site for the synthesis of the peptide bonds in vasopressin. The experimental findings are as follows: (1) After the continuous infusion of ^{35}S-cysteine into dogs for periods of from 8 to 36 hr, the specific activity of the hormone isolated from the hypothalamus was 2–3 times greater than that of neurohypophysial vasopressin (Sachs, 1960). (2) In one experiment in which a stalk section was performed prior to infusion of ^{35}S-cysteine into the third ventricle of a dog, labeled hormone was found only in the hypothalamus at the termination of the experiment.* (3) Hypothalamic-median eminence (HME) tissue of the guinea-pig was capable of *de novo* hormone biosynthesis *in vitro*. Under identical incubation conditions, isolated portions of the neurohypophysis (infundibular stem and process) did not incorporate labeled amino acids into vasopressin (Takabatake and Sachs, 1964). (4) Puromycin inhibited vasopressin biosynthesis *in vivo* or *in vitro;* these results suggest that the peptide bonds in vasopressin are constructed at sites on or resembling ribosomes. Except for mitochondrial structures (Barondes, 1966), the axonal portions of the neurosecretory cells in the posterior pituitary do not appear to contain other protein forming units requiring the participation of nucleic acids. Although considerable evidence has been accumulated in favor of the essential role of the perikaryon in the initial steps in hormone biosynthesis it should be stressed, however, that none of the data preclude the possibility that the late stages of hormone biosynthesis (e.g., release of vasopressin from a bound form) can occur within portions of the axonal elements.

Isotope experiments carried out in the intact dog have ruled out the possibility that the NSG represent the primary cellular loci for hormone biosynthesis (Sachs, 1963b). After the continuous infusion of ^{35}S-cysteine into the third ventricle of anesthetized dogs over relatively short time intervals, the vasopressin molecules associated with the NSG were always found to have the lowest specific activity compared to vasopressin found with a number of other particulate cell structures (Table 1).

Although it was reasonable to assume that nucleic acid structures (i.e., ribosomes) would constitute the primary and obligatory site for the synthesis of the polypeptide hormone, the experimental data were not in accord with such an assumption. It has been a consistent finding that after the infusion of ^{35}S-cysteine into the third ventricle of dogs for 3 to 6 hours, the most highly labeled vasopressin molecules did not follow the ribosome-rich fractions (see Table 1 and Sachs, 1963b). Instead,

---

* We are indebted to Dr. A. Rothballer for the performance of the stalk section.

TABLE 1. COMPARISON OF THE SPECIFIC ACTIVITIES OF
^{35}S VASOPRESSIN ASSOCIATED WITH CELL FRACTIONS OF
THE DOG HYPOTHALAMO-MEDIAN EMINENCE COMPLEX

^{35}S-CYSTEINE, 1.7×10^9 COUNTS/MIN, INFUSED INTO THE THIRD
VENTRICLE OF A DOG FOR 3 H

Cell fraction*	Vasopressin	
	μg	counts/min/μg
NSG	0.58	96
Cell sap	0.85	76
Nuclei, cell debris	0.36	229
Large granules	0.38	319
Microsomes	0.36	155

* Cell fractions were prepared and ^{35}S-vasopressin was isolated from each fraction and purified to constant specific activity as previously described (Sachs, 1963a, b).

^{35}S-vasopressin with the highest specific activity was found in association with particulate material which sedimented in a relatively low centrifugal field. While it cannot be excluded that these results were in part artifactual (i.e., due to distortion of pool sizes by disruption of cell structures, non-specific binding, etc.), other interpretations of the isotope results are possible. Two of these are: (a) that nucleic acid structures are not involved in vasopressin biosynthesis in analogy with the biosynthesis of the pentapeptide nucleotide of *Staphylococcus aureus* (Ito and Strominger, 1960), or gramicidin S (Bhagavan, 1966; Otani et al., 1966) or the tyrocidines (Mach et al., 1963); or (b) that the biosynthesis of vasopressin occurs on ribosomes but in a bound, biologically inactive form (i.e., as part of a macromolecule), and that labeled vasopressin first appears at a site removed from the ribosome. The results of a subsequent series of isotope experiments have provided information in support of the latter interpretation. If a biologically inactive precursor exists in significant quantities and the liberation of active hormone is relatively slow, then labeling experiments might be expected to show a lag period followed by the appearance of radioactive vasopressin at loci removed from and independent of the initial biosynthetic events. Should the formation of the precursor require the participation of nucleic acid structures, then it might be expected that puromycin would be an effective inhibitor of vasopressin biosynthesis. It is also apparent, however, that the efficacy of the puromycin inhibition would depend on the time of addition of the drug; e.g., puromycin added after the lag period (or after the formation of precursor had taken place) would not be as effective as puromycin added at the start of the experiment. These expectations have been borne out by both studies *in vivo* and *in vitro* on the incorporation of labeled amino acids into vasopressin.

Infusion of a radioactive amino acid into the third ventricle of a dog for 1.5 hours did not give rise to significant quantities of labeled hormone, whereas if the dog was permitted to survive for an additional 4.5 hours after the initial isotope infusion, considerable quantities of labeled vasopressin appeared. Furthermore, when puromycin was present from the start of the experiment, labeled hormone did not appear. If, however, puromycin was administered after the initial isotope infusion, then considerable quantities of labeled hormone were found at the end of the experiment (Sachs and Takabatake, 1964). These findings suggested that there is a lag period in vasopressin biosynthesis and that only the initial biosynthetic events in the production of hormone are puromycin sensitive. This postulate received confirmation from a series of experiments in which the release of radioactive vasopressin from some "precursor" (labeled during the initial 90 minute infusion period *in vivo*) was permitted to take place *in vitro* (Table 2). Either ^{35}S-cysteine or ^{3}H-tyrosine was infused into the third ventricle of a dog for 1.5 hours; the HME was then excised and divided in the medial plane. One half was used for the immediate isolation of vasopressin (left hand side, Table 2). The other half of the HME tissue was sliced and incubated at 37°C for 4.5 hours in a modified Krebs-Ringer buffer containing puromycin and unlabeled cysteine (or tyrosine). It can be seen (Table 2) that in each case incubation of the HME slices *in vitro* gave rise to labeled hormone under conditions which precluded *de novo* peptide bond synthesis. Furthermore, the production of radioactive hormone *in vitro* occurred only in dog HME slices which had previously been exposed to ^{35}S-cysteine or ^{3}H-tyrosine for 1.5 hours *in vivo*. Apparently, the formation of some labeled precursor took place *in vivo* during the 1.5 hour infusion period. It is also clear that whereas the initial biosynthetic events (i.e., synthesis of the precursor molecule) were inhibited by puromycin, the subsequent release (or production) of vasopressin from precursor was puromycin insensitive.

More recently Takabatake and Sachs (1964) have been able to achieve synthesis of vasopressin *de novo* by guinea pig HME tissues *in vitro*. The experimental findings *in vitro* are consistent with the isotope experiments *in vivo*. The incorporation of ^{35}S-cysteine into vasopressin *in vitro* in HME tissue taken from the guinea pig, has consistently shown a lag period

TABLE 2. PRODUCTION OF LABELED VASOPRESSIN *in vitro* BY HME SLICES TAKEN FROM DOGS WHICH WERE INFUSED WITH A RADIOACTIVE AMINO ACID FOR 1.5 HOURS PRIOR TO SACRIFICE

Exp. No.	Amino acid infused 1.5 hr *in vitro*	1/2 HME immediately after 1.5 hr infusion *in vivo**			1/2 HME, 4.5 hr incubation *in vitro**		
		Vasopressin		Protein cpm/μg	Vasopressin		Protein cpm/μg
		μg	cpm/μg		μg	cpm/μg	
1	^{35}S-cys	1.8	80	28	1.9	500	32
2	^{35}S-cys	3.0	116	123	2.3	1057	124
3	^{35}S-cys	2.9	9	44	2.8	61	25
4	^{3}H-tyr	2.4	79	33	2.7	216	27

* HME taken from dogs which were infused with either ^{35}S-cysteine (1.4×10^9 cpm, Exp. 1 and 3; 2.4×10^9 cpm, Exp. 2) or ^{3}H-tyrosine (1.4×10^9 cpm) for 1.5 hr; 1/2 HME homogenized in 10% (w/v) TCA immediately after 1.5 hr infusion *in vivo*, 1/2 HME sliced and incubated in a modifed Krebs-Ringer bicarbonate medium containing 2×10^{-4} M puromycin and either 5×10^{-3} M unlabeled cysteine (Exp. 1–3) or tyrosine (Exp. 4), respectively.

of about one hour's duration followed by the appearance of labeled hormone. Furthermore, the biosynthesis of vasopressin was completely inhibited by puromycin if the drug was present from the start of the experiment. If, however, puromycin was added after the lag period (or after the synthesis of precursor had already taken place), then it did not prevent the subsequent appearance of labeled hormone (Sachs *et al.*, 1967b).

ENZYMIC PATHWAYS OF HORMONE BIOSYNTHESIS

The presently available data regarding the nature of the enzymic steps involved in ADH and oxytocin biosynthesis are at most indirect and circumstantial. On the basis of the results of isotope studies (described in part above), Sachs and Takabatake (1964) proposed a "precursor model" for vasopressin biosynthesis (shown schematically in Fig. 1). According to this model, the biosynthesis of the peptide bonds in vasopressin would occur solely in the perikaryon, on ribosomes, via pathways common to the biosynthesis of other peptide chains (i.e., involving transfer RNA, messenger RNA, etc.). It was further proposed that the biosynthesis of vasopressin proceeds via a bound, biologically inactive form (i.e., as part of a precursor molecule) and that the appearance of the biologically active octapeptide occurs at a time and place removed from the initial biosynthetic events. Conceivably, the release of the octapeptide from the precursor molecule would take place during the formation and maturation of the NSG. The choice of the "Golgi region" for the formation of the NSG is based on the electron microscopic studies of Scharrer and Brown (1962) and Bern and Knowles (1966). The notion

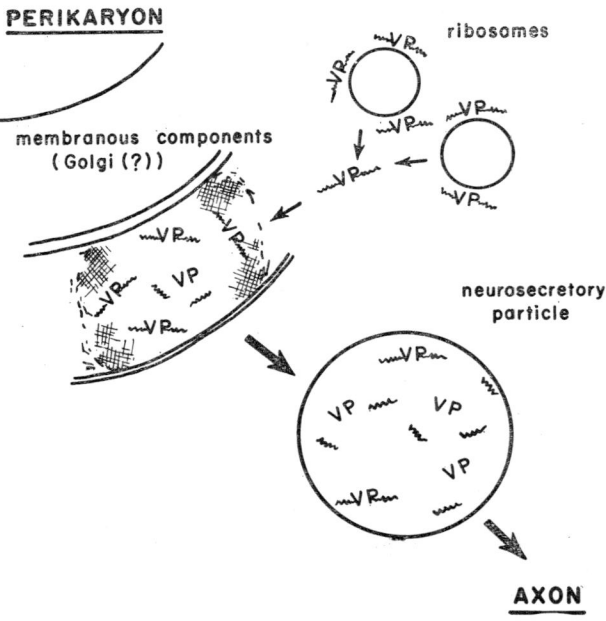

FIG. 1. A "precursor model" for vasopressin biosynthesis; (~VP~), precursor molecule containing bound, biologically inactive vasopressin; VP, biologically active octapeptide (i.e., arginine vasopressin).

that ribosomes or similar nucleic acid structures play an essential role in the initial stages of peptide bond synthesis derives from the observations that puromycin inhibits the early phase of ADH biosynthesis. Further support comes from the results of electron microscopy and chemical analysis of supraoptic neurons of rats subjected to prolonged dehydration or osmotic stimulation. Under these circumstances there are increased numbers of ribosomes and polysomes (Osinchak, 1964, Zambrano and De Robertis, 1966), increased amounts of RNA (Edström et al., 1961), and an enhanced rate of ADH biosynthesis (Takabatake and Sachs, 1964). While the overall process of ADH biosynthesis *(in vitro)* has been shown to require an energy source such as glucose, it is not known whether the energy requirement is confined entirely to the formation of the "precursor molecule". At present, there is little information regarding either the nature of the "precursor molecule" or the enzymic steps involved in the release (or production) of ADH from this "precursor". Although it is possible that the "precursor" is of small molecular weight (e.g., the $-SH$ open chain form of ADH), we are inclined to the view that a more likely candidate is a macromolecule (i.e., a protein). The formation of this molecule containing bound ADH might require a polycistronic messenger; the release of the free, biologically active hormone would conceivably involve one or more hydrolytic or ammonolytic steps. This hypothesis has a number of well-known analogies, such as the formation of angiotensin II, as well as that of enzymes involved in digestion and blood clotting. It is obvious, however, that ultimate proof of the existence of a "precursor molecule" in vasopressin biosynthesis must await its isolation and chemical characterization. Unfortunately, parallel investigations have not been carried out on oxytocin biosynthesis and virtually nothing is known about its mode of synthesis. Nevertheless, by virtue of the close similarities in chemical structure and cellular storage and release of oxytocin and ADH it would not be unreasonable to assume similar biosynthetic pathways.

SYNTHESIS OF OXYTOCIN AND VASOPRESSIN IN SEPARATE NEURONS

The available evidence, by no means conclusive, is nevertheless consistent with the view that oxytocin and vasopressin are produced, stored, and released by separate neurons. Studies on the distribution of the neurohypophysial hormones within the hypothalamus of a number of species (see Chapter 5) suggest that the neurons of the paraventricular nuclei may be especially concerned with the elaboration of oxytocin. Further support for this postulate has been obtained from studies on the effects of hypothalamic lesions. Thus in both the rat (Olivecrona, 1957) and the cat (Nibbelink, 1961), bilateral destruction of the paraventricular nuclei causes a preferential depletion of oxytocin in the pituitary. The results of ultracentrifugation of sucrose homogenates of posterior lobes have indicated that oxytocin and ADH are stored in separate NSG (Pardoe and Weatherall, 1955; Heller and Lederis, 1961; LaBella *et al.*, 1962). Recent studies by Sokol and Valtin (1967) on a strain of rats with hereditary diabetes insipidus also support the separate neuron hypothesis. This concept clearly provided the anatomical basis for the differential release of oxytocin and vasopressin observed under a variety of experimental conditions (Roberts and Share, 1966; Bisset et al., 1967).

SIMULTANEOUS BIOSYNTHESIS OF NEUROHYPOPHYSIAL HORMONES AND THEIR CARRIER PROTEINS

Oxytocin and vasopressin have been isolated from posterior pituitary extracts in the form of a noncovalently bonded hormone-protein complex (VanDyke et al., 1942). The protein moiety, termed neurophysin (or carrier protein), has now been shown to consist of several different entities, each capable of binding oxytocin and ADH to varying degrees (Ginsburg et al., 1965; Breslow and Abrash, 1966; Hope and Hollenberg, 1966). Recent studies support the concept that the neurophysins play an essential role in the storage and secretion of ADH. Thus, Ginsburg and Ireland (1966) were able to show by means of differential centrifugation of homogenates of bovine neurohypophysis that the distribution of neurophysins was similar to that of the hormones. A number of investigators (Albers and Brightman, 1959; Rennels, 1966; Friesen and Astwood, 1967) observed that prolonged dehydration led to depletion of protein and/or neurophysins as well as the neurohypophysial hormones; these results suggest the simultaneous secretion of the neurophysins and hormones. The studies of Sachs and coworkers (1967a) have demonstrated directly the release of labeled neurophysins from the neurohypophysis under circumstances which lead to the release of either one or both hormones.

Is there a synchronous and/or mutually dependent synthesis of the neurohypophysial hormones and their respective "carrier proteins"? While there is still a paucity of experimental data, the results of Friesen and Astwood (1967) and Rennels (1966) suggest an affirmative answer to this question. Their studies showed that if dehydrated rats were permitted free access to water, there occurred a repletion of neurophysins during a time period where the repletion of ADH and oxytocin was also taking place (see Moses, 1963). Of considerable interest is the finding (Friesen and Astwood, 1967) that in rats with congenital diabetes insipidus (Brattleboro strain) the concentration of neurophysins is greatly reduced; presumably the reduced quantities of neurophysins which are present in the pituitary would be associated with oxytocin. This result further supports the possibility that the biosyntheses of the neurohypophysial hormones and their respective carrier proteins are intimately related.

The development of isotope methods for the study of neurophysin biosynthesis (Fawcett and Sachs, unpublished) offers exciting prospects for future studies on this question.

THE RATES OF HORMONE BIOSYNTHESIS

The neural elements of the hypothalamo-neurohypophysial complex fulfil a number of important homeostatic and integrative functions in the intact animal (see Heller and Ginsburg, 1966). The secretory activities of these neurons are thus necessarily responsive to a variety of physiological stimuli (see Share, 1967) which may give rise to a wide range of rates of hormone secretion. As pointed out in the "Introduction", the large stores of pituitary hormones are more than sufficient to meet the needs of the organism after acute stimulation. Nevertheless, the question arises as to what extent the biosynthesis of hormone is attuned to the secretory activities of the cell. What factors are involved in the control of the rate of hormone biosynthesis?

Actual measurements (e.g., turnover studies) of the rate of either vasopressin or oxytocin biosynthesis have not been performed. Although under steady state conditions, the biosynthetic rate could be equated with the rate of secretion, precise estimates of the latter are not available. Alternatively, an estimate of the steady state (or basal) value for the rate of hormone release (and synthesis) may be calculated from measurements of the half-life time of removal of hormone from the blood, and its concentration and volume of distribution in the ECF. While there is some agreement on half-life time values, unfortunately, the estimates of the quantity of hormone in the extracellular compartment show a wide and questionable range of values (see Chapter 11).

The rate of vasopressin biosynthesis in the dog under "resting" conditions is assumed to be of the order of 1–5 mU/hr; this value is based on the work of Shannon (1942) who observed that an infusion rate of 1–5 mU ADH/hr in dogs with diabetes insipidus led to maximal antidiuresis. Estimates based on half-life time measurements give much greater values than those of Shannon (see Lauson, 1967). In the guinea-pig, a crude estimate of the capacity of hypothalamic-median eminence tissues to synthesize vasopressin *in vitro* was obtained from isotope studies (Takabatake and Sachs, 1964), and this was of the order of a few hundred microunits per hour per hypothalamus. The availability of an *in vitro* system capable of hormone biosynthesis, afforded the opportunity, however, to examine the question of whether a prolonged secretory stimulus such as dehydration leads to an enhanced synthesis of vasopressin. It has been a consistent finding that HME slices taken from guinea pigs deprived of water for 4 days incorporated 2 to 5 times more radioactivity into vasopressin than similar slices from guinea pigs with free access to water (Table 3). Analogous results have also been obtained with HME tissues of guinea pigs allowed to drink 2.0 percent sodium chloride for 10 days (exp. 4, Table 3).

TABLE 3. EFFECT OF DEHYDRATION ON THE LABELING OF VASOPRESSIN *in vitro*

Exp.*	Incuba-tion time (hr)	Control		Dehydrated	
		Vasopressin			
		cpm/μg	total cpm	cpm/μg	total cpm
1	6	17,760	3700	56,600	19,800
2	6	8200	12,500	37,000	26,400
3	4	2380	450	3400	640
4	4	4160	3255	8000	4220

* Exp. 1–3, deprived of water for 4 days; Exp. 4, "dehydrated group", consisted of guinea pigs in which 2.0% NaCl was substituted for water 10 days prior to sacrifice; all "controls" were permitted free access to water.
  Exp. 1 and 2: each flask contained hypothalamic-median eminence slices from 10 animals (either dehydrated or control guinea pigs and ^{35}S-cysteine, 5.1×10^8 cpm).
  Exp. 3 and 4: ^{3}H-tyrosine and HME slices from 8 and 10 animals per flask respectively.
  Exp. 3, 3.6×10^8 cpm per flask; Exp. 4, 1.0×10^9 cpm per flask.

What cellular mechanisms are involved in the activation of hormone biosynthesis under these circumstances? Assuming that the formation of the peptide chain constitutes the rate-limiting step and that this takes place on ribosomes, then control may be exercised at the level of either transcription, or translation, or both. Relevant to this discussion is the finding that the RNA content of the neurons of the supraoptic nuclei of rats subjected to a prolonged osmotic stimulus or dehydration is greater than that of normal rats (Edström *et al.*, 1961). Furthermore, electron micrographs of supraoptic neurons of rats subjected to chronic dehydration have shown increased numbers of ribosomes and a morphological picture indicative of enhanced activity of the protein and RNA synthesizing machinery (Osinchak, 1964, Zambrano and De Robertis, 1966). Hence, the RNA studies, the morphological observations, and the isotope experiments indicate that the chronic reception of nerve impulses effective in the release of ADH, may also be translated into an enhanced synthesis of both specific RNA molecules and entire biosynthetic units involved in polypeptide hormone biosynthesis.

What of acute stimuli? Will an intense stimulus applied over a short time interval lead to a burst of biosynthetic activity? For example, the disappearance of NSM after the application of an acute, painful stimulus (Rothballer, 1953; Barnett, 1954), and the rapid reappearance of NSM after removal of the stimulus, were taken to indicate that the neurohypophysis had discharged and resynthesized its hormonal content at a rate several orders of magnitude greater than the unstimulated rate of hormone synthesis. The studies of Moses (1963) and Daniel and Lederis (1966), however, have clearly shown that while acute stimuli lead to the loss of NSM (i.e., stainability of aggregates of NSG) and loss of osmiophilicity of the NSG, this is not synonymous with hormone depletion; and in all probability these phenomena are related to the process of secretion rather than to the biosynthetic mechanisms. Furthermore, labeling experiments carried out in the dog in our own laboratory, have thus far failed to show an enhanced uptake of ^{35}S-cysteine into vasopressin, either during or shortly after hemorrhage. Neither did electrical stimulation of HME tissues of the guinea pig enhance the incorporation of labeled amino acids into vasopressin *in vitro*. To date, there is no convincing evidence that an acute secretory stimulus leads to an immediate increase in the rate of hormone biosynthesis as in other secretory organs (e.g., the adrenal, gonads, etc.). The enhanced synthesis of vasopressin after dehydration or prolonged osmotic stress may thus be construed as an adaptive response to a set of changing environmental conditions. The nature of the cellular events which intervene between the reception of nerve impulses and enhanced RNA and hormone biosynthesis, remains a central problem in neurosecretion and neurochemistry.

In summary, an effort has been made to present some of the questions, pertinent data, and current hypotheses regarding the biosynthesis of the neurohypophysial hormones. While much of our knowledge is still rudimentary, it is clear that with the tools and information already available, we may look forward to the rapid resolution of many of the questions which have been posed.

REFERENCES

BOOKS, REVIEWS, AND MONOGRAPHS

ACHER, R. and FROMAGEOT, C. (1957). The relationship between oxytocin and vasopressin to active proteins of the posterior pituitary. *The Neurohypophysis*, pp. 39–50. Heller, H. (ed.). Butterworths, London.

BARGMANN, W. (1966) Neurosecretion. *Int. Rev. of Cytol.* **19**, pp. 183–201. Bourne, C. H. and Danielli, J. F. (eds.). Academic Press, New York.
BERN, H. and KNOWLES, F. (1966) Neurosecretion. *Neuroendocrinology*, vol. 1, pp. 139–146. Martini, L. and Ganong, W. (eds.). Academic Press, New York.
CHRIST, J. F. (1962). The early changes in the hypophysial neurosecretory fibres after coagulation. *Mem. Soc. Endocr.*, **12**: 125–142.
DE ROBERTIS, E. (1962). Ultrastructure and function in some neurosecretory systems. *Mem. Soc. Endocrin.*, **12**: 3–20.
EDSTROM, J., EICHNER, D. and SCHOR, N. (1961). Quantitative ribonucleic acid measurements in functional studies of nucleus supraopticus. *Regional Neurochemistry*, pp. 274–278. Kety, S. and Elkes, J. (eds.). Pergamon Press, New York.
HELLER, H. and GINSBURG, M. (1966). Secretion, metabolism and fate of the posterior pituitary hormones. *The Pituitary Gland*, vol. 3, pp. 330–373. Harris, G. and Donovan, B. T. (eds.). University of California Press, Berkeley.
LAUSON, H. D. (1967). Metabolism of antidiuretic hormones. *Amer. J. Med.*, **42**: 713–744.
PALAY, S. L. (1957). The fine structure of the neurohypophysis. *Ultrastructure and Cellular Chemistry of Neural Tissue*, pp. 31–44. Waelsch, H. (ed.). Hoeber-Harper, New York.
SACHS, H. (1960). Studies concerned with vasopressin biosynthesis. *Regional Neurochemistry*, pp. 264–273. Kety, S. and Elkes, J. (eds.). Pergamon Press, New York.
SACHS, H. (1966). Neurosecretion in the mammalian hypothalamo-neurohypophysial complex. *Protides of the Biological Fluids*, pp. 181–192. Peeters, H. (ed.). Elsevier, New York.
SACHS, H. (1967). Biosynthesis and release of vasopressin. *Amer. J. Med.*, **42**: 687–700.
SACHS, H., PORTANOVA, R., HALLER, E. W. and SHARE, L. (1967b). Cellular processes concerned with vasopressin biosynthesis, storage and release. *Neurosecretion* pp. 46–154. Stutinsky, F. (ed.). Strasbourg.
SCHARRER, E. and BROWN, S. (1962). Electron-microscopic studies of neurosecretory cells in Lumbricus terrestris. *Mem. Soc. Endocr.* **12**: 103–108.
SCHARRER, E. and SCHARRER, B. (1954). Hormones produced by neurosecretory cells. *Rec. Prog. Horm. Res.*, **10**: 183–240.
SHARE, L. (1967). Vasopressin, its bioassay and the physiological control of its release. *Amer. J. Med.*, **42**: 701–712.
SLOPER, J. (1966). The experimental and cytopathological investigation of neurosecretion in the hypothalamus and pituitary. *The Pituitary Gland* vol. 3, pp. 131–239. Harris, G. and Donovan, B. T. (eds.). University of California Press, Berkeley.
WEISS, P. (1961). The concept of perpetual neuronal growth and proximodistal substance convection. *Regional Neurochemistry*, pp. 220–242. Kety, S. S. and Elkes, J. (eds.). Pergamon Press, Oxford.

ORIGINAL PAPERS

ALBERS, E. and BRIGHTMAN, M. (1959). A major component of neurohypophysial tissue associated with antidiuretic activity. *J. Neurochem.*, **3**: 269–276.
BARER, R., HELLER, H. and LEDERIS, K. (1963). The isolation, identification and properties of the hormonal granules of the neurohypophysis. *Proc. Roy. Soc. (London), B*, **158**: 388–416.

BARNETT, R. J. (1954). Histochemical demonstration of disulfide groups in the neurohypophysis under normal and experimental conditions. *Endocrinology*, **55**: 484–501.

BARONDES, S. (1966). On the site of synthesis of the mitochondrial protein of nerve endings. *J. Neurochem.*, **13**: 721–727.

BHAGAVAN, N. V. (1966). The biosynthesis of gramicidin S. A restudy. *Biochemistry*, **5**: 3844–50.

BISSET, G. W., HILTON, S. M. and POISNER, A. M. (1967). Hypothalamic pathways for independent release of vasopressin and oxytocin. *Proc. Roy. Soc. (London), Ser. B*, **166**: 422–42.

BRESLOW, E. and ABRASH, L. (1966). The binding of oxytocin analogues by purified bovine neurophysins. *Proc. Nat. Acad. Sci., U.S.A.*, **56**: 640–46.

DANIEL, A. and LEDERIS, K. (1966). Effects of ether anaesthesia and hemorrhage on hormone storage and ultrastructure of the rat neurohypophysis. *J. Endocrin.*, **34**: 91–104.

FRIESEN, H. G. and ASTWOOD, E. B. (1967). Changes in neurohypophysial proteins induced by dehydration and ingestion of saline. *Endocrinology*, **80**: 278–87.

GINSBURG, M. and IRELAND, M. (1966). The role of neurophysin in the transport and release of neurohypophysial hormones. *J. Endocrin.*, **35**: 289–98.

GINSBURG, M., JAYASENA, K. and THOMAS, P. J. (1965). Subfractions from porcine neurophysin with different hormone-binding properties. *J. Physiol., Lond.*, **183**: 45P.

HELLER, H. and LEDERIS, K. (1961). Density gradient centrifugation of hormone-containing subcellular granules from rabbit neurohypophyses. *J. Physiol., Lond.*, **158**: 27–29P.

HILD, W. (1951). Experimentell-morphologische Untersuchungen über das Verhalten der "neurosekretorischen Bahn" nach Hypophysenstieldurchtrennungen, Eingriffen in den Wasserhaushalt und Belastung der Osmoregulation. *Virchows Arch. path. Anat. Physiol*, **319**: 526–46.

HILD, W. and ZETLER, G. (1953). Experimenteller Beweis für die Entstehung der sog. Hypophysenhinterlappenwirkstoffe im Hypothalamus. *Pflügers Arch. ges. Physiol.*, **257**: 169–201.

HOPE, D. B. and HOLLENBERG, M. D. (1966). Isolation of a new hormone-binding protein from the posterior lobes of bovine pituitary glands. *Biochem. J.*, **99**: 5P.

ITO, E. and STROMINGER, J. (1960). Enzymatic synthesis of the peptide in a uridine nucleotide from *Staphylococcus aureus*. *J. Biol. Chem.*, **235**: PC5.

KOENIG, E. (1967). Synthetic mechanisms in the axon. IV. *In vitro* incorporation of ^{3}H-precursors into axonal protein and RNA. *J. Neurochem.*, **14**: 437–46.

LABELLA, F., BEAULIER, G., and REIFFENSTEIN, R. (1962). Evidence for the existence of separate vasopressin and oxytocin-containing granules in the neurohypophysis. *Nature, Lond.*, **193**: 173–74.

MACH, B., RICH, E. and TATUM, E. L. (1963). Separation of the antibiotic polypeptide tyrocidine from protein synthesis. *Proc. Nat. Acad. Sci., U.S.A.*, **50**: 175–81.

MOSES, A. M., (1963). Adrenal-neurohypophysial relationships in the dehydrated rat. *Endocrinology*, **72**: 230–36.

NIBBELINK, D. W. (1961). Paraventricular nuclei, neurohypophysis and parturition. *Amer. J. Physiol.*, **200**: 1229–32.

OLIVECRONA, H. (1957). Paraventricular nucleus and pituitary gland. *Acta Physiol. Scand.*, **40**: Suppl. 136, pp. 1–178.

OSINCHAK, J. (1964). A fine structure and cytochemical study of neurosecretory cells in the rat. *Excerpta Medica Int. Congr. Ser.*, **77**: 33–4.

OTANI, S., YAMANOI, T., SAITO, Y. and OTANI, S. (1966). Fractionation of an enzyme

system responsible for gramicidin S biosynthesis. *biochem. biophys. Res. Commun.*, **25**: 590–96.
PARDOE, A. U. and WEATHERALL, M. (1955). Intracellular localisation of oxytocic and vasopressor substances in pituitary glands of rats. *J. Physiol., Lond.*, **127**: 201–212.
RENNELS, M. L. (1966). A study of proteins of the posterior pituitary of normal and dehydrated rats using disc electrophoresis. *Endocrinology*, **78**: 659–60.
ROBERTS, J., and SHARE, L. (1966). Release of oxytocin and vasopressin from guinea pig posterior pituitaries. *The Endocrine Society, 48th Meeting*, p. 36.
ROTHBALLER, A. B. (1953). Changes in the rat neurohypophysis induced with painful stimuli with particular reference to neurosecretory material. *Anat. Rec.*, **115**: 21–41.
SACHS, H. (1963a). Studies on the intracellular distribution of vasopressin. *J. Neurochem.*, **10**: 289–97.
SACHS, H. (1963b). Vasopressin biosynthesis II. Incorporation of [^{35}S] cysteine into vasopressin and protein associated with cell fractions. *J. Neurochem.*, **10**: 299–311.
SACHS, H. and TAKABATAKE, Y. (1964). Evidence for a precursor in vasopressin biosynthesis. *Endocrinology*, **75**: 943–48.
SACHS, H., FAWCETT, C. P., and HALLER, E. W. (1967a). Biosynthesis and release of neurophysin and hormonal peptides. *The Endocrine Society, 49th Meeting*, p. 77.
SHANNON, J. A. (1942). The control of the renal excretion of water. II. The rate of liberation of the posterior pituitary antidiuretic hormone in the dog. *J. Exp. Med.*, **76**: 387–99.
SLOPER, J. C. and ADAMS, C. W. M. (1956). The hypothalamic elaboration of the posterior pituitary principle in man; evidence derived from hypophysectomy. *J. Path. Bact.* **72**: 587–602.
SLOPER, J. C., ARNOTT, D. J. and KING, B. C. (1960). Sulphur metabolism in the pituitary and hypothalamus of the rat: A study of radioisotope-uptake after the injection of ^{35}S-DL-cysteine, Methionine, and sodium sulphate. *J. Endocrin.*, **20**: 9–23.
SLOPER, J. and BATESON, R. (1965). Ultrastructure of neurosecretory cells in the supraoptic nucleus of the dog and rat. *J. Endocrin.*, **31**: 139–50.
SOKOL, H. W., and VALTIN, H. (1967). Evidence for the synthesis of oxytocin and vasopressin in separate neurons. *Nature, Lond.*, **214**: 314–16.
TAKABATAKE, Y. and SACHS, H. (1964). Vasopressin biosynthesis III. *In vitro* studies. *Endocrinology*, **75**: 934–42.
VAN DYKE, H. B., CHOW, B. F., GREEP, R. O. and ROTHEN, A. J. (1942). The isolation of a protein from the pars neuralis of the ox pituitary with constant oxytocic, pressor and diuresis inhibiting effects. *J. Pharmacol. Exp. Ther.*, **74**: 190–209.
VOGT, M. (1953). Vasopressor, antidiuretic, and oxytocic activities of extracts of the dog's hypothalamus. *Brit. J. Pharmacol. Chemother.*, **8**: 193–96.
WEINSTEIN, H., MALAMED, S. and SACHS, H. (1961). Isolation of vasopressin-containing granules from the neurohypophysis of the dog. *Biochim. Biophys. Acta*, **50**: 386–89.
ZAMBRANO, D. and DE ROBERTIS, E. (1966). The secretory cycle of supraoptic neurons in the rat. *Z. Zellforsch. mikrosk. Anat.*, **73**: 414–31.

CHAPTER 7

ESTIMATION OF NEUROHYPOPHYSIAL HORMONES IN BODY FLUIDS

M. W. Smith

Agricultural Research Council Institute of Animal Physiology, Bahraham, Cambridge, England

INTRODUCTION

The original assay methods used to estimate the oxytocic, pressor and antidiuretic activities of extracts of the neurohypophysis were developed before the chemical identity of the assayed substances had been established. It followed that any substance which could either mimic or inhibit the action of oxytocin or vasopressin on the chosen assay preparation (virgin guinea pig uterus; spinal cat blood pressure, Dale and Laidlaw (1912); water-loaded rat, Burn, 1931) gave a false estimate of the potency of that particular preparation. The importance of these considerations remained more theoretical than practical so long as these assays were used to estimate the activity of neurohypophysial extracts. The high concentrations of oxytocin and vasopressin, relative to that of possible interfering substances, ensured that the error of the estimation depended only on the precision of the assay used. This consideration ceased to apply when the same assay methods were used to estimate small amounts of neurohypophysial hormones in body fluids containing large amounts of un-identified oxytocic and antidiuretic material. It was this circumstance which led first to a series of modifications to the established techniques and then to a search for more specific and sensitive assay tissues.

The purification and chemical identification of oxytocin (Pierce and du Vigneaud, 1950), vasopressin (du Vigneaud, 1956) and later vasotocin (Chauvet *et al.*, 1960b) and the synthesis of these polypeptides (du Vigneaud *et al.*, 1954; du Vigneaud, 1956; Katsoyannis and du Vigneaud, 1958) created new assay problems, for it was found that pure oxytocin had both pressor and antidiuretic activities and pure vasopressin could cause both milk-ejection and contraction of the uterus (van Dyke *et al.*, 1955). Vasotocin also had these activities, being a more potent oxytocic than vasopressin and a more powerful antidiuretic than oxytocin (Boissonnas *et al.*, 1961). To estimate one hormone in mixtures of oxytocin and vasopressin or vasotocin, allowance had to be made for the residual activities of each hormone measured on the assay tissue most specific for the other. But the gain was such that an allowance could be made with some confidence and that extraction techniques and inactivation procedures could be designed for the individual hormone under investigation. This was a great advance and it is now impossible to discuss the assay of neurohypophysial hormones in body fluids without also considering the extraction techniques used to separate these hormones from contaminating substances.

The present review emphasizes the importance of extracting oxytocin and vasopressin from body fluids before assay, and of characterizing the activities attributed to these hormones by measurement of their susceptibility to chemical and enzymic inactivators. Certain antidiuretic and milk-ejection assay methods are recommended in preference to others, and little mention is made of the absolute levels of hormones found in blood and urine, since these estimations have been notoriously unreliable in the past. Other reviews written recently from different points of view include those of van Dyke *et al.* (1955), Thorn (1958), Lauson (1960), Thorp (1962), Nielsen (1965) and Sawyer (1966).

ASSAY STANDARDS

Commercial preparations of oxytocin and vasopressin are normally standardized using the oxytocic, pressor or vasodepressor response of the rat uterus, rat blood pressure and chicken blood pressure respectively as recommended by the British Pharmacopoeia (1963) or the U. S. Pharmacopoeia (1965). Subsidiary standards are used for this purpose, assayed previously against the Third International Standard for oxytocic, vasopressor and antidiuretic substances (Bangham and Mussett, 1958). The International Standard consists of an acetone-dried powder prepared from freshly dissected bovine posterior pituitary lobes. One unit of oxytocic, vasopressor or antidiuretic activity is contained, by definition, in 0.5 mg of this powder. This standard therefore contains both oxytocin and arginine vasopressin diluted with a vast excess of unknown, but presumably pharmacologically inert, proteins. The British Pharmacopoeia (1963) describes how an equally crude preparation from ox pituitary lobes may be prepared for use as a subsidiary standard.

The pressor and antidiuretic activities of pure oxytocin are very low (Table 1, data of Boissonnas *et al.*, 1961) and the influence of oxytocin on assays for vasopressin is therefore negligible. But any estimate of oxytocin which is made using the powdered posterior pituitary lobe as standard will be affected by the vasopressin present. The extent to which arginine vasopressin interferes will depend on the assay tissue used (about 5% using the isolated rat uterus and 13% using chicken blood pressure measurements, Table 1). The overlap of activities is even greater when milk-ejection in the rabbit is used as an assay response; arginine vasopressin has 15–20% of the milk-ejecting activity of an equal weight of oxytocin (Table 1 and van Dyke et al., 1955). It is particularly ironical that the latter type of assay should be in other respects the most selective assay for oxytocin (Fitzpatrick and Walmsley, 1965) and therefore the assay of choice for the determination of oxytocin in body fluids. This difficulty can be overcome by first assaying pure oxytocin against the International Standard on the rat uterus and then using pure oxytocin as a subsidiary standard.

It might at this point be asked why pure chemical standards of oxytocin have not as yet been adopted for general use. Oxytocin can be synthesized in large amounts (Boissonnas et al., 1955) and though inactive dimers may be present (Ressler, 1958), these seem not to interfere with the biological assays used (Berde et al., 1961). The main difficulty appears to be that arginine vasopressin cannot as yet be synthesized on a commercial scale and pure preparations appear to be unstable (du Vigneaud, 1956; Heller and Lederis, 1958); lysine vasopressin is more stable than arginine vasopressin (Adamsons et al., 1958).

Pharmaceutical extracts of pituitary glands are often made from pig rather than ox pituitaries and so contain lysine rather than arginine vasopressin. The standardization of such preparations against the International Standard poses additional problems. Although lysine vasopressin is approximately equi-active with arginine vasopressin, when assayed for the initial intensity with which it inhibits water diuresis, its action is of shorter duration (Nielsen, 1958; Sawyer, 1958) and the estimated potency will therefore depend on the way in which the antidiuretic effect is measured. The result will also change with the sensitivity of the assay preparation, for the log dose–effect curves of the two vasopressins are not parallel (Berde and Cerletti, 1961). Similar but less pronounced differences can be shown when lysine vasopressin is assayed against arginine vasopressin by comparing their pressor responses in the rat (Nielsen, 1960). This problem is highlighted by the commercial production and widespread use of lysine vasopressin, but the same difficulty arises every time one of the synthetically produced peptides is assayed using oxytocin or arginine vasopressin as standard. Gross errors in potency are less likely to occur if assays are designed with consideration for the purpose to which the

TABLE 1. POTENCIES OF PURE NATURALLY OCCURRING NEUROHYPOPHYSIAL HORMONES

Name and chemical formula		
$R_2 = -CH_2-\langle\bigcirc\rangle-OH$		
H-CyS-Tyr-*Ile*-Glu(NH$_2$)-Asp(NH$_2$)-CyS-Pro-*Leu*-Gly-NH$_2$ Oxytocin	$R_3 = -\overset{CH_3}{\underset{|}{CH}}-CH_2-CH_3$	$R_8 = -CH_2-\overset{CH_3}{\underset{|}{CH}}-CH_3$
H-CyS-Tyr-*Phe*-Glu(NH$_2$)-Asp(NH$_2$)-CyS-Pro-*Lys*-Gly-NH$_2$ Lysine-vasopressin	$R_3 = -CH_2-\langle\bigcirc\rangle$	$R_8 = -CH_2-CH_2-CH_2-CH_2-NH_2$
H-CyS-Tyr-*Phe*-Glu(NH$_2$)-Asp(NH$_2$)-CyS-Pro-*Arg*-Gly-NH$_2$ Arginine-vasopressin	$R_3 = -CH_2-\langle\bigcirc\rangle$	$R_8 = -CH_2-CH_2-CH_2-NH-\overset{\overset{NH}{\|}}{C}-NH_2$
H-CyS-Tyr-*Ile*-Glu(NH$_2$)-Asp(NH$_2$)-CyS-Pro-*Arg*-Gly-NH$_2$ Arginine-vasotocin	$R_3 = -\overset{CH_3}{\underset{|}{CH}}-CH_2-CH_3$	$R_8 = -CH_2-CH_2-CH_2-NH-\overset{\overset{NH}{\|}}{C}-NH_2$

peptides are likely to be put. A clinician using one of the modified oxytocins would find the stated potency (if estimated on the blood pressure of the chicken) of no help in gauging the amount of peptide needed to induce labor. Similar considerations apply to the assay of neurohypophysial hormones in body fluids, where physiological significance is invariably attached to estimated potencies. Assays should be performed on natural target organs, preferably in the same species from which the fluid was taken, using pure chemical standards wherever this is possible. Roth (1914) proposed something similar when he suggested the use of histamine as a pure standard and the uterus as an assay tissue.

STABILITY

The stability of neurohypophysial hormones changes with the temperature, the hydrogen-ion concentration and the buffer chosen to maintain a constant pH. The stability of arginine vasopressin is also affected by its state of purity. Gaddum (1930) plotted a nomogram for oxytocin showing the amount of inactivation taking place when extracts are heated at different temperatures for different lengths of time at various hydro-

DETERMINED BY DIFFERENT METHODS OF BIO-ASSAY (FROM BOISSONNAS et al., 1961).

Oxytocin-like activities (in international units per mg)				Vasopressin-like activities (in international units per mg)			Occurs in the posterior pituitary of
rat uterus (isolated)	cat uterus (in situ)	chicken blood pressure	rabbit mammary gland	rat blood pressure	cat blood pressure	rat antidiuresis	
450±30	450±30	450±30	450±30	5±1	4±1	5±1	vertebrates
±0.5	—	40±5	60±10	270±20	306±13	~250	pig, hippopotamus
~20	—	~60	~70	~400	~400	~400	most mammals
~75	—	~150	~100	~125	—	—	non-mammalian vertebrates

gen-ion concentrations. Maximum stability was at pH 3.0–3.4 (Gaddum, 1930; Gerlough, 1930) and this was also true for vasopressin (Heller, 1939; Nielsen, 1961). The stability of oxytocin does not change when the hormone is purified (Gerlough and Bates, 1930; Adamsons et al., 1958), but arginine vasopressin becomes less stable on being purified (du Vigneaud, 1956). At pH 7.5 purified arginine vasopressin is less stable than crude arginine vasopressin or purified lysine vasopressin, but this instability is less pronounced when diethylbarbiturate is used instead of phosphate to buffer the solution (Adamsons et al., 1958). Nielsen (1961) showed also that certain buffers increased the rate of vasopressin breakdown. The optimal conditions for the storage of extracts containing neurohypophysial hormones are therefore in the cold at pH 3.0 in aqueous solution containing no buffer.

Plasma proteins bind added oxytocin and vasopressin (Heller and Lederis, 1957; Thorn and Silver, 1957). This might be responsible for an immediate drop in vasopressor activity reported by Arimura and Yamaguchi (1964), though the presence of plasma caused no loss of antidiuretic activity when assayed by the intravenous method (Heller, 1937). More serious is the long-term instability of oxytocin which can lose as much as

50% of its total activity when stored at 2° C for 40 hr in canine plasma (Adamsons et al., 1958). Vasopressin also loses activity when stored in canine plasma at 2° C and it is therefore imperative either to assay blood samples immediately after collection or to separate the hormones from plasma before storage. A particular problem arises when oxytocin estimations are to be made in the blood of lactating women, which contains an enzyme (oxytocinase) capable of destroying oxytocin. In this case blood samples, collected in pre-cooled syringes, are spun in a refrigerated centrifuge and samples stored at $-14°$ C before extraction (Fitzpatrick and Walmsley, 1965).

EXTRACTION FROM BIOLOGICAL TISSUES AND FLUIDS

Organic solvents. Various solvents can be used to separate oxytocin from vasopressin or to obtain both hormones free from interfering proteins. Melville (1937) precipitated whole blood with acidified ethanol and found antidiuretic activity in the supernatant fraction. Bisset and Walker (1954) and Bisset et al. (1956) used a similar procedure for the extraction of oxytocin from human blood. Recoveries were low and, though this was later remedied (Bisset and Lee, 1957), the method still suffered from the use of acid which has been shown to act on plasma proteins to produce oxytocic substances (Croxatto, et al., 1961). A new extraction procedure omits acid, two volumes of absolute ethanol being added to one volume of plasma to precipitate protein and extract both oxytocin and vasopressin with a 75% recovery (Bisset et al., 1967). The method can be used for very small amounts of either hormone. Oxytocin is also soluble in butan-2-ol and this solvent has been used to separate oxytocin from vasopressin by counter-current distribution (Livermore and du Vigneaud, 1949; Acher and Fromageot, 1957) and by partition chromatography (Condliffe, 1955). Vasopressin can be partitioned successfully between butan-1-ol and aqueous *p*-toluenesulfonic acid (Turner et al., 1951) and there seems every reason to suppose that butyl alcohols will extract these hormones from body fluids. Phenol has also been used to extract vasopressin from urine and blood (Jessup et al., 1961).

Oxytocin can be extracted into mixed solutions of acetic acid and acetone (Kamm et al., 1928), vasopressin and protein being left behind as an insoluble residue. The solubility of oxytocin in aqueous solutions of acetone was confirmed by Ginsburg and Smith (1958) and developed into an extraction method for oxytocin (Ginsburg and Smith, 1959; Fitzpatrick, 1961). Proteins were precipitated with ten volumes of acetone and removed by centrifugation. Acetone was later removed from the supernatant by evaporation and ether extraction. Recoveries were of the order of 80% and the method could be used to extract some of the synthetic analogues of oxytocin. Only about one-third of the vasopressin added to plasma could be recovered by this method (Smith, 1959). Acetone should not be left in contact with oxytocin for any length of time, since this can lead to the formation of acetone-oxytocin, a pharmacologically inactive complex (Yamashiro et al., 1965).

5-Hydroxytryptamine is also soluble in ethanol, butanol and acetone (Page, 1955). Blood platelets must therefore be removed from serum before solvent extraction. Specific antagonists for 5-hydroxytryptamine should be used for subsequent assays.

Dialysis and gel filtration. Early dialysis experiments were concerned to remove salts from concentrated samples of urine before assay for antidiuretic activity. Collodion and cellophane membranes were tried with variable results (Gilman and Goodman, 1937; Ham and Landis, 1942; Walker, 1939). It is now known that vasopressin added to urine (Donaldson, 1947) or plasma (Heller, 1957; Lauson, 1960) can pass through cellophane membranes on dialysis. Craig *et al.* (1964) have determined some of the factors which control the rate of dialysis for oxytocin and vasopressin. Gel filtration has now superseded membrane dialysis as one of the means by which body fluids containing neurohypophysial hormones can be desalted.

Dextran gel was introduced by Porath and Flodin (1959) to separate materials on the basis of molecular size, and one of these gels (Sephadex G25) has been used to separate oxytocin from plasma proteins (Fitzpatrick and Walmsley, 1962, 1965; Folley and Knaggs, 1965a, b). The gel was prepared in water and plasma applied directly. Development was also with water, and oxytocin was eluted, free from protein, with a 75 to 85% recovery. Columns of Sephadex in water tend to adsorb oxytocin and vasopressin slowing their elution, so that separation from salts may be incomplete (Porath and Lindner, 1961). This can be overcome by preparing the column in mixtures of acetic acid, pyridine and water (Porath and Lindner, 1961; Porath and Schally, 1962). Peptides of similar molecular size to oxytocin or vasopressin can be separated from them by preliminary filtration of the hormones attached to neurophysin (Lindner *et al.*, 1959). The complex is later disrupted with formic acid and neurophysin separated from oxytocin and vasopressin by a second filtration process. The diethylaminoethyl ether derivative of Sephadex (DEAE Sephadex) separates vasopressin from oxytocin (Porath and Lindner, 1961) and columns of dextran gel have also been used to purify both oxytocin (Yamashiro, 1964) and deamino-oxytocin (Ferrier *et al.*, 1965) by partition chromatography. The versatility of Sephadex and the mild conditions under which it may be used make this material particularly suitable for the extraction of neurohypophysial hormones from body fluids.

Neurophysin. Oxytocin and vasopressin can be extracted from the neurohypophysis in combination with a protein now called neurophysin(e) (van Dyke *et al.*, 1942). The hormone-protein complex, originally called "van Dyke protein", can be precipitated with sodium chloride (Acher *et al.*, 1958) and the bound hormones later recovered by treatment with acetic, trichloroacetic or formic acid (Acher *et al.*, 1956; Frankland *et al.*, 1966), by the addition of calcium (Smith and Thorn, 1965; Thorn, 1965; Ginsburg *et al.*, 1966) or simply by dilution (Ginsburg and Ireland, 1964). The precipitation of neurophysin-peptide complexes has been used as an important step in the extraction of neurohypophysial hormones from the pituitaries of the pollock (Heller and Pickering, 1961), the cod (Acher *et al.*, 1962) and the whale (Chauvet *et al.*, 1964). Sheep neurophysin, purified by Chauvet *et al.* (1960a), has been successfully used to extract the endogenous hormone from the pituitaries of frogs (Acher *et al.*, 1960; Acher *et al.*, 1964) and rays (Acher *et al.*, 1965). Takabatake and Sachs (1964) adsorbed vasopressin onto beef neurophysin at a late stage of purification to remove it from contaminants and Portanova and Sachs (1967) have now chemically linked beef neurophysin to cellulose, using this complex to purify radioactive vasopressin. Oxytocin is also bound to cellulose-neurophysin and this material could well prove valuable in the selective extraction of these hormones from body fluids.

Ion-exchange chromatography. Both oxytocin and vasopressin are removed by columns of cation-exchange resin (Amberlite IRC-50 XE64) or carboxymethyl cellulose (CM-cellulose) prepared in the acid form. The hormones can later be recovered by elution with increasing gradients of pH and ionic strength. Columns of IRC-50 have been used with phosphate or ammonium acetate buffers to purify vasopressin (Taylor, 1954; Sakota *et al.*, 1955), to separate oxytocin from vasopressin (Acher *et al.*, 1958) and to isolate neurohypophysial hormones from many different species (see the review by Acher, 1966). CM-cellulose can be used in a similar fashion for the purification and separation of oxytocin and vasopressin (Ward and Guillemin, 1957; Schally *et al.*, 1959) and for the identification of neurohypophysial hormones (Munsick, 1966). This type of chromatography can be used to prepare large quantities of highly purified hormones (Schally *et al.*, 1964) and to extract small amounts of hormone from biological fluids (Weinstein *et al.*, 1960; Share, 1961; Ruch, 1967).

To extract vasopressin from whole blood, proteins are first precipitated with two volumes of 15% trichloroacetic acid, the supernatant is extracted with ether and the aqueous extract passed through a small column of IRC-50 XE64 resin at pH 4.5. Vasopressin is eluted with a mixture of pyridine and acetic acid and the extract later evaporated to dryness in the presence of cystine (Weinstein *et al.*, 1960). Sixty per cent of vasopressin added to whole blood is recovered by this method. Share (1961) has slightly modified this procedure for use with smaller volumes of blood and Yoshida *et al.* (1963) have used 50% acetic acid, instead of 30% pyridine +4% acetic acid, to elute vasopressin. Cystine was omitted and the final recovery of vasopressin was about 75% of the amount added to plasma. The method becomes extremely simple when applied to urine samples, where the trichloroacetic acid and ether extraction steps are not needed. Filtered urine at pH 4.0−4.5 is passed through columns of Zeo-Carb 226 (Orr and Snaith, 1959) or IRC-50 XE64 (Ruch, 1967) and elution is with acid–ethanol or 50% acetic acid. The recovery is of the order of 80% using either of these resins. Oxytocin is also removed by these columns at a pH of 4.5 (Ruch, 1967).

Paper chromatography and electrophoresis. The technique of paper chromatography has proved most valuable for the removal of substances which might affect assay tissues and also for the identification of neurohypophysial hormones. Vogt (1954) used paper chromatography to separate sympathomimetic amines from oxytocin and von Schlichtegroll (1954) separated the two hormones in a butanol–acetic acid mixture. Heller and Lederis (1958) used a 5:1:4 mixture of n-butanol, acetic acid and water to separate several naturally occuring and synthetic hormones. They stained very small amounts of these hormones using a procedure devised by Reindel and Hoppe (1954). The proportion of butanol to acetic acid has been changed by some workers (Munsick *et al.*, 1960) and descending chromatography has been used as well as the ascending technique (Lederis, 1961). Several different solvent systems have been recently developed to characterize unknown pituitary peptides (Heller and Pickering, 1961; Follett and Heller, 1964) and thin layer chromatography has been used to separate arginine vasopressin from lysine vasopressin (Ferguson, 1965).

The original technique of Heller and Lederis successfully separated neurohypophysial hormones from each other and from other pharmacologically active substances, which might otherwise have interfered with assays for these hormones, but the recoveries were generally low and variable (Lederis, 1961; Fitzpatrick and Walmsley, 1965). The recovery of vasopressin and oxytocin in good yield after separation by glass-paper chromatography has been reported by Arimura and Dingman (1959). Minute amounts of the hormones are said to be separated in two solvent systems (butanol:ethanol:ammonium hydroxide—60:30:10 for vasopressin and n-amyl alcohol:acetic acid—80:5 saturated with water, for oxytocin). The time taken to develop these chromatograms is much shorter than for filter paper chromatography.

Paper electrophoresis has been used to separate oxytocin from vasopressin (Acher et al., 1956) and from substances which interfere with its assay on the rat mammary gland (Brovetto et al., 1967). When vasopressin is oxidized with performic acid it behaves as a neutral compound on electrophoresis at pH 6.5 and this has been used for its partial identification (Sachs, 1960).

Adsorption. Both activated charcoal and zinc ferrocyanide have been used to remove vasopressin from urine by adsorption. Grollman and Woods (1949) added activated charcoal to urine at pH 4.5–5.0, discarded the supernatant and recovered the antidiuretic activity in glacial acetic acid. The active material was precipitated from this solution with a mixture of ether and ethanol. Less than 10% of added vasopressin could be recovered by Jessup et al. (1956) when they tried to use this method and they therefore advocated the use of zinc ferrocyanide as originally suggested by Noble et al. (1939). Zinc sulphate (2 N) is added to urine at pH 5.0 (1 ml/100 ml urine) and 2.25 N potassium ferrocyanide is then added dropwise with stirring to produce a white precipitate which includes the adsorbed vasopressin. Elution is with 1% ammonia in 8% ethanol after which the solution is evaporated at 50° C. Further impurities may be removed by a second precipitation of inactive material with ethanol. Recoveries of added vasopressin are reported to be about 80%. Mayer (1960) has used this method successfully to demonstrate the presence of antidiuretic hormone in human urine, but extraction on ion-exchange columns would appear to be more specific for vasopressin and less time-consuming in operation.

ANTIDIURETIC ASSAYS

EARLY ASSAYS AND THEIR LIMITATIONS

The antidiuretic assay for vasopressin has a long history as one of the most sensitive and most easily abused methods available for the detection of this hormone in body fluids. Some of the early methods, summarized by Heller and Blackmore (1952), are given in Table 2. Those performed on conscious animals are liable to interference from endogenous vasopressin released in response to emotional stress (Rydin and Verney, 1938), a release which can be induced in dogs with the mildest of sensory stimuli (Theobald, 1934). Such interference will be at a minimum when thoroughly trained dogs are used (van Dyke et al., 1955), but it is likely to be a major complicating factor when the injection of extracts is accompanied by pain. This was one reason why the subcutaneous and intraperitoneal routes for injection in rats (Burn, 1931; Ginsburg, 1951; Birnie et al., 1950; Stein et al., 1952) were generally replaced by intravenous assays (Ginsburg and Heller, 1953a). A few workers however continued to develop methods relying on the subcutaneous or intraperitoneal injection of extracts (Crawford and Pinkham, 1954; McCreary et al., 1957; Rabasa and Bergmann, 1957). There were other reasons for preferring intravenous assays. The potencies of extracts were found to depend on the route of injection (Ames and van Dyke, 1952; Lewis, 1953) and discrepancies were aggravated by the presence of other substances which apparently retarded the absorption of vasopressin (Noble et al., 1939; Noble and Taylor, 1953). 5-Hydroxytryptamine produced a greater antidiuresis when given by intraperitoneal injection (Erspamer and Ottolenghi, 1950), though this again might have been the consequence of the pain this substance produced (Page, 1954). Antidiuretic assays in unanesthetized mice are subject to the same limitations as those performed with rats and though more sensitive to vasopressin (Heller and Blackmore, 1952), have the additional disadvantage that only small volumes can be injected at any one time.

The only assays to emerge relatively unscathed from these criticisms are those performed on the diabetes insipidus dog (Hare et al., 1945; van Dyke et al., 1955) and the ethanol-anesthetized rat (Jeffers et al., 1942). But in both these cases the water load changes throughout the assay and this may (Hart and Verney, 1934; Pickford, 1936) or may not (Ginsburg and Heller, 1953a; Gauer and Tata, 1966) change the sensitivity to vasopressin. These various difficulties have now been largely overcome, but they have been emphasized here to illustrate why so many of the values quoted for the concentration of vasopressin in biological fluids were erroneously high. It is no coincidence that the reported levels for circulating vasopressin, measured under different physiological conditions, have fallen steadily as the techniques for antidiuretic assay have improved.

TABLE 2. EARLY ASSAY METHODS FOR POSTERIOR PITUITARY

Test animal	Mode of administration	Water load
Dog (normal)	s.c.	200 ml./animal, by mouth
	i.v.	Twice 250 ml./animal, by mouth
Dog (with diab. insipidus)	i.v.	100 ml./animal, by mouth
Rabbit	i.v.	100 ml. as priming dose, then 50 ml./kg., by mouth
	i.v.	25 ml. of 20% glucose and 50 ml. saline/animal i.v.
Rat	s.c.	5 ml./100 g. by mouth,
	i.p.	3 times 3 ml./100 sq. cm. body surface at hourly intervals
	s.c.	3 times 5 ml./100 g. body weight at hourly intervals
	i.p.	2.5 ml./100 g., by mouth as priming dose, followed by 5.0 ml./100g.
	i.v.	5 ml. of 12% alcohol/100 g., by mouth followed by 3 ml. water /100 g.
Mouse	s.c.	1 ml./animal i.p.
	s.c.	1 ml./animal i.p.
	i.p.	5 ml./100 g. body weight i.p.

ANTIDIURETIC ACTIVITY (FROM HELLER AND BLACKMORE, 1952).

Experimental conditions	Sensitivity	Authors
Unanesthetized, bladder fistula	Not established	Kestranek, Molitor and Pick [1925]
Unanesthetized perineotomized bitches	0.25–0.5 mU./animal	Theobald [1934]; Samaan [1935]
Unanesthetized catheterized bitches	0.2–0.3 mU./animal	Hare, Melville, Chambers and Hare [1945]
Anesthetized, 1 ml. paraldehyde/kg.	0.5 mU./animal	Walker [1939]
Anesthetized, 3 mg. morphine sulphate and 1.56 g. urethane/kg.	0.2–0.3 mU./animal	Fugo and Aragon [1947]; Lindquist and Rowe [1949]
Unanesthetized	2–3 mU./100 g.	Burn [1931]
Unanesthetized	Not established	Birnie, Jenkins, Eversole and Gaunt [1949]
Unanesthetized	0.4 mU./100 g.	Ginsburg [1951]
Unanesthetized	0.5–1 mU./100 g.	Ham and Landis [1942]
Alcohol anesthesia, cannula in vein and bladder	0.02–0.03 mU./animal	Jeffers, Livezey and Austin [1942]
Unanesthetized	Not established	Gibbs [1930]
Unanesthetized	40 mU./animal	Glaubach and Molitor [1932]
Unanethetized	20 mU./10 g.	Nelson and Woods [1934]

ASSAYS ON THE ETHANOL-ANESTHETIZED RAT

The distinction between early and recent assays is an arbitrary one, made here because of the current widespread use of the ethanol-anesthetized rat for the assay of antidiuretic activity. Dicker (1953) made a significant advance in assay design by developing an automatic apparatus for maintaining a constant level of hydration throughout an assay (Boura and Dicker, 1953). This did not increase the sensitivity of the method (both Dicker (1953) and Jeffers *et al.* (1942) needed 20μU of vasopressin to produce a significant antidiuresis) but it did increase the stability of the preparation, which allowed the rat to be used for longer periods of time. Modifications have been made recently, both in the design of apparatus and in the treatment of rats and these will be dealt with separately. The basic technique described here takes into account the work of Dettelbach (1958), Bisset (1962) and Pliška and Rychlík (1967) as well as that of Dicker (1953).

Method. Female rats weighing 200–250 g are deprived of food but not water for 12–18 hr preceding the assay (male rats which had eaten were used by Bisset, 1962). Dettelbach (1958) has stressed the value of spayed animals and of giving increasing water loads for several days before assay. Anesthesia is induced with 50–70 ml/kg of 10–15% (v/v) ethanol given by stomach tube as a single or divided dose. Rats showing a poor diuresis should be rejected at this stage. Additional ethanol loads are given (30–50 ml/kg, 2% (v/v) ethanol) 30 to 45 min after the first dose. Inactin (sodium ethyl-(1-methylpropyl)-thiobarbitone) may also be injected intraperitoneally to complete induction of anesthesia (Thorn *et al.*, 1965). A femoral or external jugular vein is then cannulated and the bladder catheterized through the urethra or a cannula tied into the bladder and the urethra ligated. Dead space can be reduced by tying off part of the bladder. A piece of fine polythene tubing is passed into the stomach by mouth and the level of hydration finally adjusted to 60–80 ml/kg by the oral injection of 1–2% (v/v) ethanol. The rat can then be connected to an assay apparatus similar to the one used by Pliška and Rychlík (Fig. 1). The conductivity of urine is monitored (5) as it passes towards a vacuum drop divider (8). The small droplets of urine produced by this divider are then counted (10) after amplification (9) and printed out at one minute intervals (11). As the rat loses urine the balance pan on which it rests tilts, so operating a contact through a relay to switch on a micropump (3). Hydrating solution (1–2% (v/v) ethanol in a water:saline mixture (95/5)) is then pumped into the rat's stomach to restore the balance, so that the

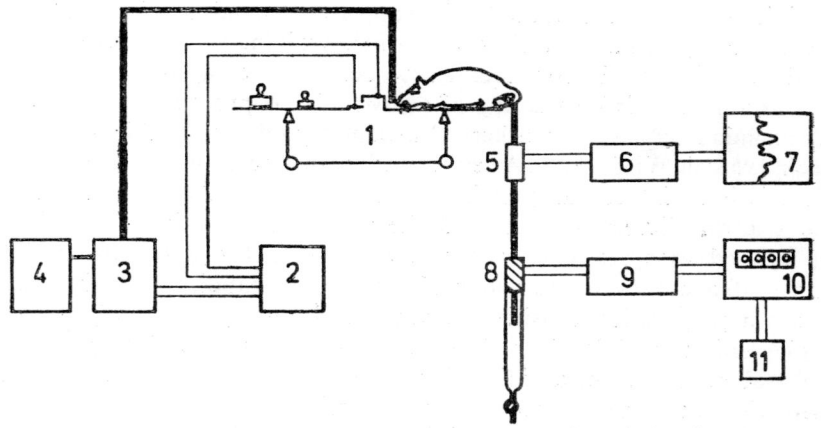

Fig. 1. Apparatus used for the antidiuretic assay of vasopressin on an ethanol-anesthetized rat. 1, Balance pan with experimental animal. 2, electromagnetic relay. 3, laboratory micropump. 4, stock of hydrating solution. 5, conductivity cell. 6, amplifier. 7, pen recorder. 8, drop divider. 9, amplifier. 10, impulse counter. 11, time relay. (From Pliška and Rychlík, 1967.)

weight of the rat never varies by more than ± 0.3 g. Volume measurements are used to express antidiuretic potencies. High and low doses of test and standard solutions should be given. The preparation responds to 5–100 μU of vasopressin.

Modifications to the apparatus. Boura and Dicker (1953) and Bisset (1962) designed their apparatus so that the collected urine should displace a second liquid of constant composition, drops of this second liquid being counted to record urine flow. This avoided changes in drop size due to changes in surface tension. In practice the surface tension of urine only changes by about 2 dyne cm^{-1} during an assay, which gives an error of about 1.5% (Pliška and Rychlík, 1967), negligible in comparison with the total error of the assay. The falling drop of urine has been used to control the flow of hydrating solution into the rat by making a momentary contact between two electrodes (de Wied, 1960), by passing a photocell (Tata and Gauer, 1966) or by displacement of a sensitive balance arm (Dyball et al., 1966). The replacement of fluid may be by the intravenous route (Clarke et al., 1955; Moran and Miltenberger, 1963; Czaczkes et al., 1964; Tata and Gauer, 1966).

Techniques devised to produce ultrasensitive preparations for the assay of vasopressin. The ability to detect small changes in urine flow following the injection of minute amounts of vasopressin, depends to a large extent on the constancy of the control flow of urine. Training rats to accept a water load by stomach tube for several days before the assay helps to produce a constant diuresis on the day of assay and this procedure has been recommended by several workers (Blackmore and Chester, 1956; Dettelbach, 1958; de Wied, 1960). A new way of producing a constant background diuresis is to infuse vasopressin at a rate of 0.5 μU/min. This reduces the control diuresis by half and the preparation retains its sensitivity to injected vasopressin (Forsling et al., 1967). The automatic maintenance of a constant water load also tends to stabilize diuresis and so create a preparation sensitive to vasopressin (10 μU—de Wied, 1960; 5 μU—Pliška and Rychlík, 1967; 2μU—Dettelbach, 1958; 1μU—Tata and Gauer, 1966). The antidiuretic assay loses much of its precision when used with such small amounts of vasopressin and two to three times the stated threshold dose has to be injected for a valid assay.

Rats have been reported to respond to as little as 1.25 μU of vasopressin if the bladder is exteriorized several days beforehand (J. Heller and Štulc, 1959). A description of the operative procedure has been given by J. Heller (1960). Czaczkes et al. (1964) confirmed this high sensitivity, showing graded effects with 0.5 to 5 μU of vasopressin with pre-operated rats whose level of hydration was maintained by intravenous infusion. Jones and Lee (1965) and Vierling et al. (1967) reported that exteriorization of the bladder had little or no effect on the subsequent sensitivity of the rat to vasopressin. Small changes in technique might be responsible for this discrepancy.

Rats with hereditary diabetes insipidus, "the Brattleboro strain", first reported by Valtin and Schroeder (1964), have recently been tested for their sensitivity to vasopressin. These rats cannot secrete vasopressin (Valtin et al., 1965) and they are reported to be twice as sensitive to vasopressin when compared with normal rats (Vierling et al., 1967; Sawyer and Valtin, 1967). This increased sensitivity has been confirmed by Jones and Lee (1967).

Choice of an assay parameter. Changes in urine osmolality have been used to estimate the potency of vasopressin solutions (Thorn et al., 1965; Thorn and Smith, 1965), and Thorn (1958) has given reasons why this response should be considered the most specific one for vasopressin. Freezing point determinations (Crawford and Pinkham, 1954), creatinine urine/plasma ratios (Hare et al., 1941) and density changes (Thorn, 1957; Baratz and Ingraham, 1959) have also been used as measures of urine water concentration. A variable amount of ethanol in the urine will complicate interpretation of these physicochemical determinations. Dyball et al. (1966) used changes in the weight of urine collected per unit time as a measure of antidiuretic activity.

The conductivity of urine is also a function of the total salt concentration and changes in this response have been used to assay vasopressin. Sawyer (1958) found conductivity measurements more variable than direct measurements of urine flow but Share (1961) concluded, after a careful comparison of both methods, that conductivity could be used as a valid assay parameter. Yoshida et al. (1963) showed a steep regression when changes in conductivity were plotted against the log dose of vasopressin and Pliška and Rychlík (1967) found that the method gave results indistinguishable from those involving direct measurements of urine flow.

Changes in the excretion of sodium and chloride ions have been used to estimate the potency of vasopressin (Anselmino et al., 1932; Ham and Landis, 1942; Ralli et al., 1950), but these changes are far too variable to be used in this way (see Pickford, 1966).

Until quite recently it was considered good assay practice to estimate the potency of vasopressin from the *maximum* effect it produced, ignoring the time taken for diuresis to return to normal. But arginine vasopressin produces a longer lasting effect than lysine vasopressin when both are given in amounts which cause the same initial effect (Sawyer, 1958; Nielsen, 1958). Some synthetic analogues of oxytocin also produce longer lasting antidiuretic effects when compared with synthetic oxytocin (Beránková-Ksandrova et al., 1966). In this situation it is obvious that potencies should be calculated from the *total* effect. This parameter can be readily obtained by including a suitable integrator in the assay apparatus. The problem of choosing which assay parameter to use in relation to the assay standard has been discussed previously.

Limitations. The rat antidiuretic assay shows great specificity for vasopressin and this, together with its high sensitivity, makes it the assay of choice when estimating vasopressin in body fluids. Several kinins will also inhibit diuresis but in larger amounts than are needed to alter the blood pressure (Bisset and Lewis, 1962). Sympathomimetic amines also produce an antidiuresis, but this response is of much shorter duration than that caused by vasopressin so that they are easily distinguished (O'Connor and Verney, 1946). There is, however, considerable individual variation in the sensitivity of the rat to vasopressin (Jones and Lee, 1967; Tata and Gauer, 1966) and seasonal variation has also been reported (Heller et al., 1957). Although ethanol is known to suppress the release of antidiuretic hormone (van Dyke and Ames, 1951; Kleeman et al., 1955), this inhibition can be overcome by both pain and hemorrhage (Tata and Buzalkov, 1966; Jones and Lee, 1967). The use of rats with diabetes insipidus overcomes problems of endogenous release but these rats are more difficult to anesthetize with ethanol, they have an enlarged urinary bladder and they show as big an individual variation in their sensitivity to vasopressin as do normal rats (Sawyer and Valtin, 1967; Jones and Lee, 1967). Prolonged overhydration is reported to decrease the sensitivity of the kidney to vasopressin in dogs (Levinsky *et al.*, 1959) and man (Jaenike and Waterhouse, 1961) and if the same applies to rats, then the water loading for several days before assay, recommended as a way to stabilize urine flow, may actually reduce the absolute sensitivity to vasopressin. Some compromise may be called for to balance these opposite effects.

OTHER ANTIDIURETIC ASSAYS

The dog has been used as its own assay animal to estimate the amount of hormone released by emotional (O'Connor, 1945; O'Connor and Verney, 1942), electrical (Fang *et al.*, 1962) and suckling stimuli (Kalliala *et al.*, 1952; Pickford, 1960), but these have been only semiquantitative. The error of the dog assay remains large even when enough material is available to design a four-point assay (van Dyke *et al.*, 1955; Munsick *et al.*, 1960). Andersson and Persson (1958) have suggested that the goat might replace the dog as an assay animal, since it is less likely to release endogenous hormone. Vasopressin has to be given to the goat in doses ranging from 2 to 6 mU to produce graded responses. The antidiuretic effect of vasotocin has been measured in the hen (Skadhauge, 1964), using intravenous hydration with a sodium chloride–glucose mixture containing sodium bicarbonate to increase the solubility of uric acid. The preparation is not easy to use but has been quoted as an assay method by Munsick *et al.* (1960).

VASOPRESSOR ASSAYS

General. Dale and Laidlaw (1912) originally standardized pituitary extracts by comparing their pressor effects with those of a standard preparation using the spinal cat. They found a developing tolerance to the repeated injection of extracts and poor discrimination between different doses and concluded that the guinea pig uterus was a more suitable assay tissue. Hogben *et al.* (1924) suggested lengthening the dose interval to avoid tachyphylaxis. The anesthetized dog on the other hand could distinguish between doses which differed by only 10% without loss of sensitivity

(Hamilton and Rowe, 1916). The dog was used successfully by Kamm et al. (1928) with chloretone in 40% ethanol as an anesthetic. Deep anesthesia was relied upon to eliminate reflex changes in the basal blood pressure. Rats were first used as assay animals by Landgrebe et al. (1946). Anesthesia was induced with a mixture of monoethyl urea, urethane and diallyl barbituric acid; vagi and associated sympathetics were cut and the lower part of the spinal cord destroyed. The basal blood pressure was more stable if sodium pentobarbital was injected and the animal respired artificially. Dekanski (1952) simplified the method by giving dibenamine (N:N-dibenzyl-β-chloroethylamine) intravenously to produce a constant low blood pressure. He used high and low doses of test and standard solutions, analysed the sources of variation in the assay, and found the approximate fiducial limits to be $\pm 5\%$ at $P=0.05$. It is his method with only slight modifications which is described below.

Method. A male rat, 250–300 g, is anesthetized by the intraperitoneal injection of a 25% (w/v) solution of urethane (5–8 ml/kg). After production of surgical anesthesia, which takes about 15 min, polythene cannulae are inserted into a femoral vein, carotid artery and the trachea. Heparin dissolved in physiological saline is injected intravenously as anticoagulant (2,000 U/kg) and the carotid cannula then connected to a sensitive mercury manometer (Condon, 1951). Dibenamine is injected intravenously (1 mg/kg) to produce a marked fall in the resting blood pressure by blockade of the α receptors to sympathomimetic amines. The injection is repeated 10 min later to ensure that inhibition is complete. Solutions for assay can then be injected in random order at intervals of 3 to 5 min. Each injection of vasopressin is immediately followed by one of saline, the total volume injected at any one time being kept constant and not more than 0.4 ml. Results are calculated from standard statistical methods as outlined in the British Pharmacopoeia (1963).

Modifications. Bisset (1962) injected atropine intraperitoneally, 1mg/kg, at the time of operation to prevent secretions into the trachea and to avoid acetylcholine-dependent changes in blood pressure. Sawyer (1966) recommends the use of high doses of atropine, 300 mg/kg, given by subcutaneous injection to ensure that the blocking effects are long-lasting. Urethane has also been given by the subcutaneous route (Dekanski, 1952; British Pharmacopoeia, 1963) but intraperitoneal injection is to be preferred because of the shorter time needed to induce anesthesia. The use of a non-volatile anesthetic can be avoided altogether by using pithed rats prepared as described by Muscholl and Vogt (1957). The sensitivity of pithed rats to vasopressin is said to be 10 times that of the urethane-anesthetized rat (Chaudhury and Joplin, 1960). This has been confirmed by Sawyer (1966) who reported graded responses to 0.4 and 0.8 mU vasopressin. Other adrenergic blocking drugs which have been used instead of dibenamine include pentolinium tartrate (Bisset, 1962), hexamethonium tartrate (British Pharmacopoeia, 1963) and phenoxybenzamine hydrochloride, given 18 hr before the assay (U. S. Pharmacopoeia, 1965).

Limitations. The pressor assay is refreshingly free from many of the disadvantages associated with other biological assays for neurohypophysial hormones. The blood pressure is extremely sensitive to acetylcholine and the sympathomimetic amines, but the availability of selective blocking agents reduces the danger of interference from these substances. Kinins also affect the blood pressure and in smaller amounts than are needed to inhibit diuresis (Bisset and Lewis, 1962). Interference from this source has probably occurred in the past (Jones and Schlapp, 1936), but this can be avoided by collecting urine or blood samples in siliconized containers, avoiding direct contact with glass or acid. It has been reported that vasopressin added to human or canine serum has a reduced activity when assayed by the rat pressor method (Arimura and Yamaguchi, 1964). Vasopressin slowly loses activity when left in contact with canine plasma for a period of days (Adamsons *et al.*, 1958) and it is an obvious precaution, either to assay solutions in plasma immediately after collection, or to extract the hormone before assay. The pressor assay using the pithed rat is still at least 10 times less sensitive than the antidiuretic assay but, if enough material can be made available, the pressor assay is recommended for its greater precision and ease of operation.

MILK-EJECTION ASSAYS

General. The discovery that an extract of posterior pituitary gland, injected intravenously into a lactating goat, increases the flow of milk from a cannulated teat (Ott and Scott, 1910) was quickly confirmed for a number of different species (Mackenzie, 1911; Schäfer and Mackenzie, 1911; Schäfer, 1913; Maxwell and Rothera, 1915 and Gaines, 1915). But the parallel discovery, that graded effects could be produced by injecting different amounts of extract (Ott and Scott, 1912) remained unexploited for the next thirty years. Turner and Cooper (1941) in the unanesthetized rabbit and Petersen (1942) using the perfused mammary gland of the cow, estimated, in a semi-quantitative way, the effects of impure preparations of oxytocin (Pitocin) and vasopressin (Pitressin), reporting that

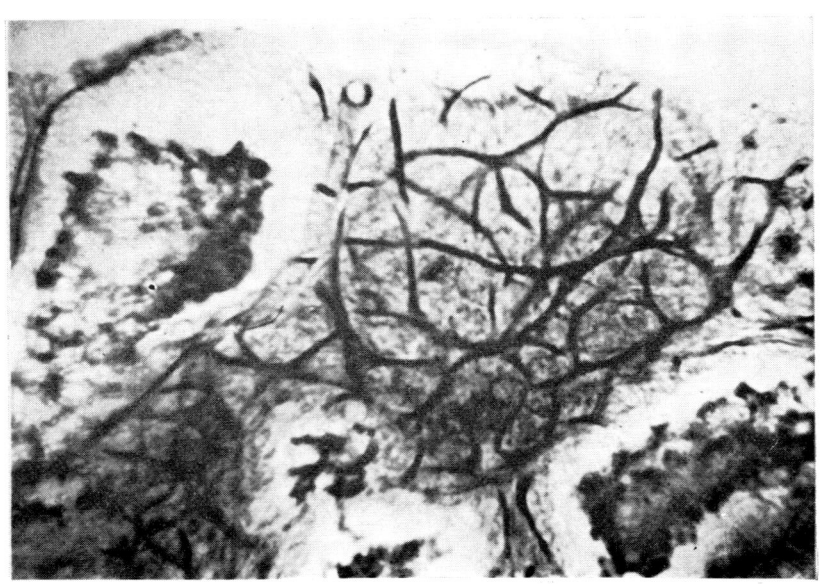

FIG. 2. Lactating mammary gland of a cat stained with silver by the method of Romanes (1950) and toned with gold chloride to show the myoepithelal cells surrounding an alveolus. Section thickness 25μ. (Courtesy of Dr. J. L. Linzell.)

oxytocin was the major factor responsible for the ejection of milk. At the same time it was realized that the oxytocin content of neurohypophysial extracts could not wholly account for the total activity, neither could the oxytocin contaminant of the vasopressin preparation explain the milk-ejecting potency of Pitressin (Cross and Harris, 1952). The problem was solved when it was discovered that highly purified vasopressin had an intrinsic milk-ejection action, about one-fifth that of oxytocin (Whittlestone, 1952; Cross and van Dyke, 1953). Many of the extraction techniques used to separate neurohypophysial hormones from body fluids do not distinguish between oxytocin and vasopressin. In these cases an additional assay must be carried out to determine the content of vasopressin (an antidiuretic assay on the ethanol-anesthetized rat would be acceptable), so that the total milk-ejecting activity of the extract can be corrected for the vasopressin present.

Before describing milk-ejection assays in detail, it is worth considering how oxytocin produces its milk-ejecting effect. An early contention (Maxwell and Rothera, 1915), disproved by Schäfer (1915), was that neurohypophysial extracts promoted the secretion rather than the expulsion of milk. Although it was later accepted that oxytocin was acting by contracting muscular structures, their identification was left in doubt for many years. The widespread distribution of myoepithelial cells around alveoli, first reported in by Richardson (1949), was extended and confirmed in other species by Linzell (1952). The typical basket-like arrangement of these cells, taken from the mammary gland of a lactating cat, is shown in Fig. 2 (Linzell, unpublished work). The anatomical distribution of these cells makes them peculiarly suited to contract alveoli. The contraction of alveoli can actually be seen after the topical application of minute amounts of oxytocin (Linzell, 1955) and since these myoepithelial cells are the only obvious contractile elements surrounding alveoli, it seems certain that these are the structures sensitive to oxytocin. Myoepithelial cells are also associated with the collecting ducts and contraction here would tend to shorten and widen individual ducts (Linzell, 1955). The mammary gland has a very few smooth muscle fibers, mostly situated close to blood vessels (Richardson, 1949) and it has been suggested that contraction of these fibers might explain the relative non-selectivity of mammary tissue used *in vitro* (van Dongen and Marshall, 1967).

INTRAVENOUS ASSAYS

It is generally agreed that oxytocin in a concentration of about $1\mu U/ml$ plasma causes milk-ejection (Cowie and Folley, 1961) but the amount of oxytocin needed to produce this concentration depends on the total blood volume of the animal. Small animals have therefore been chosen in order to develop assays specially sensitive to the milk-ejecting effect of oxytocin. The original rabbit preparation of Cross and van Dyke (1953) gave a small response to the intravenous injection of 0.5 mU oxytocin and this sensitivity has since been confirmed by several workers (van Dyke *et al.*, 1955; Berde and Cerletti, 1957; Hawker and Robertson, 1958). Four to twenty times this amount has to be injected to produce graded effects suitable for assay (Fitzpatrick, 1961). Anesthesia must be deep enough to stop the liberation of sympathomimetic amines and yet the myoepithelium loses its sensitivity to oxytocin if deprived of oxygen for any length of time (van Dyke *et al.*, 1955). It has been suggested that changes in oxygen tension affect capillary flow in mammary tissue and that this is the reason for the loss of sensitivity to oxytocin (Cross and Silver, 1961). The general procedure has been to induce anesthesia with urethane (1.25 g/kg, subcutaneous injection), to supplement this with sodium pentobarbital (10–20 mg/kg, intravenous injection) and to respire the animal artificially. Ether has been used as an initial anesthetic (Cross and Harris, 1952), but this is to be discouraged because of its ability to stimulate the neurohypophysis (Ginsburg and Heller, 1953b). One of the ducts in the rabbit nipple is cannulated, the cannula filled with 1% (w/v) sodium citrate and pressure changes then recorded with a pressure transducer. Solutions to be assayed are injected into an ear vein. The method is described in greater detail by van Dyke *et al.* (1955). Intravenous assays have also been performed on the atropinized guinea pig (Tindal and Yokoyama, 1962), in which the injection of 0.1 mU into the jugular vein produces a threshold effect and 0.3 to 1.2 mU give graded effects suitable for assay purposes. This range of sensitivity has been confirmed by Walmsley (1963). Intra-arterial assays for oxytocin are now replacing intravenous assays because of their greater sensitivity.

INTRA-ARTERIAL ASSAYS

The posterior mammary glands of the rabbit are supplied by the subcutaneous abdominal and the prepubic arteries and of these the subcutaneous abdominal artery provides the major blood supply. Retrograde injections made into the femoral artery with branches tied off, are taken straight to the ipsilateral mammary gland. This preparation responds to 100 μU oxytocin (Fitzpatrick, 1961; Gonzalez-Panizza *et al.*, 1961). Tindal and Yokoyama (1960) reported that the guinea pig can be used in a similar way to detect as little as 10 μU of oxytocin.

Fitzpatrick and Walmsley (1962) also found the guinea pig suitable for the assay of small amounts of oxytocin. The description of this method is drawn from the papers of Tindal and Yokoyama (1962), Walmsley (1963) and Folley and Knaggs (1965).

Method. A deficiency of vitamin C or E is reported to diminish the sensitivity of the myoepithelium to oxytocin and care must be taken to feed a balanced diet up to the time of assay. Primiparous guinea pigs, 2 to 4 days *post partum*, are kept apart from their litters overnight. Anesthesia is produced on the day of assay by the intraperitoneal injection of sodium pentobarbital, 50 mg/kg. Atropine sulphate is injected subcutaneously (1 mg/animal) or intraperitoneally (2 mg/kg) and the jugular vein and trachea are both cannulated. Supplementary amounts of sodium pentobarbital (15–20 mg/animal) are injected intravenously to produce deep anesthesia and the animal is respired artificially. Lysergic acid diethylamide (50 µg/animal), dibenzyline (1 mg/kg) and mepyramine maleate (10 µg/animal) can also be injected intraperitoneally at this stage to block effects from 5-hydroxytryptamine, adrenaline and histamine (Walmsley, 1963). Cinchocaine (2 ml, 0.2% (w/v) solution) can be given by paravertebral injection (L2–L3) to reduce sympathetic tone (Folley and Knaggs, 1965). The innervation and arterial supply around

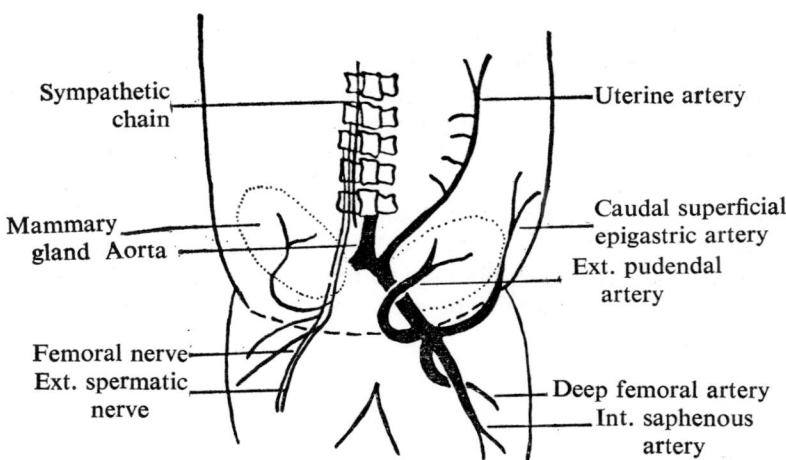

Fig. 3. Ventral aspect of nerves and arteries of a mammary region in guinea-pig. Nerves are shown on right side of the animal and arteries on left side. (From Walmsley, 1963.)

the mammary region of the guinea pig, is shown in Fig. 3. The deep femoral and caudal superficial epigastric arteries are ligated and the internal saphenous artery separated from connective tissue and branches of the external spermatic and femoral nerves, which are then cut. Local papaverine hydrochloride, (1% w/v) is used to dilate the internal saphenous artery before cannulation. Solutions injected into the cannulated internal saphenous artery, against the flow of blood, are taken directly to the ipsilateral mammary gland *via* the external pudendal artery. The animal is given 500 U heparin intravenously and the area around the arterial cannula bathed in 0.5% (w/v) cinchocaine to prevent vasoconstriction. The teat is cannulated with a blunted hypodermic needle and the cannula attached to a pressure transducer. High and low doses of solutions to be assayed are injected every 2 to 3 min and the volume of injection is kept constant. The preparation responds initially to 5–10 μU of oxytocin (30 μU—Fitzpatrick and Walmsley, 1965) and four-point assays can be carried out with doses of oxytocin in the range 15–60 μU. The approximate fiducial limits ($P = 0.05$) are $\pm 20\%$ (Tindal and Yokoyama, 1962); $\pm 26\%$ (Walmsley, 1963).

Limitations. The assay is not very accurate but is reasonably selective for oxytocin. Vasopressin is the main exception and, as stated previously, the vasopressin content of extracts should be known when oxytocin is assayed by this method. Acetylcholine, bradykinin, angiotensin II, 5-hydroxytryptamine, histamine, adenosine triphosphate and adrenaline can all interfere with the assay (Folley and Knaggs, 1965), but in practice the amounts of polypeptides other than oxytocin and vasopressin, needed to produce an effect, are far larger than would be normally expected to occur in extracts of body fluids (Fitzpatrick *et al.*, 1962). The effects of other substances can be inhibited by the use of selective blocking agents (Fitzpatrick and Walmsley, 1965). The method is recommended as the best means now available for the assay of small amounts of oxytocin, but the guinea pig may be replaced in time by the rat, since this animal has been shown to be even more sensitive to oxytocin (Bisset *et al.*, 1967).

ASSAYS *in vitro*

A piece of lactating mammary gland, cut out as a cylinder and suspended in a physiological saline solution, gives graded increases in tension in response to increasing concentrations of oxytocin (Mendez-Bauer *et al.*, 1960). Although this response may show a variable sensitivity to oxytocin

(Manunta and Albergoni, 1962a, b), it can be used with a precision that compares favorably with the other methods of milk-ejection assay (approximate fiducial limits ($P = 0.05$) on the rat mammary strip of $\pm 15\%$, Smith, 1961; $\pm 11\%$, Rydén and Sjöholm, 1962). An unusual characteristic of the response is the linear relation between dose and response (Sjöholm and Rydén, 1962, rat; Moore and Zarrow, 1965, rabbit). Rabbit mammary strips give graded effects to concentrations of oxytocin from 500 to 7000 μU/ml (Mendez-Bauer et al., 1960; Moore and Zarrow, 1965), while strips from rats respond to 200–400 μU/ml (Smith, 1961); 5–100 μU/ml (Rydén and Sjöholm, 1962). Conditions which change the sensitivity of the rabbit strip to oxytocin have been investigated by Moore and Zarrow (1965), who concluded that 32°C was the optimal temperature. It is surprising that the myoepithelium used *in vitro* should be so insensitive to oxytocin. Mammary strips also respond to adrenaline, noradrenaline, acetylcholine, 5-hydroxytryptamine and histamine. The rat mammary strip appears more sensitive to interference from these substances (Rydén and Sjöholm, 1962) than does that from the rabbit (Moore and Zarrow, 1965), but the rat is in any case more sensitive to oxytocin, so that the difference in selectivity may be more apparent than real. The ability of vasopressin to contract the mammary strip is 15% that of an equal amount of oxytocin when measured in the rabbit (Moore and Zarrow, 1965) but is only 3% in the rat (Smith, 1961) and 8% in the mouse (Linzell, 1955). A different method for recording responses to oxytocin *in vitro*, introduced by van Dongen and Hays (1964), measures the time taken for strips of lactating rat mammary gland to eject milk. The response, which occurred at 15°C in the presence of as little as 1×10^{-4} μU oxytocin/ml medium, was directly related to the concentration of oxytocin (van Dongen and Hays, 1966), but the selectivity was poor when measured at 5°C (van Dongen and Marshall, 1967). Rat mammary gland slices have also been used by Anderson et al. (1966) to assay oxytocin, though no details of their method are given. The methods of assay *in vitro* may prove useful but they need investigating further before being adopted for the routine assay of small amounts of oxytocin.

OTHER MILK-EJECTION ASSAYS

A number of workers have demonstrated the sensitivity of the human mammary gland to oxytocin. Both Beller et al. (1958) and Friedman (1960) found a threshold effect after the intravenous injection of 10 mU oxytocin and Wiederman and Stone (1962) found the response to be linearly related to the intravenous dose over the range 2–50 mU oxytocin. This response is particularly interesting because oxytocinase is present in the blood of lactating women and, if oxytocin is to be used clinically to encourage milk-ejection, this is the test which will give relevant information on the effective dose. Althabe et al. (1966) found the human mammary gland even more sensitive to intravenous oxytocin, 1.2 and 3.2 mU giving graded increases in intramammary pressure.

Lactating animals have also been used to assay oxytocin released from their own posterior pituitary glands by a variety of stimuli. Debackere and Peeters (1960) matched the ejection of milk caused by distension of a cow's vagina with the intravenous injection of oxytocin and later repeated this type of estimation using a cross-circulation technique to show that stimulation of the seminal vesicles of a ram or of the vagina of an ewe released oxytocin, which then caused milk-ejection in a parabiotic lactating ewe (Debackere et al., 1961; Peeters et al., 1965). Such an estimate must be subject to very large errors considering that a properly designed assay for milk-ejection has an error of about $\pm 20\%$. The lactating anesthetized mouse has been used to detect oxytocin (Vorherr, 1965). Intravenous injection of oxytocin is followed by pups behaving in a characteristic manner if milk-ejection has occurred. The method therefore gives all or no effects; responses can be obtained with about 120 μU oxytocin.

There have been various reports about milk-ejection assays performed on large animals. Whittlestone (1954) suggested the use of the lactating sow and Jones (1967) the lactating ewe, but the insensitivity of both methods means that they have little value for the determination of oxytocin in body fluids.

CHICKEN DEPRESSOR ASSAY

General. Paton and Watson (1912) were the first to show that extracts of the pituitary lobe lowered the avian blood pressure. This activity was found to be localized in the pars nervosa of the gland (Hogben, 1925) and to be mainly due to oxytocin (Gaddum, 1928). Coon (1939) developed this response into a quantitative assay for oxytocin and it is basically his method which is described in the latest editions of the British and U. S. Pharmacopoeias. The statistical treatment was improved by Smith and Vos (1943) using the assay design of Schild (1942). Thompson (1944) found the method accurate using the less conventional treatment of Vos (1943), where one dose of standard is alternated with three different doses of the unknown extract. Different values have been reported for the precision of the assay using high and low doses of test and standard. Elmqvist (1957) compared 12 doses of test and standard, 24 doses in all, and calculated the approximate fiducial limits as $\pm 20\%$ ($P=0.05$). Stewart (1949) found the method more precise ($\pm 10\%$, $P=0.05$).

Method. White Leghorn chickens, weighing about 2 kg, are anesthetized by the intravenous injection of sodium phenobarbitone, 180–200 mg/kg. The breed of chicken is important, Rhode Island Reds are insensitive to the depressor action of oxytocin (Stewart, 1950; Thorp, 1962). The crural or brachial vein is cannulated for injection of oxytocin solutions and the blood pressure is recorded from the ischiadic or popliteal artery using a mercury or membrane manometer (Coon, 1939; Thompson, 1944) or a strain gauge transducer of the type described by Bisset (1962) for the rat. Sodium citrate, 8.5% (w/v), or heparin is used as anticoagulant and doses of oxytocin are injected every 3 to 10 min. The method is described in greater detail by Thorp (1962).

Limitations. The sensitivity of the assay is low, 40 to 100 mU are normally needed to produce graded responses and discrimination between oxytocin and vasopressin is poor. The degree of discrimination depends on the concentration of magnesium in chicken serum (Smith, 1942). Pronounced tachyphylaxis is a feature of the assay which can only be avoided if small amounts of oxytocin are given at long intervals (Woolley and Waring, 1958). Adrenaline raises the blood pressure of birds (Paton and Watson, 1912) and vasopressin can exert a pressor as well as a depressor action, the former becoming more pronounced after the development of tachyphylaxis to oxytocin (Strahan and Waring, 1954). Substance P lowers the blood pressure (van Dyke et al., 1955). The lack of sensitivity of this method precludes its general use unless oxytocin or vasotocin are first extracted from body fluids and then concentrated before assay.

OXYTOCIC ASSAYS

THE ISOLATED UTERUS

General. The virgin guinea pig uterus, introduced by Dale and Laidlaw (1912) for the standardization of pituitary extracts by a method described in detail by Burn and Dale (1922), can be used with approximate fiducial limits at $P=0.01$ of $\pm 20\%$ (Gaddum, 1938). However it is difficult to obtain uteri which give reproducible results and attempts to modify the method by using a quantal response (Morrell et al., 1940), by making repeated measurements (Hamburger, 1945) or by changing the magnesium and calcium concentrations and injecting animals with stilbestrol (Stewart,

1949), have been only partly successful in improving the technique. The guinea pig uterus is still included in the U. S. Pharmacopoeia (1965) for determination of the oxytocic potency of Injection of Vasopressin, and Rorie and Newton (1965) recommend the estrogen-progesterone treated guinea pig for the assay of oxytocin by recording intrauterine pressure changes, but the rat uterus is now generally preferred for its greater stability. Beauvillain (1943) first used the rat uterus, adding drops of extract to be assayed to the bath solution until a threshold concentration was reached and the uterus gave a series of contractions. Holton (1948) used the rat uterus in the low calcium suspension fluid of Garcia de Jalon *et al.* (1945) to reduce spontaneous activity of the uterus, and an assay design was followed which permitted an analysis of variance. The method of Holton (1948) is also described in the British Pharmacopoeia (1963) and the details of description are acceptable except that uteri in proestrus or estrus are now known to be more sensitive to oxytocin and reliable in performance than those in diestrus (Schneider and Stumpf, 1953; Flatters, 1954; Guerné and Stutinsky, 1961; Chan *et al.*, 1963).

Method. The rat uterus is suspended in an organ both containing Locke's solution with half the usual amount of glucose (0.25g/l) and one quarter the usual amount of calcium (0.06g/l), aerated with $95\% \; O_2 + 5\% \; CO_2$ at a constant temperature of 32° C. The uterus should be in pro-estrus or estrus: this may be verified by taking vaginal smears or guaranteed by the intramuscular injection of stilbestrol diproprionate, 25–50 μg/kg, 17–18 hr before assay (Gaddum, 1953; Fitzpatrick, 1961). Three daily injections of 100 μg stilbestrol are reported to cause more than a ten-fold increase in sensitivity to oxytocin (Follett and Bentley, 1964). A large dose of oxytocin should be added to the organ bath as soon as possible as this helps to reduce spontaneous activity. Isotonic contractions are usually recorded with a frontal writing lever as described by Schild (1947), so that the shortening of muscle is recorded in a linear manner. More recently isometric recordings have been adopted (Munsick and Jeronimus, 1965; Krejčí *et, al.* 1966) and these, or auxotonic recordings (Paton, 1957), give more information if the log dose–effect curves are to be compared (Paton, 1961). Doses of oxytocin can be given every 3 or 4 min, high and low doses of test and standard being chosen to give between 30% and 70% of the maximal contraction. The approximate fiducial limits at $P=0.05$ are $\pm 9.6\%$ (Holton, 1948) and $\pm 5\%$ (Smith, 1959). The minimum effective concentration using the multiple stilbestrol treatment of Follett and Bentley (1964) is about 15 μU/ml and the uterus can be suspended adequately in a 2 ml bath.

Modifications. The bicarbonate-phosphate medium of van Dyke and Hastings (1928) provides a greater buffering capacity than the modified Locke solution used by Holton (1948), but the magnesium it contains has been reported to potentiate the action of oxytocin and vasopressin in a differential and sometimes unpredictable way (Fraser, 1939; Stewart, 1949). Munsick (1960) therefore suggested that van Dyke-Hastings solution should be used without magnesium. Relatively high magnesium concentrations can however be used to improve the sensitivity of the uterus to small amounts of oxytocin, provided the calcium concentration remains low (Heller and Lederis, 1959). Bentley (1965b) found that manganese as well as magnesium increased the sensitivity of the rat uterus to oxytocin. Assays with and without magnesium have proved useful for distinguishing pituitary hormones which resemble oxytocin from oxytocin itself (Munsick et al., 1960; Heller et al., 1961).

Periodic electrical stimulation of uterine strips produces a steady baseline response on which the effect of added oxytocin can clearly be seen. When this technique is used with strips of parturient rabbit uterus, the recorded tension increases in proportion to the log dose of oxytocin (Coutinho and Csapo, 1960); electrically stimulated rat uteri have also been successfully used to estimate oxytocin (see below). The total response to oxytocin (tension $\times$ time) may be computed for normally responding or electrically driven uteri and this may help to separate real responses from spontaneous contractions (Styles and Sullivan, 1962).

Other uteri which have been used in an isolated organ bath, besides those listed in the section on vasotocin assays, include that of the cat (Robson and Schild, 1938; Berde et al., 1957), the mouse (Wang, 1964) and strips of human uterus (Berde and Saameli, 1959). The sensitivity of the rat uterus to oxytocin is said to increase after treatment with hyaluronidase (Fendler et al., 1963).

Limitations. The isolated rat uterus assay is the most accurate method available for the assay of oxytocin. Unfortunately it probably also shows less selectivity for oxytocin than any other assay tissue. Anomalous oxytocic effects have been reported from urine (Jones and Schlapp, 1936; Aujard et al., 1954), blood (Bell and Robson, 1935; Bisset and Walker, 1954; Hawker and Robertson, 1958; Hawker et al., 1961) and cerebrospinal fluid (van Dyke et al., 1929) and in each case the activity could have been caused by one of a number of oxytocic polypeptides or lipids. Bradykinin is equi-active with oxytocin on the isolated uterus (Bisset and Lewis, 1962), angiotensin is very potent (Bisset et al., 1966), so is substance P (Cleugh et al., 1964) and other kinins (Armstrong et al., 1957;

Croxatto et al., 1961). Similar oxytocic kinins can be found in colostrum (Werle, 1960) and in urine (Horton, 1960) and they are particularly liable to arise in blood collected during labor (Armstrong and Stewart, 1960). Prostaglandins, present in a number of tissues (Vogt, 1958), have been found to be oxytocic, their potency depending on their chemical configuration (Horton and Main, 1966). Oxytocic lipids are also present in the amniotic fluid (Hawkins, 1962). Apart from these possibilities, the rat uterus is known to contract to acetylcholine and 5-hydroxytryptamine and to relax in the presence of small amounts of adrenaline and noradrenaline or large amounts of histamine. The sensitivity of the rat uterus to oxytocin can be improved by superfusion, but the problem of non-specific responses remains unchanged.

THE SUPERFUSED UTERUS

The technique of suspending a tissue in air in a constant stream of physiological saline at a constant temperature, was first introduced by Gaddum (1953) to improve the sensitivity of tissues to drugs. The stream is stopped for the application of the solution to be tested and the flow restarted after a few seconds. Oxytocin in a concentration of 100 μU/ml causes contraction of the rat uterus (Gaddum, 1953). Superfused uteri in proestrus are more sensitive to oxytocin (Fitzpatrick, 1961). The sensitivity of a uterus to histamine can be increased by replacing part of the sodium in the Ringer solution with sucrose (Hughes et al., 1956) and this has also been found to increase the sensitivity of the rat uterus to oxytocin (Smith, 1959). But spontaneous contractions sometimes make the assay difficult and the limits of error at $P=0.05$ are $\pm 20\%$ (Smith, 1959) compared with $\pm 5\%$ by the method of Fitzpatrick (1961).

The superfused uterus can be stimulated electrically and oxytocin then included in the superfusion fluid to produce an increase in tension (Fielitz et al., 1960). When this technique is used with a uterus in a solution low in calcium, the preparation shows little spontaneous activity and responds to oxytocin with graded increases in tension over the concentration range 5–50 μU/ml (Wiqvist et al., 1962).

A novel way of using the superfused rat uterus, suggested by Siddiqi and Walker (1960), was to allow rabbit arterial blood to flow directly over the uterus. The response to 5-hydroxytryptamine was blocked with dibenamine. The threshold sensitivity to endogenously released oxytocin was reduced by the slow infusion of oxytocin.

THE UTERUS *in situ*

The importance of estimating oxytocic substances on the uterus *in situ* increased when it was realized that synthetic analogues of oxytocin were more potent (on a unitage basis) when assayed in this way. This was true when the intensity of the initial contraction was used as an assay parameter (Berde *et al.*, 1957; Smith and Ginsburg, 1961) and was even more noticeable when the total effect was used for comparison (Bisset *et al.*, 1966). The usefulness of this type of assay increased still further when it was found that the rat uterus showed a greater specificity for oxytocin *in situ* when compared against bradykinin (Bisset *et al.*, 1966).

The early method used for recording isotonic contractions *in situ* was simple but rather insensitive (Bell and Robson, 1937). The technique has been improved by recording isometric contractions through a strain gauge transducer from a cannulated uterine horn filled with saline (Bisset *et al.*, 1966). The preparation is relatively insensitive to bradykinin, angiotensin and 5-hydroxytryptamine, but the sensitivity to oxytocin is equal to that of preparations *in vitro*. A similar insensitivity to bradykinin had been reported previously in man (Berde and Saameli, 1961), and in the cat and rabbit (Stürmer and Berde, 1963). The total response as recommended by Beránková-Ksandrova *et al.* (1966) and Bisset *et al.* (1966) should be used in these preparations.

The uteri of various species have been used *in situ* to match the effect caused by the endogenous release of oxytocin with intravenous injections of standard solutions. Using this technique, Abrahams and Pickford (1954) estimated the amount of oxytocin released by a variety of stimuli and Fuchs and Wagner (1963) have matched uterine contractions recorded during suckling with intravenous injections of oxytocin. Recordings have also been made from one horn of a pregnant rabbit uterus near term (Fuchs, 1966), but any estimate made of the amount of oxytocin released can only be semi-quantitative in such uncontrolled circumstances.

Another estimate of oxytocic potency has been made by counting the number of rabbits born within 60 min of injecting the solution to be assayed into a number of pregnant rabbits (Berde and Cerletti, 1958). The number of animals needed for such a test limits its use in all but the wealthiest of laboratories.

ASSAYS FOR ARGININE VASOTOCIN

General. The fact that arginine vasotocin (vasotocin) is distributed widely within the vertebrate class is a relatively recent discovery (see Heller, 1964) and assays for this hormone have until now, been designed to identify this hormone in pituitary extracts of various species rather than for the study of its physiological importance by estimation in body fluids. The pituitary glands of vertebrates which contain vasotocin usually also elaborate one or more additional oxytocic peptides and this makes the rat uterus assay impractical without previous separation of the hormones. Fortunately these additional peptides have negligible pressor effects (see Berde and Boissonnas, 1966), and it is therefore generally considered valid to estimate vasotocin in crude extracts by using the pressor effect in the rat as assay parameter (Follett, 1963).

Another approach to the assay of vasotocin has been to seek out tissues which respond selectively to the hormone and the first test to be used in this way was the frog water-balance assay of Heller (1941). This assay has since been used to identify vasotocin in the pituitary glands of cold-blooded vertebrates (Pickering and Heller, 1959; Sawyer *et al.*, 1959); the use of this test has been described again recently (Heller and Pickering, 1961). Other assay tissues which have been chosen for their relative selectivity to vasotocin include the frog bladder (Sawyer, 1960; Bentley, 1963) and various avian, reptilian and amphibian oviducts (Munsick *et al.*, 1960; Heller *et al.*, 1967).

Water-balance assay. Frogs are kept in shallow water overnight and weighed the following morning. Weighings are repeated every hour, the urinary bladders being emptied before each weighing. Vasotocin is injected into the lymph sac 3 hr after the first weighing. The weighings are continued until there is no further change, when the assay response is taken as the percentage increase in body weight. Synthetic oxytocin has been used as a standard but pure vasotocin would now seem preferable. The method can be used with high and low doses of test and standard. The assay is reasonably selective, vasotocin is about seven times more active than oxytocin when compared on a molar basis (Heller and Pickering, 1961). The assay is not very sensitive and takes a long time to complete.

Isolated frog skin, prepared as described by Maetz *et al.* (1959) to record short-circuit current, shows a fivefold discrimination between vasotocin and oxytocin on a weight basis (Heller *et al.*, 1961), which is not too different from that of the whole animal. The isolated skin is insensitive to hormones in winter (Heller et al., 1961) and the same is probably true for the whole frog.

Frog bladder assay. The urinary bladder of *Rana esculenta* is tied on to a piece of glass tubing, 0.8 ml of Ringer's solution is placed inside, and the whole assembly is immersed in 30 ml of aerated Ringer's solution maintained at 25° C. The potential difference across the bladder wall is recorded through agar bridges and calomel half cells and the current needed to reduce this potential to zero periodically measured by shunting the potentiometer across a standard resistance (Bentley, 1960) and a source of current. Vasotocin is added to the bath immediately after a reading of short-circuit current and three more readings are then taken at 5 min intervals. The bladder is then placed in fresh Ringer solution and the baseline current measured 20 min later. The response is taken as the average increase in short-circuit current measured while the hormone is in contact with the bladder. The error of the assay, using 2 high and 2 low doses of oxytocin, is 25% (Bentley, 1963). Oxytocin was found to be nearly equiactive with vasotocin when compared on a weight basis but Heller et al. (1961) reported a much greater selectivity to vasotocin. The sensitivity of the frog bladder varies with the time of year and there is a considerable individual variation.

Vasotocin also increases the permeability of the bullfrog bladder to water (Sawyer, 1960) and this response is nearly thirty times more sensitive to vasotocin than oxytocin (Munsick et al., 1960).

Hen oxytocic assay. Munsick et al. (1960) used the hen oviduct as one of several tissues sensitive to vasotocin. Strips of the uterine portion were cut and suspended in the medium of van Dyke and Hastings (1928) with 0.15 mM calcium, 0.5 mM magnesium and 1 mg glucose/ml at a temperature of 43° C. The same assay method, but using isometric recordings with a strain gauge transducer, has been described by Munsick (1964). Heller and Pickering (1961) used a low sodium medium (Heller and Lederis, 1960) at a temperature of 40° C. The assay design is as described by Holton (1948). Vasotocin is twenty to fifty times more active than oxytocin in this preparation (Munsick et al., 1960; Heller and Pickering, 1961).

Other oviduct preparations which have been or are being developed for the assay of vasotocin include those of the turtle (Munsick et al., 1960); the viviparous reptiles (LaPointe, personal communication) and the amphibia (Heller et al., 1967).

FURTHER ASSAY POSSIBILITIES

Mention has already been made of the frog water-balance assay for vasotocin. A similar assay for vasopressin using the hydrated toad has been reported by Buchborn (1955). The toads *(Bufo bufo)* are left in water for 8 hours before assay and are given an additional hydrating dose of hypotonic saline equal to 50 ml/kg at the time of assay. Graded inhibitions of diuresis were produced by the injection of 5–50 μU vasopressin/kg b.w. (Buchborn, 1957). The assay could not be repeated at this dose level by Reineck *et al.* (unpublished data cited by Tata and Gauer, 1966), though Lauber *et al.* (1959) found a similar method successful when vasopressin was injected into *Bufo marinus* (5–1000 μU/toad).

Neurohypophysial hormones produce several other effects which could be developed into assay methods. The proximal part of the guinea-pig colon is sensitive to vasopressin but not to oxytocin (Botting, 1965). Vasotocin raises the blood glucose concentration of toads when injected in amounts similar to those needed to produce a water-balance effect (Bentley, 1965a). Small amounts of oxytocin increase the utilization of glucose by rat epididymal adipose tissue *in vitro* (Mirsky and Perisutti, 1962) and decrease the plasma levels of free fatty acids when injected into dogs (Mirsky, 1963).

An important criterion on which assays for neurohypophysial hormones can be judged is the degree to which methods can differentiate between the hormone to be assayed and other pharmacologically active substances. The antigen-antibody reaction is known to be extremely specific and there is therefore great interest in developing an immunochemical assay for oxytocin and vasopressin. Rabbit antibodies have been formed to oxytocin (Gilliland and Prout, 1965) and to lysine vasopressin linked to bovine serum albumin (Permutt *et al.*, 1966) and both groups of workers claim high specificity, judged from binding and competition studies with hormones labeled with radioactive iodine. Holländer *et al.* (1966) have also reported preliminary results on the production of antibodies to oxytocin–albumin and lysine vasopressin–albumin complexes and though there is some evidence to suggest inactivation of oxytocin by the anti-oxytocin antibody, there is no doubt that this type of work will yield interesting results in the future.

INHIBITION AND INACTIVATION STUDIES

An elegant way to establish the identity of a neurohypophysial hormone is to block its assay response with a specific inhibitor. Such inhibitors are now being synthesized and though far from perfect, information gained from their use and from the use of chemical and enzymic inactivators, besides helping to identify hormones, allows the reliability of extraction and assay techniques to be judged with greater confidence.

Inhibitors. [2-*O*-methyltyrosine]-oxytocin (methyloxytocin), synthesized by Law and du Vigneaud (1960), inhibits the rat vasopressor response to arginine vasopressin when both are injected together (30 µg methyloxytocin + 0.008 µg arginine vasopressin). This analogue sometimes shows a small oxytocic effect on the rat uterus (Law and du Vigneaud, 1960; Bisset, 1962), but at the same time inhibits the action of oxytocin on this tissue (Beránková *et al.*, 1961; Bisset, 1962). The inhibition is probably competitive, the analogue showing a high affinity but little or no intrinsic activity for the oxytocin receptor (Rudinger and Krejčí, 1962). Methyloxytocin does not inhibit the milk-ejecting response to oxytocin (Bisset, 1962), but it has been reported to block the vasoconstrictor and vasodilator effects of oxytocin in rats and dogs (Pickford, in a discussion of a paper by Krejčí *et al.*, 1966). The effects of methyloxytocin have been re-evaluated recently by Krejčí *et al.* (1966, 1967b), who found that the inhibitory effect depended on the ionic composition of the fluid used to bathe the uterus and on whether the uterus had been pretreated with estrogen and progesterone. Various 2-*O*-alkyltyrosine analogues of oxytocin and lysine vasopressin inhibit the pressor action of vasopressin in rats (Krejčí *et al.*, 1967a).

The avian depressor effect of oxytocin is antagonized by glycyloxytocin (du Vigneaud *et al.*, 1960), the simultaneous injection of 0.68 µg glycyloxytocin and 0.04 µg oxytocin producing half the response from 0.04 µg oxytocin injected alone. This analogue also inhibits the milk-ejection response to oxytocin (Bisset, 1963) but not the oxytocic effect (du Vigneaud *et al.*, 1960). Two other synthetic analogues of oxytocin having substitutions on one half of the cystine residue, tested by Bisset (1963), antagonized the milk-ejection response to oxytocin in the lactating guinea-pig.

Thioglycollate inactivates oxytocin and vasopressin by reduction of the S–S link which each of these polypeptides contains (van Dyke *et al.*, 1942). Recently however Martin and Schild (1962, 1965) showed that, though this reaction took place, it was too slow to account for the rapid loss of oxytocic and milk-ejecting activities and they suggested that thioglycollate may antagonize the actions of these hormones at the receptor level. Another thiol, α-thioglycerol, antagonized the effect of oxytocin on the rat uterus without producing chemical degradation of the molecule.

Chemical inactivation. The reduction of vasopressin and oxytocin molecules with thioglycollate has proved a useful way of demonstrating the presence of vasopressin in blood (Ames and van Dyke, 1952) and in urine (Ames et al., 1950) and of separating the effect of oxytocin from that of other oxytocic substances in blood (Hawker, 1961). Reduction with sodium borohydride is also effective in abolishing the antidiuretic effect of vasopressin (Share, 1962). Electrolytic reduction causes a less pronounced inactivation (Gulland and Randall, 1935a) and there is some difference of opinion as to whether cysteine causes loss of activity (Sealock and du Vigneaud, 1935; Audrain and Clauser, 1958). The method for incubating extracts containing neurohypophysial hormones with neutralized thioglycollic acid has been described by Ames and van Dyke (1951) and by Vogt (1953). However, the reaction is not specific for these hormones: any disulfide-containing polypeptide will be affected by this reagent. The disulfide bridges of oxytocin and vasopressin can also be oxidized with various agents. Sachs (1960) oxidized vasopressin with performic acid to identify this hormone after extraction from posterior pituitary glands and Gulland and Randall (1935b) reported that oxytocin could be destroyed at pH 3.5 by aqueous solutions of iodine or chlorine. Neurohypophysial hormones are also inactivated in solutions of strong acid or alkali (pH 1 or 10) by boiling for 30 to 60 min.

Enzymic inactivation. Care must be taken to obtain enzymes of the highest purity before attempting experiments on the enzymic stability of neurohypophysial hormones. Some of the earlier experiments could not be repeated when pure enzymes were used. Both oxytocin and vasopressin are destroyed by incubation with *tyrosinase* (de la Maza and Croxatto, 1944; Croxatto and de la Maza, 1945; Fraser, 1950). The time course of this inactivation has been determined by Bisset (1962) using synthetic oxytocin and vasopressin. One hundred micrograms of tyrosinase incubated with 0.5 ml extract, in 0.9% (w/v) sodium chloride solution for 60 min at 37°C, destroys both oxytocin and vasopressin (Beleslin et al., 1967). *Trypsin* inactivates vasopressin but not oxytocin (Lawler and du Vigneaud, 1953) and this enzyme has been used for the partial identification of antidiuretic activity in rat blood (Thorn and Silver, 1957). Small amounts of vasopressin are inactivated by incubation with 50 μg trypsin in sodium bicarbonate solution for a period of 2–3 hr at room temperature (Share, 1962). Both vasopressin (Croxatto et al., 1942) and oxytocin (du Vigneaud et al., 1954) are inactivated by *chymotrypsin*. Another peptidase, *oxytocinase*, present in human pregnancy serum and having the specificity of an *aminopeptidase* acting on substrates with an amino terminal half-cystine residue, inactivates both vasopressin and oxytocin (Tuppy, 1960). This enzyme has recently been purified by Tuppy and Wintersberger (1960). Any or all of the above enzymes may be used to determine whether a particular biological activity is due to oxytocin or vasopressin. It may also be valuable to know that both these hormones remain unaffected when incubated with *pepsin* or *carboxypeptidase*.

STATISTICAL TREATMENT OF RESULTS

Most biological responses to drugs show a log-normal distribution (Gaddum, 1945) and plots of log dose-effect curves produce lines which can usually be assumed to be straight over a chosen range of doses. But the log dose–effect line will cease to be straight for very small and very large responses and may show significant curvature at intermediate dose ranges. An index of curvature may be calculated over the dose range to be used (Gaddum, 1953) and if significant curvature exists, a transformation can be applied to straighten the curve. Such a transformation was used by J. Heller and Štulc (1959) to convert the percentage antidiuretic response–log dose curve to a straight line. Milk ejection assays *in vitro* apparently provide an exception to the log-normal distribution rule, the contractile response being linearly related to the dose of oxytocin (Rydén and Sjöholm, 1962; Moore and Zarrow, 1965); when the latent period is used as an assay parameter (van Dongen and Hays, 1966), $\log t$ is found to be directly related to log-dose oxytocin. This is in agreement with the general formula $\log t = a - b \log X$, given by Gaddum (1953) for this type of response.

Once a linear relationship has been established between dose and effect, the assay should be designed as suggested by Schild (1942) so that the accuracy of the result can be calculated from the assay itself. In this method, (2+2) design assay, high and low doses of test and standard solutions are chosen to give between 10% and 90% of the maximum response. The dose ratio should be the same for test and standard and be sufficiently large to cause a consistent difference in size of response. The four doses are given in random order in blocks of four and the potency calculated graphically or from the formula given by Schild (1942). An analysis of variance can then be carried out to determine the causes for variation in response. The use of different doses should account for most of the variation and differences between the slopes of the two dose–effect curves must be statistically insignificant for the assay to be valid. This last point is particularly important where mixed standards (i.e. International Standard) or impure extracts are used to produce the assay response. The variation which cannot be accounted for can then be converted into fiducial limits and these values have been quoted in this review as a measure of the precision of assay methods. The values depend, however, both on the skill of the experimentor and on the number of responses which are used to calculate the limits, and they should not be assumed to hold under all conditions. The accuracy of each assay should therefore be re-checked by anyone wishing to use it for the routine assay of neurohypophysial hormones. Holton (1948) has described in detail how such a calculation can be made for the assay of oxytocin on the rat uterus and the same principle can be applied to any other properly designed assay.

The accuracy of an assay may also be calculated as an index of precision (λ), estimated from the ratio s/b (Gaddum, 1931), where s is the standard deviation of a single response, calculated from the residual variation in an analysis of variance, and b is the slope of the log dose–response line (dose-response or log dose–log response lines for milk-ejection assays *in vitro*). Gaddum (see Cleugh *et al.*, 1961) preferred to use the reciprocal of λ which he called Woolf's index, denoted by the symbol L. The index of precision is independent of the number of responses measured and it therefore gives an absolute estimate of precision. Indices of precision for a number of biological assays, varying from 0.033 to 0.2, have been tabulated by Gaddum (1953). The rat antidiuretic assay has been used with a λ of 0.08 (Yoshida *et al.*, 1963) to assay vasopressin, and oxytocin has been assayed on rat mammary strips with a λ of 0.109 (Rydén and Sjöholm, 1962).

If there is only enough unknown material to give one response, an assay can still be completed by bracketing this dose with doses of standard solution giving smaller and larger responses. But it has to be assumed in this case that the log dose–effect curve is straight and the error of the estimate cannot be calculated from the internal evidence of such an assay. The method for calculating results from such assays is given by Gaddum (1953), who points out that the error will be least when the doses of standard approach that of the unknown. It is advisable, wherever possible, to use the four-point $(2+2)$ assay design.

REFERENCES

BOOKS, REVIEWS, AND MONOGRAPHS

Acher, R. (1966). Chemistry of neurohypophysial hormones. *The Pituitary Gland*, Vol. 3, pp. 269–287. Harris, G. W. and Donovan, B. T. (eds.). Butterworths, London.

Acher, R. and Fromageot, C. (1957). The relationship of oxytocin and vasopressin to active proteins of posterior pituitary origin. *The Neurohypophysis*, pp. 39–50. Heller, H. (ed.). Butterworths, London.

Berde, B. and Boissonnas, R. A. (1966). Synthetic analogues and homologues of the posterior pituitary hormones. *The Pituitary Gland*, Vol. 3 pp. 624–661. Harris, G. W. and Donovan, B. T. (eds.). Butterworths, London.

BERDE, B., CERLETTI, A. and KONZETT, H. (1961). The biological activity of a series of peptides related to oxytocin. *Oxytocin*, pp. 247–265. Caldeyro-Barcia, R. and Heller, H. (eds.). Pergamon Press, London.

BISSET, G. W., HALDAR, J. and LEWIN, J. E. (1966). Actions of oxytocin and other biologically active peptides on the rat uterus. *Mem. Soc. Endocr.* **14**: 185–198.

COWIE, A. T. and FOLLEY, S. J. (1961). The mammary gland and lactation. *Sex and Internal Secretions* 3rd ed., pp. 590–602. Young, W. C. (ed.). The Williams and Wilkins Co., Baltimore.

CROXATTO, H., PEREDA, T. and ZAMORANO, B. (1961). Oxytocic substances in blood serum. *Oxytocin*, pp. 412–424. Caldeyro-Barcia, R. and Heller, H. (eds.). Pergamon Press, London.

DYKE, H. B. VAN, ADAMSONS, K. JR. and ENGEL, S. L. (1955). Aspects of the biochemistry and physiology of the neurohypophysial hormones. *Recent Prog. Horm. Res.*, **11**: 1–41.

FITZPATRICK, R. J. (1961). The estimation of small amounts of oxytocin in blood. *Oxytocin*, pp. 358–379. Caldeyro-Barcia, R. and Heller, H. (eds.). Pergamon Press, London.

FITZPATRICK, R. J. and WALMSLEY, C. F. (1965). Release of oxytocin during parturition. *Advances in Oxytocin Research*, pp. 51–73. Pinkerton, J. H. M. (ed.). Pergamon Press, London.

FOLLEY, S. J. and KNAGGS, G. S. (1965). Oxytocin levels in the blood of ruminants with special reference to the milking stimulus. *Advances in Oxytocin Research*, pp. 37–49. Pinkerton, J. H. M. (ed.). Pergamon Press, London.

FUCHS, A-R. (1966). The physiological role of oxytocin in the regulation of myometrial activity in the rabbit. *Mem. Soc. Endocr*, **14**: 229–248.

GADDUM, J. H. (1953). Bioassays and mathematics. *Pharmac. Rev.*, **5**: 87–134.

GONZALEZ-PANIZZA, V. H., SICA-BLANCO, Y. and MENDEZ-BAUER, C. (1961). The fate of injected oxytocin in the pregnant woman near term. *Oxytocin*, pp. 347–357. Caldeyro-Barcia, R. and Heller, H. (eds.). Pergamon Press, London.

HAWKER, R. (1961). Oxytocin and an unidentified oxytocic substance in extracts of blood. *Oxytocin*, pp. 425–436. Caldeyro-Barcia, R. and Heller, H. (eds.). Pergamon Press, London.

HELLER, H. (1957). The state and concentration of the neurohypophysial hormones in the blood. *Ciba Fdn Colloq. Endocr.*, **11**: 3–14.

HELLER, H. (1964). Class and species differences in the distribution of hypothalamo-neurohypophysial peptides. *Comparative Neurochemistry*, pp. 303–312. Richter, D. (ed.). Pergamon Press, London.

HORTON, E. W. (1960). Urinary kinin. *Polypeptides which affect Smooth Muscles and Blood Vessels*, pp. 263–265. Schachter, M. (ed.). Pergamon Press, London.

HORTON, E. W. and MAIN, I. H. M. (1966). The relationship between the chemical structure of prostaglandins and their biological activity. *Mem. Soc. Endocr.*, **14**: 29–36.

KREJČI, I., POLÁČEK, I. and RUDINGER, J. (1966). The effect of an oxytocin analogue on the uterus and its dependence on the functional state of the myometrium. *Mem. Soc. Endocr.*, **14**: 171–184.

LAUSON, H. D. (1960). Vasopressin and oxytocin in the plasma of man and other mammals. *Hormones in Human Plasma, Nature and Transport*, pp. 225–293. Antoniades, H. N. (ed.). Little, Brown & Co., Boston.

NIELSEN, A. T. (1965). Hypofysebaglaphormoner. Styrkebestemmelse, Standardpraeparater og Stabilitet. *Dansk. Tidsskr. Farm.*, **39**: 1–96.
PAGE, I. H. (1954). Serotonin (5-hydroxytryptamine). *Physiol. Rev.*, **34**: 563–588.
PEETERS, G., DEBACKERE, M., LAURYSSENS, M. and KÜHN, E. (1965). Studies on the release of oxytocin in domestic animals. *Advances in Oxytocin Research*, pp. 75–81. Pinkerton, J. H. M. (ed.). Pergamon Press, London.
PICKFORD, M. (1960). The release of oxytocin and vasopressin. *Polypeptides which Affect Smooth Muscles and Blood Vessels*, pp. 42–48. Schachter, M. (ed.). Pergamon Press, London.
PICKFORD, M. (1966). Neurohypophysis and kidney function. *The Pituitary Gland*, Vol. 3, pp. 374–398. Harris, G. W. and Donovan, B. T. (eds.). Butterworths, London.
SAWYER, W. H. (1966). Biological assays for neurohypophysial principles in tissues and in blood. *The Pituitary Gland*, Vol. 3 pp. 288–306. Harris, G. W. and Donovan, B. T. (eds.). Butterworths, London.
SMITH, M. W. (1959). The fate of oxytocins in the rat. Ph. D. Thesis, University of Bristol.
THORN, N. A. (1958). Mammalian antidiuretic hormone. *Physiol. Rev.*, **38**: 169–195.
THORP, R. H. (1962). Posterior pituitary hormones. *Methods in Hormone Research*, Vol. 2, pp. 495–516. Dorfman, R. I. (ed.). Academic Press, London.
TUPPY, H. (1960). Enzymic inactivation and degradation of oxytocin and vasopressin. *Polypeptides which Affect Smooth Muscles and Blood Vessels*, pp. 49–58. Schachter, M. (ed.). Pergamon Press, London.
VOGT, W. (1958). Naturally occuring lipid-soluble substances of pharmacologica interest. *Pharmac. Rev.*, **10**: 407–435.
WALMSLEY, C. F. (1963). The concentration of oxytocin in blood in relation to reproduction. M.Sc. Thesis, University of Bristol.
WERLE, E. (1960). Kallikrein, Kallidin and related substances. *Polypeptides which Affect Smooth Muscles and Blood Vessels*, pp. 199–209. Schachter, M. (ed.). Pergamon Press, London.

ORIGINAL PAPERS

ABRAHAMS, V. C. and PICKFORD, M. (1954). Simultaneous observations on the rate of urine flow and spontaneous uterine movements in the dog, and their relationship to posterior lobe activity. *J. Physiol., Lond.*, **126**: 329–346.
ACHER, R., CHAUVET, J., CHAUVET, M. T. and CREPY, D. (1962). Isolement d'une nouvelle hormone neurohypophysaire, l'isotocine, présente chez les poissons osseux. *Biochim. Biophys. Acta*, **58**: 624–625.
ACHER, R., CHAUVET, J., CHAUVET, M. T. and CREPY, D. (1964). Phylogénie des peptides neurohypophysaires: Isolement de la mesotocine (Ileu$_8$-ocytocine) de la grenouille, intermèdiare entre la Ser$_4$-Ileu$_8$-ocytocine des poissons osseux et l'ocytocine des mammifères. *Biochim. Biophys. Acta*, **90**: 613–615.
ACHER, R., CHAUVET, J., CHAUVET, M. T. and CREPY, D. (1965). Phylogénie des peptides neurohypophysaires: Isolement d'une nouvelle hormone, la glumitocin (Ser$_4$-Glu$_8$-ocytocine) présente chez un poisson cartilagineux, la Raie *(Raia clavata)*. *Biochim. Biophys. Acta*, **107**: 393–396.
ACHER, R., CHAUVET, J., LENCI, M. T., MOREL, F. and MAETZ, J. (1960). Presence

d'une vasotocine dans la neurohypophyse de la grenouille *(Rana esculenta L.)*. *Biochim. Biophys. Acta*, **42**: 379–380.
ACHER, R., CHAUVET, J. and OLIVRY, G. (1956). Sur l'existence éventuelle d'une hormone unique neurohypophysaire. 1. Relations entre l'ocytocine, la vasopressine et la protéine de van Dyke extraites de la neurohypophyse du boeuf. *Biochim. Biophys. Acta*, **22**: 421–427.
ACHER, R., LIGHT, A. and DU VIGNEAUD, V. (1958). Purification of oxytocin and vasopressin by way of a protein complex. *J. Biol. Chem.*, **233**: 116–120.
ADAMSONS, K. JR., ENGEL, S. L. and VAN DYKE, H. B. (1958). The stability of natural and synthetic neurohypophysial hormones *in vitro*. *Endocrinology*, **63**: 679–687.
ALTHABE, O. JR., ARNT, I. C., BRANDA, L. A. and CALDEYRO-BARCIA, R. (1966). Comparison of the milk-ejecting potencies of oxytocin and deamino-oxytocin in lactating women. *J. Endocr.*, **36**: 7–14.
AMES, R. G. and VAN DYKE, H. B. (1951). Thioglycollate inactivation of posterior pituitary antidiuretic principle as determined in the rat. *Proc. Soc. Exp. Biol. Med.*, **76**: 576–578.
AMES, R. G. and VAN DYKE, H. B. (1952). Antidiuretic hormone in the serum or plasma of rats. *Endocrinology*, **50**: 350–360.
AMES, R. G., MOORE, D. H. and VAN DYKE, H. B. (1950). The excretion of posterior pituitary antidiuretic hormone in the urine and its detection in the blood. *Endocrinology*, **46**: 215–227.
ANDERSON, R. R., KUMARESAN, P. and TURNER, C. W. (1966). Bioassay for oxytocic activity in posterior pituitary glands of cattle and rats. *J. Anim. Sci.*, **25**: 917–918.
ANDERSSON, B. and PERSSON, N. (1958). Intravenous assay of antidiuretic hormone using the goat. *Acta Physiol. Scand.*, **42**: 257–261.
ANSELMINO, K. J., HOFFMANN, F. and KENNEDY, W. P. (1932). Relation of hyperfunction of posterior lobe of hypophysis to eclampsia and nephropathy of pregnancy. *Edinb. Med. J.*, **39**: 376–388.
ARIMURA, A. and DINGMAN, J. F. (1959). Specific and sensitive assay method for vasopressin and oxytocin using glass-paper chromatography. *Nature, Lond.*, **184**: 1874–1875.
ARIMURA, A. and YAMAGUCHI, T. (1964). Serum protein-vasopressin binding and its influence on the pressor activity of the hormone. *Jap. J. Physiol.*, **14**: 90–101.
ARMSTRONG, D. A. J., JEPSON, J. B., KEELE, C. A. and STEWART, J. W. (1957). Pain-producing substance in human inflammatory exudates and plasma. *J. Physiol., Lond.*, **135**: 350–370.
ARMSTRONG, D. A. J. and STEWART, J. W. (1960). Spontaneous plasma kinin formation in human plasma collected during labour. *Nature, Lond.*, **188**: 1193.
AUDRAIN, L. and CLAUSER, H. (1958). Relation entre l'activité physiologique de l'ocytocine et l'état de son pont disulfure. *Biochim. Biophys. Acta*. **30**: 191–192.
AUJARD, C., CSANYI, E. and LE BRETON, E. (1954). Recherches sur l'activité ocytocique des urines. *Archs Sci. Physiol.*, **9**: 71–82.
BANGHAM, D. R. and MUSSETT, M. W. (1958). Third International Standard for posterior pituitary (re-named Third International Standard for Oxytocic, Vasopressor and Antidiuretic substances in 1956). *Bull. Wld. Hlth. Org.*, **19**: 325–340.
BARATZ, R. A. and INGRAHAM, R. C. (1959). Sensitive bioassay method for measuring antidiuretic hormone in mammalian plasma. *Proc. Soc. Exp. Biol. Med.*, **100**: 296–299.
BEAUVILLAIN, A. (1943). Titrage des préparations post-hypophysaires par leur seuil d'action sur l'utérus isolé de rat adulte. *C. R. séanc Soc. Biol.*, **137**: 284–285.

BELESLIN, D., BISSET, G. W., HALDAR, J. and POLAK, R. L. (1967). The release of vasopressin without oxytocin in response to haemorrhage. *Proc. Roy. Soc.*, B **166**: 443–458.
BELL, G. H. and ROBSON, J. M. (1935). Oxytocic properties of blood extracts and their physiological significance. *J. Physiol., Lond.*, **84**: 351–361.
BELL, G. H. and ROBSON, J. M. (1937). The effect of certain hormones on the activity of the uterine muscle of the guinea-pig. *J. Physiol., Lond.*, **88**: 312–317.
BELLER, F. K., KRUMHOLZ, K. H. and ZEININGER, K. (1958). Vergleichende Oxytocinbestimmungen gemessen durch den lactagogen Effect der Milchdrüse (Milkejection). *Acta Endocr. Copnh.*, **29**: 1–8.
BENTLEY, P. J. (1960). The effects of vasopressin on the short-circuit current across the wall of the isolated bladder of the toad, *Bufo marinus*. *J. Endocrin.*, **21**: 161–170.
BENTLEY, P. J. (1963). A method for the detection and estimation of small amounts of arginine-vasotocin. *J. Endocrin.*, **26**: 295–296.
BENTLEY, P. J. (1965a). Hyperglycaemic effect of vasotocin in toads. *Nature, Lond.*, **206**: 1053–1054.
BENTLEY, P. J. (1965b). The potentiating action of magnesium and manganese on the oxytocic effect of some oxytocin analogues. *J. Endocrin.*, **32**: 215–222.
BERÁNKOVÁ, Z., JOŠT, K., RYCHLÍK, I., RUDINGER, J. and ŠORM, F. (1961). Inhibition of the uterus-contracting effect of oxytocin by O-methyloxytocin. *Colln. Czech. Chem. Commun.*, **26**: 2673–2675.
BERÁNKOVÁ-KSANDROVÁ, Z., BISSET, G. W., JOŠT, K., KREJČÍ, I., PLIŠKA, V., RUDINGER, J., RYCHLÍK, I. and ŠORM, F. (1966). Synthetic analogues of oxytocin acting as hormonogens. *Brit. J. Pharmac. Chemotherap.*, **26**: 615–632.
BERDE, B. and CERLETTI, A. (1957). Démonstration expérimentale de l'action de l'ocytocine sur la glande mammaire. *Gynaecologia*, **144**: 275–278.
BERDE, B. and CERLETTI, A. (1958). Quantitative comparison of substances related to oxytocin: a new test. *Acta Endocr. Copnh.*, **27**: 314–324.
BERDE, B. and CERLETTI, A. (1961). Über die antidiuretische Wirkung von synthetischen Lysin-Vasopressin. *Helv. Physiol. Pharmac. Acta*, **19**: 135–150.
BERDE, B., DOEPFNER, W. and KONZETT, H. (1957). Some pharmacological actions of four synthetic analogues of oxytocin. *Brit. J. Pharmac. Chemotherap.*, **12**: 209–214.
BERDE, B. and SAAMELI, K. (1959). The action of the synthetic polypeptide valyl-oxytocin on the human uterus *in vitro* and *in vivo*. *Acta Endocr. Copnh.*, **32**: 391–398.
BERDE, B. and SAAMELI, K. (1961). Effect of bradykinin on uterine activity. *Nature, Lond.*, **191**: 83.
BIRNIE, J. H., EVERSOLE, W. J., BOSS, W. R., OSBORN, C. M. and GAUNT, R. (1950). An antidiuretic substance in the blood of normal and adrenalectomized rats. *Endocrinology*, **47**: 1–12.
BIRNIE, J. H., JENKINS, R., EVERSOLE, W. J. and GAUNT, R. (1949). An antidiuretic substance in the blood of normal and adrenalectomized rats. *Proc. Soc. Exp. Biol. Med.*, **70**: 83–85.
BISSET, G. W. (1962). Effect of tyrosinase preparations on oxytocin, vasopressin and bradykinin. *Brit. J. Pharmac. Chemotherap.*, **18**: 405–420.
BISSET, G. W. (1963). Synthetic analogues of oxytocin acting as antagonists. *J. Physiol., Lond.*, **165**: 69–71P.
BISSET, G. W., CLARK, B. J., HALDAR, J., HARRIS., M. C., LEWIS, G. P. and ROCHA E SILVA, M. (1967). The assay of milk-ejecting activity in the lactating rat. *Brit. J. Pharmac. Chemother.*, **31**: 537–549.

BISSET, G. W., HILTON, S. M. and POISNER, A. M. (1967). Hypothalamic pathways for independent release of vasopressin and oxytocin. *Proc. Roy. Soc.*, B **166**: 422–442.
BISSET, G. W. and LEE, J. (1957). An improved method for extracting oxytocic and antidiuretic hormones from blood. *Lancet*, **i**: 1173–1174.
BISSET, G. W., LEE, J. and BROMWICH, A. F. (1956). Oxytocic and antidiuretic activity in blood from the internal jugular vein in man. *Lancet*, **ii**: 1129–1132.
BISSET, G. W. and LEWIS, G. P. (1962). A spectrum of pharmacological activity in some biologically active peptides. *Brit. J. Pharmac. Chemother.*, **19**: 168–182.
BISSET, G. W. and WALKER, J. M. (1954). Assay of oxytocin in blood. *J. Physiol., Lond.*, **126**: 588–595.
BLACKMORE, W. P. and CHESTER, H. T. (1956). Assay of antidiuretic substance in plasma of normal and diabetes insipidus dogs. *Endocrinology*, **59**: 493–494.
BOISSONNAS, R. A., GUTTMANN, ST., BERDE, B. and KONZETT, H. (1961). Relationships between the chemical structures and the biological properties of the posterior pituitary hormones and their synthetic analogues. *Experientia*, **17**: 377–390.
BOISSONNAS, R. A., GUTTMANN, ST., JAQUENOUD, P. A. and WALLER, J. P. (1955). Une nouvelle synthèse de l'ocytocine. *Helv. Chim. Acta*, **38**: 1491–1501.
BOTTING, J. H. (1965). An isolated preparation with a selective sensitivity to vasopressin. *Brit. J. Pharmac. Chemother.*, **24**: 156–162.
BOURA, A. and DICKER, S. E. (1953). An apparatus for the maintenance of a constant water load and the recording of urine flow in rats. *J. Physiol., Lond.*, **122**: 144–148.
BROVETTO, J., OLHABERRY, J., GIOIA DE COCH, M. N., CODA, H., FIELITZ, C., CABOT, H. M., FRAGA, A. and COCH, J. A. (1967). Chromatographic and electrophoretic separation of oxytocin from the substances that interfere with its biological assays on the isolated rat mammary gland. *J. Endocr.*, **38**: 355–356.
BUCHBORN, E. (1955). Ein quantitativer biologischer Adiuretin–(Vasopressin)–nachweis an der Kröte. *Z. ges. exp. Med.*, **125**: 614–625.
BUCHBORN, E. (1957). Plasma level of antidiuretic hormone and serum osmolarity in normal human adults. *Endocrinology*, **61**: 375–379.
BURN, J. H. (1931). Estimation of the antidiuretic potency of pituitary (posterior lobe) extract. *Quart. J. Pharm. Pharmac.*, **4**: 517–529.
BURN, J. H. and DALE, H. H. (1922). On the physiological standardisation of extracts of the posterior lobe of the pituitary body. Reports on Biological standards. M. R. C. Special Reports Ser. No. 69, 1–52.
CHAN, W. Y., O'CONNELL, M. and POMEROY, S. R. (1963). Effects of the estrous cycle on the sensitivity of rat uterus to oxytocin and desamino-oxytocin. *Endocrinology*, **72**: 279–282.
CHAUDHURY, R. R. and JOPLIN, G. F. (1960). Preliminary observations on the release of oxytocin and vasopressin in human subjects. *J. Endocr.*, **21**: 125–128.
CHAUVET, J., CHAUVET, M. T. and ACHER, R. (1964). Les hormones neurohypophysaires des mammifères: Isolement et charactérisation de l'ocytocine et de la vasopressine de la baleine (*Balaenoptera physalus* L.). *Bull. Soc. Chim. Biol.*, **45**: 1369–1378.
CHAUVET, J., LENCI, M. T. and ACHER, R. (1960a). L'ocytocine et la vasopressine du mouton: reconstitution d'un complexe hormonal actif. *Biochim. Biophys. Acta*, **38**: 266–272.
CHAUVET, J., LENCI, M. T. and ACHER, R. (1960b). Présence de deux vasopressines dans la neurohypophyse du poulet. *Biochim. Biophys. Acta.*, **38**: 571–573.
CLARKE, N. P., ZUIDEMA, G. D. and REEVES, J. L. (1955). Modification of technique for assay of antidiuretic substance in urine. *Amer. J. Physiol.*, **183**: 603P.

CLEUGH, J., GADDUM, J. H., HOLTON, P. and LEACH, E. (1961). Assay of substance P on the fowl rectal caecum. *Brit. J. Pharmac. Chemother.*, **17**: 144–158.

CLEUGH, J., GADDUM, J. H., MITCHELL, A. A., SMITH, M. W. and WHITTAKER, V. P. (1964). Substance P in brain extracts. *J. Physiol., Lond.*, **170**: 69–85.

CONDLIFFE, P. G. (1955). Partition chromatography of oxytocin and vasopressin. *J. Biol. Chem.*, **216**: 455–464.

CONDON, N. E. (1951). A modification of the conventional mercury manometer for blood-pressure recordings. *Brit. J. Pharmac. Chemother.* **6**, 19–20. An addendum to the paper by T. B. B. Crawford and A. S. Outschoorn. *Brit. J. Pharmac. Chemother.*, **6**: 8–20.

COON, J. M. (1939). A new method for the assay of posterior pituitary extracts. *Archs Int. Pharmacodyn. Thér.*, **62**: 79–99.

COUTINHO, E. M. and CSAPO, A. (1960). The effect of oxytocics on the "Ca—deficient" uterus. A measure of oxytocic potency. *J. Gen. Physiol.*, **43**: 13–27.

CRAIG, L. C., HARFENIST, E. J. and PALADINI, A. C. (1964). Dialysis studies 7. Behaviour of angiotensin, oxytocin, vasopressin and some of their analogs. *Biochemistry*, **3**: 764–769.

CRAWFORD, J. D. and PINKHAM, B. (1954). An assay method for antidiuretic hormone based on a more sensitive response index. *Endocrinology*, **55**: 521–529.

CROSS, B. A. and VAN DYKE, H. B. (1953). The effects of highly purified posterior pituitary principles on the lactating mammary gland of the rabbit. *J. Endocr.*, **9**: 232–235.

CROSS, B. A. and HARRIS, G. W. (1952). The role of the neurohypophysis in the milk-ejection reflex. *J. Endocr.*, **8**: 148–161.

CROSS, B. A. and SILVER, I. A. (1961). Mammary oxygen tension and the milk-ejection mechanism. *J. Endocr.*, **22**: xxxiii.

CROXATTO, H., CROXATTO, R., ILLANES, G. and SALVESTRINI, H. (1942). Accion de la quimotripsina y de la pepsitensina por la aminopolipeptidasa. *Rev. Méd. y alimen., Chile*, **5**: 300.

CROXATTO, H. and DE LA MAZA, J. (1945). Accion de la Tirosinasa (extractos *psalliota campestris*) sobre la vasopressina. *Boln. Soc. Biol. Santiago Chile*, **2**: 46–48.

CZACZKES, J. W., KLEEMAN, C. R. and KOENIG, M. (1964). Physiologic studies of antidiuretic hormone by its direct measurement in human plasma. *J. Clin. Invest.*, **43**: 1625–1640.

DALE, H. H. and LAIDLAW, P. P. (1912). A method of standardising pituitary (infundibular) extracts. *J. Pharmac. exp. Ther.*, **4**: 75–95.

DEBACKERE, M. and PEETERS, G. (1960). The influence of vaginal distension on milk ejection and diuresis in the lactating cow. *Archs Int. Pharmacodyn. Thér.*, **123**: 462–471.

DEBACKERE, M., PEETERS, G. and TUYTTENS, N. (1961). Reflex release of an oxytocic hormone by stimulation of genital organs in male and female sheep studied by a cross-circulation technique. *J. Endocr.*, **22**: 321–334.

DEKANSKI, J. (1952). The quantitative assay of vasopressin. *Brit. J. Pharmac. Chemother.* **7**: 567–572.

DE LA MAZA, J. and CROXATTO, H. (1944). Accion de la Tirosinasa sobre la ocitocina. *Boln. Soc. Biol. Santiago, Chile*, **2**: 23–25.

DETTELBACH, H. R. (1958). A method for assaying small amounts of antidiuretic substances with notes on some properties of vasopressin. *Amer. J. Physiol.*, **192**: 379–386.

DE WIED, D. (1960). A simple automatic and sensitive method for the assay of anti-

diuretic hormone with notes on the antidiuretic potency of plasma under different experimental conditions. *Acta Physiol. Pharmac. Néerl.*, **9**: 69–81.
DICKER, S. E. (1953). A method for the assay of very small amounts of antidiuretic activity with a note on the antidiuretic titre of rat's blood. *J. Physiol., Lond.*, **122**: 149–157.
DONALDSON, W. (1947). The dialyzability of the pressor and antidiuretic activities of pitressin. *J. Clin. Invest.*, **26**: 1023–1025.
DU VIGNEAUD, V. (1956). The isolation and proof of structure of the vasopressins and the synthesis of octapeptide amides with pressor-antidiuretic activity, pp. 49–54. In *Proc. 3rd Int. Congr. Biochem., Brussels*. Academic Press, New York.
DU VIGNEAUD, V., FITT, P. S., BODANSZKY, M. and O'CONNELL, M. (1960). Synthesis and some pharmacological properties of a peptide derivative of oxytocin: glycyloxytocin. *Proc. Soc. Exp. Biol. Med.*, **104**: 653–656.
DU VIGNEAUD., V., RESSLER, C., SWAN, J. M., ROBERTS, C. W. and KATSOYANNIS, P. G. (1954). The synthesis of oxytocin. *J. Amer. Chem. Soc.*, **76**: 3115–3121.
DYBALL, R. E. J., LANE, G. J. and MORRIS, R. G. (1966). A simplified automatic device for the performance of antidiuretic assays. *J. Physiol., Lond.*, **186**: 43–44P.
ELMQVIST, A. (1957). Synpunkter po bestämning av Felgränser vid biologisk styrkebestämning av oxytocin. *Svensk. farm. Tidskr.*, **61**: 657–661.
ERSPAMER, V. and OTTOLENGHI, A. (1950). Antidiuretic action of enteramine. *Experientia*, **6**: 428.
FANG, H. S., LIU, H. M. and WANG, S. C. (1962). Liberation of antidiuretic hormone following hypothalamic stimulation in the dog. *Amer. J. Physiol.*, **202**: 212–216.
FENDLER, K., ENDROCZI, E. and LISSAK, K. (1963). Einfluss der Hyaluronidase auf die Oxytocinempfindlichkeit des Rattenuterus *in vitro* und *in vivo*. *Endokrinologie*, **44**: 153–156.
FERGUSON, D. R. (1965). Separation of mammalian neurohypophysial hormones by thin-layer chromatography. *J. Endocr.*, **32**: 119–120.
FERRIER, B. M., JARVIS, D. and DU VIGNEAUD, V. (1965). Deamino-oxytocin, its isolation by partition chromatography on Sephadex and crystallization from water, and its biological activities. *J. Biol. Chem.*, **240**: 4264–4266.
FIELITZ, C. A., GONZALEZ-PANIZZA, V. H. and CALDEYRO-BARCIA, R. (1960). Effect of low concentrations of oxytocin on the uterine response to electrical stimulation. *Acta physiol. latinoa.*, **10**: 201–204.
FITZPATRICK, R. J., MORRIS, A. and WALMSLEY, C. F. (1962). Oxytocin-like activity of the blood of cows in labour. *Proc. 22nd Int. Congr. Physiol., Leiden*, vol. 2. Abstract No. 522.
FITZPATRICK, R. J. and WALMSLEY, C. F. (1962). The concentration of oxytocin in bovine blood during parturition. *J. Physiol., Lond.*, **163**: 13–14P.
FLATTERS, M. (1954). Über die Vorzüge der Verwendung von Rattenuteri im Proöstrus zur Auswertung von Oxytocin. *Arch. Exp. Path. Pharmak.*, **221**: 171–176.
FOLLETT, B. K. (1963). Mole ratios of the neurohypophysial hormones in the vertebrate neural lobe. *Nature, Lond.*, **198**: 693–694.
FOLLETT, B. K. and BENTLEY, P. J. (1964). Bioassay of oxytocin: increased sensitivity of the rat uterus in response to serial injections of stilboestrol. *J. Endocr.*, **29**: 277–282.
FOLLETT, B. K. and HELLER, H. (1964). The neurohypophysial hormones of bony fishes and cyclostomes. *J. Physiol., Lond.*, **172**: 74–91.
FOLLEY, S. J. and KNAGGS, G. S. (1965). Levels of oxytocin in the jugular vein blood of goats during parturition. *J. Endocr.*, **33**: 301–315.

FORSLING, M. L., JONES, J. J. and LEE, J. (1967). A change of sensitivity to neurohypophysial hormones induced by their intravenous infusion in the rat. *J. Physiol., Lond.*, **191**: 127–128P.

FRANKLAND, B. T. B., HOLLENBERG, M. D., HOPE, D. B. and SCHACTER, B. A. (1966). Dissociation of oxytocin and vasopressin from their carrier protein by chromatography on Sephadex G-25. *Brit. J. Pharmac. Chemother.*, **26**: 502–510.

FRASER, A. M. (1939). Effect of Mg on response of uterus to posterior pituitary hormones. *J. Pharmac. Exp. Ther.*, **66**: 85–94.

FRASER, A. M. (1950). The effect of arginase and of tyrosinase on the activity and composition of posterior pituitary extracts. *Revue Can. Biol.*, **9**: 54–61.

FRIEDMAN, E. A. (1960). Direct measurement of milk ejection pressure in unanaesthetized lactating humans. *Amer. J. Obst. Gynec.*, **80**: 119–123.

FUCHS, A. R. and WAGNER, G. (1963). Quantitative aspects of release of oxytocin by suckling in unanaesthetized rabbits. *Acta Endocr. Copenh.*, **44**: 581–592.

FUGO, N. W. and ARAGON, G. T. (1947). The utilization of an old technique for a sensitive antidiuretic assay. *Fedn. Proc. Fedn Am. Socs Exp. Biol.*, **6**: 330–331.

GADDUM, J. H. (1928). Some properties of the separated active principles of the pituitary (posterior lobe). *J. Physiol., Lond.*, **65**: 434–440.

GADDUM, J. H. (1930). The stability of watery solutions of the oxytocic principle of the pituitary gland. *Biochem. J.*, **24**: 939–944.

GADDUM, J. H. (1931). The determination of vitamin A in cod liver oils. Statistical examination of results. *Biochem. J.*, **25**: 1113–1119.

GADDUM, J. H. (1938). The error of the oxytocic assay of post-pituitary extracts. *Quart. J. Pharm. and Pharmacol.*, **11**: 697–699.

GADDUM, J. H. (1945). Lognormal distributions. *Nature, Lond.*, **156**: 463–466.

GAINES, W. L. (1915). A contribution to the physiology of lactation. *Amer. J. Physiol.*, **38**: 285–312.

GARCIA DE JALON, P., BAYO BAYO, J. and GARCIA DE JALON, M. (1945). Sensible y nuevo metodo de valoracion de adrenalina en utero aislado de Rata. *Farmacoter. Act.*, **11**: 313–318.

GAUER, O. H. and TATA, P. S. (1966). Vasopressin studies in the rat. II. The amount of water reabsorbed by the rat kidney after a single i.v. injection of vasopressin: the vasopressin water equivalent. *Pflügers Arch. ges. Physiol.*, **290**: 286–293.

GERLOUGH, T. D. (1930). The rate of thermal decomposition at 100° of the oxytocic principle of the posterior lobe of the pituitary gland. I. The effect of hydrogen-ion concentration. *J. Amer. Chem. Soc.*, **52**: 824–834.

GERLOUGH, T. D. and BATES, R. W. (1930). The rate of thermal decomposition of the oxytocic principle of the posterior lobe of the pituitary gland. II. The effect of temperature. *J. Amer. Chem. Soc.*, **52**: 1098–1102.

GIBBS, O. S. (1930). A practical test for the antidiuretic action of the pituitary. *J. Pharmac. Exp. Ther.*, **40**: 129–137.

GILLILAND, P. F. and PROUT, T. E. (1965). Immunological studies of octapeptides II. Production and detection of antibodies to oxytocin. *Metabolism*, **14**: 918–923.

GILMAN, A. and GOODMAN, L. (1937). The secretory response of the posterior pituitary to the need for water conservation. *J. Physiol., Lond.*, **90**: 113–124.

GINSBURG, M. (1951). A method for the assay of antidiuretic activity. *Brit. J. Pharmac. Chemother.*, **6**: 411–416.

GINSBURG, M. and HELLER, H. (1953a). The antidiuretic assay of vasopressin by intravenous injection into unanaesthetized rats. *J. Endocr.*, **9**: 267–273.

GINSBURG, M. and HELLER, H. (1953b). Antidiuretic activity in blood obtained from various parts of the cardiovascular system. *J. Endocr.*, **9**: 274–282.
GINSBURG, M. and IRELAND, M. (1964). Binding of vasopressin and oxytocin to protein in extracts of bovine and rabbit neurohypophyses. *J. Endocr.*, **30**: 131–145.
GINSBURG, M., JAYASENA, K. and THOMAS, P. J. (1966). Preparation and properties of porcine neurophysin and the influence of calcium on the hormone-neurophysin complex. *J. Physiol, Lond.*, **184**: 387–401.
GINSBURG, M. and SMITH, M. W. (1958). The disappearance of oxytocin from the circulation of rats. *J. Physiol., Lond.*, **143**: 13P.
GINSBURG, M. and SMITH, M. W. (1959). The fate of oxytocin in male and female rats. *Brit. J. Pharmac. Chemother.*, **14**: 327–333.
GLAUBACH, S. and MOLITOR, H. (1932). Vergleich der Auswertungsmethoden von Gesamtextracten des Hypophysenhinterlappens am isolierten Meerschweinchen und an der Diuresehemmung von Hunden, Ratten und Mäusen. *Arch. Exp. Path. Pharmak.*, **166**: 243–264.
GROLLMAN, A. and WOODS, B. (1949). A new procedure for the detection of the antidiuretic principle in the urine. *Endocrinology*, **44**: 409–414.
GUERNÉ, J. M. and STUTINSKY, F. (1961). Étude in vivo des variations de la sensibilité à l'ocytocine de l'uterus de la ratte cyclique. *J. Physiol., Paris*, **53**: 357–358.
GULLAND, J. M. and RANDALL, S. S. (1935a). The oxytocic hormone of the posterior lobe of the pituitary gland. V. Recognition as an oxidation-reduction system. *Biochem. J.*, **29**: 378–390.
GULLAND, J. M. and RANDALL, S. S. (1935b). The oxytocic hormone of the posterior lobe of the pituitary gland. VI. Further studies of the action of oxidising and reducing agents. *Biochem. J.*, **29**: 391–396.
HAM, G. C. and LANDIS, E. M. (1942). A comparison of pituitrin with the antidiuretic substance found in human urine and placenta. *J. Clin. Invest.*, **21**: 455–470.
HAMBURGER, C. (1945). Modification of the standardization of posterior pituitary extract after Dale's principle. *Acta Pharmac. Tox.*, **1**: 112–119.
HAMILTON, H. C. and ROWE, L. W. (1916). Pituitary standardisation. *J. Lab. Clin. Med.*, **2**: 120–129.
HARE, K., HICKEY, R. C. and HARE, R. S. (1941). The renal excretion of an antidiuretic substance by the dog. *Amer. J. Physiol.*, **134**: 240–244.
HARE, K., MELVILLE, E. V., CHAMBERS, G. H. and HARE, R. S. (1945). The assay of antidiuretic material in blood and urine. *Endocrinology*, **36**: 323–331.
HART, P. D. and VERNEY, E. B. (1934). Observations on the rate of water loss by man at rest. I. Description of a constant temperature and humidity room. II. 'Spontaneous' diuresis during prolonged rest. *Clin. Sci.*, **1**: 367–396.
HAWKER, R. W. and ROBERTSON, P. A. (1958). Some properties of an oxytocic substance found in blood extracts. *Endocrinology*, **63**: 242–249.
HAWKER, R. W., WALMSLEY, C. F., ROBERTS, V. S., BLACKSHAW, J. K. and DOWNES, J. C. (1961). Oxytocic activity of blood in parturient and lactating women. *J. Clin. Endocr. Metab.* **21**: 985–995.
HAWKINS, D. F. (1962). Oxytocic lipids in human amniotic fluid. *Nature, Lond.*, **194**: 975–976.
HELLER, H. (1937). The state in the blood and the excretion by the kidney of the antidiuretic principle of posterior pituitary extracts. *J. Physiol., Lond.*, **89**: 81–95.
HELLER, H. (1939). The effect of the hydrogen-ion concentration on the stability of the antidiuretic and vasopressor activities of posterior pituitary extracts. *J. Physiol., Lond.*, **96**: 337–347.

HELLER, H. (1941). Differentiation of an (amphibian) water balance principle from the antidiuretic principle of the posterior pituitary gland. *J. Physiol., Lond.*, **100**: 125–141.

HELLER, H. and BLACKMORE, K. E. (1952). The assay of small amounts of antidiuretic activity by intravenous injections into mice. *J. Endocr.*, **8**: 224–228.

HELLER, H., FERRERI, E. and LEATHERS, D. H. G. (1967). The effect of neurohypophysial hormones on the amphibian oviduct. *J. Endocr.*, **37**: xxxix.

HELLER, H., HERDAN, G. and ZAIDI, S. M. A. (1957). Seasonal variations in the response of rats to the antidiuretic hormone. *Brit. J. Pharmac. Chemother.*, **12**: 100–103.

HELLER, H. and LEDERIS, K. (1957). Unpublished data cited by H. Heller in The state and concentration of the neurohypophysial hormones in the blood. *Ciba Fdn Colloq. Endocr.*, **11**: 3–14.

HELLER, H. and LEDERIS, K. (1958). Paper chromatography of small amounts of vasopressins and oxytocins. *Nature, Lond.*, **182**: 1231–1232.

HELLER, H. and LEDERIS, K. (1959). Maturation of the hypothalamo-neurohypophysial system. *J. Physiol., Lond.*, **147**: 299–314.

HELLER, H. and LEDERIS, K. (1960). Posterior pituitary hormones of the hippopotamus. *J. Physiol., Lond.*, **151**: 47–49P.

HELLER, H. and PICKERING, B. T. (1961). Neurohypophysial hormones of non-mammalian vertebrates. *J. Physiol., Lond.*, **155**: 98–114.

HELLER, H., PICKERING, B. T., MAETZ, J. and MOREL, F. (1961). Pharmacological characterization of the oxytocic peptides in the pituitary of a marine teleost *(Pollachius virens)*. *Nature, Lond.*, **191**: 670–671.

HELLER, J. (1960). A simple method for determination of renal function in small laboratory animals. *Physiologia bohemoslov.*, **9**: 150–156.

HELLER, J. and ŠTULC, J. (1959). Physiology of the antidiuretic hormone. I. A simple titration method. *Physiologia bohemoslov.*, **8**: 558–564.

HOGBEN, L. T. (1925). Studies on the pituitary — V. The avian depressor response. *Quart. J. Exp. Physiol.*, **15**: 155–161.

HOGBEN, L. T., SCHLAPP, W. and MACDONALD, A. D. (1924). Studies on the pituitary — IV. Quantitative comparison of pressor activity. *Quart. J. Exp. Physiol.*, **14**: 301–318.

HOLLANDER, L. P., FRANZE, J. and BERDE, B. (1966). An attempt to produce antibodies to oxytocin and vasopressin. *Experientia*, **22**: 325–328.

HOLTON, P. (1948). A modification of the method of Dale and Laidlaw for standardization of posterior pituitary extract. *Brit. J. Pharmac. Chemother.*, **3**: 328–334.

HUGHES, F. B., MCDOWELL, R. J. S. and SOLIMAN, A. A. I. (1956). Sodium chloride and smooth muscle. *J. Physiol., Lond.*, **134**: 257–263.

JAENIKE, J. R. and WATERHOUSE, C. (1961). The renal response to sustained administration of vasopressin and water in man. *J. Clin. Endocr. Metab.*, **21**: 231–242.

JEFFERS, W. A., LIVEZEY, M. M. and AUSTIN, J. H. (1942). A method for demonstrating an antidiuretic action of minute amounts of pitressin: statistical analysis of results. *Proc. Soc. Exp. Biol. Med.*, **50**: 184–188.

JESSUP, D. C., CARROLL, K. K. and NOBLE, R. L. (1961). Recovery of vasopressin from urine and blood by phenol extraction. *Can. J. Biochem.*, **39**: 1647–1649.

JESSUP, D. C., TAYLOR, N. B. G. and NOBLE, R. L. (1956). A comparison of methods for extracting pituitary antidiuretic substance from urine. *Endocrinology*, **60**: 6–12.

JONES, A. M. and SCHLAPP, W. (1936). The action and fate of injected posterior pituitary extracts in the decapitated cat. *J. Physiol., Lond.*, **87**: 144–157.

Jones, J. J. and Lee, J. (1965). The value of the pre-operated rat in the bioassay of vasopressin. *J. Endocr.*, **33**: 329–330.
Jones, J. J. and Lee, J. (1967). The value of rats with hereditary hypothalamic diabetes insipidus for the bioassay of vasopressin. *J. Endocr.*, **37**: 335–344.
Jones, R. C. (1967). Milk ejection by lactating ewes after the intramuscular injection of synthetic oxytocin. *J. Endocr.*, **37**: 233–234.
Kalliala, H., Karvonen, M. J. and Leppänen, V. (1952). Release of antidiuretic hormone during nursing in dog. *Ann. Med. Exp. Biol. Fenn.*, **30**: 96–107.
Kamm, O., Aldrich, T. B., Grote, I. W., Rowe, L. W. and Bugbee, E. F. (1928). The active principles of the posterior lobe of the pituitary gland. I. The demonstration of the presence of two active principles. II. The separation of the two principles and their concentration in the form of potent solid preparations. *J. Amer. Chem. Soc.*, **50**: 573–601.
Katsoyannis, P. G. and du Vigneaud, V. (1958). Arginine-vasotocin, a synthetic analogue of the posterior pituitary hormones containing the ring of oxytocin and the side chain of vasopressin. *J. Biol. Chem.*, **233**: 1352–1354.
Kestranek, W., Molitor, H. and Pick, E. P. (1925). Determination of the strength of pituitary extracts by their antidiuretic properties. *Biochem. Z.*, **164**: 34–43.
Kleeman, C. R., Rubin, M. E., Lambdin, E. and Epstein, F. H. (1955). Studies on alcohol diuresis II. The evaluation of ethyl alcohol as an inhibitor of the neurohypophysis. *J. Clin. Invest.*, **34**: 448–455.
Krejčí, I., Kupkova, B. and Vávra, I. (1967a). The effect of some 2-O-alkyltyrosine analogues of oxytocin and lysine vasopressin on the blood pressure of the rat, rabbit, and cat, *Brit. J. Pharmac. Chemother.*, **30**: 497–505.
Krejčí, I., Poláček, I. and Rudinger, J. (1967b). The action of 2-O-methyltyrosine-oxytocin on the rat and rabbit uterus: effect of some experimental conditions on change from agonism to antagonism. *Brit. J. Pharmac. Chemother.*, **30**: 506–517.
Landgrebe, F. W., Macauley, M. H. I. and Waring, H. (1946). The use of rats for pressor assays of pituitary extracts with a note on response to histamine and adrenaline. *Proc. Roy. Soc. Edinb.*, **62**: 202–210.
Lauber, J. K., Eversole, W. J. and Childs, W. A. (1959.) The use of the toad for bioassay of mammalian antidiuretic hormone (vasopressin). *Endocrinology*, **64**: 316–318.
Law, H. D. and du Vigneaud, V. (1960). Synthesis of 2-p-methoxyphenylalanine oxytocin (O-methyl-oxytocin) and some observations on its pharmacological behavior. *J. Amer. Chem. Soc.*, **82**: 4579–4581.
Lawler, H. C. and du Vigneaud, V. (1953). Enzymatic evidence for intrinsic oxytocic activity of pressor antidiuretic hormone. *Proc. Soc. Exp. Biol. Med.*, **84**: 114–116.
Lederis, K. (1961). Vasopressin and oxytocin in the mammalian hypothalamus. *Gen. Comp. Endocr.*, **1**: 80–89.
Levinsky, N. G., Davidson, D. G. and Berliner, R. W. (1959). Changes in urine concentration during prolonged administration of vasopressin and water. *Amer. J. Physiol.*, **196**: 451–456.
Lewis, A. G. (1953). Control of renal excretion of water. *Ann. Roy. Coll. Surg. (Sci. Edn).*, **13**: 36–54.
Lindner, E. B., Elmqvist, A. and Porath, J. (1959). Gel filtration as a method for purification of protein-bound peptides exemplified by oxytocin and vasopressin. *Nature, Lond.*, **184**: 1565–1566.
Lindquist, K. M. and Rowe, L. W. (1949). The antidiuretic activity of the posterior pituitary and its quantitative evaluation. *J. Amer. Pharm. Ass.*, **38**: 227–231.

LINZELL, J. L. (1952). The silver staining of myoepithelial cells, particularly in the mammary gland, and their relation to the ejection of milk. *J. Anat.*, **86**: 49–57.
LINZELL, J. L. (1955). Some observations on the contractile tissue of the mammary glands. *J. Physiol., Lond.*, **130**: 257–267.
LIVERMORE, A. H. and DU VIGNEAUD, V. (1949). Preparation of high potency oxytocic material by the use of counter-current distribution. *J. Biol. Chem.*, **180**: 365–373.
MACKENZIE, K. (1911). An experimental investigation of the mechanism of milk secretion. *Quart. J. Exp. Physiol.*, **4**: 305–330.
MAETZ, J., MOREL, F. and RACE, B. (1959). Mise en évidence dans la neurohypophyse de *Rana esculenta* L. d'un facteur hormonal nouveau stimulant le transport actif de sodium à travers la peau. *Biochim. Biophys. Acta (Amst.)*, **36**: 317–326.
MANUNTA, G. and ALBERGONI, V. (1962a). Sulla contrazione *in vitro* del mioepitelio mammario di coniglia ed oxytocina. *Boll. Soc. Ital. Biol. sper.*, **38**: 1263–1265.
MANUNTA, G. and ALBERGONI, V. (1962b). Contrazione *in vitro* del mioepitelio mammario di cavalla, vacca, asina, capra, pecora, cagna, gatta, cavia e ratta. *Boll. Soc. Ital. Biol. sper.*, **38**: 1266–1267.
MARTIN, P. J. and SCHILD, H. O. (1962). Effects of thiols on oxytocin and vasopressin receptors. *Nature, Lond.*, **196**: 382–383.
MARTIN, P. J. and SCHILD, H. O. (1965). The antagonism of disulphide polypeptides by thiols. *Brit. J. Pharmac. Chemother.* **25**: 418–431.
MAXWELL, A. L. I. and ROTHERA, A. C. H. (1915). The action of pituitrin on the secretion of milk. *J. Physiol., Lond.*, **49**: 483–491.
MAYER, F. S. (1960). Identification of the antidiuretic substance in human urine. *Acta Endocr. Copnh.*, **35**: 568–574.
MCCREARY, A. B., ADAMS, J. Q. and OVERMAN, R. R. (1957). A bioassay technique for plasma antidiuretic activity. *J. Lab. Clin. Med.*, **49**: 626–629.
MELVILLE, K. I. (1937). Antidiuretic pituitary substances in blood, with special reference to toxaemia of pregnancy. *J. Exp. Med.*, **65**: 415–429.
MENDEZ-BAUER, C., CABOT, H. M. and CALDEYRO-BARCIA, R. (1960). New test for the biological assay of oxytocin. *Science, N. Y.*, **132**: 299–300.
MIRSKY, I. A. (1963). Relative effects of insulin, oxytocin and vasopressin on the free fatty acid concentration of the plasma of nondiabetic and diabetic dogs. *Endocrinology*, **73**: 613–618.
MIRSKY, I. A. and PERISUTTI, G. (1962). Action of oxytocin and related peptides on epididymal adipose tissue of the rat. *Endocrinology*, **71**: 158–163.
MOORE, R. D. and ZARROW, M. X. (1965). Contraction of the rabbit mammary strip *in vitro* in response to oxytocin. *Acta Endocr. Copnh.*, **48**: 186–198.
MORAN, W. H. and MILTENBERGER, F. W. (1963). Use of the intravenous route for maintenance of water balance in the alcoholized rat bioassay of vasopressin. *Fedn Proc. Fedn Am. Socs Exp. Biol.* **22**: 386.
MORRELL, C. A., ALLMARK, M. G. and BACHINSKI, W. M. (1940). On the biological assay of the oxytocic activity of pituitary extract (posterior lobe). *J. Pharmac. Exp. Ther.*, **70**: 440.
MUNSICK, R. A. (1960). The effect of magnesium on the response of the rat uterus to neurohypophysial hormones and analogues. *Endocrinology*, **66**: 451–457.
MUNSICK, R. A. (1964). Neurohypophysial hormones of chickens and turkeys. *Endocrinology*, **75**: 104–112.
MUNSICK, R. A. (1966). Chromatographic and pharmacological characterization of the neurohypophysial hormones of an amphibian and a reptile. *Endocrinology*, **78**: 591–599.

MUNSICK, R. A. and JERONIMUS, S. C. (1965). Effect of diethyl-stilboestrol and magnesium on the rat oxytocic potencies of some neurohypophysial hormones and analogues. *Endocrinology*, **76**: 90–96.

MUNSICK, R. A., SAWYER, W. H. and VAN DYKE, H. B. (1960). Avian neurohypophysial hormones: pharmacological properties and tentative identification. *Endocrinology*, **66**: 860–871.

MUSCHOLL, E. and VOGT, M. (1957). The concentration of adrenaline in the plasma of rabbits treated with reserpine. *Brit. J. Pharmac. Chemother.*, **12**: 532–535.

NELSON, E. E. and WOODS, G. G. (1934). The diuretic-antidiuretic activity of posterior pituitary extracts. *J. Pharmac. Exp. Ther.*, **50**: 241–253.

NIELSEN, A. T. (1958). A note on the relative antidiuretic potency of beef and hog vasopressin. *Acta Endocr. Copnh.*, **29**: 561–564.

NIELSEN, A. T. (1960). Dissimilarity between arginine- and lysine vasopressin in rat pressor assays. *Acta Endocr. Copnh.*, **35**: 299–311.

NIELSEN, A. T. (1961). Om stødpudekatalyse of inaktiveringen of vasopressin ved opvarmning. *Dansk. Tidsskr. Farm.*, **35**: 21–35.

NOBLE, R. L., RINDERKNECHT, H. and WILLIAMS, P. C. (1939). The apparent augmentation of pituitary antidiuretic action by various retarding substances. *J. Physiol., Lond.*, **96**: 293–301.

NOBLE, R. L. and TAYLOR, N. B. G. (1953). Antidiuretic substances in human urine after haemorrhage, fainting, dehydration and acceleration. *J. Physiol., Lond.*, **122**: 220–237.

O'CONNOR, W. J. (1945). The effect of section of the supraoptico-hypophyseal tracts on the inhibition of water diuresis by emotional stress. *Quart. J. Exp. Physiol.*, **33**: 149–162.

O'CONNOR, W. J. and VERNEY, E. B. (1942). The effect of the removal of the posterior lobe on the inhibition of water diuresis by emotional stress. *Quart. J. Exp. Physiol.*, **31**: 393–408.

O'CONNOR, W. J. and VERNEY, E. B. (1946). The effect of increased activity of the sympathetic system in the inhibition of water-diuresis by emotional stress. *Quart. J. Exp. Physiol.*, **33**: 77–90.

ORR, J. and SNAITH, A. H. (1959). A method for the estimation of antidiuretic hormone in urine. *J. Endocr.*, **18**, xvi.

OTT, I. and SCOTT, J. C. (1910). The action of infundibulum upon the mammary secretion. *Proc. Soc. Exp. Biol. Med.*, **8**: 48–49.

OTT, I. and SCOTT, J. C. (1912). The action of various agents upon the secretion of milk. *Proc. Soc. Exp. Biol. Med.*, **9**: 63.

PATON, D. N. and WATSON, A. (1912). The actions of pituitrin, adrenalin and barium on the circulation of the bird. *J. Physiol., Lond.*, **44**: 413–424.

PATON, W. D. M. (1957). A pendulum auxotonic lever. *J. Physiol., Lond.*, **137**: 35–36P.

PATON, W. D. M. (1961). A theory of drug action based on the rate of drug-receptor combination. *Proc. Roy. Soc.*, **B 154**: 21–69.

PERMUTT, M. A., PARKER, C. W. and UTIGER, R. D. (1966). Immunochemical studies with lysine vasopressin. *Endocrinology*, **78**: 809–814.

PETERSEN, W. E. (1942). Effect of certain hormones and drugs on the perfused mammary gland. *Proc. Soc. Exp. Biol. Med.*, **50**: 298–300.

PICKERING, B. T. and HELLER, H. (1959). Chromatographic and biological characteristics of fish and frog neurohypophysial extracts. *Nature, Lond.*, **184**: 1463–1464.

PICKFORD, M. (1936). The inhibition of water diuresis by pituitary (posterior lobe) extract and its relation to the water load of the body. *J. Physiol., Lond.*, **87**: 291–297.
PIERCE, J. G. and DU VIGNEAUD, V. (1950). Studies on high potency oxytocic material from beef posterior lobes. *J. Biol. Chem.*, **186**: 77–84.
PLIŠKA, V. and RYCHLÍK, I. (1967). Determination of antidiuretic activity in the rat for structural analogues of the neurohypophysial hormones. *Acta Endocr. Copnh.*, **54**: 129–140.
PORATH, J. and FLODIN, P. (1959). Gel filtration: a method for desalting and group separation. *Nature, Lond.*, **183**: 1657–1659.
PORATH, J. and LINDNER, E. B. (1961). Separation methods based on molecular sieving and ion exclusion. *Nature, Lond.*, **191**: 69–70.
PORATH, J. and SCHALLY, A. V. (1962). Gel filtration of posterior pituitary hormones. *Endocrinology*, **70**: 738–742.
PORTANOVA, R. and SACHS, H. (1967). A specific adsorbent for vasopressin: the purification of labeled hormone. *Endocrinology*, **80**: 527–529.
RABASA, S. L. and BERGMANN, F. (1957). A method to reduce the individual variation in an antidiuretic assay. *Endocrinology*, **60**: 597–601.
RALLI, E. P., RAISZ, L. G., LESLIE, S. H., DUMM, M. E. and LAKEN, B. (1950). Evidences for more than one antidiuretic substance in pitressin. *Amer. J. Physiol.*, **163**: 141–147.
REINDEL, F. and HOPPE, W. (1954). Über eine Färbemethode zum Anfärben von Aminosäuren, Peptiden und Proteinen auf Papier Electropherogrammen. *Chem. Ber.*, **87**: 1103–1107.
RESSLER, C. (1958). Inactivations of oxytocins suggesting peptide denaturation. *Science, N. Y.*, **128**: 1281–1282.
RICHARDSON, K. C. (1949). Contractile tissues in the mammary gland, with special reference to myoepithelium in the goat. *Proc. Roy. Soc.*, **B 136**: 30–45.
ROBSON, J. M. and SCHILD, H. O. (1938). Response of the cat's uterus to the hormones of the posterior pituitary lobe. *J. Physiol., Lond.*, **92**: 1–8.
ROMANES, G. J. (1950). The staining of nerve fibres in paraffin sections with silver. *J. Anat.*, **84**: 104–115.
RORIE, D. and NEWTON, M. (1965). New method for the quantitative estimation of oxytocin. *Anat. Rec.*, **151**: 407.
ROTH, G. B. (1914). A new standard for the determination of the strength of pituitary extract. *J. Pharmac. Exp. Ther.*, **5**: 559–570.
RUCH, W. (1957). Estimation of antidiuretic hormone in the urine of healthy subjects and patients with inappropriate secretion of vasopressin (Schwartz-Bartter syndrome). *Acta Endocr. Copnh.*, **54**: 113–121.
RUDINGER, J. and KREJČÍ, I. (1962). Dose-response relations for some synthetic analogues of oxytocin and the mode of action of oxytocin on the isolated uterus. *Experientia*, **18**: 585–595.
RYDÉN, G. and SJÖHOLM, I. (1962). Assay of oxytocin by rat mammary gland *in vitro*. *Brit. J. Pharmac. Chemother.*, **19**: 136–141.
RYDIN, H. and VERNEY, E. B. (1938). The inhibition of water-diuresis by emotional stress and by muscular exercise. *Quart. J. Exp. Physiol.*, **27**: 343–374.
SACHS, H. (1960). Vasopressin biosynthesis – I. *In vivo* studies. *J. Neurochem.*, **5**: 297–303.
SAKOTA, N., TSUKUDA, T. and SASAI, T. (1955). Posterior pituitary hormones, I. Chromatographic separation of oxytocic and pressor activities on the ion-exchange column. *J. Biochem., Tokyo*, **42**: 465–469.

SAMAAN, A. (1935). The effect of pituitary (posterior lobe) extract upon the urinary flow in non-anaesthetized dogs. *J. Physiol., Lond.*, **85**: 37–46.

SAWYER, W. H. (1958). Differences in the antidiuretic response of rats to the intravenous administration of lysine and arginine vasopressins. *Endocrinology*, **63**: 694–698.

SAWYER, W. H. (1960). Increased water permeability of the bullfrog *(Rana catesbiana)* bladder *in vitro* in response to synthetic oxytocin and arginine vasotocin and to neurohypophysial extracts from non-mammalian vertebrates. *Endocrinology*, **66**: 112–120.

SAWYER, W. H., MUNSICK, R. A. and VAN DYKE, H. B. (1959). Pharmacological evidence for the presence of arginine vasotocin and oxytocin in neurohypophysial extracts from cold-blooded vertebrates. *Nature, Lond.*, **184**: 1464–1465.

SAWYER, W. H. and VALTIN, H. (1967). Antidiuretic responses of rats with hereditary hypothalamic diabetes insipidus to vasopressin, oxytocin and nicotine. *Endocrinology*, **80**: 207–210.

SCHÄFER, E. A. (1913). On the effect of pituitary and corpus luteum extracts on the mammary gland in the human subject. *Quart. J. Exp. Physiol.*, **6**: 17–19.

SCHÄFER, E. A. (1915). Note on preceding paper by Simpson and Hill: "The mode of action of pituitary extract on the mammary gland". *Quart. J. Exp. Physiol.*, **8**: 379–381.

SCHÄFER, E. A. and MACKENZIE, K. (1911). The action of animal extracts on milk secretion. *Proc. Roy. Soc.*, B **84**: 16–22.

SCHALLY, A. V., BOWERS, C. Y., CARTER, W. H. and HEARN, I. C. (1964). Isolation of gram amounts of arginine vasopressin, oxytocin and α-MSH. *Archs Biochem. Biophys.*, **107**: 332–335.

SCHALLY, A. V., LIPSCOMB, H. S. and GUILLEMIN, R. (1959). Chromatographic separation of oxytocin and vasopressin on carboxymethylcellulose. *Biochem. Biophys. Acta*, **31**: 252–254.

SCHILD, H. O. (1942). A method of conducting a biological assay on a preparation giving repeated graded responses illustrated by the estimation of histamine. *J. Physiol., Lond*, **101**: 115–130.

SCHILD, H. O. (1947). pA, a new scale for the measurement of drug antagonism. *Brit. J. Pharmac. Chemother.*, **2**: 189–206.

SCHNEIDER, W. and STUMPF, C. (1953). Über den Einfluss des Sexualcyclus auf Hypophysenhinterlappenextrakt—Auswertungen nach der Methode von P. Holton. *Archs Int. Pharmacodyn. Thér.*, **94**: 406–415.

SEALOCK, R. R. and DU VIGNEAUD, V. (1935). Studies on the reduction of pitressin and pitocin with cysteine. *J. Pharmac. Exp. Ther.*, **54**: 433–437.

SHARE, L. (1961). Acute reduction in extracellular fluid volume and the concentration of antidiuretic hormone in blood. *Endocrinology*, **69**: 925–933.

SHARE, L. (1962). Vascular volume and blood level of antidiuretic hormone. *Amer. J. Physiol.*, **202**: 791–794.

SIDDIQI, S. and WALKER, J. M. (1960). Oxytocic activity of rabbits blood applied directly to superfused rat uterus. *J. Physiol., Lond.*, **152**: 381–390.

SJÖHOLM, I. and RYDÉN, G. (1962). Improved method for quantitative estimation of oxytocin. *Nature, Lond.*, **193**: 77–78.

SKADHAUGE, E. (1964). Effects of unilateral infusion of arginine-vasotocin into the portal circulation of the avian kidney. *Acta Endocr. Copnh.*, **47**: 321–330.

SMITH, M. W. (1961). Some properties of rat mammary tissue. *Nature, Lond.*, **190**: 541–542.

SMITH, M. W. and GINSBURG, M. (1961). Fate of synthetic oxytocin analogues in the rat. *Brit. J. Pharmac. Chemother.*, **16**: 244–252.
SMITH, M. W. and THORN, N. A. (1965). The effects of calcium on protein-binding and metabolism of arginine vasopressin in rats. *J. Endocr.*, **32**: 141–151.
SMITH, R. B. JR. (1942). A comparison of the official and the chicken methods for the oxytocic bioassay of posterior pituitary preparations. *J. Pharmac. Exp. Ther.*, **75**: 342–349.
SMITH, R. B. JR. and VOS, B. J. JR. (1943). The biological assay of posterior pituitary solution. *J. Pharmac. Exp. Ther.*, **78**: 72–78.
STEIN, M., JINKS, R. and MIRSKY, I. A. (1952). The bioassay of pitressin and antidiuretic substances in blood and urine. *Endocrinology*, **51**: 492–503.
STEWART, G. A. (1949). An examination of factors affecting the precision of the assay of the oxytocic hormone in posterior pituitary lobe preparations. *J. Pharm. Pharmac.*, **1**: 436–453.
STEWART, G. A. (1950). The assay of posterior lobe extracts. *Analyst*, **75**: 452–550.
STRAHAN, R. and WARING, H. (1954). The effect of pituitary posterior lobe extracts on the blood pressure of the fowl. *Aust. J. Exp. Biol. Med. Sci.*, **32**: 193–206.
STÜRMER, E. and BERDE, B. (1963). A comparative pharmacological study of synthetic eledoisin and synthetic bradykinin. *J. Pharmac. Exp. Ther.*, **140**: 349–355.
STYLES, P. R. and SULLIVAN, T. J. (1962). Measurement of uterine activity *in vitro* by integrating muscle tension. *Brit. J. Pharmac. Chemother.*, **19**: 129–135.
TAKABATAKE, Y. and SACHS, H. (1964). Vasopressin biosynthesis III. *In vitro* studies. *Endocrinology*, **75**: 934–942.
TATA, P. S. and BUZALKOV, R. (1966). Vasopressin studies in the rat. III. Inability of ethanol anaesthesia to prevent ADH secretion due to pain and haemorrhage. *Pflügers Arch. ges. Physiol.*, **290**: 294–297.
TATA, P. S. and GAUER, O. H. (1966). Vasopressin studies in the rat. I. A sensitive bioassay for exogenous vasopressin. *Pflügers Arch. ges. Physiol.*, **290**: 279–285.
TAYLOR, S. P. (1954). Ion-exchange chromatography of oxytocin, arginine-vasopressin and lysine-vasopressin. *Proc. Soc. Exp. Biol. Med.*, **85**: 226–228.
THEOBALD, G. W. (1934). The repetition of certain experiments on which Molitor and Pick base their water-centre hypothesis, and the effect of afferent nerve stimuli on water diuresis. *J. Physiol., Lond.*, **81**: 243–254.
THOMPSON, R. E. (1944). Biological assay of posterior pituitary. *J. Pharmac. Exp. Ther.*, **80**: 373–382.
THORN, N. A. (1957). A densimetric method for assay of small amounts of antidiuretic hormone. *J. Exp. Med.*, **105**: 585–590.
THORN, N. A. (1965). Role of calcium in the release of vasopressin and oxytocin from posterior pituitary protein. *Acta Endocr. Copnh.*, **50**: 357–364.
THORN, N. A. and SILVER, L. (1957). Chemical form of circulating antidiuretic hormone in rats. *J. Exp. Med.*, **105**: 575–583.
THORN, N. A. and SMITH, M. W. (1965). Renal excretion of synthetic arginine-vasopressin injected into dogs. *Acta Endocr. Copnh.*, **49**: 388–392.
THORN, N. A., SMITH, M. W. and SKADHAUGE, E. (1965). The antidiuretic effect of intravenous and intracarotid infusion of calcium chloride in hydrated rats. *J. Endocr.* **32**: 161–165.
TINDAL, J. S. and YOKOYAMA, A. (1960). Bioassay of milk-ejection hormone (oxytocin) in body fluids in relation to the milk-ejection reflex. *Rep. Natn Inst. Res. Dairy*, 52–53.
TINDAL, J. S. and YOKOYAMA, A. (1962). Assay of oxytocin by the milk-ejection response in the anaesthetized lactating guinea pig. *Endocrinology*, **71**: 196–202.

TUPPY, H. and WINTERSBERGER, E. (1960). Zone electrophoresis of aminopeptidases on starch columns. *Monatsh. Chem.*, **91**: 406–411.
TURNER, C. W. and COOPER, W. D. (1941). Assay of posterior factors which contract the lactating mammary gland. *Endocrinology*, **29**: 320–323.
TURNER, R. A., PIERCE, J. G. and DU VIGNEAUD, V. (1951). The purification and the amino acid content of vasopressin preparations. *J. Biol. Chem.*, **191**: 21–28.
VALTIN, H., SAWYER, W. H. and SOKOL, H. W. (1965). Neurohypophysial principles in rats homozygous and heterozygous for hypothalamic diabetes insipidus (Brattleboro strain). *Endocrinology*, **77**: 701–706.
VALTIN, H. and SCHROEDER, H. A. (1964). Familial hypothalamic diabetes insipidus in rats (Brattleboro strain). *Amer. J. Physiol.*, **206**: 425–430.
VAN DONGEN, C. G. and HAYS, R. L. (1964). Bio-assay for oxytocic activity in untreated blood plasma. *J. Anim. Sci.*, **23**: 1229.
VAN DONGEN, C. G. and HAYS, R. L. (1966). Sensitive *in vitro* assay for oxytocin. *Endocrinology*, **78**: 1–5.
VAN DONGEN, C. G. and MARSHALL, J. M. (1967). Effect of various hormones on the milk ejection response of tissue isolated from the rat mammary gland. *Nature, Lond.*, **213**: 632–633.
VAN DYKE, H. B., and AMES, R. G. (1951). Alcohol diuresis. *Acta Endocr., Copnh.* **7**: 110–121.
VAN DYKE, H. B., BAILEY, P. and BUCY, P. C. (1929). Oxytocic substance of cerebrospinal fluid. *J. Pharmac. Exp. Ther.*, **36**: 595–610.
VAN DYKE, H. B., CHOW, B. F., GREEP, R. O. and ROTHEN, A. (1942). The isolation of a protein from the pars neuralis of the ox pituitary with constant oxytocic, pressor, and diuresis-inhibiting activites. *J. Pharmac. Exp. Ther.*, **74**: 190–209.
VAN DYKE, H. B. and HASTINGS, A. B. (1928). The response of smooth muscle in different ionic environments. *Amer. J. Physiol.*, **83**: 563–577.
VIERLING, A. F., LITTLE, J. B. and RADFORD, E. P. JR. (1967). Antidiuretic hormone bio-assay in rats with hereditary hypothalamic diabetes insipidus (Brattleboro strain). *Endocrinology*, **80**: 211–214.
VOGT, M. (1953). Vasopressor, antidiuretic and oxytocic activities of extracts of the dog's hypothalamus. *Brit. J. Pharmac. Chemother.*, **8**: 193–196.
VON SCHLICHTEGROLL, A. (1954). Vasopressorische und oxytocische Wirkung in Hypothalamus und Hypophysenhinterlappenextrakten. *Naturwissenschaften*, **41**: 188–189.
VORHERR, H. (1965). Eine neue Methode zum Oxytocin-Nachweis an der lactierenden Maus. *Arch. Exp. Path. Pharmak.*, **251**: 123.
VOS, B. J. JR. (1943). Use of the latent period in the assay of ergonovine on the isolated rabbit uterus. *J. Amer. Pharm. Ass. (Sci. Edn.)*, **32**: 138–141.
WALKER, A. M. (1939). Experiments upon the relation between the pituitary gland and water diuresis. *Amer. J. Physiol.*, **127**: 519–540.
WANG, S. M. (1964). Bioassay method for pituitary (posterior lobe) extract using the mouse uterus. *Acta Pharm. Sin.*, **11**: 626–628.
WARD, D. N. and GUILLEMIN, R. (1957). A simple method for preparation of highly purified vasopressin. *Proc. Soc. Exp. Biol. Med.*, **96**: 568–570.
WEINSTEIN, H., BERNE, R. M. and SACHS, H. (1960). Vasopressin in blood: effect of hemorrhage. *Endocrinology*, **66**: 712–718.
WHITTLESTONE, W. G. (1952). The milk-ejecting activity of extracts of the posterior pituitary gland. *J. Endocr.*, **8**: 89–95.
WHITTLESTONE, W. G. (1954). Intramammary pressure changes in the lactating sow. I. The effect of oxytocin. *J. Dairy Res.*, **21**: 19–29.

WIEDERMAN, J. and STONE, M. L. (1962). Effect of oxytocin on myoepithelium of the breast. *J. Appl. Physiol.*, **17**: 539–542.

WIQVIST, N., WIQVIST, I., FIELITZ, C. A. and CALDEYRO-BARCIA, R. (1962). Effects of oxytocin on the uterine response to electrical stimulation. *Acta Endocr. Copnh.* **41**: 161–169.

WOLLEY, P. and WARING, H. (1958). Responses of the perfused fowl leg to posterior lobe pituitary extracts. *Aust. J. Exp. Biol. Med. Sci.*, **36**: 447–456.

YAMASHIRO, D. (1964). Partition chromatography of oxytocin on 'Sephadex'. *Nature, Lond.*, **201**: 76–77.

YAMASHIRO, D., AANING, H. L. and DU VIGNEAUD, V. (1965). Inactivation of oxytocin by acetone. *Proc. Natn. Acad. Sci. U.S.A.*, **54**: 166–171.

YOSHIDA, S. K., MOTOHASHI, K., IBAYASHI, H. and OKINAKA, S. (1963). Method for the assay of antidiuretic hormone in plasma with a note on the antidiuretic titer of human plasma. *J. Lab. Clin. Med.*, **62**: 279–285.

CHAPTER 8 (a)

RENAL EFFECTS OF POSTERIOR PITUITARY PEPTIDES AND THEIR DERIVATIVES*

Georges Peters and Françoise Roch-Ramel

*Institut de Pharmacologie de l'Université de Lausanne
Lausanne, Switzerland*

INTRODUCTION AND TERMINOLOGY

The two major and definitely established renal effects of posterior pituitary peptides are either antidiuresis or diuresis. Both effects may occur simultaneously. This apparently paradoxical statement is due to the customary usage, in which "antidiuresis" is usually taken to mean a decrease in the clearance of free water (C_{H_2O}) occurring in an animal "in water diuresis", i.e. excreting a hypotonic urine, while "diuresis" designates an enhanced excretion of sodium and other solutes. Unless accompanied by a simultaneous increase of the flow of the isotonic component of a dilute urine (osmotic clearance = C_{osm}), a decrease in C_{H_2O} will usually result in a decrease in urine flow ($V = C_{H_2O} + C_{osm}$), which is often recorded instead of the more appropriate C_{H_2O} for reasons of experimental expedience. The "antidiuretic" effect of posterior pituitary peptides, which should preferably be called "antidilutional" or "concentrating" effect, may under certain circumstances occur simultaneously with an enhanced renal excretion of solutes. The terms "antidilutional", "concentrating" and "antidiuretic" will, however, be used interchangeably in this review.

For historical reasons the term "diuretic effect" is usually used as a synonym of "natriuretic effect". The simultaneous occurrence of an antidilutional effect and natriuresis may result in an increase, a decrease or no change in urine flow.

In contrast to drugs like 5-hydroxytryptamine (Van Arman, 1956) or [Val[5]]-angiotensin-II-amide (Bonjour *et al.*, 1967, 1968), posterior pitu-

---

*Most of the authors' work mentioned in this review was supported by Fonds National Suisse de la Recherche Scientifique (Grants No. 2966–4190).

itary peptides do not depress sodium excretion or glomerular filtration rate in mammals (see Sawyer, 1967). A number of older reports on the occurrence of anuria after the administration of more or less purified posterior pituitary hormones are to be ascribed to non-specific side-effects of the large doses given. A consistent depression of glomerular filtration rate (GFR) and renal sodium, chloride and total solute output has, however, been reported to occur in pregnant women in the 34th to 40th week of gestation, after intravenous injection or infusion of 50 to 100 mU per hr of a purified vasopressin preparation (Assali et al., 1960). This peculiar vascular antidiuretic and antinatriuretic effect of vasopressin disappeared after confinement and could not be elicited in non-pregnant women.

Depression of GFR and a consequent fall of renal sodium excretion by posterior pituitary peptides occurs to a lesser degree in amphibia (Jard et al., 1960; Jard and Morel, 1963) and to a large extent in reptiles (Heller and Bentley, 1965; Dodd et al., 1966): thus, in a species of the latter group, the water snake *Natrix sipedon*, very small doses of synthetic arginine-vasotocin (3 ng/kg) have been shown to depress GFR and sodium excretion (Dantzler, 1967).

ANTIDILUTIONAL EFFECTS: GENERAL CONSIDERATIONS

When occurring in animals excreting hypotonic urine at a rapid rate, the antidilutional action of the posterior pituitary peptides results in a marked decrease of urine flow. The same concentrating effect entails much less conspicuous antidiuretic effects in animals excreting either an isotonic or a hypertonic urine.

Any increase in urinary osmolar concentration induced by these hormones must, however, slow the urine flow, unless it is accompanied by an increased excretion of solutes, i.e. of sodium and the corresponding anions. Thus, the observation that vasopressin is not "antidiuretic" in rats (Sawyer, 1952; Brunner et al., 1956a; Kellog et al., 1954) or mice (Stelter, 1959) loaded with isotonic or hypertonic salt solutions is readily explained by the simultaneous occurrence of a natriuretic and a concentrating effect (Fig. 1).

In any given experimental or physiological condition, the concentrating effect of the vasopressins or other posterior pituitary hormones is limited by the maximal urinary osmolarity attainable in the presence of maximal doses of antidiuretic hormones. The maximal urinary osmolarity is generally identical with the osmolarity of papillary interstitial tissue

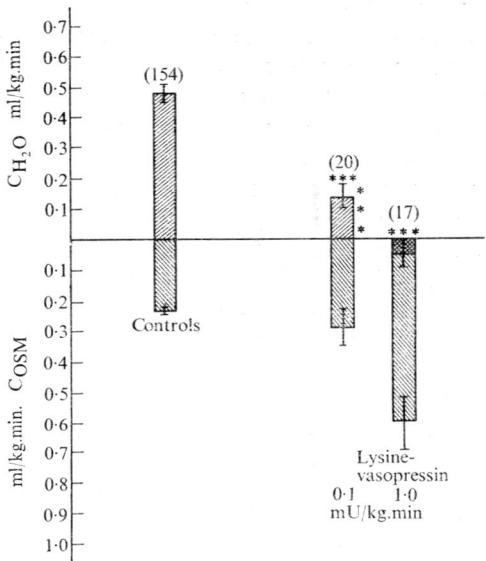

Fig. 1. Clearance of free water (C_{H_2O}) and osmotic clearance (C_{OSM}), as influenced by infusion of vasopressin. Rats prehydrated with 50 ml water/kg by gavage, and infused with 1.0 ml/kg of a hypotonic glucose–fructose solution. Numbers of experimental animals in brackets. Asterisks above columns indicate significance of differences of C_{H_2O} between controls and treated groups (*** = $P < 0.001$). Asterisks at the right side of columns indicate significance of differences in urine flow ($C_{H_2O} + C_{OSM} = V$) between treated and control groups ($^*_*$ = $P < 0.001$). The smaller dose of vasopressin causes a smaller depression of C_{H_2O}, but a greater depression of urine flow than the larger dose.

water. Apparent refractoriness to the antidilutional action of antidiuretic hormones may, thus be due to low medullary and papillary osmolarity rather than to a truly refractory state.

The comparative pharmacology of antidilutional effects is discussed in Chapters 3, 4 and 9, and structure-activity relationships (Sawyer *et al.*, 1962; Sawyer, 1967) are the topic of Chapter 4.

SITE AND MECHANISM OF THE ANTIDILUTIONAL EFFECT

There is no doubt that the antidilutional effects of posterior pituitary peptides are direct effects on the kidney (Berliner and Bennett, 1967).

While their major renal effect appears to be an increase of the permeability to water of certain segments of the nephron, this permeability increasing activity may not be the sole component of the antidilutional effects.

Conclusions about the mode of action of these peptides are usually based on a comparison of tubular fluid and urinary osmolarity, or electrolyte (or urea) concentration, between non-diuretic or dehydrated animals assumed to secrete large amounts of vasopressin, and animals in water diuresis after loading with hypotonic fluid assumed to secrete little or no vasopressin. Some of the major concepts have been confirmed by studies in untreated animals with surgically produced, or congenital, hypothalamo-pituitary diabetes insipidus. Only the latter type of study allows definite conclusions about the mechanism of action of the vasopressins, since there is no doubt that dehydration induces a number of changes in the composition and in the functions of the kidney, which may be unrelated to the presence of large amounts of vasopressin, or may be remote consequences of the long-continued presence of large amounts of vasopressin rather than imediate effects (Miles et al., 1954; West et al., 1955; Jones and de Wardener, 1956; Dicker, 1957; Senay and Christensen, 1965; Harrington and Valtin, 1965).

Since posterior pituitary antidilutional peptides are necessary for the elaboration of a concentrated urine, a knowledge of the steps of urinary concentration in the nephron is necessary for the understanding of the action of these peptides. There is general agreement on the major steps in the production of a concentrated urine, i.e. urine hypertonic to body fluids (Berliner and Bennett, 1967). As originally suggested by Wirz and his colleagues (Wirz et al., 1951; Wirz, 1956a, b, c), the urine is generally thought to become concentrated on its way through the medullary collecting ducts by passive outward movement of water into the strongly hypertonic medullary interstitium. Only one investigator (Marsh, 1966) thinks, that an active outward transport of water from the collecting ducts could contribute to urinary concentration. The active transport of water, in his model, is thought to be coupled to sodium transport. However, though thermodynamically possible, such an outward transport of water seems very improbable (Berliner and Bennett, 1967). The hypertonicity of the medullary and papillary interstitial tissue water is thought to be due to a primary accumulation of sodium and chloride and a secondary accumulation of urea.

High medullary concentrations of sodium and chloride are generally thought to be due to a specific function of Henle's loop which is thought to operate as a countercurrent-multiplier system (Gottschalk and Mylle, 1959; Berliner and Bennett, 1967). There is, as yet, no final proof that the

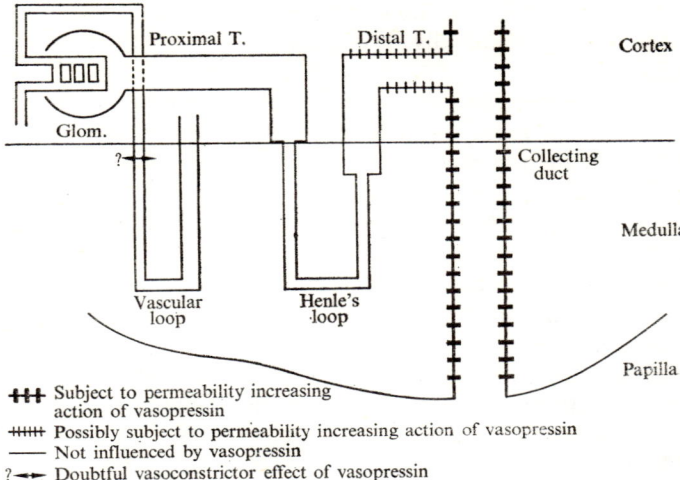

+++ Subject to permeability increasing action of vasopressin
+++++ Possibly subject to permeability increasing action of vasopressin
— Not influenced by vasopressin
?→ Doubtful vasoconstrictor effect of vasopressin

FIG. 2. Sites of action of antidilutional (antidiuretic) hormones in the mammalian nephron.

loop of Henle acts in this manner, though the steadily increasing osmolarity and sodium concentration along the course of the descending branch of Henle's loop and a similar decrease along the ascending limb, together with a lower osmolarity in the corresponding sites of the ascending limb (Jamison et al., 1967) are most suggestive.

There is no valid support for the hypothesis (Lever, 1965), that Henle's loop acts as a countercurrent-exchanger, while the actual countercurrent-multiplier system is located in the vascular loop (Fig. 2) (Berliner and Bennett, 1967).

It is puzzling that the primary effect multiplied by the countercurrent-multiplier system of Henle's loop is not known with certainty. As originally suggested by Kuhn and Ramel (1959), the primary effect is most probably an active transport of sodium ions out of the ascending limb of Henle's loop (Berliner and Bennett, 1967). Transport of sodium out of the ascending limb could not be directly demonstrated in experiments in which a drop of salt solution was squeezed between two columns of oil into the lumen of this tiny structure (Marsh and Solomon, 1965). This negative result may witness the limited tolerance of the thin walls of the ascending limb to rather brutal manipulations rather than the actual absence of an outward transport. The fact that proximal as well as distal tubular walls, after similar mistreatment, maintain their ability to transport sodium does not automatically show a lack of sensitivity of the much thinner ascending limb.

Thus the nature of the primary effect in the countercurrent-multiplier system of Henle's loop, has not been elucidated completely, but this has no bearing on the mechanism of action of antidiuretic hormones, since it is generally agreed that they do not influence the countercurrent-multiplier system. The basis for this belief is the finding, made originally by Wirz (1956 a, b, c), and subsequently confirmed by many investigators using micropuncture techniques, that early distal tubular fluid is strongly hypotonic to plasma in the presence as well as in the absence of antidiuretic hormones.

The events involved in the conversion of a large volume of iso-osmotic glomerular filtrate to a much smaller volume of hypertonic urine may be summarized by quoting a recent authoritative review (Berliner and Bennett, 1967): "In the proximal tubule, as a consequence of the active removal of salt in a highly water-permeable segment, the volume of fluid is markedly reduced without change in its osmotic pressure. A variable fraction of the glomerular filtrate enters the medulla in the thinwalled descending limb of the loop of Henle. As it flows into the hyperosmotic medulla, the fluid becomes progressively concentrated by (1) loss of water to its highly concentrated surrounding, (2) inward diffusion of urea from the urea-rich interstitium, and (3) possibly some entry of sodium chloride. Somewhere between the bend of the loop and re-entry of the nephron into the cortex, the permeability of the loop to water diminishes and outward transport of sodium and chloride dilutes the fluid that remains in the tubule lumen; thus, when the fluid arrives in the distal convoluted tubule, it is markedly hypotonic to plasma. The salt, that has been removed in this dilution process, remains behind to raise the osmolarity of the interstitial fluid and blood in the medulla. In the presence of antidiuretic hormones, the fluid flowing through the distal nephron loses its excess water by passive re-equilibration with its surroundings before (considerably reduced in volume) it re-enters the medulla in the collecting ducts. As it traverses the collecting ducts, it gives up water to reach the same hyperosmotic state as the surrounding medullary interstitial fluid".

It is generally assumed that the major effect of antidiuretic hormones in the concentrating mechanism is exerted by their action of increasing the water permeability of the walls of the distal tubules and of the collecting ducts (see Berliner and Bennett, 1967).

That the antidiuretic hormones cannot notably increase the permeability of the ascending limb of Henle's loops supposed to be relatively impermeable to water, devolves from the constant finding of a hypotonic tubular fluid in the early distal tubule mentioned above. This finding does not completely exclude the possibility that the antidiuretic posterior pituitary peptides exert an action on the countercurrent-multiplier system responsible for the establishment of high sodium and chloride concentrations in the medulla, since medullary sodium and chloride concentrations and osmolarity are much lower in water diuresis than in non-diuretic or dehydrated animals.

Following a suggestion by Berliner (1961), these low sodium concentrations in water diuresis are generally attributed to an increased rate of water passage through the medullary interstitium towards the medullary blood vessels in water diuresis, while the rate of the deposition of sodium is assumed to remain constant (Roch-Ramel and Peters, 1967). One cannot, however, fail to be somewhat disturbed by the finding that in rats, in water diuresis, medullary sodium concentration (R. B. Cross, 1964) as well as the amount of sodium per unit of dry weight of papilla (R. B. Cross and Sherrington, 1965) increase within as short a time as 15 min after the injection of an antidiuretic dose of vasopressin. If the only action of vasopressin consisted in increasing the permeability of collecting duct epithelium, one would expect a decrease rather than an increase of medullary salt concentration immediately after an injection of a single dose of vasopressin. This observation seems to point to the possibility of a direct enhancement of the establishment of the cortico-medullary sodium concentration gradient by vasopressin. The mechanism of such an action would be difficult to explain. One hypothesis would be a vasoconstrictor action of vasopressin on the descending limb of the vascular loop which would result in more effective trapping of salt in medullary tissue. In spite of the difficulty of measuring medullary blood flow accurately, it is suggestive that two groups of investigators (Thurau et al., 1960; Lilienfield and Maganzini, 1961) using different methods, found a lower medullary blood flow in non-diuretic animals as compared to animals in water diuresis. The increase in medullary blood flow in diuretic animals could be secondary to an increased passage of water from a collecting duct to the blood vessels, as suggested by Berliner and Bennett (1967), but could also be due to the disappearance of a primary vasoconstrictor action of the peptides. Another possibility would be a decrease of the water permeability of the ascending limb of Henle's loop under the influence of vasopressin. Though such an effect would contrast strangely with the effect of the peptide on the collecting duct, this possibility receives some support from recent micropuncture observations by Schnermann et al. (1967) who found a decrease of the amount of water reabsorbed from

Henle's loop, when vasopressin was injected into rats with hereditary pituitary diabetes insipidus.

The major action of vasopressin in the elaboration of a concentrated urine is, however, certainly an increase in the permeability to water of the walls of the collecting ducts and possibly also of the walls of the distal convoluted tubules. While a comparison of late distal tubular and urinary osmolarities shows an increased permeability to water in the collecting ducts of all species of mammals so far studied, the evidence in favor of an effect of the peptide on the distal tubules is far more contradictory. In the dog, vasopressin does not appear to exert any action on the water permeability of distal tubules: in hydropenic animals the tubular fluid is just as dilute at the end of the tubules as at their beginning (Clapp and Robinson, 1966) while the inulin concentration does not increase notably (Berliner and Bennett, 1967). The distal tubules, thus, appear quite impermeable to water in the dog in a state in which there is maximal secretion of vasopressin. In water diuresis, i.e. in the presumed absence of endogenous vasopressin, the osmolarities in the distal tubular fluid of dogs are slightly lower than those in the dehydrated animal: the difference can, however, be explained by the slightly lower urea concentrations during water diuresis (Clapp and Robinson, 1966). Similarly, vasopressin does not influence the water permeability of the distal tubule in the rhesus monkey (Berliner and Bennett, 1967).

In contrast to the findings in the dog and in the monkey, an action of vasopressin on the water-permeability of the distal tubule of the rat appears to be established by the classical observations of Wirz (1956a) and of Gottschalk and Mylle (1959). According to their results, the luminal fluid in distal tubules in water diuresis remains dilute and hypotonic throughout the whole length of the distal convolution, while in the non-diuretic or dehydrated state, i.e. in the presence of endogenous vasopressin the osmotic gradient in early distal tubular fluid is dissipated before the distal tubule re-enters the medulla. A considerable increase in the inulin concentration in distal tubular fluid of the non-diuretic rat (Ullrich *et al.*, 1963; Roch-Ramel *et al.*, 1968) equally argues for major water losses through distal tubules whose permeability has been increased by vasopressin.

There are some doubts about the validity of these findings which could be artefacts due to the partial re-aspiration of collecting duct fluid along an inadequate oil block, which did not completely close the distal tubular lumen downstream from the site of puncture (Morel *et al.*, 1966). However, a change in the permeability to water of the distal tubule has also been found when passing from the non-diuretic state to water diuresis in experiments which are not subject to the possible error of re-aspiration of collecting duct fluid. In these experiments the water permeability of the tubular walls was directly measured by microperfusion of the tubules with hypotonic or hypertonic solutions and by measuring the rate at which the perfused solutions became isotonic to plasma (Ullrich et al., 1964). Such experiments allow a calculation of "filtration permeability" of the tubular walls which in the majority of all experiments on animals in water diuresis was found to decrease to one third or less of its value in the non-diuretic state. These experiments leave little doubt that the water permeability of the distal convoluted tubules is greater in the non-diuretic rat than in water diuresis, while the water permeability of proximal tubules is the same in both states. This difference could be due to factors other than vasopressin. Only experiments on rats in water diuresis or with diabetes insipidus, in the presence or in the absence of additional exogenous vasopressin, could definitely establish an effect of vasopressin on the water-permeability of the distal convoluted tubule in this species.

Doubts about a direct action of antidiuretic hormones on the permeability of the distal tubule in the rat are reinforced by the observation of similar mean distal tubular concentration factors (TF/P) for inulin in non-diuretic rats and in animals with diabetes insipidus induced by hypothalamic lesions (Gertz et al., 1964).

While there are some doubts about the distal tubule, it is certain that vasopressin increases considerably the water permeability of the medullary collecting ducts (Fig. 1). This has been most clearly demonstrated by tracer microinjection of tritiated water (Morel et al., 1965). The circumscribed action of vasopressin might be due to selective sensitivity of the collecting ducts (and perhaps the distal tubules) or to selective localization. Autoradiographic observations on isolated nephrons from the kidneys of rats injected with ^{131}I-vasopressin (Darmady et al., 1960), showed selective localization of ^{131}I in the distal convoluted tubules and in the upper two thirds of the collecting ducts. Since ^{131}I-labelled diodotyrosine selectively stained the proximal tubules, a selective localization of vasopressin was suggested.

The permeability-increasing action of vasopressin on collecting ducts has also been demonstrated in segments of isolated rabbit collecting tubules perfused *in vitro* (Grantham and Burg, 1966). Addition of very low and probably "physiological" amounts of vasopressin to the contraluminal side of such tubules caused an approximately three-fold increase in the permeability to water: the relative changes in "diffusion permeability" measured with tritiated water were approximately the same as the changes in "filtration permeability" (rate of net water movement in response to an osmotic gradient). Addition of vasopressin to the luminal side of the collecting tubule had no influence on water permeability. Thus, in analogy to its action on amphibian membranes, vasopressin in the nephron appears to increase permeability only when added to the blood side but not when present on the epithelial side (Leaf, 1965). This conclusion is strengthened, insofar as nephrons of warm-blooded animals are concerned, by two findings: on the one hand, vasopressin forced by retrograde injection into the collecting ducts of rats in water diuresis did not exert an antidiuretic action (Skadhauge, 1964a); on the other hand the avian antidiuretic hormone vasotocin caused unilateral antidilutional effects when infused through a leg vein into the renal portal circulation of chickens (Skadhauge, 1964b).

Almost all observations on the renal site and mechanism of action of posterior pituitary peptides possessing an antidilutional effect have been made with either arginine or lysine vasopressin in mammals. The generally accepted inference that other neurohypophysial peptides have an analogous effect in lower vertebrates (including birds) requires further experimental support.

In view of the important, although not completely understood role of urea in the elaboration of a concentrated urine, observations demonstrating indirectly an increase in the permeability to urea of collecting duct walls in dog under the influence of vasopressin (Jaenike, 1961) are of great interest and seemed to be confirmed by the experiments of Gardner and Maffly (1963): perfusion with urea-containing solutions of isolated papillae obtained from rats in either water diuresis, or after an injection of vasopressin showed a much larger accumulation of urea in the papillae from the vasopressin-treated animals. However, no increase in permeability to urea could be shown in isolated perfused collecting ducts of rabbits (Grantham and Burg, 1966). In distal and in proximal tubules, microperfusion experiments in the rat (Čapek et al., 1966) failed to show a difference in the permeability to urea in the antidiuretic state and in water diuresis. It is thus doubtful, whether antidiuretic posterior pituitary peptides influence the urea permeability of the collecting ducts, and certain that they do not influence the permeability to urea of more proximal segments of the nephron.

MECHANISM OF THE WATER PERMEABILITY-INCREASING EFFECT OF POSTERIOR PITUITARY ANTIDILUTIONAL HORMONES

Since it is technically much easier to study transport across amphibian membranes than across renal tubular walls, most attempts to elucidate the permeability increasing action of posterior pituitary peptides were made by studying such membranes (see Chapters 9 and 10). The applicability of these results to the mammalian nephron remains in doubt, as long as the identity of effects on amphibian membranes and on mammalian tubules has not been conclusively demonstrated. It may be useful to point out the differences between the amphibian membranes and the mammalian tubular walls (mainly those of the collecting ducts), which, in the reviewers' opinion, are sufficiently large to shed considerable doubt on the applicability of conclusions evolved from studies in amphibian membranes to the mammalian kidney (Table 1).

One hypothesis concerned with the mechanism of action of antidiuretic hormones on mammalian renal tubules which is not derived from studies on amphibian membranes is that of Ginetzinsky, originally based on the finding that the urinary excretion of hyaluronidase activity in man varied inversely with the rate of urine flow (Ginetzinsky et al., 1954). Similar variations were subsequently found in the urine of other species when urine flow was varied either by the administration of water, by dehydration or by exogenous antidiuretic hormone, (Ginetzinsky and Ivanova, 1958; Ginetzinsky, 1958, 1961). Originally not confirmed by Berlyne (1960), these observations were later fully confirmed and amplified in man by Dicker and Eggleton (1960) who found that water and saline diuresis were regularily accompanied by a decrease in the urinary excretion of hyaluronidase, while a depression of urine flow in water diuresis, under the influence of vasopressin or of progressive dehydration, was accompanied by an increased urinary excretion. Similar observations were also made in rats. In patients with kidneys non-responsive to the concentrating action of exogenous vasopressin ("nephrogenic diabetes insipidus"), vasopressin did not increase urinary hyaluronidase activity. It thus appears, that the concentrating action of posterior pituitary peptides in mammals is associated with an increased passage of hyaluronidase into the urine. It is, however, quite uncertain whether this increased excretion of hyaluronidase is causally connected with the establishment of vasopressin-induced antidiuresis or merely accompanies it, Ginetzinsky et al. (1958) concluded from histological observations, which could not

TABLE 1. SIMILARITIES AND DIFFERENCES IN THE RESPONSE OF AMPHIBIAN MEMBRANES AND THE MAMMALIAN NEPHRON TO POSTERIOR PITUITARY PEPTIDES

Effect	Frog skin or toad bladder	Mammalian nephron: *in situ*, or isolated collecting duct
Enhancement of "osmotic flow" of water ("Filtration permeability")	+++ [1, 2, 3, 4]	+++ [6, 7, 8]
Simple diffusion of water molecules ("Diffusion permeability")	+ [1, 2, 3, 4]	+++ [8] ++ [9, 10]
Potency of different peptides	Vasotocin > oxytocin > vasopressin (see above)	Arg-vasopressin > lys-vasopressin > vasotocin > oxytocin (see above)
Enhancement of sodium transport and of short circuit-current	+++ [1, 2, 3, 4]	0 [7, 11]
Enhancement of permeability to urea (and some closely related solutes)	+++ [1, 2]	0 – ? (see above)
Simulation of antidiuretic hormone effect by cyclic adenosine-3', 5'-phosphate	+++ [3, 5]	0 (diuretic kidney) [12] +++ (isolated collecting duct) [8]
Simulation of effect by (high concentrations of) theophylline	++ [3, 5]	0 [3]
Simulation of permeability effect by angiotensin II – amide	0 [1]	+ [13]
Inhibition of sodium transport	0 [1]	+++ (see below)

References in brackets
1. Leaf (1965). 2. Ussing (1960) 3. Leaf (1967) 4. Orloff and Handler (1967). 5. Orloff *et al.* (1962). 6. Berliner and Bennett (1967). 7. Berliner (1961). 8. Grantham and Burg (1966). 9. Morel *et al.* (1965). 10. Ullrich *et al.* (1964). 11. Berliner (1961). 12. Alexander (1965). 13. Bonjour *et al.* (1967).

be confirmed (J. Heller and Lojda, 1960), that vasopressin and other antidiuretic hormones act by stimulating the secretion of hyaluronidase by a process of apocrine secretion from the cells of the collecting ducts. The hyaluronidase was supposed to act on a hyaluronic acid-containing intercellular cement and thus to open the pores necessary for an enhanced back-diffusion of water along the osmotic gradient. However, even if the basis of this reasoning had not been shaken by J. Heller and Lojda's findings, this interpretation is physico-chemically highly unlikely in view of the considerable disproportion between the size of pores needed for back-flow of water and the size of the intercellular clefts shown by Ginetzinsky *et al.*, as well as for many other reasons (Orloff and Handler, 1964). These arguments do not exclude the possibility that a liberation of hyaluronidase from cellular elements in the kidney plays a role in the causation of the antidiuretic effects of vasopressin. In ethanol-anesthetized rats in water diuresis intravenous injections of large doses of purified hyaluronidase have been shown to exert an antidiuretic effect correlated with the hyaluronidase activity excreted in the urine (Thorn et al., 1961).

FACTORS FAVORING THE CONCENTRATING EFFECT OF POSTERIOR PITUITARY PEPTIDES

The concentrating effect of drugs may be measured as the decrease of C_{H_2O}. Under particularily suitable circumstances the decrease of urine flow in water diuresis may be taken to reflect the decrease of C_{H_2O}. In conditions other than water diuresis, the concentrating effect should be expressed as the increase of $T^c_{H_2O}$, or, grossly, by the increase in urinary osmolarity. Its extent, according to the foregoing discussion, depends on four factors.

Intrinsic activity and affinity. The intrinsic activity of a drug or hormone in enhancing the permeability of the collecting ducts to water, and its affinity for the receptors are primary determinants of this action. Both parameters could be measured directly by microperfusion experiments. Little information is available on factors augmenting the permeability-increasing action of antidilutional hormones on renal tubules. This action may be influenced by the calcium concentration in tubular fluid. In dogs and in rats various posterior pituitary peptides have been found to enhance the urinary excretion of calcium (Thorn, 1961). There was a correlation between the antidiuretic and the calciuretic effects of arginine vasopressin, lysine vasopressin, lysine vasotocin and oxytocin. This observation was interpreted as indicating a role of intratubular calcium in the action of antidiuretic hormones. Other investigators (Fisch et al., 1965) did not find any change in renal calcium excretion after the injection of strongly antidiuretic doses of lysine vasopressin or arginine vasopressin into hydrated normal human subjects.

In microperfusion studies in the rat (Lassiter et al., 1965), addition of calcium to solutions circulated through the distal nephron resulted in a decrease in the water permeability of the tubular walls, i.e. in an action opposite to that of the antidiuretic hormones. The water permeability of proximal tubules proved completely insensitive to additions of calcium to the perfusing fluid. Lack of calcium in distal tubular fluid could, therefore, have the opposite effect and enhance the permeability-increasing effect. No experimental data are available on this point.

In contrast to the effect expected from these observations, the intravenous injection of moderate doses of calcium ions into hydrated rats induces a pronounced antidiuretic effect (Thorn et al., 1965). Since this effect is more pronounced when the calcium ions are injected into the carotid artery than after an intravenous injection, it may be assumed to be due to an enhanced secretion of vasopressin rather than to a direct renal action of calcium. Many observations, which cannot be discussed here, point to a role of calcium ions in the mechanism of vasopressin liberation from the posterior pituitary gland (see Chapter 5). Thus, the liberation of vasopressin from isolated posterior pituitary glands *in vitro* by increasing the potassium concentration of the medium ("depolarization"), occurs only in the presence of calcium ions (Douglas, 1963).

Lack of glucocorticosteroids has recently been shown to increase the water permeability of distal tubules in the rat (Wiederholt and Hierholzer, 1967). This effect could result in an enhanced permeability-increasing effect of antidiuretic hormones. A large number of arguments against the hypothesis of an antagonism between glucocorticosteroids and vasopressin (Peters, 1960) speak against this possibility.

The as yet unexplained observation that rats are more sensitive to the antidiuretic effect of vasopressin in spring and in summer than in autumn and in winter (H. Heller et al., 1957), may reflect changes in the permeability response to the hormones, but may also be due to other factors.

The same uncertainty prevails about the enhancement of the antidiuretic response to vasopressin by an acid load, i.e. by the infusion of a hypotonic solution of NH_4Cl in the dog and in man (Ullmann et al., 1965; Curtis and de Wardener, 1963), which contrasts with the depression of the antidiuretic response caused by an infusion of sodium bicarbonate. The observation, that sodium bicarbonate does not depress the so-called $Tm^c_{H_2O}$ measured under maximal mannitol infusion, is not necessarily a valid argument against the assumption of a change in the permeability response of the tubules. Loading with sodium bicarbonate also lowers the maximal urinary osmolarity in the dehydrated rat (Goodman and Levitin, 1965).

Ethanol anesthesia is frequently used in bioassays for antidilutional peptides in body fluids. This procedure, initiated by Jeffers et al. (1942) and popularized by Ames and van Dyke (1952), is based on observations which show an impairment of the secretion of vasopressin by ethanol (Jeffers et al., 1942; Ames and van Dyke, 1952; van Dyke and Ames, 1951). However, vasopressin release in response to such stimuli as hemorrhage or even pain, is not necessarily impaired by ethanol anesthesia (Ginsburg and Brown, 1956; Tata and Buzalkov, 1966). Ethanol anesthesia is supposed to prevent interference by endogenous vasopressin with the assay of antidiuretic activity in exogenous materials, and thus to enhance the specificity of bioassays. Several investigators have stated, however, that ethanol anesthesia also increased the sensitivity of water-loaded rats to the antidilutional effect of vasopressin (Ames and van Dyke, 1952; Czakes et al., 1964; Tata and Gauer, 1966). Ethanol-anesthetized water-loaded rats are approximately ten times more sensitive to exogenous vasopressin than similarly loaded unanesthetized animals (Fig. 3). The increase in sensitivity did not seem to have been related to

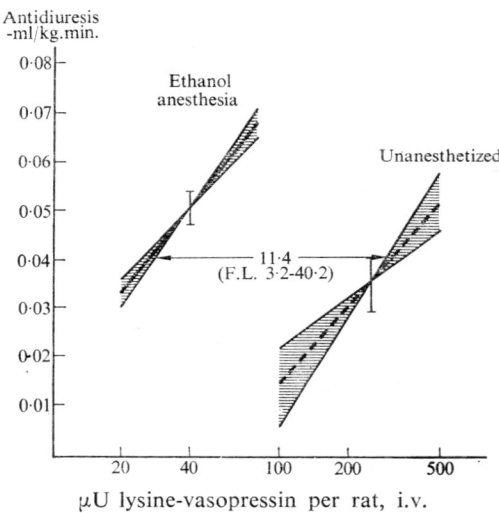

FIG. 3. Effect of ethanol anesthesia on the antidiuretic action of lysine vasopressin in rats. The shaded areas represent ± S.E. of the regression lines. The sensitization by ethanol has been calculated as a potency ratio which is shown, with its 95% fiducial limits, between the two regression lines (from Bonjour et al., 1967).

the level of endogenous vasopressin in the experiments summarized in Fig. 3, since both groups of animals, prior to the injection of vasopressin, excreted equal amounts of an equally dilute urine and, thus, presumably secreted endogenous vasopressin at the same rate. Furthermore, rats with hereditary hypothalamic diabetes insipidus ("Brattleboro rats"), anesthetized with ethanol, are twice as sensitive to exogenous vasopressin as ethanol-anesthetized normal rats (Sawyer and Valtin, 1967; Vierling et al., 1967; Valtin, 1967). Since ethanol anesthesia apparently also enhances the sensitivity of Brattleboro rats, which do not secrete vasopressin, its sensitizing effect cannot be due to the suppression of vasopressin secretion. Ethanol, therefore, must be assumed to increase the antidiuretic effect of vasopressin by another mechanism which may well be an enhancement of the permeability-increasing action of the antidiuretic hormone.

Medullary osmolarity. The efficacy of the mechanism responsible for the establishment of high sodium concentrations in medullary and papillary interstitial tissue water limits the maximal urinary osmolarity attained under the influence of vasopressin. If this mechanism is countercurrent-multiplication of sodium transport out of the ascending limb of Henle's loop, its performance would primarily depend on the rate of this transport, or on the permeability of the descending limb to sodium.

The efficacy of the medullary sodium-trapping mechanism may be assessed from experiments involving tissue analysis, or by measuring $T^c_{H_2O}$, i.e. the amount of water abstracted from fluid in the collecting ducts in excess of solute, in the presence of maximal amounts of antidilutional hormones, and of an adequate response to these compounds. $T^c_{H_2O}$ must, furthermore, be measured at a given rate of solute excretion and also at a given rate of sodium excretion (Berliner and Bennett, 1967).

An enhanced accumulation of sodium in medullary tissues due to an increased transport of sodium out of the ascending limb was originally thought to be responsible for the stimulation of the urinary concentrating effect of vasopressin by pretreatment with aldosterone in normal man (Crabbé, 1961). This effect of pretreatment with aldosterone may, however, quite as well be due to enhanced solute reabsorption from distal tubules and collecting ducts and a consequent decrease in volume flow through the collecting ducts (Crabbé, 1962; Berliner and Bennett, 1967). Unfortunately, it is not known whether exogenous aldosterone stimulates sodium reabsorption from collecting ducts of non-adrenalectomized mammals. Aldosterone re-establishes normal sodium reabsorption in the distal tubule of the rat after adrenalectomy (Hierholzer *et al.*, 1966), but does not accelerate sodium reabsorption in the non-adrenalectomized animal (Wiederholt *et al.*, 1966).

Similarly, an enhanced concentrating effect of vasopressin observed under certain circumstances as a result of a reduction in GFR was originally ascribed to more efficient medullary trapping of sodium as a consequence of more favorable rates of flow in the countercurrent-multiplier system of Henle's loop (Levinsky *et al.*, 1959a). Its real cause is, however, probably a reduction in volume flow through the concentrating segments of the nephrons (Berliner and Bennett, 1967). While relatively slight depressions of GFR enhance the urinary concentrating effect of vasopressin, large decreases have the opposite effect which must then probably be ascribed to a disturbance of the functions of the countercurrent-multiplier systems (Levinsky et al., 1959a).

Volume flow of fluid entering the medullary collecting ducts. The amount of water which can be abstracted from water-permeable collecting tubules is a function of the velocity of the establishment of high medullary sodium concentrations. For a given velocity of accumulation, the concentration of the final urine must therefore decrease with increasing rates of volume flow through the collecting ducts. This flow in turn, depends on the rate of entry of fluid into the distal tubules, the rate of abstraction of water from the distal tubules (if and when such an abstraction takes place), and finally, as pointed out by Berliner and Bennett (1967) as well as by Crabbé (1962), on the rate of solute reabsorption from the collecting tubules. Volume flow through the collecting ducts can be measured indirectly in micropuncture experiments.

Reduction of the volume of fluid running through the collecting ducts per unit time is probably responsible for the enhancement of the urinary concentrating effects of vasopressin by aldosterone. The same interpretation can be given to the improved antidiuretic effect of posterior pituitary hormones at low rates of GFR. As shown in the classical experiments of Berliner and Davidson (1957), reduction of GFR may result in the production of a slightly hypertonic urine even in the absence of endogenous vasopressin. This fact has many times been confirmed in human patients with pituitary diabetes insipidus, in whom GFR was depressed by dehydration (Coggins and Leaf, 1967). Similar observations were made in dogs (White and Heinbecker, 1938; Shannon, 1942a) and in rats (Fusco et al., 1966) with surgically induced hypothalamic diabetes insipidus. In rats with hereditary hypothalamic diabetes insipidus, dehydration may increase the concentration of the urine to values above 1100 mOsm/kg H_2O (Valtin, 1967). One is, however, somewhat disturbed by the finding that papillary and medullary interstitial osmolarity under these circumstances increases to a much greater extent than urinary osmolarity (Valtin, 1966, 1967). While this difference may be due to a smaller rate of passage of water through the medullary tissue, it could also denote an improved functioning of the countercurrent mechanism. Dehydration enhances the urinary concentrating effect of vasopressin in normal mammals of all the species investigated (Jones and de Wardener, 1956; Dicker, 1957; Orloff et al., 1958; Macfarlane et al., 1963; Roch-Ramel and Peters, 1967).

Concentration of urea in medullary and papillary interstitial tissue and amount of urea excreted in the urine. The maximal urinary concentrating effect of posterior pituitary peptides depends on the presence of adequate amounts of urea in medullary interstitial tissue which reach this site presumably from the collecting ducts. The back-diffusion of urea allows the urinary urea to be excreted largely in water already required for the excretion of other urinary solutes (Berliner *et al.*, 1958). There are, however, some doubts (Roch-Ramel and Peters, 1967), whether the whole amount of the medullary urea is freely diffusible and available for osmotic equilibration.

Besides this role of urea, high urinary concentrations of urea, for reasons not yet understood, allow non-urea solute to be concentrated (Gamble *et al.*, 1934; Crawford, Doyle and Probst, 1959; Bray and Preston, 1961). An increase in the renal excretion of urea considerably enhances the concentrating effect of vasopressin in states where the basic urea excretion is abnormally low, as e.g. in newborn infants, who normally excrete little urea because of their high nitrogen needs for protein anabolism (Edelmann *et al.*, 1960), or in men or animals fed on a protein-deficient diet (Epstein *et al.*, 1957 a, b). In the latter case the urinary urea excretion may be increased either by feeding protein or by giving urea by mouth. In normal dogs the enhancement of the urinary concentrating effect of vasopressin by urea is much smaller.

FACTORS DEPRESSING THE CONCENTRATING EFFECT OF NEUROHYPOPHYSIAL PEPTIDES

These factors may be considered in relation to their known or presumed mechanisms of action:

Factors depressing the intrinsic activity or the affinity of the peptides in relation to their ability to increase the water permeability of tubular walls. Removal of the sites of action of antidiuretic hormones by excision of the renal papilla in the rat (Kroon *et al.*, 1962) or in the golden hamster (Miller *et al.*, 1961) abolishes the ability to elaborate a concentrated urine.

A factor which should clearly affect the intrinsic activity or the affinity of the concentrating peptides for their membrane-receptors is the presence of specific antagonists, i.e. drugs which abolish the specific action without exerting themselves an opposite effect. A fairly large number of possibly specific antagonists to concentrating posterior pituitary principles has been proposed or described, but a specific antagonism against the action of vasopressin to increase the water permeability of parts of the mammalian nephron has not been demonstrated. Most "antagonists" have only been shown to depress or to abolish the decrease in urine flow induced by antidiuretic peptides. Such a depression may be due to the fact that "antagonists" inhibit tubular sodium reabsorption and thus increase urine flow without interfering with the tubular effect of the antidiuretic hormone. A pronounced natriuretic effect of "antagonists" may even depress the fall in C_{H_2O} induced by antidiuretic hormones, not by interfering with the permeability-increasing action, but by increasing volume flow through the concentrating sites of the nephron. An apparent "antagonist" may also act by interfering in other ways with the elaboration of a concentrated urine. Evidence on the antagonism to the antidiuretic action of posterior pituitary peptides is thus of doubtful value, as long as it has not been obtained by direct measurement of tubular water permeability by microperfusion techniques.

The antidiuretic action of arginine- or lysine-vasotocin in the frog is inhibited by 10–700 times higher doses of oxytocin, [1-Mercaptopropionic acid]-oxytocin (1-deamino-oxytocin), [Ile^8]-oxytocin or [Val^3]-oxytocin, i.e. peptides with a ring structure similar to that of vasotocin, whereas lysine-vasopressin, [Phe^3]-oxytocin (oxypressin) or [Phe^2, Lys^8]-vasopressin are ineffective in this respect (Morel and Jard, 1963). With the exception of oxytocin, the antagonistic peptides increase GFR and sodium excretion in frogs, so that their apparent antagonistic action may be related to this effect. Oxytocin itself could be a specific antagonist to the action of vasotocin in the frog, where it also antagonizes the antinatriuretic effect of the vasotocins. As discussed previously anti-natriuretic effects of posterior pituitary peptides do not occur in mammals.

The possibility of an antagonistic action of oxytocin against the antidilutional effects of vasopressin in mammals has aroused considerable interest in view of the evidence that the secretion of vasopressin may be accompanied by that of larger amounts of oxytocin. In non-anesthetized hydrated rats, oxytocin injected in doses two to eight times larger than those of vasopressin, given simultaneously or sometimes later, depressed the antidiuretic response measured by the decrease in urine flow (Brunner et al., 1956b). Given in a one to one ratio, oxytocin did not antagonize vasopressin antidiuresis (Ginsburg, 1956). An "antagonism" in relationship to urine flow was also observed in unanesthetized dogs (Pickford, 1961). In rats in ethanol anesthesia, the antidiuretic response to vasopressin was not depressed by oxytocin (Vorherr, 1964). The observed "antagonistic" responses to oxytocin were, presumably all related to its natriuretic activity: in man oxytocin neither elicits a natriuretic response (Brunner et al., 1957; Chalmers et al., 1951; Pickford, 1961), nor does it antagonize vasopressin antidiuresis (Vorherr, 1964). There is, thus, no evidence in favor of an antagonistic action against the primary permeability-increasing effect of antidilutional pituitary peptides.

Vasopressin-antagonists would be therapeutically important in the treatment of states of dilutional hyponatremia induced by inappropriate secretion of vasopressin. The testing of possible vasopressin antagonists has sometimes been limited to the search for an action against the pressor effect of vasopressin (Moyle and Chern, 1963). On the other hand, a series of derivatives of 2-amino-4-azido-6-phenyl-pyrimidine has been investigated systematically for their ability to reverse obliguria induced by exogenous vasopressin in the alcohol-saline-loaded rat (Hofmann, 1966). Among these derivatives the 5-ethoxyethyl-derivative (SC-16102) and the 5-(2)propionyl-derivative (SC-16100) caused a 50% reversal of vasopressin antidiuresis at doses lower than 1 mg/kg (Hofmann, 1966). Though other diuretics (e.g. hydrochlorothiazide) were ineffective as vasopressin antagonists in these tests, the antagonism of these phenylpyrimidine compounds did not appear to be specific, since both compounds had marked natriuretic and diuretic effects of their own.

In dogs, the antidiuretic effect of vasopressin is consistently depressed by pyrogens (Brandt et al., 1955). The nature of this antagonism is unknown. Some tranquillizers have been shown to increase urine flow in antidiuresis caused by dehydration in rats at doses which had no influence on urine flow after water-loading. This effect may represent an antagonism to the action of vasopressin or, more probably, to the secretion of vasopressin, or may be a phenomenon unrelated to vasopressin. The tranquillizers found effective were chlorpromazine, prochlorperazine, perphenazine, triflupromazine, trifluoperazine, fluphenazine, thioridazine, chlorprothixene and tetrabenazine. Large doses of phenobarbital had the same effect, while reserpine, meprobamate, chlordiazepoxide and diazepam were ineffective. An anti-concentrating effect was also shown by antidepressants like imipramine, desimipramine, amytryptiline, nortryptiline or the antidepressant monoamine-oxidase-inhibitors (Boris and Stevenson, 1967).

In dogs some cytostatic drugs suppress the antidiuretic effect of vasopressin by an unknown mechanism: thus cyclophosphamide and nor-nitrogen mustard have been shown to antagonize vasopressin antidiuresis, but also to exert a diuretic effect by themselves (Zedeck et al., 1966). In dogs with diabetes insipidus, an injection of a small dose of ethyleneimine has been shown to suppress the antidiuretic effect of exogenous vasopressin for 24 hr (Goldblatt et al., 1966). This response which might be an instance of a true and specific antagonism has not yet been further investigated. In man diphenylhydantoin enhances water excretion and C_{H_2O}, and lowers urinary osmolarity after a water load given to patients suffering from inappropriate secretion of vasopressin. In normal dehydrated subjects, it increases urine flow and depresses urinary osmolarity and $T^c_{H_2O}$. The drug probably inhibits the release, but may also antagonize the antidilutional effect of endogenous vasopressin (Fichman, 1966).

It is, thus, uncertain whether the so-called ADH (antidiuretic hormone) antagonists affect the water permeability-increasing effects. There are other factors which may do so. Overhydration, induced in man by drinking 5–10 liters of water per day for 3–10 days, results in an inadequate concentrative response to endogenous or to exogenous vasopressin during an ensuing period of dehydration (de Wardener and Herxheimer, 1957; Epstein et al., 1957a; Yoon and Hong, 1961; Habener et al., 1964). The hypothesis that hypo-osmolarity of body fluids may directly affect the permeability of tubular cells, is possibly supported by the observation of a decreased effect of vasopressin on osmotically induced water transport across the toad bladder when the serosal side of the tissue is bathed in a hypotonic solution (Hays and Leaf, 1961). In contrast to the observations in man, progressively increasing overhydration in rats, continued for 3 weeks with a daily water intake equal to the body weight during the last week, did not depress the maximal urinary osmolarity attained in a subsequent 72 hr period of dehydration and under the influence of large doses of exogenous vasopressin (Peters and Roch-Ramel, 1967). This may not represent a species difference: it could be due to the disappearance of the disturbance caused by overhydration during the period of dehydration. In man the disturbance caused by a 9 day course of overhydration proved readily reversible within 2 days (Yoon and Hong, 1961). While a primary effect of overhydration on tubular water permeability appears probable, the disturbance in concentrating ability could also be due to a washout of corticomedullary sodium- and urea-gradients by the long-continued water diuresis (Roch-Ramel and Peters, 1967).

An apparent "escape" from the urinary concentrating effect of vasopressin occurs in dogs (Davis et al., 1954; Levinsky et al., 1959b) or in man (Leaf et al., 1953) after long term treatment with vasopressin (given twice daily or daily as vasopressin tannate in oil), while the usual water intake is maintained by forced drinking or by infusions or gavage. In this situation the urine remains concentrated for 3–12 days: the subject retains water, gains weight and develops dilutional hyponatremia. After this initial period, the urine concentration decreases rapidly and the subject may come into water balance again despite the continued administration of vasopressin. That this train of events is no true "escape" phenomenon, is shown by the permanently elevated urinary osmolarity of dogs, given similar doses of vasopressin but drinking only as much water as they want (Levinsky et al., 1959b). The loss of the concentrating effect of vasopressin under these circumstances is probably due to the same mechanism as in simple overhydration. It appears improbable that enhanced secretion of aldosterone as a consequence of salt depletion contributes to the non-responsiveness to vasopressin, as originally supposed (Levinsky et al., 1959b), since excess aldosterone favors rather than depresses the antidilutional effect of vasopressin (Crabbé, 1961, 1962). An effect resembling that of chronic vasopressin administration plus water-loading in intact dogs may be produced more rapidly in an isolated dog kidney perfused from a normal donor animal (McDonald and de Wardener, 1965). Infusion of vasopressin, together with large amounts of either isotonic saline, or saline plus bovine albumin, into the donor dog induces the excretion of a hypotonic urine during periods of rising or of falling solute excretion by the isolated kidney.

The decrease in antidiuretic response to vasopressin induced in dogs (Ullmann et al., 1965) or in patients with pituitary diabetes insipidus (Czakes et al., 1961) by the infusion of bicarbonate solutions, may or may not represent a change in the permeability response of collecting ducts.

Old rats concentrate their urine less efficiently than younger animals. While some observers think that this deficiency is due to a decrease in vasopressin release in response to hyper-osmolarity (Friedman et al., 1960), others (Dicker and Nunn, 1958) demonstrated a depression of the antidiuretic response to exogenous as well as to endogenous vasopressin secreted at a normal rate in response to hypertonic stimuli. The mechanism of the renal non-responsiveness may possibly be a change in tubular permeability characteristics.

Factors interfering with the establishment of high medullary sodium concentration. Newborn infants (H. Heller, 1944, 1951, 1958; Thomson, 1944; Barnett et al., 1948; Ames, 1953; Calcagno et al., 1954; Edelmann et al., 1960; Poláček et al., 1965) or newborn rats (H. Heller, 1951, 1952, 1958; Dlouha et al., 1965; Dlouha, 1965; Yunibhand and Held, 1965) cannot concentrate their urine efficiently when dehydrated. The maximal urinary osmolarity in newborn infants is about half that in adults under similar conditions of dehydration (H. Heller, 1958), and still smaller in newborn rats. The main cause for this inability is a deficient response to the concentrating action of endogenous vasopressin which is practically ineffective in newborn infants or animals, reaches a measurable concentrating effect a short time after birth, but in rats attains its adult level only 23 days after birth and several months after birth in man. The lack of response to vasopressin is probably partly due to a deficient operation of the medullary sodium-concentrating system, i.e. presumably sodium transport out of the ascending limb or countercurrent-multiplication in Henle's loop. Medullary sodium concentrations in newborn and very young rats are considerably lower than in older or grown-up animals (Yunibhand and Held, 1965). The deficiency may be related to the relative shortness of Henle's loop in newborn mammals. The urea concentration in medullary tissue water is lowered much more conspicuously than the sodium concentration, when compared to adult values (Yunibhand and Held, 1965). While this depression of the urea concentration may be partly secondary to a disturbance of the sodium-concentrating mechanism, it is probably primarily and largely due to the low amount of urea excreted in the urine of newborn mammals, who use all their alimentary amino-nitrogen for their own protein anabolism. In newborn infants, the urinary concentration-response to dehydration and/or to exogenous vasopressin may be increased considerably, although not to normal adult values, by high protein-diets or by the feeding or the infusion of urea (Edelmann et al., 1960). By contrast, a restriction of fluid-intake does not improve the urinary concentrating ability in newborn infants. There is no reason to assume that non-responsiveness to vasopressin in newborn mammals could be due to an immaturity of the tubules, which would preclude an increase of permeability under the influence of exogenous vasopressin. If there is any immaturity of the tubules of the newborn infant, the deviation from the adult state should rather be in the sense of an increased permeability to water, since water diuresis is equally impaired in the newborn state. It is, however, quite possible that the inability of the terminal nephron walls to become impermeable to water in this state, is due to a lack of glucocorticosteroid secretion from the adrenals (H. Heller, 1958).

Potassium depletion is known to depress urinary concentrating ability in response to antidiuretic hormones (Brokaw, 1953; Dustan et al.,1956; Relman and Schwartz, 1956, 1958; Welt et al., 1960). The disturbance has often been ascribed to a decrease in water permeability of the collecting duct walls (Giebisch and Lozano, 1959; Rubini, 1961) partly because the most conspicuous pathological changes in potassium-depleted rats occur in the collecting ducts (Oliver et al., 1957; Spargo et al., 1960). The finding of osmotic equilibration between papillary interstitium and collecting duct fluid, both in the non-diuretic state and in mannitol diuresis, in K^+-depleted rats, excludes defective water permeability (Gottschalk et al., 1965; Bank and Aynedjian, 1964). In the dog and in man, potassium depletion may, however, depress the water permeability of collecting ducts (Jones et al., 1965).

Manitius *et al.* (1960a) and Levitin *et al.* (1960) found a considerable decrease in medullary and papillary tissue-sodium as well as urea-concentrations in potassium deficient rats which was sufficient to account for a depressed reabsorption of water from the collecting ducts. The deficient functioning of the medullary concentrating mechanism could not be due to a disturbance of ascending limb-sodium reabsorption: in potassium-depleted rats early distal tubular osmolarity was as low or lower than that in normal rats (Bank and Aynedjian, 1964; Gottschalk *et al.*, 1965). A greater rise in inulin concentrations along the proximal (and the distal) convolutions and an increased loss of urea from proximal tubular fluid (Jones *et al.*, 1965) of potassium-depleted rats point to an inadequate delivery of sodium, and presumably also of urea, to Henle's loop. A decrease in GFR in potassium depletion may contribute to this disturbance. Overhydration may also contribute to the urinary concentrating deficiency and the polyuria: potassium deficiency causes considerable thirst, presumably by direct chemical stimulation of thirst centers (Fourman and Leeson, 1959; Hollander *et al.*, 1957).

Renal disturbances in many ways comparable to those due to potassium depletion may be induced by hypercalcemia due to treatment with vitamin D (Epstein *et al.*, 1958; Sanderson, 1959) or with high acid phosphate—high calcium diets (Sanderson, 1959) in rats or to overtreatment with parathyroid extract in dogs (Epstein *et al.*, 1959). Similar changes occur in the so-called "hyperabsorption hypercalciuria", in hypercalciuria with sarcoidosis, in idiopathic hypercalciuria, in primary or iatrogenic hyperparathyroidism (Gill and Bartter, 1962) or osteolytic infiltration of bone, in the "milk-and-alkali"-syndrome, or finally in vitamin D-intoxication (Fourman and Leeson, 1959) in man. The concentrating deficiency may be related to the action of calcium ions, which antagonize the water permeability increasing effect of vasopressin on renal tubules. As in potassium deficiency, the major morphological lesions are found in the collecting ducts (Epstein *et al.*, 1958; Cohen *et al.*, 1957), but analysis of renal tissue showed a decrease in medullary sodium and urea concentrations (Manitius *et al.*, 1960b) smaller than that found in experimental potassium depletion. Hypercalcemia is also accompanied by considerably increased thirst.

Experimental protein deficiency, besides impairing water diuresis in rats, may also impair urinary concentrating ability: a decrease in urinary osmolarity was found in protein-deficient rats after 24 hr of dehydration (Dicker *et al.*, 1946), but could possibly have been due to a depressed secretion of vasopressin rather than to an impairment of the renal response to antidiuretic hormones, since other investigators (Guggenheim and Hegsted, 1953) found a prolonged antidiuretic response to exogenous vasopressin in protein-deficient rats.

On the other hand, protein-deficiency was found to cause histological lesions in the thick part or the ascending limb of Henle's loop, which might account for a primarily renal lack of response to vasopressin. Acute short periods of hunger, in rats, induce a lack of response to antidilutional hormones which results in a decrease in maximal urinary osmolarity after dehydration, even when exogenous vasopressin is given (Bauman et al., 1964).

While the urinary concentrating ability of adrenalectomized rats, maintained on isotonic saline, is not impaired (Peters, 1959a), hypophysectomy results in a concentrating deficiency apparently due mainly to non-responsiveness to antidilutional hormones (Bauman, 1965). The non-responsiveness may be due to an inadequate functioning of the medullary sodium-concentrating mechanism, which could be a consequence of the low values of GFR in hypophysectomized animals.

Severe salt restriction for 5 days in normal human subjects had no effect on maximal urinary concentration (Levitt et al., 1959), but salt deprivation, continued for more than one week in dogs, depressed maximal urinary osmolarity in the presence of exogenous vasopressin, and $T^c_{H_2O}$ measured during the infusion of exogenous vasopressin (Levinsky et al., 1959a; Goldsmith et al., 1961). The concentrating deficiency appears to be caused by inadequate concentration of sodium in medullary tissue due to decreased GFR.

Concentrating defects occur in patients with cirrhosis of the liver. These defects have been described (Vaamonde et al., 1965) as decreases in "$Tm^c_{H_2O}$" during mannitol infusion, with an undisturbed response of urinary osmolarity to dehydration as well as in precisely the opposite manner, i.e. as a decrease in maximal urinary osmolarity during dehydration and vasopressin administration with normal values for $T^c_{H_2O}$ (Jick et al., 1964). There is, thus, possibly more than one type of concentrating defect in cirrhosis of the liver, in which the secretion and metabolism of vasopressin is thought to be normal (Chaudhury et al., 1961).

A particular type of concentrating defect observed in patients with sickle cell anemia is thought to be due to a failure of the mechanism responsible for the establishment of high sodium concentrations in medullary interstitial tissue (Levitt et al., 1960).

Non-responsiveness to antidilutional hormones due to accelerated flow of fluid into and through the collecting ducts. Increased volume flow through the concentrating sites in the collecting ducts is presumably responsible for the well-known decrease in urinary osmolarity with increasing rates of solute excretion (Rapoport et al., 1949; Raisz et al., 1959; Giebisch et al., 1964). In osmotic diuresis induced by mannitol or by urea, the concentrating defect is furthermore enhanced by interference with sodium reabsorption from the ascending limb (Berliner and Bennett, 1967), while this factor should not intervene, when solute excretion is raised by infusions of hypertonic sodium chloride (Giebisch et al., 1964). Increased volume flow through the collecting ducts must be held responsible for all depressed responses to antidiuretic hormones in states of increased solute excretion per unit time.

A mechanism analogous to that of osmotic diuresis is thought to be responsible for the concentrating defect observed in many types of human renal disease (Bricker et al., 1959), as well as in the case of toxic destruction of renal tissue. In these states, in which a part of the nephron population is eliminated with a resulting increase in blood urea concentration, the remaining nephrons may show solute diuresis due to an increased load of filtered urea. Whenever the blood urea concentration or the ratio solute excretion: GFR is considerably increased, depressed antidilutional responses may be due to "osmotic" acceleration of volume flow through the collecting ducts.

Inadequate antidilutional responses due to an insufficient contribution of urea to urinary concentration. The contribution of urea to urinary concentration becomes inadequate, when the amount of urea delivered to the concentrating sites decreases substantially, or, when the permeability of collecting duct walls to urea falls to levels too low to allow a rapid equilibration. A decrease in the delivery of urea to the collecting ducts is thought to be responsible for the concentrating deficiency in rats (Hendrikx and Epstein, 1958) and in dogs (Levinsky and Berliner, 1959) fed on protein-deficient diets, as well as in normal newborn infants (Edelmann et al., 1960) or animals. A decrease in the collecting duct-permeability to urea is thought to be partially responsible for a particular type of concentrating deficiency observed in rats intoxicated with aristolochic acid (Peters and Hedwall, 1963). In this type of toxic renal damage, a decrease in GFR and a consequent decrease in delivery of sodium to the loops may contribute to the low osmolarity of medullary tissue.

If medullary tissue urea is partially bound or unavailable for diffusional exchanges because of sequestration into as yet unidentified compartments (Roch-Ramel and Peters, 1967), changes in the rate or in the type of sequestration might also cause considerable changes in the response to antidilutional hormones.

NATRIURETIC EFFECTS: GENERAL CONSIDERATIONS

Diuretic (Magnus and Schäfer, 1901) as well as antidiuretic effects of posterior pituitary extracts were discovered in an early period of endocrinology, in which a hormone had to be a pure messenger with a single message to transmit. When an antidiuretic action of posterior pituitary extracts had been established the diuretic action described by previous observers had to be false, because there could be only one true effect. This mental attitude is still expressed in Homer W. Smith's classical monograph of 1951, in which there are two separate discussions on the (enhancing) effects of the posterior pituitary extracts on electrolyte excretion, which is discussed as an established phenomenon, and on "the alleged diuretic action of Pitressin", which is rejected as uninterpretable. Such authoritative statements certainly blocked investigation. A more serious argument against studies on the natriuretic effect of neurohypophysial peptides may be doubts about the physiological role of these effects. The solution of this problem depends mainly on the answers to two questions:

Are the concentrations of posterior pituitary hormones in blood sufficiently large to produce natriuretic effects? The answer to this question depends on the evaluation of contradictory data and on additional assumptions. The results of most investigators appear to show that in the rat (Brunner *et al.*, 1956b, 1957; Peters, 1959b; Fraser, 1942; Croxatto and Labarca, 1958; Kuschinsky and Bundschuh, 1939) and in the dog (Brooks and Pickford, 1956; Abrahams and Pickford, 1954; Baird and Pickford, 1958; Pickford, 1956, 1960, 1961; Horster *et al.*, 1959), oxytocin is a markedly more potent natriuretic agent than the vasopressins. Figure 4 shows a comparison of natriuretic and antidiuretic potencies of oxytocin and vasopressin in hydrated rats under conditions, in which the natriuretic effect of vasopressin is exaggerated by acute overloading with water. Under these circumstances, oxytocin appears to be about ten times more potent than vasopressin as a natriuretic agent. In view of the great difference of the types of the natriuretic responses to both compounds, such comparisons are, however, somewhat arbitrary. By selecting other conditions one may very well arrive at the conclusion that the natriuretic potencies of oxytocin and vasopressin in the rat (Sawyer, 1952) or in the dog (Chan and Sawyer, 1961) are equal, but that both peptides differ in the type of the response which they elicit. One group of observers (Kramar *et al.*, 1966) described diuretic and chloruretic effects after such minute i.v. doses as 0.005–0.04 μU/rat of either natural or synthetic arginine-vasopressin, while larger doses induced the well known antidilutional and antidiuretic effects. The effects of such doses have not been studied by other investigators.

Oxytocin being probably the more important natriuretic hormone, the following considerations will be limited to this peptide. According to the observers quoted above, natriuretic doses of oxytocin in rats or in dogs vary from 5–100 mU/kg as a single intravenous or subcutaneous

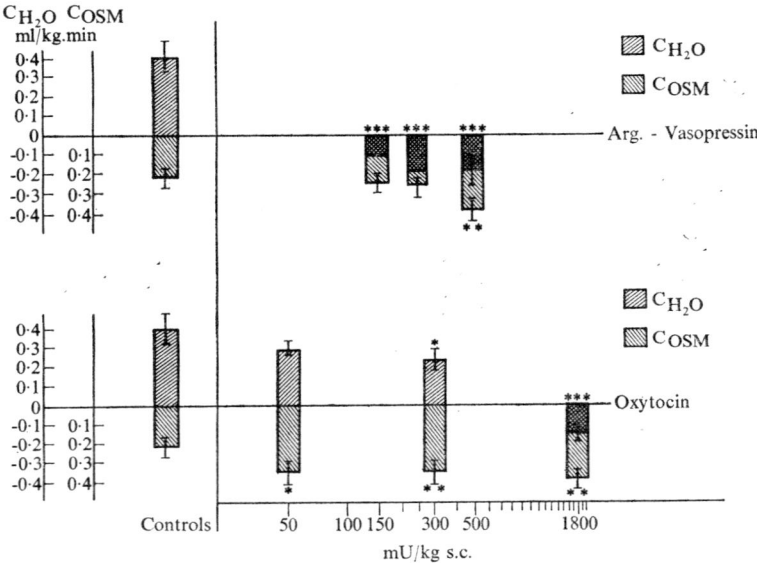

FIG. 4. Effects of arginine vasopressin and oxytocin on the excretion of free water and solutes in rats in water diuresis. Columns are means ±S.E. If C_{H_2O} is positive, urine flow $= C_{OSM} + C_{H_2O}$. If C_{H_2O} is negative, urine flow $= C_{OSM} - T^C_{H_2O}$. Single subcutaneous injections of natural arginine vasopressin or of synthetic oxytocin. Water diuresis induced by 50 ml water/kg by stomach tube, followed by 0.2 ml/rat/min of 0.3% glucose +0.1% NaCl i.v. Urine collection periods 60 min. after injections.

injection. Assuming distribution in the extra-cellular space and a fairly rapid inactivation, resulting in approximately half of the zero time concentration of oxytocin in blood throughout the ensuing period of urine collection, the oxytocin concentration necessary for inducing a natriuretic effect would range from 10–250 μU/ml plasma. Considering that the natriuretic effect of oxytocin may be considerably enhanced by pretreatment with cortisone in rats (Peters, 1959), and thus possibly also by over-secretion of endogenous corticosteroids, still lower concentrations may be sufficient to induce natriuresis and diuresis. Even without invoking such potential enhancing factors, one may state confidently, that the lower range of concentrations mentioned is well within limits that may be attained under physiological conditions. In view of the lack of sensitivity of the usual methods, there are few data on the oxytocin concentration in peripheral blood, in the absence of a stimulation of the neurohypophysis. Measurements in peripheral blood after different types of stimuli such as suckling and other mammary stimuli, the intracarotid or intravenous injection of hypertonic NaCl-solutions or the injection of nicotine into rabbits (B. A. Cross, 1951; Harris, 1947; Chaudhury and Walker, 1960) or in the dog (Abrahams and Pickford, 1954; Baird and Pickford, 1956, 1958, 1960), or else measurements of the concentration of both hormones in jugular vein blood of non-stimulated or stimulated men (Bisset et al., 1956; Bisset and Lee, 1957b) showed, that a given amount of released vasopressin was accompanied by a far greater amount of oxytocin. The relation of oxytocic to vasopressor-antidiuretic activity found by different investigators varied from 4 : 1 in the peripheral blood of human subjects stimulated by nicotine (Chaudhury and Walker, 1960), to 15-35:1 in the peripheral blood of rabbits after stimulation by narcotics or in dogs after the intracarotid injection of hypertonic saline (Abrahams and Pickford, 1954; Baird and Pickford, 1958), or under certain conditions in jugular vein blood of conscious human subjects (Bisset and Lee, 1957b), and up to 100 : 1 in jugular vein blood of man (Bisset et al., 1956), or in suckling antidiuresis in rabbits (B. A. Cross, 1951). The secretion and the peripheral concentrations of oxytocin, thus, appeared to exceed those of vasopressin in many conditions. However, there is also evidence in favor of a differential secretion of oxytocin and vasopressin. Thus, hemorrhage in rats raised the antidiuretic activity of blood without much effect on its oxytocic potency (Ginsburg and Smith, 1959). In thirsty rabbits the depletion of vasopressin from the posterior lobe was much greater than that of oxytocin (Lederis, 1962). In man (Gaitan et al., 1964) suckling and mammary duct dilatation appear to favor the secretion of oxytocin and to increase the oxytocin: vasopressin ratio in blood, while injections of hypertonic solutions or of nicotine favor the secretion of vasopressin and lower this ratio. If the concentration of vasopressin in peripheral blood is taken to be of the order of 3–5 μU/ml of plasma (Share, 1967), the concentration of oxytocin could lie somewhere between 10–50 μU/ml, i.e. in the natriuretic range, under conditions favoring the secretion of oxytocin. The natriuretic range may not be reached under conditions of preferential release of vasopressin.

Could the secretion of posterior pituitary peptides, and mainly of oxytocin, contribute to the regulation of the renal excretion of sodium and chloride? Could oxytocin play the role of a physiological natriuretic hormone? The *prima facie* answer to this question is negative: loss of posterior pituitary secretion induces diabetes insipidus, but has not been shown to induce sodium retention. Similarly, no conspicuous differences in sodium metabolism have been described between the states of surgically induced hypothalamic diabetes insipidus, in which both oxytocin and vasopressin secretion are suppressed, and hereditary hypothalamic diabetes insipidus of rats, in which no vasopressin is secreted, but oxytocin is thought to be secreted at least at a normal rate (Valtin, 1967). This statement, however, does not exclude a contribution of oxytocin to the maintenance of a normal balance of sodium in the organism, by enhanced urinary excretion of salt. It is clear from the present evidence that both major and auxiliary systems contribute to the regulation of renal sodium excretion. Major systems are the secretion of aldosterone from the adrenal cortex, and the possible production of a sodium excretory humoral factor of unknown nature in response to distension of the extracellular space. Modulating factors are renin and angiotensin which enhance sodium excretion in the presence of a distension of the extracellular space (Bonjour *et al.*, 1968), as well as various minor influences of glands with internal secretion as for example, the gonads, the thyroid and the parathyroids, and finally central nervous influences. Oxytocin, which in the rat (Brunner *et al.*, 1956b) as well as in normal (Horster *et al.*, 1959) or in hypophysectomized (Heidenreich *et al.*, 1966a, b) dogs has a greater relative natriuretic effect in a state of thirst and water deprivation than in the hydrated animal, may be an auxiliary factor contributing to the defense of body fluid osmolarity in states of dehydration. Its efficacy in this respect could be tested by studying the fate of oxytocin-deficient animals, as compared to oxytocin treated or normal animals during water deprivation. On the other hand, the physiological significance of an auxiliary regulating system can also be judged by experiments on animals deprived of their major regulating systems. As long as such experiments have not been done, it is difficult to evaluate the role of the renal natriuretic effect of oxytocin. Similar considerations apply to the natriuretic effect of larger doses of vasopressin which in some respects resemble those of angiotensin.

Since there are marked differences between the natriuretic effects of oxytocin and of vasopressin, the two hormones will be discussed separately. There are very few data on natriuretic effects of other natural or synthetic posterior pituitary peptides. In conscious dogs, the vasotocins, i.e. [Arg^8]- or [Lys^8]-oxytocin were found to have an oxytocin-like, although somewhat weaker natriuretic effect (Chan and Sawyer, 1961), while oxypressin, i.e. [3-phenylalanine]-oxytocin like arginine-vasopressin had very little natriuretic effect.

NATRIURETIC EFFECTS OF OXYTOCIN

Oxytocin may influence sodium and water excretion both by an ill-understood vascular effect which results in an increase in GFR and by a more commonly observed tubular action on sodium reabsorption.

Renal vascular effects of oxytocin. A renal vascular effect of oxytocin has been observed by Demunbrun *et al.* (1954) in dogs in which GFR and renal plasma flow had fallen very considerably in the chronic stage of diabetes insipidus induced by neurohypophysectomy. In such animals, oxytocin caused a rise in RPF and in GFR to normal values, while these parameters were not influenced by oxytocin in normal dogs. Similarly, Heidenreich *et al.* (1966a) found a considerable increase of GFR and RPF in totally hypophysectomized dogs, after injecting 15 to 150 mU/kg of oxytocin. These doses, again, had no effect in normal animals. The natriuretic effect of oxytocin was also much more conspicuous in hypophysectomized than in normal dogs (Heidenreich *et al.*, 1966b). Totally hypophysectomized dogs never show any symptoms of diabetes insipidus.

Though Demunbrun *et al.* (1954) interpreted their results in this sense, it appears improbable that oxytocin plays a major role in the maintenance of a normal value of renal blood flow and of GFR. Other investigators, who induced diabetes insipidus in dogs either by placing hypothalamic lesions or by neurohypophysectomy, and clinicians observing human pituitary diabetes insipidus, found that the state of diabetes insipidus was not accompanied by a reduction in GFR (Pickford and Ritchie, 1945; Shannon, 1942a). According to Shannon, GFR in diabetes insipidus dogs regularily fell as a result of dehydration and could be brought back to normal values by rehydration. On the other hand, Handley and Keller (1950) found a regular fall in both renal plasma flow and GFR in diabetes insipidus induced either by hypothalamic lesions or by neurohypophysectomy (Demunbrun *et al.*, 1954). This fall was attributed by Smith (1951) to either inadvertent dehydration of the experimental animals, or else to concomitant lesions of the anterior pituitary.

Though oxytocin then may not play an important role in the maintenance of normal blood flow in the kidney, it can apparently restore normal blood flow and GFR in dogs in which both values are lowered by loss of *anterior* pituitary secretions. The mechanism of this vascular action which by the token of an increase in GFR also increases sodium excretion, remains obscure for the time being. It is doubtful, whether a similar effect occurs in other species. In hypophysectomized rats, the clearance of endogenous creatinine is not significantly increased by oxytocin; in adrenalectomized rats there may be a slight but highly questionable increase; in adrenalectomized rats pretreated with cortisone, oxytocin causes a small (approximately 15%) increase in the excretion of endogenous creatinine (Peters, 1959a).

Less certain vascular effects of oxytocin were observed in species other than the dog under different conditions: Dicker and Heller (1946) found increases in the renal clearances of inulin (GFR) and of Diodone (RPF) in rats injected s.c. with 30 mU/rat of oxytocin. Since similar increases occurred after subcutaneous injections of 3 mU/kg of vasopressin, these increases which could not be reproduced under different conditions (unpublished observations), may have been due to the vasopressin-component of the pituitary extracts used in these experiments. In normal man (Mertz, 1960), intravenous injection of 3 U of oxytocin has been reported to increase the renal clearance of PAH by 30% in approximately one half of the subjects, without influencing GFR or the excretion of sodium and of water.

Tubular natriuretic effects of oxytocin. Tubular natriuretic and diuretic effects of oxytocin have been observed in the rat and in the dog, but neither in the mouse (Stelter, 1959) nor in man (Brunner et al., 1957; R. B. Cross et al., 1960; Mertz, 1960; Thomson, 1960). Curiously enough, oxytocin has been reported to increase the clearance of free water when given simultaneously with either ACTH or with glucocorticosteroids to patients suffering from inappropriate secretion of vasopressin due to a malignant tumor (Bernard-Weil, 1966). The increase in the clearance of free water obtained in these cases, was not accompanied by an enhanced excretion of sodium and was thought to be due to a depression of the secretion of vasopressin rather than to a renal effect.

In the rat, diuretic and natriuretic effects of oxytocin lasting one to three hours have been observed after the subcutaneous injection of 10–500 mU/kg of either purified natural or synthetic oxytocin (Fraser, 1937; Kuschinsky and Bundschuh, 1939; Fraser, 1942; Sawyer, 1952; Brunner et al., 1956a; Jacobson and Kellog, 1956; Berde and Cerletti, 1956; Croxatto and Labarca, 1958). Shorter-lasting effects are observed after single intravenous injections of the peptides, while continuous intravenous infusion of appropriate doses induced the same or more marked effects than the subcutaneous injection (unpublished observations). The additional urine excreted under the influence of the peptide tends to be isotonic or moderately hypertonic: urinary sodium and chloride concentrations generally increase moderately in rats in water diuresis, but decrease in dehydrated animals. The absolute increase in urine flow produced by oxytocin has been reported to attain its largest degree in animals hydrated with 0.05 M NaCl solutions (Sawyer, 1952), while the largest relative increases are observed in rats denied access to water for 6 hr or slightly longer (Brunner *et al.*, 1956a). Moderate dehydration enhances the relative, but not the absolute natriuretic and diuretic effect of oxytocin (Fraser, 1937; Brunner *et al.*, 1956a). Long-continued dehydration may depress or abolish the diuretic effect (Fraser, 1942).

When given to animals in water diuresis, moderate doses of oxytocin increase urinary solute output without depressing the clearance of free water (Fig. 4). According to classical concepts this observation should point to an inhibitory action of oxytocin on sodium reabsorption in the proximal tubules. The natriuretic action of oxytocin has not been studied with micropuncture methods until now. With larger doses of oxytocin, in water diuresis there is a simultaneous natriuretic and antidilutional action, the latter being due to an inherent weak "vasopressin-like" effect of oxytocin.

In the rat, the natriuretic action of oxytocin, thus, resembles that of angiotensin because of the "proximal" type of response in water diuresis (Bonjour *et al.*, 1968), as well as by an often isotonic increment in urine excretion. It differs markedly from that of angiotensin by its occurrence in the non-hydrated and even in the dehydrated state. While angiotensin, as well as vasopressin, has a natriuretic and diuretic effect only in animals overloaded with water and salt and with an expanded extracellular space (Bonjour *et al.*, 1968) and may, therefore, be supposed to exert their action by favoring the diuretic response to an expansion of the extracellular space, the action of oxytocin on the renal tubules appears to be independent of the control system responsible for maintaining the volume of the total extra-cellular space (Peters, 1967). Like the diuretic effect of angiotensin (Gross *et al.*, 1964) the tubular action of oxytocin in the rat depends on the presence of the adrenal glands (Peters, 1959a), but is not mediated through an enhanced secretion of glucocorticosteroids, which may exert natriuretic effects in rats. In adrenalectomized animals, the diuretic action of angiotensin can easily be restored by glucocorticosteroids (Gross *et al.*, 1964), while the restoration of the natriuretic effect of oxytocin is somewhat less easy (Peters, 1959), and may depend on treatment with glucocorticosteroids as well as on a partial repletion of salt losses.

The natriuretic and diuretic action of oxytocin in the dog resembles the effects observed in the rat by its occurrence in the dehydrated animal

(Horster et al., 1959; Abrahams and Pickford, 1954; Baird and Pickford, 1958; Brooks and Pickford, 1958; Chan and Sawyer, 1961; Heidenreich et al., 1966a, 1966b), as well as by the usually isotonic increment in urine excretion. A notable difference to the effect in the rat is seen in water diuresis, when the sodium excreting effect of oxytocin appears to be considerably depressed in comparison to that observed in animals loaded with moderate amounts of saline or in non-prehydrated animals (Abrahams and Pickford, 1954; Baird and Pickford, 1958; Brooks and Pickford, 1958; Pickford, 1961; Karvonen et al., 1953; Heidenreich et al., 1966a, b), though it may not be completely abolished (R. B. Cross, 1959). In dogs with surgically induced diabetes insipidus, oxytocin has been found to lose its diuretic and natriuretic activity (Brooks and Pickford, 1958). There are no comparable data in rats. Like in man, oxytocin in the dog apparently increases renal plasma flow as measured by the renal clearance of para-aminohippurate (Brooks and Pickford, 1958; Baird and Pickford, 1958; Pickford, 1961) without necessarily increasing GFR. Other observers found a consistent increase in GFR with higher doses of oxytocin (Ali, 1958). It is not clear, whether there are any relations between the increase in the renal clearance of para-aminohippurate and the presumably tubular natriuretic effect of oxytocin in the dog.

The statement that the natriuretic and diuretic effects of oxytocin are apparently independent of the natriuretic reaction to expansion of the extra-cellular space, does not mean that oxytocin acts directly on the kidneys. There are no reported observations on the effect of unilateral injections or infusions of oxytocin into one renal artery which could demonstrate such an action. On the contrary, Brooks and Pickford (1958) found in dogs that small doses of oxytocin, which did not elicit any notable action when given by the intravenous route, had a pronounced natriuretic and diuretic effect when injected into the carotid artery. The diuretic action of the peptide could, thus, be due to the liberation of an as yet unidentified diuretic principle. The marked diuretic effect of oxytocin injected in cats into the cerebrospinal fluid (Vaneček et al., 1960) may support this interpretation.

A very different role is, however, ascribed to oxytocin by Cort and his collaborators (Cort and Lichardus, 1963a, b; Cort et al., 1966) who studied the renal functions of cats during occlusion of the carotid artery. The well-known carotid sinus pressor reflex, in this species, is accompanied by a very marked tubular natriuretic and diuretic effect which occurs simultaneously with a slight increase in GFR. Both effects may, however, be dissociated experimentally. Like the tubular natriuretic and diuretic effect of an expansion of the intravascular space by infusions of dextran-solutions (Cort and Lichardus, 1963c), the diuretic response to carotid occlusion is abolished by cervical, but not by subdiaphragmatic section of the vagus. The diuretic response to carotid occlusion is abolished by lesions in the posterior nucleus of the hypothalamus, but may not be elicited by stimulation of this structure (Cort and Lichardus, 1963b). The posterior nucleus of the hypothalamus is, thus, thought to maintain a normal rate of tubular sodium reabsorption and to be inhibited by occlusion of the carotid artery. It may possibly exert its sodium-conserving function by restraining the secretion of oxytocin from the posterior pituitary. In favor of this assumption is the finding that the natriuretic response to carotid occlusion in the cat may be inhibited by some peptides which are partial specific antagonists of oxytocin, such as [2-O-methyltyrosine]-oxytocin, [2-O-ethyltyrosine]-oxytocin or [2-p-ethylphenylalanine]-oxytocin (Cort et al., 1966). Oxytocin did not depress the natriuretic effect to carotid occlusion, but exerted by itself an analogous natriuretic effect. Some peptides like [2-phenylalanine]-oxytocin, [2-p-aminophenylalanine]-oxytocin, or [2-O-methyltyrosine, 8-lysine]-vasopressin had the same effects as oxytocin. This interpretation which is based on fairly indirect evidence would suggest that oxytocin is a physiological diuretic and natriuretic principle. The arguments in favor and against this possibility have already been discussed (pp. 255–258).

Other renal effects of oxytocin. In rats pretreated and "sensitized" by estrogens and progesterone or estrogens alone, intravenous injections of diuretic doses of oxytocin induce extensive renal cortical necrosis which, histologically, looks like multiple cortical infarction (Byrom and Pratt, 1959). This particular vascular toxic action does not depend on the presence of the adrenals, and can also be elicited in adrenalectomized animals, treated first with estrogens and then injected with either oxytocin or a non-purified posterior pituitary extract (Kovács and Dávid, 1963). It never occurs in normal non-pretreated rats, but curiously enough may also be produced by pretreatment with corticotrophin followed by injections of posterior pituitary extracts (Kovács and Dávid, 1963).

NATRIURETIC AND DIURETIC EFFECTS OF VASOPRESSIN

From countless observations in non-hydrated and dehydrated mammals and man, it is quite clear that small, moderate and even high doses of vasopressin do not increase urine flow or sodium excretion. Similarly, in a large number of studies designed to measure "$Tm^c_{H_2O}$" and carried out usually after some dehydration, vasopressin has never been observed to enhance sodium excretion. In the absence of overhydration, vasopressin, thus, does not appear to exert an inhibitory effect on tubular sodium reabsorption.

A natriuretic and chloruretic effect of vasopressin, often accompanied by an enhanced excretion of potassium, appears, however, often, though not under all circumstances in water-loaded mammals. The doses of vasopressin necessary to elicit this effect are generally higher than the smallest antidilutional doses: thus it might be argued that the natriuretic effect of vasopressin is "pharmacological".

Natriuretic effects in animals loaded or overloaded with water or hypotonic solutions have been demonstrated in the rat (Sawyer, 1952; Brunner et al., 1956a; Jacobson and Kellog, 1956; Kramar et al., 1966), and in the dog (Karvonen et al., 1953; Davis et al., 1954; Chan and Sawyer 1961; Baisset et al., 1959a, b; Perlmutt, 1961). As shown by Chan and Sawyer, the occurrence or non-occurrence of a natriuretic effect of a given dose of vasopressin depends on the rate of water diuresis: while arginine vasopressin proved markedly natriuretic in brisk water diuresis, there was no such effect at low rates of urine flow after water loading. Since the rate of urine flow in water diuresis depends directly on the volume of the water load administered, this relationship probably is an expression of the dependence of the natriuretic effect of vasopressin on the prior or simultaneous expansion of the extra-cellular space and other body compartments. Natriuretic effects of vasopressin in water diuresis were also demonstrated in sheep (Kuehn and Peeters, 1965) and in man (Leaf et al 1953; Jaenike and Waterhouse, 1961; Barraclough and Jones, 1962; Schroeder et al., 1966). In man, the continued administration of relatively small doses of vasopressin (1 U/12 hr, as Pitressin tannate in oil) first induces water retention without natriuresis; on the 2nd or on the 3rd day of water retention, urinary sodium and chloride excretion increase considerably, while after cessation of vasopressin administration, there is first a large water diuresis followed by a fall of the urinary sodium and chloride excretions below the control level (Leaf et al., 1953). These results were interpreted to mean that "the increased excretion of sodium and chloride is the result of water retention, and not a direct effect of Pitressin". The data do not warrant this conclusion. In fact, it was shown by these experiments, that the natriuretic effect of vasopressin depends on prior water retention, but not that it is due to the water retention and would have occurred even in the absence of vasopressin. The events after cessation of vasopressin administration in such experiments show the contrary.

Thus, the natriuretic effect of vasopressin in rats, dogs, sheep and in man appears to depend on a preliminary retention of water, or of water and salt like the natriuretic effect of angiotensin in the rat. Like angiotensin, vasopressin might act by facilitating the natriuretic response to an expansion of the extra-cellular space. This action may, on the one hand, facilitate the maintenance of water and salt homeostasis under conditions of overloading with salt, but will, on the other hand, facilitate the occurrence of dilutional hyponatremia in cases of inappropriate secretion of vasopressin. It has also been shown in man, that vasopressin, like angiotensin, has a much more pronounced natriuretic effect in hypertensive than in normal subjects (Barraclough and Jones, 1962). This natriuretic effect in hypertensive subjects results in a smaller gain in weight and in larger urine volumes, in a greater fall in plasma sodium concentration and in more marked symptoms of water intoxication than in normal subjects (Barraclough and Jones, 1962).

That expansion of the extra-cellular space rather than of other body compartments may be the prerequisite of the natriuretic action of vasopressin is suggested by observations in the rat, which show that the natriuretic action of vasopressin is enhanced to a greater degree by loading with isotonic saline solutions than by loading with water or hypotonic solutions (Brunner et al., 1956a; Jacobson and Kellog, 1956). It has been shown that loading with equal volumes of an isotonic saline solution and of hypotonic solutions results in a much greater expansion of the extra-cellular space with the isotonic than with the hypotonic loading fluid (Bonjour et al., 1968).

While depending on a preliminary expansion of the extracellular space, the natriuretic action of angiotensin in the rat is also influenced by the rate of sodium excretion before the administration of the peptide. The natriuretic effect is greater at high rates of sodium excretion than at low rates (Bonjour et al., 1968). Though vasopressin has not been studied under comparable conditions, some observations suggest that vasopressin is also more natriuretic under conditions of high sodium excretion. Thus, pituitary extracts have been shown to enhance considerably the sodium excretion, to prevent a rise in serum sodium concentrations, and to prolong the survival of rats and dogs chronically overloaded with hypertonic sodium chloride solutions (Baïsset et al., 1958a, b, 1959a, b). Similarly, sodium excretion is enhanced, the rise of serum sodium concentration diminished and the subjective well-being improved in human volunteers submitted to simulated "drinking of sea-water" (Baïsset et al., 1959c). While enhanced sodium excretion was clearly demonstrated in these experiments, the amount of expansion of the extracellular space cannot be judged from the published data. Since these experiments were done with posterior pituitary extracts, the oxytocin present in these extracts may have contributed to a greater or a smaller extent to the observed natriuretic effects. Vasopressin, thus, exerts natriuretic effects which resemble those of angiotensin. These effects are often overshadowed by the very potent antidilutional effect which angiotensin does not share, save under exceptional circumstances (Bonjour *et al.*, 1968). Even under conditions favoring the natriuretic action of vasopressin, small doses usually do not exert a natriuretic action. A report on natriuretic effects of very small doses in rats (Kramar *et al.*, 1966) contradicts this statement, but needs confirmation.

REFERENCES

BOOKS, REVIEWS, AND MONOGRAPHS

BERLINER, R. W. (1961). Mechanisms involved in the formation of diluted and concentrated urine. *Néphrologie. C. R. du 1er Congrès International de Néphrologie à Genève et Evian*, pp. 5–12. Richet, G. (ed.). Karger, Basle.

DODD, J. M., PERKS, A. M. and DODD, M. H. I. (1966). Physiological functions of neurohypophysial hormones in sub-mammalian vertebrates. *The Pituitary Gland*, vol. 3. pp. 578–623. Harris, G. W. and Donovan, B. T. (eds.). Butterworths, London.

HELLER, H. (1951). The water metabolism of newborn infants and animals. *Archs Dis. Childh.*, **26**: 195–204.

HELLER, H. (1958). Die Hypophysenhinterlappen- und Nebennierenrindenhormone während der ersten Lebenszeit im Zusammenhang mit der Regulation des Wasserhaushaltes. *Mschr., Kinderheilk.*, **106**: 81–87.

LEAF, A. (1965). Transepithelial transport and its hormonal control in toad bladder. *Ergebn. Physiol.*, **56**: 216–263.

LEAF, A. (1967). Membrane effect of antidiuretic hormone. *Amer. J. Med.*, **42**: 745–756.

LEDERIS, K. (1962). The distribution of vasopressin and oxytocin in hypothalamic nuclei. *Mem. Soc. Endocr.*, **12**: 227–244.

LILIENFELD, L. S. and MANGANZINI, H. C. (1961). Regulation of medullary blood flow. *Néphrologie. C. R. du 1er Congrès International de Néphrologie à Genève et Evian*, pp. 562–563. Richet, G. (ed.). Karger, Basle.

ORLOFF, J. and HANDLER, J. S. (1967). The role of adenosine-3′5′-phosphate in the action of antidiuretic hormone. *Amer. J. Med.*, **42**: 757–768.

PETERS, G. (1960). *Nebennierenrinden-Inkretion und Wasser-Elektrolythaushalt. Befunde und Deutungen*. G. Thieme, Leipzig.

PICKFORD, M. (1956). Antidiuresis. *Modern Views on the Secretion of Urine. The Cushny Memorial Lectures*, pp. 128–147. Winton, F. R. (ed.). Churchill, London.

PICKFORD, M. (1961). Some extrauterine actions of oxytocin. *Oxytocin*, pp. 68–79. Caldeyro-Barcia, R. and Heller, H. (eds.). Pergamon Press, Oxford.

SAWYER, W. H. (1967). Evolution of antidiuretic hormones and their functions. *Amer. J. Med.* **42**: 678–686.

SMITH, H. W. (1951). *The Kidney. Structure and Function in Health and Disease* pp. 262–263, 284–286. Oxford University Press, New York.

VALTIN, H. (1967). Hereditary hypothalamic diabetes insipidus in rats (Brattleboro strain). A useful experimental model. *Amer. J. Med.*, **42**: 814–827.
WIRZ, H. (1956b). The location of antidiuretic action in the mammalian kidney. *The Neurohypophysis*, pp. 157–169. Heller, H. (ed.). Butterworths, London.

ORIGINAL PAPERS

ABRAHAMS, V. C. and PICKFORD, M. (1954). Simultaneous observations on the rate of urine flow and spontaneous uterine movements in the dog and their relationship to posterior lobe activity. *J. Physiol., Lond.*, **126**: 329–346.
ALEXANDER, C. S., (1965). The effect of 3′-5′-cyclic AMP and other nucleotides on urine flow and hemodynamics in the rat. (Abstract). *J. Clin. Invest.*, **44**: 1025.
ALI, M. N. (1958). A comparison of some activities of arginine vasopressin and lysine vasopressin on kidney function in conscious dogs. *Brit. J. Pharmacol. Chemother.*, **13**: 131–137.
AMES, R. G. (1953). Urinary water excretion and neurohypophysial function in full term and premature infants shortly after birth. *Pediatrics*, **12**: 272–281.
AMES, R. G. and VAN DYKE, H. B. (1952). Antidiuretic hormone in the serum and plasma of rats. *Endocrinology*, **50**: 350–359.
ASSALI, N. S., DIGNAM, W. J. and LONGO, L. (1960). Renal function in human pregnancy. III. Effects of antidiuretic hormone (ADH) on renal hemodynamics and water and electrolyte excretion near term and post partum. *J. Clin. Endocrinol. Metab.*, **20**: 581–592.
BAIRD, S. and PICKFORD, M. (1958). The simultaneous occurrence of certain changes in uterine and renal activity in dogs and the role of oxytocin in these phenomena. *J. Physiol., Lond.*, **144**: 80–91.
BAÏSSET, A., DEMONTE, H. and MONTASTRUC, P. (1958a) Rôle favorable des extraits posthypophysaires dans la surcharge sodique. Nouveaux arguments. *C. R. Séance Soc. Biol.*, **152**: 1593–1597.
BAÏSSET, A., DEMONTE, H. and MONTASTRUC, P. (1958b). Effets de l'extrait posthypophysaire chez l'Homme en surcharge saline. *C. R. Séanc. Soc. Biol.*, **152**: 1813–1816.
BAÏSSET, A., DEMONTE, H. and MONTASTRUC, P. (1959a). Action des extraits posthypophysaires et de la désoxycorticostérone dans la surcharge sodique. *Path. Biol., Paris*, **7**: 815–827.
BAÏSSET, A., DEMONTE, H. and MONTASTRUC, P. (1959b). Recherches sur l'hormone antidiurétique. *Toulouse Méd.*, **60**: 71–91.
BAÏSSET, A., MONTASTRUC, P. and DEMONTE, H. (1959c). L'homme peut-il boire de l'eau de mer? Mise en évidence de l'action favorable des extraits posthypophysaires sur le naufragé de laboratoire. *Nature, Paris*, **1959c**: 307–311.
BANK, N. and AYNEDJIAN, H. S. (1964). A micropuncture study of the renal concentrating defect of potassium depletion. *Amer. J. Physiol.*, **206**: 1347–1354.
BARNETT, H. L., HARE, K., NAMARA, H. M. and HARE, R. (1948). Measurement of glomerular filtration rate in premature infants. *J. Clin. Invest.*, **27**: 691–699.
BARRACLOUGH, M. A. and JONES, N. F. (1962). Effect of fluid retention following vasopressin on sodium excretion by hypertensive subjects. *Clin. Sci.*, **23**: 433–440.
BAUMAN, J. W. JR. (1965). Effect of hypophysectomy on the renal concentrating ability of the rat. *Endocrinology*, **77**: 496–500.

BAUMAN, J. W. JR., GUYOT-JEANNIN, C. and DOBROWOLSKI, J. (1964). Nutritional state and urine concentrating ability in the rat. *J. Endocrinol.*, **30**: 147–148.
BERDE, B. and CERLETTI, A. (1956). Über die antidiuretische und diuretische Wirkung von synthetischem Oxytocin im Wasserdiureseversuch an Ratten. *Helv. Physiol. Pharmac. Acta*, **14**: 129–134.
BERLINER, R. W. and BENNET, C. M. (1967). Concentration of urine in the mammalian kidney. *Amer. J. Med.*, **42**: 777–789.
BERLINER, R. W. and DAVIDSON, D. G. (1957). Production of hypertonic urine in the absence of pituitary antidiuretic hormone. *J. Clin. Invest.*, **36**: 1416–1427.
BERLINER, R. W., LEVINSKY, N. G., DAVIDSON, D. G. and EDEN, M. (1958). Dilution and concentration of the urine and the action of antidiuretic hormone. *Amer. J. Med.*, **24**: 730–744.
BERLYNE, G. M. (1960). Urinary hyaluronidase. *Nature, Lond.*, **185**: 389–390.
BERNARD-WEIL, E. (1966). Effets de l'oxytocine dans les syndromes de sécrétion inappropriée d'hormone antidiurétique, et en particulier chez les malades cancéreux. *Schweiz. med. Wschr.*, **96**: 212–217.
BISSET, G. W. and LEE, J. (1957a). An improved method for extracting oxytocin and antidiuretic hormones from blood. *Lancet*, **i**: 1173–1174.
BISSET, G. W. and LEE, J. (1957b). Oxytocic and antidiuretic activity in blood from the conscious subject. *Lancet*, **ii**: 770–772.
BISSET, G. W., LEE, J. and BROMWICH, A. F. (1956). Oxytocic and antidiuretic activity in blood from the internal jugular vein in man. *Lancet*, **ii**: 1129–1132.
BONJOUR, J. PH., PETERS, G., CHOMETY, F. and REGOLI, D. (1967). Renal effects of val_5-angiotensin II-amide, vasopressin and diuretics in the rat, as influenced by water diuresis and by ethanol anesthesia. *Eur. J. Pharmac.*, **2**: 88–105.
BONJOUR, J. PH., REGOLI, D., ROCH-RAMEL, F. and PETERS, G. (1968). Prerequisites for the natriuretic effect of val_5-angiotensin II-amide in the rat. *Amer. J. Physiol*, **215**: 1133–1138.
BORIS, A. and STEVENSON, R. H. (1967). The effects of some psychotropic drugs on dehydration-induced antidiuretic hormone-activity in the rat. *Archs Int. Pharmacodyn. Thér.*, **166**: 486–498.
BRANDT, J. L., RUSKIN, H. D., ZUMOFF, B., CASTLEMAN, L. and ZUCKERMAN, S. (1955). Inhibition of renal tubular responsiveness to antidiuretic hormone by pyrogens. *Proc. Soc. Exp. Biol. Med.*, **88**: 451–453.
BRAY, G. A. and PRESTON, A. S. (1961). Effect of urea on urine concentration in the rat. *J. Clin. Invest.*, **40**: 1952–1960.
BRICKER, N. S., DEWEY, R. R., LUBOWITZ, H., STOKES, J. and KIRKENSGAARD, T. (1959). Observations on the concentrating and diluting mechanism of the diseased kidney. *J. Clin. Invest.*, **38**: 516–523.
BROKAW, H. (1953). Renal hypertrophy and polydipsia in potassium-deficient rats. *Amer. J. Physiol.*, **172**: 333–346.
BROOKS, F. P. and PICKFORD, M. (1956). The influence of posterior lobe hormones on the excretion of Na and K in the conscious dog. *J. Physiol., Lond.*, **131**: 33P.
BROOKS, F. P. and PICKFORD, M. (1958). The effect of posterior pituitary hormones on the excretion of electrolytes in dogs. *J. Physiol., Lond.* **142**: 468–493.
BRUNNER, H., KUSCHINSKY, G., MÜNCHOW, O. and PETERS, G. (1957). Der Einfluss von natürlichem und synthetischem Oxytocin auf endogene Kreatinin-Clearance, Salzausscheidung und Säureausscheidungsfähigkeit der Ratte und auf die Diurese des Menschen. *Arch. Exp. Path. Pharmak.*, **230**: 80–89.
BRUNNER, H., KUSCHINSKY, G. and PETERS, G. (1956a). Die Wirkung von Vasopressin

auf die renale Wasser- und Salzausscheidung der Ratte bei Veränderungen der Salzkonzentration des Trinkwassers und nach Nierenparenchymresektionen. *Arch. Exp. Path. Pharmak.*, **228**: 434–456.
BRUNNER, H., KUSCHINSKY, G. and PETERS, G. (1956b). Der Einfluss von Oxytocin auf die renale Wasser- und Salzausscheidung der Ratte. *Arch. Exp. Path. Pharmak.*, **228**: 457–473.
BYROM, F. B. and PRATT, O. E. (1959). Oxytocin and renal cortical necrosis. *Lancet*, **1**: 753–755.
CALCAGNO, P. L., RUBIN, M. I. and WEINTRAUB, D. H. (1954). Studies on the renal concentrating and diluting mechanisms in the premature infant. *J. Clin. Invest.*, **33**: 91–96.
ČAPEK, K., FUCHS, G., RUMRICH, G. and ULLRICH, K. J. (1966). Harnstoffpermeabilität der corticalen Tubulusabschnitte von Ratten in Antidiurese und Wasserdiurese. *Pflügers Arch. ges. Physiol.*, **290**: 237–249.
CHALMERS, T. M., LEWIS, A. A. G. and PAWAN, G. L. S. (1951). The effect of posterior pituitary extracts on the renal excretion of sodium and chloride in man. *J. Physiol., Lond.*, **112**: 238–242.
CHAN, W. Y. and SAWYER, W. H. (1961). Saluretic activity of neurohypophysial peptides in conscious dogs. *Amer. J. Physiol.*, **201**: 799–803.
CHAUDHURY, R. R., CHUTTANI, H. K. and RAMALINGASWAMI, V. (1961). The antidiuretic hormone and liver damage. *Clin. Sci.*, **21**: 199–203.
CHAUDHURY, R. R. and WALKER, J. M. (1960). The fate of injected oxytocin in the rabbit. *J. Endocrinol.*, **19**: 189–192.
CLAPP, J. R. and ROBINSON, R. R. (1966). Osmolarity of distal tubular fluid in the dog. *J. Clin. Invest.*, **45**: 1847–1853.
COGGINS, C. H. and LEAF, A. (1967). Diabetes insipidus. *Amer. J. Med.*, **42**: 807–813.
COHEN, S. I., FITZGERALD, M. G., FOURMAN, P., GRIFFITHS, W. J. and DE WARDENER, H. E. (1957). Polyuria in hyperparathyroidism. *Quart. J. Med.*, **26**: 423–431.
CORT, J. H. and LICHARDUS, B. (1963a). The effect of the carotid sinus pressor reflex on renal function and electrolyte excretion. On the nature of the afferent signal. *Physiologia bohemoslov.*, **12**: 291–299.
CORT, J. H. and LICHARDUS, B. (1963b). The role of the hypothalamus in the renal response to the carotid sinus pressor reflex. *Physiologia bohemoslov.*, **12**: 389–396.
CORT, J. H. and LICHARDUS, B. (1963c). The effect of cervical vagotomy and posterior hypothalamic lesions on the saluretic response to dextran infusion. *Physiologia bohemoslov.*, **12**: 300–303.
CORT, J. H., RUDINGER, J., LICHARDUS, B. and HAGEMANN, I. (1966). Effects of oxytocin antagonists on the saluresis accompanying carotid occlusion. *Amer. J. Physiol.*, **210**: 162–168.
CRABBÉ, J. (1961). Stimulation by aldosterone of sodium transport in the loops of Henle. *Nature, Lond.*, **191**: 817.
CRABBÉ, J. (1962). The role of aldosterone in the renal concentration mechanism in man. *Clin. Sci.*, **23**: 39–46.
CRAWFORD, J. D., DOYLE, A. P. and PROBST, J. H. (1959). Service of urea in renal water conservation. *Amer. J. Physiol.*, **196**: 545–548.
CROSS, B. A. (1951). Suckling antidiuresis in rabbits. *J. Physiol., Lond.*, **114**: 447–453.
CROSS, R. B. (1959). Quoted by M. PICKFORD (1961).
CROSS, R. B. (1964). The effects of osmotic diuresis and vasopressin on the distribution of sodium, potassium and urea in the rat kidney. *Aust. J. Exp. Biol. Med. Sci.*, **42**: 523–527.

Cross, R. B., Dicker, S. E., Kitchin, A. H., Lloyd, S. and Pickford M. (1960). The effect of oxytocin on the urinary excretion of water and electrolytes in man. *J. Physiol., Lond.*, **153**: 553-561.
Cross, R. B. and Sherrington, L. A. (1965). The effect of vasopressin on water distribution in the rat kidney. *Austr. J. Exp. Biol. Med. Sci.*, **43**: 505-510.
Croxatto, H. and Labarca, E. (1958). Die Wirkung von synthetischem Oxytocin (Syntocinon) und Acetazolamid auf die Ausscheidung von Wasser, Natrium und Kalium. *Experientia*, **14**: 339-341.
Curtis, J. R. and de Wardener, H. E. (1963). Effect of urinary pH on the changes in urine concentration produced by vasopressin. *Clin. Sci.*, **24**: 159-166.
Czakes, J. W., Eliakim, M. and Ullmann, T. D. (1961). Diminished antidiuretic response to pitressin in diabetes insipidus during the infusion of sodium bicarbonate solution. *J. Lab. Clin. Med.*, **57**: 938-945.
Czakes, J. W., Kleeman, C. R. and Koenig, M. (1964). Physiological studies of antidiuretic hormone by its direct measurement in human plasma. *J. Clin. Invest.*, **43**: 1625-1640.
Dantzler, W. H. (1967). Glomerular and tubular effects of arginine vasotocin in water snakes *(Natrix sipedon)*. *Amer. J. Physiol.*, **212**: 83-91.
Darmady, E. M., Durant, J., Matthews, E. R. and Stranack, F. (1960). Location of ^{131}I-pitressin in the kidney by autoradiography. *Clin. Sci.*, **19**: 229-241.
Davis, B. B., Knox, F. G. and Berliner, R. W. (1967). Effect of vasopressin on proximal tubular sodium reabsorption in the dog. *Amer. J. Physiol.*, **212**: 1361-1364.
Davis, J. O., Hallowell, D. S. and Hyatt, R. E. (1954). Effect of chronic pitressin administration on electrolyte excretion in normal dogs and dogs with experimental ascites. *Endocrinology*, **55**: 409-416.
Demunbrun, T. W., Keller, A. D., Levkoff, A. H. and Purser, R. M. Jr. (1954). Pitocin restoration of renal hemodynamics to preneurohypophysectomy levels. Effect of administering neurohypophysial extraction products upon the reduced renal functions associated with neurohypophysectomy. *Amer. J. Physiol.*, **179**: 429-442.
de Wardener, H. E. and Herxheimer, A. (1957). The effect of a high water intake on the kidney's ability to concentrate urine in man. *J. Physiol., Lond.*, **139**: 42-52.
Dicker, S. E. (1957). Urine concentration in the rat during acute and prolonged dehydration. *J. Physiol., Lond.*, **139**: 108-122.
Dicker, S. E. and Eggleton, M. G. (1960). Hyaluronidase and antidiuretic activity in urine of man. *J. Physiol., Lond.*, **154**: 378-384.
Dicker, S. E. and Heller, H. (1946). The renal action of posterior pituitary extract and its fractions as analyzed by clearance experiments in rats. *J. Physiol., Lond.*, **104**: 353-360.
Dicker, S. E., Heller, H. and Hewer, T. F. (1946). Renal effects of protein-deficient vegetable diets: a functional and histological study. *Brit. J. Exp. Pathol.*, **27**: 158-169.
Dicker, S. E. and Nunn, J. (1958). Antidiuresis in adult and old rats. *J. Physiol., Lond.*, **141**: 332-336.
Dlouha, H. (1965). A comparison of the antidiuretic and pressor effects of vasopressin in infant and adult rats. *Physiol. bohemoslov.*, **14**: 225-227.
Dlouha, H., Kreček, J., Kraus, M. and Pliška, V. (1965). Sensitivity of rats to vasopressin in the weaning period. *Physiol. bohemoslov.*, **14**: 217-224.
Douglas, W. W. (1965). A possible mechanism of neurosecretion: release of vasopressin by depolarization and its dependence on calcium. *Nature, Lond.*, **197**: 81-12.

DUSTAN, H. P., CORCORAN, A. C. and PAGE, I. H. (1956). Renal function in primary aldosteronism. *J. Clin. Invest.*, **35**: 1357–1363.
EDELMANN, C. M. JR., BARNETT, H. L. and TROUPKOU, V. (1960). Renal concentrating mechanisms in newborn infants. Effect of dietary protein and water-content, role of urea and responsiveness to antidiuretic hormone. *J. Clin. Invest.*, **39**: 1062–1069.
EPSTEIN, F. H., BECK, D., CARONE, F. A., LEVITIN, H. and MANITIUS, A. (1959). Changes in renal concentrating ability produced by parathyroid extract. *J. Clin. Invest.* **38**: 1214–1221.
EPSTEIN, F. H., KLEEMAN, C. R. and HENDRIKX, A. (1957a). The influence of bodily hydration on the renal concentrating process. *J. Clin. Invest.*, **36**: 629–634.
EPSTEIN, F. H., KLEEMAN, C. R., PURSEL, S. and HENDRIKX, A. (1957b). The effect of feeding protein and urea on the renal concentrating process. *J. Clin. Invest.*, **36**: 635–641.
EPSTEIN, F. H., RIVERA, M. J. and CARONE, F. A. (1958). The effect of hypercalcemia induced by calciferol upon renal concentrating ability. *J. Clin. Invest.*, **37**: 1702–1709.
FICHMAN M. P. (1966). Inhibition of antidiuretic hormone by diphenylhydantoin. *Clin. Res.*, **14**: 376.
FISCH, L., MILLER, L. H. and KLEEMAN, C. R. (1965). Effect of vasopressin on calcium and sodium excretion in hydrated normal subjects. *Proc. Soc. Exp. Biol. Med.*, **119**: 719–722.
FOURMAN, P. and LEESON, P. M. (1959). Thirst and polyuria. With a note on the effects of potassium deficiency and calcium excess. *Lancet*, i: 268–271.
FRASER, A. M. (1937). The diuretic action of the oxytocic hormone of the pituitary gland and its effect on the assay of pituitary extracts. *J. Pharmacol. Exp. Ther.* **60**: 89–95.
FRASER, A. M. (1942). The action of the oxytocic hormone of the pituitary gland on urine secretion. *J. Physiol., Lond.*, **101**: 236–245.
FRIEDMAN, S. M., FRIEDMAN, C. L. and NAKASHIMA, M. (1960). Effect of pitressin on old age changes of salt and water metabolism in the rat. *Amer. J. Physiol.*, **199**: 35–38.
FUSCO, M., MALVIN, R. L. and CHURCHILL, P. (1966). Alterations in fluid, electrolyte and energy balance in rats with median eminence lesions. *Endocrinology*, **79**: 301–308.
GAITAN, E., COBO, E. and MIZRACHI, M. (1964). Evidence for the differential secretion of oxytocin and vasopressin in man. *J. Clin. Invest.*, **43**: 2310–2322.
GAMBLE, J. L., MCKHANN, C. F., BUTLER, A. M. and TUTHILL, E. (1934). An economy of water in renal function referable to urea. *Amer. J. Physiol.*, **109**: 139–154.
GARDNER, K. D. JR., and MAFFLY, R. H. (1963). The effect of vasopressin on rat collecting tubule permeability to urea studied *in vitro*. *Clin. Res.*, **11**: 241.
GERTZ, K. H., KENNEDY, G. C. and ULLRICH, K. J. (1964). Mikropunktionsuntersuchungen über die Flüssigkeitsrückresorption aus den einzelnen Tubulusabschnitten bei Wasserdiurese (Diabetes insipidus). *Pflügers Arch. ges. Physiol.*, **278**: 513–519.
GIEBISCH, G., KLOSE, R. M. and WINDHAGER, E. E. (1964). Micropuncture study of hypertonic sodium chloride loading in the rat. *Amer. J. Physiol.*, **206**: 687–693.
GIEBISCH, G. and LOZANO, R. (1959). The effects of adrenal steroids and potassium depletion on the elaboration of an osmotically concentrated urine. *J. Clin. Invest.*, **38**: 843–853.

GILL, J. R. JR. and BARTTER, F. C. (1962). On the impairment of renal concentrating ability in prolonged hypercalcemia and hypercalciuria in man. *J. Clin. Invest.*, **41**: 716–722.

GINETZINSKY, A. G. (1958). Role of hyaluronidase in the reabsorption of water in renal tubules: the mechanism of action of the antidiuretic hormone. *Nature, Lond.*, **182**: 1218–1219.

GINETZINSKY, A. G. (1961). Relationship between urinary hyaluronidase and diuresis. *Nature, Lond.*, **189**: 235–236.

GINETZINSKY, A. G., BROYTMAN, A. J. and IVANOVA, L. N. (1954). The hyaluronidase activity of human urine (Russian). *Bjul. eksp. biol. med.*, **38**: 37–40.

GINETZINSKY, A. G. and IVANOVA, L. N. (1958). The role of the system hyaluronic acid-hyaluronidase in the process of water reabsorption in tubules of the kidney (Russian). *Dokl. Akad. Nauk. SSSR.* **119**: 1043–1045.

GINETZINSKY, A. G., ZAKS, M. G. and TITOVA, L. K. (1958). The mechanism of action of the antidiuretic hormone (Russian). *Dokl. Akad. Nauk. SSSR.* **120**: 216–220.

GINSBURG, M. (1956). Antidiuretic activity of postpituitary preparations *Brit. J. Pharmacol. Chemother.*, **11**: 245–247.

GINSBURG, M. and BROWN, L. M. (1956). Effects of anaesthetics and haemorrhage on the release of neurohypophysial antidiuretic hormone. *Brit. J. Pharmacol. Chemother.*, **11**: 236–244.

GINSBURG, M. and SMITH, M. W. (1959). The fate of oxytocin in male and female rats. *Brit. J. Pharmacol. Chemother.*, **14**: 327–33.

GOLDBLATT, E. L., KLAUKER, M. L., HARE, R. S. and HARE, K. (1966). Effect of ethyleneimine on renal action of vasopressin. *Proc. Soc. Exp. Biol. Med.*, **123**: 845–847.

GOLDSMITH, C., BEASLEY, H. K., WHALLEY, P. J., RECTOR, F. C. JR. and SELDIN, D. W. (1961). The effect of salt deprivation on the urinary concentrating mechanism of the dog. *J. Clin. Invest.*, **40**: 2043–2052.

GOODMAN, A. and LEVITIN, H. (1965). Effect of urinary pH on the renal concentrating mechanism. *Amer. J. Physiol.*, **208**: 847–851.

GOTTSCHALK, C. W. and MYLLE, M. (1959). Micropuncture study of the mammalian urinary concentrating mechanism: evidence for the countercurrent hypothesis. *Amer. J. Physiol.*, **196**: 927–936.

GOTTSCHALK, C. W., MYLLE, M., JONES, N. F., WINTERS, R. W. and WELT, L. G. (1965). Osmolarity of renal tubular fluids in potassium depleted rodents. *Clin. Sci.*, **29**: 249–260.

GRANTHAM, J. J. and BURG, M. B. (1966). Effect of vasopressin and cyclic AMP on permeability of isolated collecting tubules. *Amer. J. Physiol.*, **211**: 255–259.

GROSS, F., SCHAECHTELIN, G., BRUNNER, H. and PETERS, G. (1964). The role of the renin-angiotensin system in blood pressure regulation and kidney function. *Canad. Med. Ass. J.*, **90**: 258–262.

GUGGENHEIM, K. and HEGSTED, D. M. (1953). Effect of desoxycorticosterone and posterior pituitary hormones on water and electrolyte metabolism in protein deficiency. *Amer. J. Physiol.*, **172**: 23–28.

GYERMEK, L. and FEKETE, G. (1955). On the vasopressor and antidiuretic activities of synthetic oxytocin. *Experientia*, **11**: 238.

HABENER, J. F., DASME, A. M. and SOLOMON, D. H. (1964). Response of normal subjects to prolonged high fluid intake. *J. Appl. Physiol.*, **19**: 134–136.

HANDLEY, C. A. and KELLER, A. D. (1950). Changes in renal functions associated with diabetes insipidus precipitated by anterior hypothalamic lesions. *Amer. J. Physiol.*, **160**: 321–324.

HARRINGTON, A. R. and VALTIN, H. (1965). Vasopressin effect on urinary concentration in rats with hereditary hypothalamic diabetes insipidus (Brattleboro strain) *Proc. Soc. Exp. Biol. Med.*, **118**: 448–450.
HARRIS, G. W. (1947). The innervation and actions of the neurohypophysis: an investigation using the method of remote-control stimulation. *Phil. Trans. Roy. Soc., Ser. B*, **232**: 285–441.
HAYS, R. M. and LEAF, A. (1961). The problem of clinical vasopressin resistance: *in vitro* studies. *Ann. Int. Med.*, **54**: 700–709.
HEIDENREICH, O., KOOK, Y., LING, V. and MENZEL, H. (1966a). Der Einfluss von Oxytocin auf die Nierendurchblutung und die Grösse des Glomerulusfiltrats bei normalen und totalhypophysektomierten Hunden. *Arch. Exp. Path. Pharmak.*, **239**: 328–335.
HEIDENREICH, O., KOOK, Y., LING, V. and MENZEL, H. (1966b). Die diuretische Wirkung von Oxytocin bei totalhypophysektomierten Hunden während verschiedener Diureseformen. *Arch. Exp. Path. Pharmak.*, **239**: 336–344.
HELLER, H. (1944). The renal function of newborn infants. *J. Physiol., Lond.*, **102**: 429–435.
HELLER, H. (1952). The action and fate of vasopressin in newborn and infant rats. *J. Endocrinol.*, **8**: 214–223.
HELLER, H. and BENTLEY, P. J. (1965). Phylogenetic distribution of the effects of neurohypophysial hormones on water and sodium metabolism. *Gen. Comp. Endocr.*, **5**: 96–108.
HELLER, H., HERDAN, G. and ZAIDI, S. M. A. (1957). Seasonal variations in the response of rats to the antidiuretic hormone. *Brit. J. Pharmacol. Chemother.*, **12**: 100–103.
HELLER, H. and LOJDA, Z. (1960). The physiology of the antidiuretic hormone. VII. Histological notes on Ginetzinsky's theory of the action of antidiuretic hormone. *Physiol. bohemoslov.*, **9**: 504–509.
HENDRIKX, A. and EPSTEIN, F. H. (1958). Effect of feeding protein and urea on renal concentrating ability in the rat. *Amer. J. Physiol.*, **195**: 539–542.
HIERHOLZER, K., WIEDERHOLT, M. and STOLTE, H. (1966). Hemmung der Natriumresorption im proximalen und distalen Konvolut adrenalektomierter Ratten. *Pflügers Arch. ges. Physiol.*, **291**: 43–62.
HOFMANN, L. (1966). SC-16 102, SC-16 100: Anti-ADH diuretics in the rat. *Pharmacologist*, **8**: 179.
HOLLANDER, W. JR., WINTERS, R. W., WILLIAMS, T. F., BRADLEY, J., OLIVER, J. and WELT, L. G. (1957). Defect in the renal tubular reabsorption of water associated with potassium depletion in rats. *Amer. J. Physiol.*, **189**: 557–563.
HORSTER, F. A., KUSCHINSKY, G. and PETERS, G. (1959). Die diuretische Wirkung von Oxytocin beim Hund. *Arch. Exp. Path. Pharmak.*, **237**: 241–246.
JACOBSON, H. N. and KELLOG, R. H. (1956). Isotonic NaCl diuresis in rats. Antidiuresis and chloruresis produced by posterior pituitary extracts. *Amer. J. Physiol.*, **184**: 376–389.
JAENIKE, J. R. (1961). The influence of vasopressin on the permeability of the mammalian collecting duct to urea. *J. Clin. Invest.*, **40**: 144–151.
JAENIKE, J. R. and WATERHOUSE, C. (1961). The renal response to sustained administration of vasopressin and water in man. *J. Clin. Endocr. Metab.*, **21**: 231–242.
JAMISON, R. L., BENNETT, C. M. and BERLINER, R. W. (1967). Countercurrent multiplication by the thin loops of Henle. *Amer. J. Physiol.*, **212**: 357–366.
JARD, S., MAETZ, J. and MOREL, F. (1960). Action de quelques analogues de l'oxyto-

cine sur différents récepteurs intervenant dans l'osmorégulation de Rana esculenta. *C. R. hebd. Séanc. Acad. Sci., Paris*, **251**: 788–790.
JARD, S. and MOREL, F. (1963). Actions of vasotocin and some of its analogues on salt and water excretion by the frog. *Amer. J. Physiol.*, **204**: 222–226.
JEFFERS, W. A., LIVEZEY, M. M. and AUSTIN, J. M. (1942). A method for demonstrating an antidiuretic action of minute amounts of pitressin: statistical analysis of results. *Proc. Soc. Exp. Biol. Med.*, **50**: 184–188.
JICK, H. C., KAMM, D. E., SNYDER, J. G., MORRISON, R. S. and CHALMERS, T. C. (1964). On the concentrating defect in cirrhosis of the liver. *J. Clin. Invest.*, **43**: 258–266.
JONES, N. F., MYLLE, M. and GOTTSCHALK, C. W. (1965). Renal tubular microinjection studies in normal and potassium-depleted rats. *Clin. Sci.*, **29**: 261–275.
JONES, R. V. H. and DE WARDENER, H. E. (1956). Urine concentration after fluid deprivation or pitressin tannate in oil. *Brit. Med. J.*, i: 271–273.
KARVONEN, M. J., LEPPÄNEN, V. and PITKÄNEN, M. E. (1953). The effect of pituitrin, pitressin and pitocin on urinary sodium and potassium excretion in dogs. *Ann. Med. Exp. Biol. Fenn.*, **31**: 117–128.
KELLOG, R. H., BURACK, W. R. and ISSELBACHER, K. J. (1954). Comparison of diuresis produced by isotonic saline solutions and by water in rats studied by a steady-state method. *Amer. J. Physiol.*, **177**: 27–37.
KOVÁCS K. and DÁVID, M. A. (1963). Effect of corticotrophin on the renal response to posterior pituitary extract in rats. *Lancet*, ii: 417–418.
KRAMAR, J., GRINNELL, E. H. and DUFF, W. M. (1966). Observations on the diuretic activity of antidiuretic hormone. *Amer. J. Med. Sci.*, **252**: 53–61.
KROON, D. B., JONGKIND, J. F. and WISE, J. H. (1962). Resection of renal papillae in rats. *Experientia*, **18**: 581–583.
KUEHN, E. and PEETERS, G. (1965). Influence de l'arginine-vasopressine sur l'excrétion d'électrolytes chez le mouton. *Archs Internat. Pharmacodyn. Thér.*, **155**: 455–458.
KUHN, W. and RAMEL, A. (1959). Aktiver Salztransport als möglicher (und wahrscheinlicher) Einzeleffekt bei der Harnkonzentrierung in der Niere. *Helv. Chim. Acta*, **42**: 628–660.
KUSCHINSKY, G. and BUNDSCHUH, E. (1939). Über eine diuretische und Kochsalz ausschwemmende Substanz in Hypophysenhinterlappen-Präparaten. *Arch. Exp. Path. Pharmak.*, **192**: 683–700.
LASSITER, W. E., FRICK, A., RUMRICH, G. and ULLRICH, K. J. (1965). Influence of ionic calcium on the water permeability of proximal and distal tubules in the rat kidney. *Pflügers Arch. ges. Physiol.*, **285**: 90–95.
LEAF, A., BARTTER, F. C., SANTOS, R. F. and WRONG, D. (1953). Evidence in man that urinary electrolyte loss induced by pitressin is a function of water retention. *J. Clin. Invest.*, **32**: 868–878.
LEVER, A. F. (1965). The vase recta and countercurrent multiplication. *Acta Med. Scand.*, **178**: Suppl. 434, 1–43.
LEVINSKY, N. G. and BERLINER, R. W. (1959). The role of urea in the urine concentrating mechanism. *J. Clin. Invest.*, **38**: 741–748.
LEVINSKY, N. G., DAVIDSON, D. G. and BERLINER, R. W. (1959a). Effects of reduced glomerular filtration on urine concentration in the presence of antidiuretic hormone. *J. Clin. Invest.*, **38**: 730–740.
LEVINSKY, N. G., DAVIDSON, D. G. and BERLINER, R. W. (1959b). Changes in urine concentration during prolonged administration of vasopressin and water. *Amer. J. Physiol.*, **196**: 451–456.

LEVITIN, H., MANITIUS, A. and EPSTEIN, F. H. (1960). Urinary dilution in potassium deficiency. *Yale J. Biol. Med.*, **32**: 390–396.
LEVITT, M. F., HAUSER, D., LEVY, M. S. and POLIMEROS, D. (1960). The renal concentrating defect in sickle cell anemia. *Amer. J. Med.*, **19**: 611–622.
LEVITT, M. F., LEVY, M. S. and POLIMEROS, D. (1959). The effect of a fall in filtration rate on solute and water excretion in hydropenic man. *J. Clin. Invest.*, **38**: 843–853.
MACFARLANE, W. V., MORRIS, R. J. H. and HOWARD, B. (1963). Turn-over and distribution of water in desert camels, sheep, cattle and kangaroos. *Nature, Lond.*, **197**: 270–271.
MAGNUS, R. and SCHAFER, E. A. (1901). The action of pituitary extracts upon the kidney. *J. Physiol., Lond.* **27**: ix.
MANITIUS, A., LEVITIN, H., BECK, D. and EPSTEIN, F. H. (1960a). On the mechanism of impairment of renal concentrating ability in potassium deficiency. *J. Clin. Invest.*, **39**: 684–692.
MANITIUS, A., LEVITIN, H., BECK, D. and EPSTEIN, F. H. (1960b). On the mechanism of impairment of renal concentrating ability in hypercalcemia. *J. Clin. Invest.*, **39**: 693–697.
MARSH, D. J. (1966). Hypo-osmotic reabsorption due to active salt transport in perfused collecting ducts of the rat renal medulla. *Nature, Lond.*, **210**: 1179–1180.
MARSH, D. J. and SOLOMON, S. (1965). Analysis of electrolyte movements in Henle's loops of hamster papilla. *Amer. J. Physiol.*, **208**: 1119–1128.
MCDONALD, S. J. and DE WARDENER, H. E. (1965). Some observations on the production of a hypo-osmotic urine during the administration of 0.9% saline and vasopressin in the dog. *Clin. Sci.*, **28**: 445–459.
MERTZ, D. P. (1960). Ueber die akute Wirkung von synthetischem Oxytocin auf die Nierenhämodynamik und renale Elektrolytausscheidung beim Menschen. *Arch. Exp. Path. Pharmak.*, **239**: 410–424.
MILES, B. E., PATON, A. and DE WARDENER, G. E. (1954). Maximum urine concentration. *Brit. Med. J.*, **ii**: 901–904.
MILLER, T. B., MARSHALL, S. and FARAH, A. (1961). Effect of papillectomy on the process of urine concentration in the golden hamster. *Pharmacologist.*, **1**: 58.
MOREL, F., DE ROUFFIGNAC, C. and LECHÊNE, C. (1966). Personnal communication.
MOREL, F. and JARD, S. (1963). Inhibition of frog (Rana esculenta) antidiuretic action of vasotocin by some analogues. *Amer. J. Physiol.*, **204**: 227–232.
MOREL, F., MYLLE, M. and GOTTSCHALK, C. W. (1965). Tracer microinjection studies of effect of ADH on renal tubular diffusion of water. *Amer. J. Physiol.*, **209**:179–187.
MOYLE, C. L. and CHERN, D. M. (Dow Chem. Corp.). U.S. Patent 3075991 (1.20.60/ 1.29.63).
OLIVER, J., MACDOWEL, M., WELT, L. G., HOLLIDAY, M. A., HOLLANDER, W., JR., WINTERS, W. R., WILLIAMS, F. T. and SEGAR, W. E. (1957). The renal lesions of electrolyte imbalance. I. The structural alterations in potassium-depleted rats. *J. Exp. Med.*, **106**: 563–573.
ORLOFF, J. and HANDLER, J. S. (1964). The cellular mode of action of antidiuretic hormone. *Amer. J. Med.*, **36**: 686–697.
ORLOFF, J., HANDLER, J. S. and PRESCOTT, A.S. (1962). The similarity of effects of vasopressin, adenosine-3′,5′-phosphate (cyclic AMP) and theophylline on the toad bladder. *J. Clin. Invest.*, **41**: 702–709.
ORLOFF, J., WAGNER, H. N. JR., and DAVIDSON, D. G. (1958). The effect of variations in solute excretion and vasopressin dosage on the excretion of water in the dog. *J. Clin. Invest.*, **37**: 458–464.

PERLMUTT, J. H. (1961). Renal activity of vasopressin in anesthetized dogs. *Amer. J. Physiol.* **200**: 400–404.

PETERS, G. (1959a). Der Einfluss von Nebennierenrindenhormonen, auf die renale Wasser- und Elektrolytausscheidung bei adrenalektomierten und normalen Ratten nach Gabe von Wasser oder isotonischer NaCl-Lösung und im Durst. *Arch. Exp. Path. Pharmakol.*, **235**: 155–184.

PETERS, G. (1959b). Nebennieren und renale Oxytocinwirkungen bei der Ratte. *Arch. Exp. Path. Pharmakol.*, **235**: 335–343.

PETERS, G. (1967). Régulation de l'excrétion rénale d'eau et d'électrolytes. *Bull. Schweiz. Acad. Med. Wiss.*, **23**: 313–337.

PETERS, G. and HEDWALL, P. R. (1963). Aristolochic acid intoxication: a new type of impairment or urinary concentrating ability. *Archs Internat. Pharmacodyn. Thér.*, **145**: 334–355.

PETERS, G. and ROCH-RAMEL, F. (1967). Unpublished observations.

PICKFORD, M. (1960). Factors affecting milk release in the dog and the quantities of oxytocin liberated by suckling. *J. Physiol., Lond.*, **152**: 515–526.

PICKFORD, M. and RITCHIE, A. E. (1945). Experiments on the hypothalamic-pituitary control of water excretion in dogs. *J. Physiol., Lond.*, **104**: 105–128.

POLACEK, E., VOGEL, J., NEUGEBAUEROVA, L., SEBKOVA, M. and VECHETOVA, E. (1965). The osmotic concentrating ability in healthy infants and children. *Archs Dis. Childh.*, **40**: 291–295.

RAISZ, L. G., AU, W. Y. W. and SCHEER, R. L. (1959). Studies on the renal concentrating mechanism. IV. Osmotic diuresis. *J. Clin. Invest.*, **38**: 1725–1732.

RAPOPORT, S., BRODSKY, W. A., WEST, C. D. and MACKLER, B. (1949). Urinary flow and excretion of solutes during osmotic diuresis in hydropenic man. *Amer. J. Physiol.*, **156**: 433–441.

RELMAN, A. S. and SCHWARTZ, W. B. (1956). The nephropathy of potassium depletion. A clinical and pathological entity. *New Engl. J. Med.*, **255**: 195–203.

RELMAN, A. S. and SCHWARTZ, W. B. (1958). The kidney in potassium depletion. *Amer. J. Med.*, **24**: 764–773.

ROCH-RAMEL, F., CHOMÉTY, F., and PETERS, G. (1968). Urea concentrations in tubular fluid and in renal tissue of nondiuretic rats *Amer. J. Physicol.*, **215**: 429–438.

ROCH-RAMEL, F. and PETERS, G. (1967). Intrarenal urea and electrolyte concentrations as influenced by water diuresis and by hydrochlorothiazide. *Eur.J. Pharmac.*, **1**: 124–139.

RUBINI, M. E. (1961). Water excretion in potassium-deficient man. *J. Clin. Invest.*, **40**: 2215–2224.

SANDERSON, P. H. (1959). Functional effects of renal calcification in rats. *Clin. Sci.*, **18**: 67-69.

SAWYER, W. H. (1952). Posterior pituitary extracts and excretion of electrolytes by the rat. *Amer. J. Physiol.*, **169**: 583–587.

SAWYER, W. H., CHAN, W. Y. and VAN DYKE, H. B. (1962). Antidiuretic responses to neurohypophysical hormones and some of their synthetic analogues in dogs and rats. *Endocrinology*, **71**: 536–540.

SAWYER, W. H. and VALTIN H. (1967). Antidiuretic responses of rats with hereditary hypothalamic diabetes insipidus to vasopressin, oxytocin and nicotine. *Endocrinology*, **80**: 207–210.

SCHNERMANN, J., VALTIN, H., FISCHBACH, H., NAGEL, W., HORSTER, M., LIEBAU, G., TABOR, M., GELTINGER, A. and THURAU, K. (1967). Tubuläre Natrium- und Wasserresorption bei Ratten mit hereditärem hypothalamischen Diabetes insipidus vor und nach ADH-Gabe (Mikropunktionsversuche). Paper read at the 5th Symposium of the Gesellschaft für Nephrologie, Lausanne, Sept. 23, 1967.

SCHROEDER, R., BUSCHMANN, H. J. and EHRENTAL, K. (1966). Die Wirkung von Tonephin auf die renale Elektrolyt- und Harnstoffausscheidung bei Infusion von Glucose und Serofundin. *Klin. Wschr.*, **44**: 943-951.

SENAY, L. C. JR. and CHRISTENSEN, M. L. (1965). Changes in blood plasma during progressive dehydration. *J. Appl. Physiol.*, **20**: 1136-1140.

SHANNON, J. A. (1942a). The control of the renal excretion of water. 1. The effects of variations in the state of hydration on water excretion in dogs with diabetes insipidus. *J. Exp. Med.*, **76**: 371-386.

SHANNON, J. A. (1942b). The control of the renal excretion of water. II. The rate of liberation of the posterior pituitary antidiuretic hormone in the dog. *J. exp. Med.*, **76**: 387-399.

SHARE, L. (1967). Vasopressin, its bioassay and the physiological control of its release. *Amer. J. Med.*, **42**: 701-712.

SKADHAUGE, E. (1964a). Effects of retrograde injections of vasopressin into the upper urinary tract of hydrated rats. *Proc. Soc. Exp. Biol. Med.*, **117**: 807-810.

SKADHAUGE, E. (1964b). Effects of unilateral infusion of arginine-vasotocin into the portal circulation of the avian kidney. *Acta Endocr., Copnh.*, **47**: 321-330.

SPARGO, B., STRAUS, F. and FITCH, F. (1960). Zonal renal papillary droplet change with potassium depletion. *Archs Pathol.*, **70**: 599-613.

STELTER E. (1959). Die Diurese der Maus nach oraler Gabe von Wasser oder NaCl-Lösungen und ihre Beeinflussung durch Hypophysenhinterlappenhormone. *Arch. Exp. Path. Pharmak.*, **237**: 409-422.

TATA, P. S. and BUZALKOV, R. (1966). Vasopressin studies in the rat. III. Inability of ethanol anesthesia to prevent ADH secretion due to pain and hemorrhage. *Pflügers Arch. ges. Physiol.*, **290**: 294-297.

TATA, P. S. and GAUER, O. H. (1966). Vasopressin studies in the rat. I. A sensitive bioassay for exogenous vasopressin. *Pflügers Arch. ges. Physiol.*, **290**: 279-285.

THOMSON, J. (1944). Observations on the urine of the newborn infant. *Archs Dis. Childh.*, **19**: 169-177.

THOMSON, W. B. (1960). The effect of oxytocin and vasopressin and of phenylalanyl-oxytocin on the urinary excretion of water and electrolytes in man. *J. Physiol., Lond.*, **150**: 284-294.

THORN, N. A. (1961). Correlation between antidiuretic hormone effects and changes in renal excretion of calcium in rats and dogs. *Acta Endocr., Copnh.*, **38**: 563-570.

THORN, N. A., KNUDSEN, P. J. and KOEFOED, J. (1961). Antidiuretic effect of large doses of bovine testicular hyaluronidase in rats. *Acta Endocr., Copnh.*, **38**: 571-576.

THORN, N. A., SMITH, M. W. and SKADHAUGE, E. (1965). The antidiuretic effect of intravenous and intracarotid infusion of calcium chloride in hydrated rats. *J. Endocr.*, **32**: 161-165.

THURAU, K., DEETJEN, P. and KRAMER, K. (1960). Hämodynamik des Nierenmarks. II. Mitteilung. Wechselbeziehung zwischen vaskulärem und tubulärem Gegenstromsystem bei arteriellen Drucksteigerungen, Wasserdiurese und osmotischer Diurese. *Pflügers Arch. ges. Physiol.*, **270**: 270-285.

ULLMANN, T. D., CZAKES, W. J. and MENCZEL, J. (1965). Modification of the antidiuretic effect of vasopressin by acid and alkaline loads. *J. Clin. Invest.*, **44**: 754-764.

ULLRICH, K. J., RUMRICH, G. and FUCHS, G. (1964). Wasserpermeabilität und transtubulärer Wasserfluss corticaler Nephronabschnitte bei verschiedenen Diuresezuständen. *Pflügers Arch. ges. Physiol.*, **280**: 99-119.

ULLRICH, K. J., SCHMIDT-NIELSEN, B., O'DELL, R., PEHLING, G., GOTTSCHALK, C. W., LASSITER, W. E. and MYLLE, M (1963). Micropuncture study of composition of proximal and distal tubular fluid in rat kidney. *Amer. J. Physiol.*, **204**: 527–531.
USSING, H. H. (1960). The frog skin potential. *J. Gen. Physiol.*, **43**: Suppl. 1: 135–147.
VAAMONDE, C. A., VAAMONDE, L. S., MOROSI, H. J., KLINGLER, L. JR. and PAPPER, S. (1965). Renal concentrating ability in cirrhosis of the liver. *Clin. Res.*, **13**: 316.
VALTIN, H. (1966). Sequestration of urea and non-urea solutes in renal tissues of rats with hereditary hypothalamic diabetes insipidus: effect of vasopressin and dehydration on the countercurrent mechanism. *J. Clin. Invest.*, **45**: 337–345.
VAN ARMAN, C. G. (1956). The antidiuretic effect of 5-hydroxytryptamine in the rat as influenced by dibenamine. *Archs Internat. Pharmacodyn. Thér.*, **108**: 356–365.
VAN DYKE, H. B. and AMES, R. G. (1951). Alcohol diuresis. *Acta Endocr., Copnh.*, **7**: 110–121.
VAN DYKE, H. B., ENGEL, S. L. and ADAMSONS, K. JR., (1956). Comparison of pharmacological effects of lysine and arginine vasopressins. *Proc. Soc. Exp. Biol. Med.*, **91**: 484–486.
VANEČEK, J., KÜCHEL, D., ŠPAČKOVÁ, M. and KUCHAROVÁ, M. (1960). Zur Wirkung von Pituitrin und synthetischem Oxytocin bei intrazerebraler Applikation. *Acta Biol. Med. Germ.*, **4**: 278–282.
VIERLING A. F., LITTLE, J. B. and RADFORD, E. P. JR. (1967). Antidiuretic hormone bioassay in rats with hereditary hypothalamic diabetes insipidus (Brattleboro strain). *Endocrinology*, **80**: 211–214.
VORHERR, H. (1964). Zur Frage des Oxytocin-Vasopressin-Antagonismus an der Diurese bei Mensch und Tier. *Klin. Wschr.*, **42**: 198–201.
WELT, L. G., HOLLANDER, W., JR. and BLYTHE, W. B. (1960). The consequences of potassium depletion. *J. Chron. Dis.*, **11**: 213–254.
WEST, C. D., TRAEGER, J. and KAPLAN, S. A. (1955). A comparison of the relative effectiveness of hydropenia and of Pitressin^R in producing a concentrated urine. *J. Clin. Invest.*, **34**: 887–898.
WHITE, H. L. and HEINBECKER, P. (1938). Observations on creatinine and urea clearances, on responses to water ingestion, and on concentrating power of kidneys in normal, diabetes insipidus and hypophysectomized dogs. *Amer. J. Physiol.*, **123**: 566–576.
WIEDERHOLT, M. and HIERHOLZER, K. (1967). Personnal communication.
WIEDERHOLT, M., STOLTE, H., BRECHT, J. P. and HIERHOLZER, K. (1966). Mikropunktionsuntersuchungen über den Einfluss von Aldosteron, Cortison und Dexamethason auf die renale Natriumresorption adrenalektonierter Ratten. *Pflügers Arch. ges. Physiol.*, **292**: 316–333.
WIRZ, H. (1956a). Der osmotische Druck in den corticalen Tubuli der Rattenniere *Helv. Physiol. Pharmac. Acta*, **14**: 353–362.
WIRZ, H. (1956b). Die Wirkung des antidiuretischen Hormones in der Säugetierniere. *Schweiz. med. Wschr.*, **86**: 1261.
WIRZ, H., HARGITAY, B. and KUHN, W. (1951). Lokalisation des Konzentrierungsprozesses in der Niere durch direkte Kryoskopie. *Helv. Physiol. Pharmac. Acta*, **9**: 196–207.
YOON, M. O. and HONG, S. K. (1961). Effect of prolonged bodily hydration on the renal concentrating operation. *J. Appl. Physiol.*, **16**: 815–818.
YUNIBHAND, P. and HELD, U. (1965). Nierenmark und Urinosmolalität nach der Geburt bei der Ratte unter Flüssigkeitsentzug. *Helv. Physiol. Pharmac. Acta*, **23**: 91–96.
ZEDECK, M. S., MELLETT, L. B. and CAFRUNY, E. J. (1966). The diuretic effect of cyclophosphamide and nor-nitrogen mustard: relationship to antidiuretic hormone. *J. Pharm. Exp. Ther.*, **153**: 550–561.

CHAPTER 8 (b)

PHYSIOLOGICAL AND PHARMACOLOGICAL EFFECTS OF NEUROHYPOPHYSIAL HORMONES AND THEIR SYNTHETIC ANALOGUES: UTERINE ACTION

Robert A. Munsick

Department of Obstetrics and Gynecology, University of New Mexico School of Medicine, 2211 Lomas Boulevard, N.E., Albuquerque, New Mexico, 87106, U.S.A.

INTRODUCTION AND HISTORY

Sir Henry Dale's discovery of the uterotonic effect of posterior pituitary extract resulted, like many other important findings, from serendipity. He was studying the sympatholytic effect of ergot on the pressor response to epinephrine in cats. Reasoning that the ergot-induced reversal of the pressor response to epinephrine might be specific for the adrenal medullary hormone he tested this hypothesis by injecting another potent pressor material, posterior pituitary extract, into a cat which had e en treated with ergot. His theory was documented—ergot did not block or reverse the pressor response. But Dale noted an unusual phenomenon in this cat. There was a most remarkable contraction of its uterus. In his paper of 1906, Dale gave only peremptory attention to this observation but subsequently he and his collaborators went on to investigate in detail the oxytocic effect of posterior lobe extracts (see Dale, 1957).

Nr ow more than sixty years after Dale's discovery, utilizing vastly imp oved assay methods, electronic equipment undreamed of in 1906, and pure synthetic neurohypophysial hormones and analogues, we understand considerably more about the effects of these peptides on the uterus. It is amazing, however, how much we still have to learn. The present emphasis on cell biology, with synchronization of work by electrophysiologists, biochemists, membrane transport physiologists, ultramicroscopists and cell-oriented pharmacologists will, in the next decade, doubtlessly lead to many answers to the questions which will be raised in the following chapter.

UTERINE CONTRACTILITY

The uterine smooth muscle or myometrium is specialized for several functions. The cardinal one is its ecbolic function—contracting rhythmically and strongly to expel ova or products of conception at a time usually advantageous to the particular species under consideration. It is probable, however, that the contractile mechanism serves other physiological purposes which are less well understood, e.g. ovum transport prior to nidation, transport of spermatozoa, etc. The myometrial fibers must therefore have several peculiar characteristics: they must be capable not only of contracting, but should have controls to prevent or increase contractility at appropriate times depending upon the animal's reproductive status, and they should also be capable of acting in a coordinated, organ-directed manner.

Like most other mammalian smooth muscle fibers, myometrial cells depend for their contractility on complex proteins, including acto-myosin, which, given the proper energy sources, ionic constituents, and enzymes, undergo altered molecular orientation in such a way as to become foreshortened, thus causing cellular contraction. Because these aspects of myometrial contractility do not appear to be directly governed by the neurohypophysial peptides, they will not be given further consideration in this chapter. The subject of the biochemistry of the myometrium has recently been extensively reviewed by Needham and Shoenberg (1967). Most evidence indicates that the principal site of action of the neurohypophysial peptides is on the myometrial cell membrane. Thus, a brief account of this important anatomical and physiological entity will follow.

Myometrial cells are electrically charged. This charge appears to be a membrane-dependent and localized phenomenon derived from the presence in or near the membrane of Na^+ and K^+ pumps which are probably coupled. The active external transport of Na^+ and internal transport of K^+ results in an intracellular ionic milieu which differs markedly from extracellular fluid. Casteels and Kuriyama (1965), for example, have found that the estrous rat's intramyometrial cellular fluid has the following ionic concentrations: Na^+ 58, K^+ 106, and Cl^- 68 meq/l cell water. Kao (1967) believes there is sufficient evidence to suggest that there is also active Cl^- transport from without to within the cell.

The myometrial cell has an electrical charge which is positive outside and negative inside, caused by the active transport of the above ions. Hence, the myometrial cell has a resting potential of about 50 mv, negative inside (see Fig. 1). For normal, physiological myometrial contractions to occur, action potentials are required. Each spike discharge or action potential involves a rapid change of the membrane potential toward electrical neutrality. When threshold is reached and a spike discharge occurs, Na$^+$ rushes into the cell and the cell rapidly becomes less electronegative. A spike discharge therefore has a positive direction (see Fig. 1). It is of short duration, lasting about 0.1 sec, and has a magnitude of 30–70 mv, depending upon the resting membrane potential and other factors. Spikes are thought to be caused by a sudden increase in membrane permeability to Na$^+$. Each spike may cause an individual twitch of a cell, but bursts of spike activity are required for measurable myometrial contractions to occur. In this physiological tetanic system, the periodicity of the bursts of spike activity determines the frequency of overt uterine contractions. The frequency and number of spike discharges controls the intensity of individual contractions (see Fig. 1).

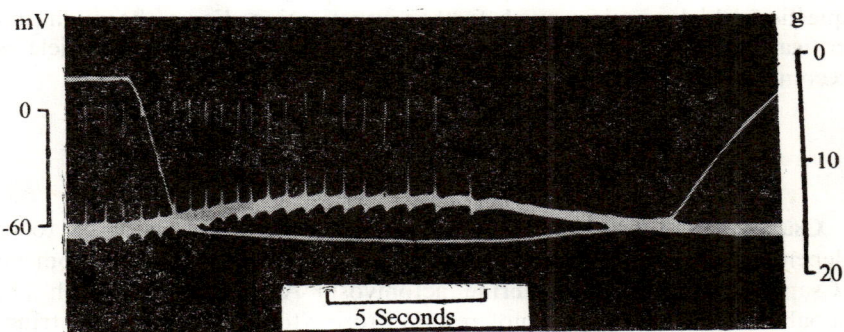

Fig. 1. Relationship between whole muscle tension (upper tracing, with downward displacement indicating contraction) and the discharge of a burst of action potentials or spikes in single muscle fiber (lower tracing). Note that the burst of spike activity precedes the contraction and ends before the muscle relaxes in spontaneous contraction from an estrogen-treated rat uterus. From J. M. Marshall (1959).

The contractile system described above has been called the tetanic system. A second system, known as the tonic system, depends upon sustained membrane depolarization, and leads to maintained contraction, known as contracture. Jung (1961) believes that contracture is caused by increased permeability of the membrane to K$^+$.

The membrane electrophysiological properties, and, consequently, contractile characteristics, are profoundly affected by sex steroids. In castrated rats, the resting potential is about -35 mv and there is little or no spontaneous contractile activity. Estrogen treatment increases the resting potential to −57 mv and causes an increase in the size and number of action potentials. Therefore, spontaneous contractions are more frequent and more powerful (Marshall, 1959). Although progesterone treatment has been found to alter the membrane potential very little if at all in castrated animals, some observers, e.g. Marshall (1959), have found that progesterone with or following estrogen treatment causes a further increase in the resting membrane potential. This observation has not been uniform, however, and Kao (1967) believes that the weight of evidence does not support the fact that progesterone causes further increase of the resting membrane potential. The mechanism by which progesterone appears to disturb intercellular impulse conduction and to cause desynchronization of spike discharges is not known. Whether or not it is progesterone which causes alterations in the contractility and membrane electrical behavior of the myometrium of pregnant animals is another question which requires much further investigation. For a thorough and critical discussion of these phenomena, Kao's (1967) review article is recommended.

ACTION OF NEUROHYPOPHYSIAL PEPTIDES ON MEMBRANE POTENTIAL

Csapo and others have shown that the oxytocic action of oxytocin depends predominantly, or entirely, on its effect on membrane phenomena (Csapo, 1961). Isolated uterine actomyosin–ATP systems, which are capable of contraction, do not respond to oxytocin. In the myometrium depolarized by K^+, oxytocin is ineffectual in causing typical spike discharges or contractions, whereas an electrical stimulus still causes maximal contractions.

Accepting the fact that oxytocin modifies the membrane in such a way as to facilitate spike discharges, how does it accomplish this? If one examines the effects of small doses of oxytocin on the resting and spike potentials of the membrane, several changes can be seen (Kao 1967). Spike production is initiated, the frequency of burst discharges is increased, the number of spikes per burst is increased and spike amplitude is increased. None of these effects is surprising, for all are consonant with the fact that the hormone is causing contractile responses, and we have accepted the fact that it is the tetanic system which governs the usual contractile mechanism. Based on several types of experiment, Marshall (1963) has concluded that oxytocin facilitates the entry of sodium into the cell during or preceeding spike potentials (see Fig. 2), and that this action is mediated by a release of Ca^{++} from the membrane by oxytocin.

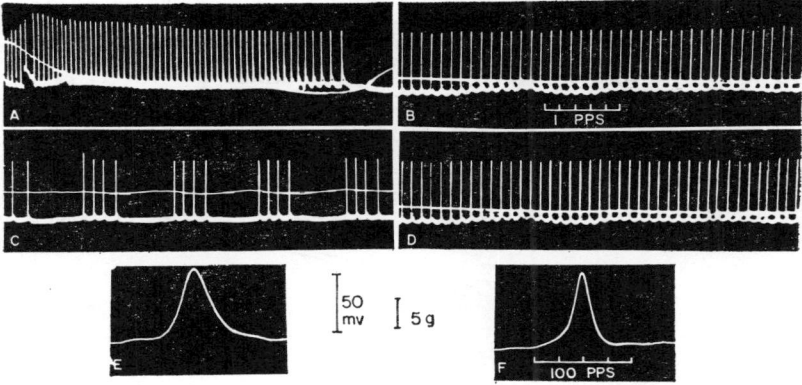

FIG. 2. In A, a spontaneous contraction is shown with the muscle in a solution containing 143.3 mM Na^+; in B, after 10 min at a Na^+ concentration of 35.8 mM (difference made up with LiCl); in C, after 150 min in same solution; in D, continuation of same tracing, 2 min after addition of oxytocin (50 μU/ml in bath). E and F are rapid time base tracings of individual action potentials from C and D, respectively. Note that oxytocin restores spike discharges nearly to normal even in the presence of a low sodium environment. Rat uterus. From J. M. Marshall (1963)

Indeed, various investigators have suggested that it is this Ca^{++} liberation which characterizes the basic action of oxytocin. Utilizing this hypothesis, it has even been proposed that the difference in oxytocin responsiveness between estrogen and progesterone dominated uteri is due to an altered binding of Ca^{++} caused by the sex steroids. Although these hypotheses are attractive, they cannot as yet be accepted as proved (Kao, 1967). Kao believes that alteration of the resting potential is not requisite for the action of oxytocin, but thinks that neurohypophysial peptides act by providing more sodium channels in the membrane (see Fig. 3).

So far only the effects on the electrical and contractile properties of the myometrium stimulated by neurohypophysial peptides have been mentioned and the possible way in which these effects are mediated. Another important matter which requires attention is the receptor-site for these peptides and how the activation of this site influences Na^+ channels through the membrane. Unfortunately, very little is known about these aspects.

It has been known for years that several receptor-sites are involved which activate uterine contractions in response to different drugs and hormones. In the rat uterus, for example, atropine blocks acetylcholine-induced contractions but does not influence sensitivity to oxytocin. Similar results have been obtained with inhibitors of 5-hydroxytryptamine.

Bentley (1964) and Martin and Schild (1965) have implicated interaction of SH and S-S groups at the neurohypophysial peptide receptor sites. Recently, Taira and Marshall (1967) have studied the effects of three oxytocin inhibitors, thioglycollate, N-ethylmaleimide, and an analogue of oxytocin, $[(O\text{–Me})\text{Tyr}^2]$-oxytocin, on both contractility and electrical behavior. They found that thioglycollate and $[(O\text{–Me})\text{Tyr}^2]$-oxytocin apparently acted in the same way. Their inhibitory effects were reversible

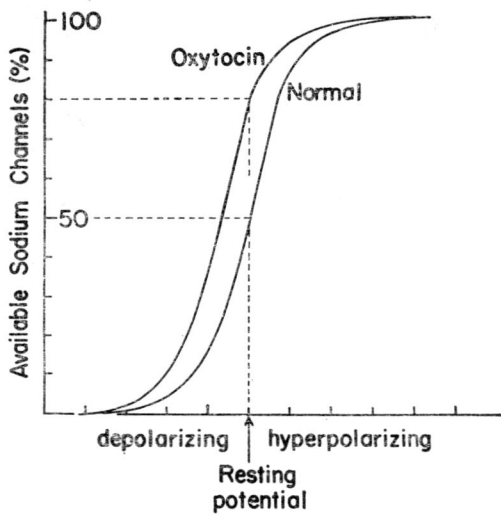

FIG. 3. Kao's (1967) diagram showing the hypothetical action of oxytocin on myometrium, assuming that at a resting potential of -50 mv means that 50% of all Na$^+$ channels are available for spike production. Increasing or decreasing resting potential by 10 mv will result in 80% or 15% availability of Na$^+$ channels, respectively. According to Kao's theory, oxytocin shifts this curve to the left, thereby increasing available Na$^+$ channels for spike production independent of the resting membrane potential.

with time and increased dose of oxytocin, the resting membrane potential was unaltered and those action potentials which did occur were normal. Neither compound inhibited spontaneous or acetylcholine or bradykinin induced contractions. Their findings are therefore in agreement with those of Bentley (1964) and Martin and Schild (1965) and support the assumption that neurohypophysial peptide receptor sites are occupied by these antagonists. N-ethylmaleimide, on the other hand, profoundly affected all types of contractile activity, whether spontaneous, or drug or electrically induced. Nevertheless, the resting membrane potential was not greatly affected. Again, these results are in agreement with those of others. Apparently this potent sulfhydryl blocking agent affects the biochemical mechanism of contraction at various sites in the cell and not exclusively at receptor sites.

Although disruption of the disulfide bond of oxytocin abolishes oxytocic activity, it is possible that the resultant opening of the ring, and not the loss of the disulfide group *per se*, is responsible for the loss of activity. Analogues of oxytocin, in which selenium has replaced sulfur, have potent oxytocic activity (see Chapter 4; Chan and Kelley, 1967). Several groups of workers have studied the relationship between peptide structure and receptor by indirectly analyzing the peptide's affinity for the receptor and the intrinsic activity of the peptide on the receptor. Results in the studies of Rudinger and Krejčí (1962) and of Chan and Kelley (1967) are in agreement. The latter investigators, basing their conclusions on cumulative dose–response curves, studied analogues of oxytocin in which the six functional groups had been modified. They found that the 5-carboxamide group was essential for intrinsic activity. The 4-carboxamide group affects affinity for the receptor, and the 9-carboxamide and phenolic hydroxyl groups affect both affinity and intrinsic activity. The terminal amino group probably influences affinity only. The significance of the disulfide group is mentioned elsewhere.

Very recently, W. Y. Chan, R. Fear and V. du Vigneaud (unpublished results) have found that [1-L-penicillamine]-oxytocin and [1-deamino-L-penicillamine]-oxytocin are extremely potent inhibitors of oxytocin and other neurohypophysial peptides. Despite the inhibition of all the neurohypophysial peptides studied, there was no inhibition of spontaneous contractions, or of angiotensin or bradykinin induced contractions. This evidence strongly supports the theory that there are distinct, specific, uterine receptors for the neurohypophysial peptides.

OXYTOCIC ASSAYS

Many methods of assaying oxytocic activity have been devised. There are inherent differences between various assay methods and these differences may profoundly influence potency estimates. In the following section certain aspects of some commonly used assay methods will be discussed.

Several points need emphasis concerning assays *in vitro*. First, one is substituting for blood plasma and extracellular fluid a surrogate whose composition is of extreme importance. Potencies derived by identical assay methods may differ significantly because of differences in the ionic composition of the bath solution. Secondly, variations in the alkalinity of the solution can result from varying the HCO_3^- concentration or the HCO_2 of the gas used to oxygenate the solution. Thirdly, without a buffer of sufficient strength, the addition of test solutions can dramatically alter the pH of the bath and, thus, the potency estimate of the unknown sample. Lastly, oxytocic assays *in vitro* are not suitable for assaying neurohypophysial hormones in blood or blood derivatives.

What are the effects of changing the concentrations of different ions in the bath solution? Most alterations were studied by van Dyke and Hastings (1928) in the isolated guinea pig uterus. They found that contractile responses to posterior pituitary extract were directly, but not necessarily proportionately, related to the concentrations of Na^+, K^+ or Ca^{++}, i.e., lowering the concentration of any one of these cations diminished the response; increasing the concentration increased the response. They found that this was also true for Mg^{++}, but that increasing the Mg^{++} concentration well above normal plasma levels caused a decreased response. Abarbanel (1945) has confirmed this finding in an excellent clinical study.

In studying the effects of ions on peptide potency, magnesium has been most extensively investigated. There are probably two reasons for this: (1) magnesium can be completely omitted from the bath fluid without seriously impeding the assay, and (2) magnesium has had much use and attention in obstetrics. Table 1 shows data for the naturally occurring neurohypophysial peptides, showing potency ratios in bath solutions containing 0.5 mM and no Mg^{++}. Utilizing magnesium ratios, it has been possible to characterize tentatively several oxytocin-like peptides from natural sources (see Sawyer, 1968). Munsick and Jeronimus

TABLE 1. MAGNESIUM RATIOS OF KNOWN, NATURALLY OCCURRING NEUROHYPOPHYSIAL PEPTIDES IN ISOLATED RAT UTERUS ASSAY. THE RATIO ($R_{Mg^{++}}$) IS EXPRESSED AS POTENCY WITH 0.5 mM Mg^{++}: POTENCY WITHOUT Mg^{++} IN BATH SOLUTION

Peptide	$R_{Mg^{++}}$	Reference
Oxytocin	0.97	Munsick and Jeronimus (1965)
[Ile⁸]-oxytocin	1.3	Munsick (1966)
[Arg⁸]-oxytocin	2.0	Munsick and Jeronimus (1965)
[Ser⁴,Ile⁸]-oxytocin	2.9	Follett and Heller (1964)
[Ser⁴,Glu⁸]-oxytocin	about 10	Acher et al. (1965)
[Arg⁸]-vasopressin	2.3	Munsick and Jeronimus (1965)
[Lys⁸]-vasopressin	2.6	Munsick (1960)

(1965) showed that the magnesium effect on the potencies of neurohypophysial peptides is not correlated with the effects of estrogen. Until recently, no adequate explanation existed for the variable augmentation of potency caused by magnesium ions. Recently, Chan and Kelley (1967), like Bentley (1965), have concluded that Mg^{++} probably acts by increasing the affinity of the peptide for its receptor site. How magnesium ion produces this effect and why there should be marked variations in the degree to which it does, depending both on the particular peptide and the magnesium concentration, are questions which are still unanswered.

Another divalent cation which has recently received attention is manganese (Bentley, 1965). Bentley found that 0.1 mM Mn^{++} was generally more effective than 0.5 mM Mg^{++} in potentiating potencies and that augmentation was discernible at concentrations as low as 0.01 mM Mn^{++}. The augmentation is believed by Bentley to be due either to altered steric configuration of the receptor site or to a decreased rate of removal of the peptide from the receptor site.

It is evident that cations markedly influence oxytocic responses; most anions appear not to be so important. Van Dyke and Hastings (1928) concluded that phosphate ions have some potentiating action. This is a difficult ion to study, however, because Ca^{++} is precipitated when phosphate concentrations are high. The same investigators studied the relationships between pCO_2, HCO_3^-, H^+, and $CO_3^=$ concentrations. They concluded that the $CO_3^=$ ion is most directly related to uterine responsiveness, the concentration being related inversely to responsiveness. Bentley and Dicker (1955) have shown that lowering the pH of the bath solution sensitizes the uterus to neurohypophysial peptides for as long as 30 min. This fact and the others mentioned above should serve to emphasize that the bath solution is extremely important in assay work. For a variety of reasons, the author has advocated the use of a modified van Dyke–Hastings solution for oxytocic assays (Munsick, 1960).

Oxytocic assays of neurohypophysial peptides have also been devised by means of *in situ* preparations. If one's interest in the assay result relates predominantly to the clinical or *in vivo* potency of a peptide, these methods are of value. However, the methods so far described are somewhat cumbersome, expensive, and time-consuming, and they present problems in obtaining an adequate degree of precision. The *in vivo* rat preparation described by Chan and Kelley (1967) holds promise for the future and does diminish the expense and magnitude of the required animal facilities usually necessary for assays *in vivo*. It should be emphasized, however, that assays on the uterus of animals *in situ* may give results which correlate poorly with clinical experience and assays in human subjects *in vivo*. Several problems arise: (1) what parameter should be chosen for determining the oxytocic response, (2) what species of animal should be used, and (3) in what phase of the reproductive cycle or of pregnancy should the assay be performed? Berde and Saameli (1966) have discussed many of these problems in their review.

Different results have been obtained from oxytocic assays on the rat uterus *in vivo* and *in vitro*. Berde, Doepfner and Konzett (1957) found that [3-valine]-oxytocin was 3.6 times as potent in the assays *in vivo*. Munsick (1960) found that the $R_{Mg^{++}}$ (potency with 0.5 mM Mg^{++} divided by potency without Mg^{++} in the bath) for this analogue was also 3.6. He stated then that "...it is possible that the reported differences between *in vitro* and *in vivo* potencies are largely attributable to the absence of magnesium from the bath solution used for the *in vitro* assay". The recent findings of Chan and Kelley (1967), who studied several different neurohypophysial peptides, support this conclusion (see Table 2). Hence, the bath solution for future *in vitro* assays might well be designed to replicate the Mg^{++} and Ca^{++} concentrations of plasma if close correlation with results *in vivo* is desired.

TABLE 2. POTENCIES AND POTENCY RATIOS FOR SEVERAL NEUROHYPOPHYSIAL PEPTIDES. NOTE THAT THE RATIO ($R_{Mg^{++}}$) POTENCY 1.0 mM Mg^{++} : POTENCY 0.0 mM Mg^{++} IS APPROXIMATELY EQUAL TO THE RATIO (R) POTENCY *in vivo*: POTENCY *in vitro*, 0.0 mM Mg^{++}. FROM CHAN AND KELLEY (1967). SEE TEXT AND ORIGINAL ARTICLE FOR DETAILS.

Peptide	Rat oxytocic potency in U.S.P. U/mg ± S.E.			Ratios	
	In vitro		*In vivo*	$R_{Mg^{++}}$	R
	0.0 mM Mg^{++}	1.0 mM Mg^{++}			
Oxytocin	546 ± 18	420 ± 10	468 ± 35	0.77	0.86
Deamino-oxytocin (amorphous)	451 ± 17	476 ± 15	487 ± 41	0.86	0.88
[Phe²]-deamino-oxytocin	21 ± 1	105 ± 3	104 ± 10	5.0	5.0
4-Decarboxamido-oxytocin	72 ± 2	337 ± 18	344 ± 24	4.7	4.8
[Lys⁸]-vasopressin	4.8 ± 0.3	35 ± 2	48 ± 5	7.3	10.0

Even if the differences between oxytocic potencies determined *in vitro* and *in vivo* can be minimized or nullified, there are still the problems of species variation and of the sex hormone-induced changes in uterine sensitivity to neurohypophysial peptides. Saameli (1964) has studied some of the differences in potencies found in different species and preparations and has included results from assays on the human post-partum uterus (see Table 3). Chan, O'Connell and Pomeroy (1963) demonstrated the profound influence which the estrous cycle in the rat *in vitro* has on the oxytocic potencies of oxytocin and deamino-oxytocin (Table 4), and Munsick and Jeronimus (1965) have shown the distinct effects of estrogen and magnesium ion on several neurohypophysial peptides (Table 5).

TABLE 3. OXYTOCIN-LIKE ACTIVITIES OF NEUROHYPOPHYSIAL PEPTIDES BY DIFFERENT ASSAY METHODS. VALUES ARE MEANS ± S.E. VALUES IN ITALICS ARE THOSE CORRESPONDING MOST CLOSELY TO RESULTS ON THE HUMAN UTERUS. OXYTOCIN USED FOR STANDARD. FROM K. SAAMELI (1964)

Peptide	Potency (U/mg)				
	Rat uterus *in vitro*	Avian depressor	Rabbit milk-ejection	Cat oxytocic (*in situ*)	Human oxytocic (post partum *in situ*)
Oxytocin	450	450	450	450	450
[Val^3]-oxytocin	59±8	58±4	207±14	*226±17*	227±65
[Ile^8]-oxytocin	289±21	498±37	*328±21*	563±74	365±70
[Asp^4]-oxytocin	108±29	202±12	300±128	335±75	150±40
Deamino-oxytocin	360±55	710±60	440±15	*900±130*	1,030±300
[Ser^4, Ile^8]-oxytocin	150±12	*320±15*	300±15	250±40	335±95

TABLE 4. OXYTOCIC POTENCIES DETERMINED ON ISOLATED RAT UTERUS DURING DIFFERENT PHASES OF THE ESTROUS CYCLE. FROM CHAN, O'CONNELL AND POMEROY (1963)

Peptide	Oxytocic potency U/mg ± S.E.			
	Diestrus	Proestrus	Estrus	Metestrus
Oxytocin	497±14	483±13	546±18	533±28
Deamino-oxytocin	771±36	564±17	551±17	899±24

TABLE 5. RATIOS ($R_{Mg^{++}}$) ± S.E. FOR ISOLATED RAT UTERUS IN DIETHYLSTIL-BESTROL-TREATED AND METESTROUS RATS. $R_{Mg^{++}}$ = POTENCY WITH 0.5 mM Mg^{++} : POTENCY WITHOUT Mg^{++}. FROM MUNSICK AND JERONIMUS (1965).

Peptide	Diethylstilbestrol $R_{Mg^{++}}$	Metestrous $R_{Mg^{++}}$
Oxytocin	0.97±0.011	0.86±0.009
Deamino-oxytocin	0.88±0.021	1.01±0.02
[Arg^8]-vasopressin	3.32±0.09	2.20±0.13
[Arg^8]-oxytocin	1.98±0.06	1.23±0.04

If oxytocic potencies are to be meaningful from the clinical standpoint, it is obvious from the above discussion that oxytocic assays should be performed in women. If the results are to be applied to pregnant women at term, then the assays should be performed at that time. It is doubtful, however, whether there is justification for using these peptides in pregnant women; for the liability to uterine contracture which sometimes results from excessive dosage, even of a known peptide such as oxytocin, might be dangerous to the mother and fetus. Embrey (1965) has shown that the results of external tokographic measurements used by him and Saameli (1964) in women *post partum* agree, at least for deamino-oxytocin, with findings obtained *ante partum*. Hence, this type of assay may have the requisite qualities to justify its use in clinical pharmacologic investigations.

Space does not permit discussion of the effects of neurohypophysial peptides on non-mammalian oviducal smooth muscle. Here, species differences markedly affect structure–activity relationships. For further information on this subject see Chapter 9.

STRUCTURE–ACTIVITY RELATIONSHIPS

In Chapter 4 Pickering has tabulated many of the published results concerned with the oxytocic potency of oxytocin analogues; Berde and Boissonnas (1966) also have reported many such measurements in great detail.

If one notes the structure of oxytocin (see Chapter 2) it is easy to see that the number of changes which can be made in the structure of an oxytocin molecule are almost unlimited. So far, chemists have principally concentrated on synthesizing analogues with alterations of the functional groups, substitutions of single amino acids, and lengthened and shortened side chains and rings. Many more compounds must be studied before we can thoroughly understand how peptide structure influences oxytocic potency. Also, far more must be learned concerning the mechanism of the oxytocic response and the membrane receptors which initiate it. However, some generalizations seem justifiable:

N-terminal substitution of organic radicals and amino acids on oxytocin appears inevitably to result in diminished activity, total loss of activity, or in the creation of inhibitory compounds.

Deamination, resulting in deamino-oxytocin or deamino-oxytocin-like peptides affects activity very little and may even increase it. The increased potency can partly be explained by diminished tissue inactivation of the peptide.

The functional necessity of the disulfide bond, as mentioned earlier, is still unknown. Its disruption undoubtedly abolishes potency; however, this disruption also involves opening of the ring, and it is still not known to what extent the disulfide bond, *per se*, is required.

The ring structure of oxytocin has slight intrinsic activity (Ressler, 1956). Addition of the next two amino acids of the side chain, proline and leucine, does not markedly increase activity, but addition of the glycine-amide residue, creating oxytocin, increases it dramatically. Hence, it appears that the side chain has a requisite length for optimal activity.

Just as disruption of the ring destroys activity completely, lengthening or shortening it by only one methylene group can markedly reduce activity and can even produce substances with inhibitory properties. Amino acid substitutions, with very few exceptions, diminish activity. Some of the effects of altering the functional groups have already been described previously in connection with the results of Chan and Kelley (1967). Flouret and du Vigneaud (1965) have synthesized D-oxytocin, the enantiomer of oxytocin. It is devoid of activity on the rat uterus.

CONCLUSIONS

It appears that the neurohypophysial polypeptides and their analogues act on the myometrium principally by altering the electrical properties of the cell membrane. The nature of this effect on the cell membrane is unknown, but most investigators agree with the concept that sodium channels are opened. Whether mobilization of calcium from the membrane is responsible for this action is still unknown. Although the sex steroids profoundly affect the ability of the myometrium to respond to neurohypophysial peptides and alter the potencies of various peptides quite variably, the manner by which they do this is still unknown. An exact definition of the receptor sites for neurohypophysial peptides is not currently available, but recent studies are contributing significantly to our knowledge of them. It appears that these receptors are specific for the neurohypophysial peptides, for their blockade by inhibitors does not affect the uterine response to angiotensin, bradykinin or acetylcholine.

As more attention has been directed to assay methods, greater sophistication and enlightenment have resulted. When assays *in vitro* are desired, the assay preparation and the bath fluid have to be chosen with great care, for many factors can markedly affect potency. *In vivo* assay techniques in *post-partum* women hold promise for the evaluation of the effect of these peptides on the human uterus *in situ*.

REFERENCES

BOOKS, REVIEWS, AND MONOGRAPHS

BERDE, B. and BOISSONNAS, R. A. (1966). Synthetic analogues and homologues of the posterior pituitary hormones. *The Pituitary Gland*, pp. 624–661. Harris, G. W. Donovan, B. T. (eds.). Butterworths, London.

BERDE, B. and SAAMELI, K. (1966). Evaluation of substances acting on the uterus, *Methods in Drug Evaluation*, p. 481. North-Holland Publishing Co., Amsterdam.

CSAPO, A. (1961). The effects of oxytocic substances on the excitability of the uterus. *Oxytocin*, pp. 100–121. Caldeyro-Barcia, R. and Heller, H. (eds.). Pergamon Press, New York.

DALE, H. H. (1957). Evidence concerning the endocrine function of the neurohypophysis and its nervous control. *The Neurohypophysis*, pp. 1–9. Heller, H. (ed.). Academic Press Inc., New York.

JUNG, H. (1961). The effect of oxytocin on the mechanism of uterine excitation. *Oxytocin*, pp. 87–99. Caldeyro-Barcia, R. and Heller, H. (eds.). Pergamon Press, New York.

KAO, C. Y. (1967). Ionic basis of electrical activity in uterine smooth muscle. *Cellular Biology of the Uterus*, pp. 386-448. Wynn, R. M. (ed.). Appleton-Century-Crofts, New York.

NEEDHAM, D. M. and SHOENBERG, C. F. (1967). The biochemistry of the myometrium. *Cellular Biology of the Uterus*, pp. 291–352. Wynn, R. M. (ed.). Appleton-Century-Crofts, New York.

SAWYER, W. H. (1968). Phylogenetic aspects of the neurohypophysial hormones. *Neurohypophysial Hormones and Similar Polypeptides, Handbuch der Experimentellen Pharmakologie*, Vol. 23, pp. 717–747. Berde, B. (ed.). Springer-Verlag, New York.

ORIGINAL PAPERS

ABARBANEL, A. R. (1945). The spasmolysant action of magnesium ions on the tetanically contracting human gravid uterus. *Amer. J. Obstet. Gynec.*, **49**: 473–483.

ACHER, R., CHAUVET, J., CHAUVET, M. T. and CREPY, D. (1965). Phylogenie des peptides neurohypophysaires: Isolement d'une nouvelle hormone, la glumitocine (Ser_4-Gln_8-ocytocine) presente chez un poisson cartilagineux, la raie *(Raia clavata)*. *Biochim. Biophys. Acta*, **107**: 393–396.

BENTLEY, P. J. (1964). The effects of N-ethylmaleimide and glutathione on the isolated rat uterus and frog bladder with special reference to the action of oxytocin. *J. Endocr.*, **30**: 103–113.

BENTLEY, P. J. (1965). The potentiating action of magnesium and manganese on the oxytocic effect of some oxytocin analogues. *J. Endocr.*, **32**: 215–222.

BENTLEY, P. J. and DICKER, S. E. (1955). Effects of transient changes of acidity on the isolated rat's uterus, with reference to the assay of oxytocic activity. *Brit. J. Pharmacol., Chemother.*, **10**: 424–428.

BERDE, B., DOEPFNER, W. and KONZETT, H. (1957). Some pharmacological actions of four synthetic analogues of oxytocin. *Brit. J. Pharmac. Chemother.*, **12**: 209–214.

CASTEELS, R., and KURIYAMA, H. (1965). Membrane potential and ionic content in pregnant and non-pregnant rat myometrium. *J. Physiol., Lond.*, **177**: 263–287.

CHAN, W. Y., O'CONNELL, M. and POMEROY, S. R. (1963). Effect of the estrous cycle on the sensitivity of rat uterus to oxytocin and desamino-oxytocin. *Endocrinology*, **72**: 279–282.

CHAN, W. Y. and KELLEY, N. (1967). A pharmacologic analysis of the significance of the chemical functional groups of oxytocin to its oxytocic activity and on the effect of magnesium on the *in vitro* and *in vivo* activity of neurohypophysial hormones. *J. Pharmacol. Exp. Ther.*, **156**: 150–158.

EMBREY, M. P. (1965). The action of desamino-oxytocin on the human pregnant uterus. *J. Endocr.*, **31**: 185–189.

FLOURET, G., and DU VIGNEAUD, V. (1965). The synthesis of D-oxytocin, the enantiomer of the posterior pituitary hormone, oxytocin. *J. Amer. Chem. Soc.*, **87**: 3775–3776.

FOLLETT, B. K. and HELLER, H. (1964). The neurohypophysial hormones of lungfishes and amphibians. *J. Physiol., Lond.*, **172**: 92–106.

MARSHALL, J. (1959). Effects of estrogen and progesterone on single uterine muscle fibers in the rat. *Amer. J. Physiol.*, **197**: 935–942.

MARSHALL, J. (1963). Behaviour of uterine muscle in Na-deficient solutions; effects of oxytocin. *Amer. J. Physiol.*, **204**: 732–738.

MARTIN, P. J. and SCHILD, H. O. (1965). The antagonism of disulphide polypeptides by thiols. *Brit. J. Pharmacol. Chemother*, **25**: 418–431.

MUNSICK, R. A. (1960). Effect of magnesium ion on the response of the rat uterus to neurohypophysial hormones and analogues. *Endocrinology*, **66**: 451–457.

MUNSICK, R. A. (1966). Chromatographic and pharmacologic characterization of the neurohypophysial hormones of an amphibian and a reptile. *Endocrinology*, **78**: 591–599.

MUNSICK, R. A. and JERONIMUS, S. C. (1965). Effects of diethylstilbestrol and magnesium on the rat oxytocic potencies of some neurohypophysial hormones and analogues. *Endocrinology*, **76**: 90–96.

RESSLER, C. (1956). The cyclic disulfide ring of oxytocin. *Proc. Soc. Exp. Biol. Med.*, **92**: 725–730.

RUDINGER, J. and KREJČÍ, I. (1962). Dose-response relations for some synthetic analogues of oxytocin, and the mode of action of oxytocin on the isolated uterus. *Experientia*, **18**: 585–588.

SAAMELI, K. (1964). Quantitative comparison between oxytocin and four related neurohypophysial peptides on the human uterus *in situ*. *Brit. J. Pharmacol.*, **23**: 176–183.

TAIRA, N. and MARSHALL, J. M. (1967). Action of oxytocin antagonists on electrical and mechanical activity of the uterus. *Amer. J. Physiol.*, **212**: 725–731.

VAN DYKE, H. B. and HASTINGS, A. B. (1928). The response of smooth muscle in different ionic environments. *Amer. J. Physiol.*, **83**: 563–577.

CHAPTER 8 (c)

PHYSIOLOGICAL AND PHARMACOLOGICAL EFFECTS: MAMMARY ACTION

S. J. Folley and G. S. Knaggs

*National Institute for Research in Dairying,
Shinfield, Reading, England*

INTRODUCTION

The best known mammary action of the neurohypophysial hormones, particularly oxytocin, is the abrupt rise in intramammary pressure after their introduction into the blood stream, sometimes called the galactokinetic or galactobolic effect. Other less well-characterized effects have been described; these include a galactopoietic action on repeated injections, an influence on the permeability of the mammary parenchymal cells to electrolytes and other substances and, finally, effects on the carbohydrate metabolism of mammary tissue *in vitro*. By virtue of its action in increasing intramammary pressure oxytocin has a vital physiological role in the withdrawal of milk from the mammary gland and it is with this function that most of this review is concerned.

THE ROLE OF NEUROHYPOPHYSIAL HORMONES IN THE MILK-EJECTION REFLEX

EFFECT ON INTRAMAMMARY PRESSURE

In order to obtain the full yield of milk during suckling or milking (by hand or machine), a reflex contraction of the mammary alveoli must be evoked. This reflex, once believed to have a purely nervous arc, is now known to be a neuroendocrine reflex involving the release from the neurohypophysis of oxytocin into the blood which circulates to the mammary gland and causes contraction of its target tissue, the myoepithelial cells surrounding the alveoli. This results in a rise in intramammary pressure as the alveolar milk is forced into the larger ducts and sinuses, or cisterns if present, from which it can be readily withdrawn. Physiologists in the U.S.S.R. believe that the neuroendocrine phase of the milk-ejection reflex* is preceded by a segmental neural reflex which alters the tone of the smooth muscle elements in the walls of the larger ducts and milk cisterns thereby facilitating the action of the neuroendocrine milk-ejection reflex (see Barȳshnikov, 1959; Zaks, 1962). The role of the neurohypophysial hormones, particularly oxytocin, in the milk-ejection reflex has been reviewed by Cowie and Folley (1957), Harris (1958), Cross (1961, 1966), Denamur (1965) and Benson and Fitzpatrick (1966).

The intramammary pressure rise characteristic of the milk-ejection reflex may be mimicked by the administration of posterior pituitary extract, synthetic oxytocin or synthetic vasopressin. The milk-ejection activity of synthetic vasopressin, however, is only 15–20% of that of oxytocin (Boissonnas et al., 1961; Berde, 1963; Folley and Knaggs, 1965). Oxytocin is by far the most active natural milk-ejecting substance known and there is now a great accumulation of evidence summarized in the above-mentioned reviews which makes it virtually certain that oxytocin is the natural milk-ejection hormone.

The amount of i.v. injected oxytocin required to simulate a normal milk-ejection pressure response in the various species studied is given in Table 1.

TABLE 1. THE AMOUNT OF INTRAVENOUSLY INJECTED OXYTOCIN REQUIRED TO MATCH A NORMAL MILK-EJECTION PRESSURE RESPONSE

Species	Oxytocin (mU)	Reference
Cow	1000	Donker, 1958; Peeters, Stormorken and Vanschoubroek, 1960.
	100	Cleverley, 1967.
Sow	1000	Whittlestone, 1954a; Cross, Goodwin and Silver, 1958.
Goat	1000	Cowie, cited by Folley, 1952; Denamur and Martinet, 1953.
Rabbit	50–100	Cross, 1955a; Fuchs and Wagner, 1963.
Bitch	10–20	Pickford, 1960.
Woman	10	Beller, Krumholz and Zeininger, 1958; Theobald, 1959.

* In this article the terms lactation, milk secretion, milk-ejection reflex and milk removal are used in the special sense defined by Cowie et al. (1951).

The mammary gland has a very low threshold sensitivity to oxytocin; doses as small as 1×10^{-6} μU *in vitro* (van Dongen and Hays, 1966) or 1–10 μU after close intra-arterial injection in the guinea-pig (Tindal and Yokoyama, 1962) are sufficient to induce alveolar contraction. Within certain limits of dosage there is a positive correlation between intramammary pressure response and the dose of oxytocin and, the dose–

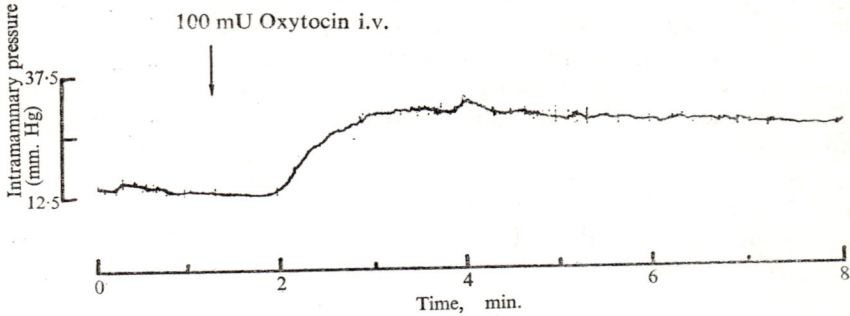

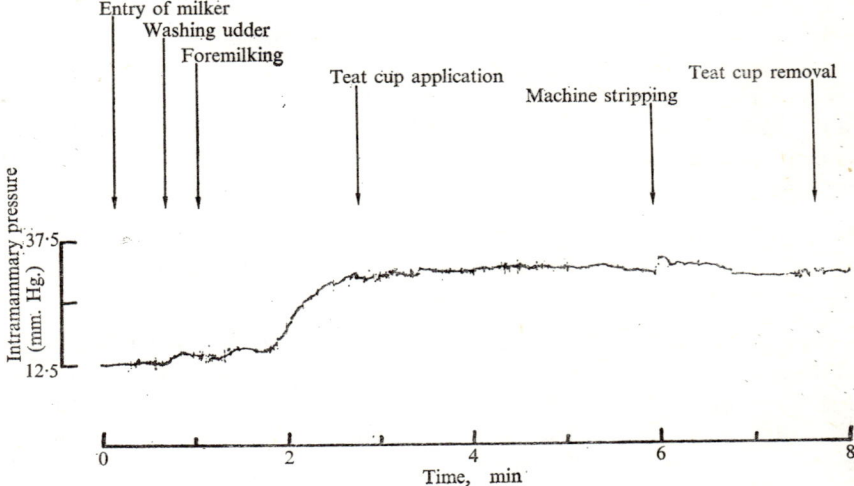

Fig. 1. Polygraph records of the intramammary pressure in the right hind quarter of cow S 61. (a) Effect of rapid injection of 100 mU synthetic oxytocin (Pitocin, Parke Davis & Co.) into the external jugular vein. (b) Effect of the various stimuli associated with a machine milking routine.

response relationship has been determined for several species as follows: *in vivo* for the guinea-pig (Tindal and Yokoyama, 1962), sow (Whittlestone, 1954a) and woman (Wiederman and Stone, 1962; Sala, 1965), and *in vitro* for the rat (Rydén and Sjöholm, 1962; van Dongen and Hays, 1966) and rabbit (Méndez-Bauer, Cabot and Caldeyro-Barcia, 1960; Moore and Zarrow, 1965).

Milk-ejection pressure recordings in several species have shown that the nature of the intramammary pressure response varies according to the species, and the amount and route of administration of the oxytocin. Usually, a single intravenous injection or the reflex release of the hormone at suckling or milking brings about a considerable but short-term increase in the intramammary pressure in the rabbit (van Dyke, Adamsons and Engel, 1955), goat (Martinet and Denamur, 1960) and guinea-pig (Tindal and Yokoyama, 1962). With higher doses of oxytocin a series of rhythmic pressure increases of diminishing intensity often occur (see Berde and Cerletti, 1960, for the rabbit; Martinet and Denamur, 1960, for the goat); similar rhythmic intramammary pressure changes are frequently observed in women during suckling (Caldeyro-Barcia, 1961). Slow intravenous infusions, intramuscular and intranasal application of oxytocin induce either rhythmic series of contractions or a tonic pressure rise without significant fluctuations which returns gradually to normal (see Berde and Cerletti, 1960, for the rabbit; Caldeyro-Barcia, 1961 and Wiederman and Stone, 1962, for women). This type of tonic reaction is also noted after very large intravenous doses of the hormone (Bisset, 1964). In the cow (see Fig. 1) the intravenous injection of "physiological" doses of oxytocin (100 mU) gives an intramammary pressure rise of long duration, closely resembling that observed during machine milking (Cleverley, 1967).

NATURE OF THE EFFECTOR CONTRACTILE TISSUE OF THE MAMMARY GLAND

The nature of the effector contractile tissue of the mammary gland was still uncertain at the time the neurohumoral theory of milk ejection was first proposed (Ely and Petersen, 1941). The earlier views that contraction of smooth muscle (Schäfer, 1898; Gaines, 1915) or udder vascular erection (Hammond, 1936) were responsible for milk ejection were refuted when Richardson (1949, 1951) clearly demonstrated the presence of myoepithelial cells around the alveoli and along the finer milk ducts in the goat and human mammae. The classical observations of Richardson were later confirmed in other species by Linzell (1952) and Silver (1954).

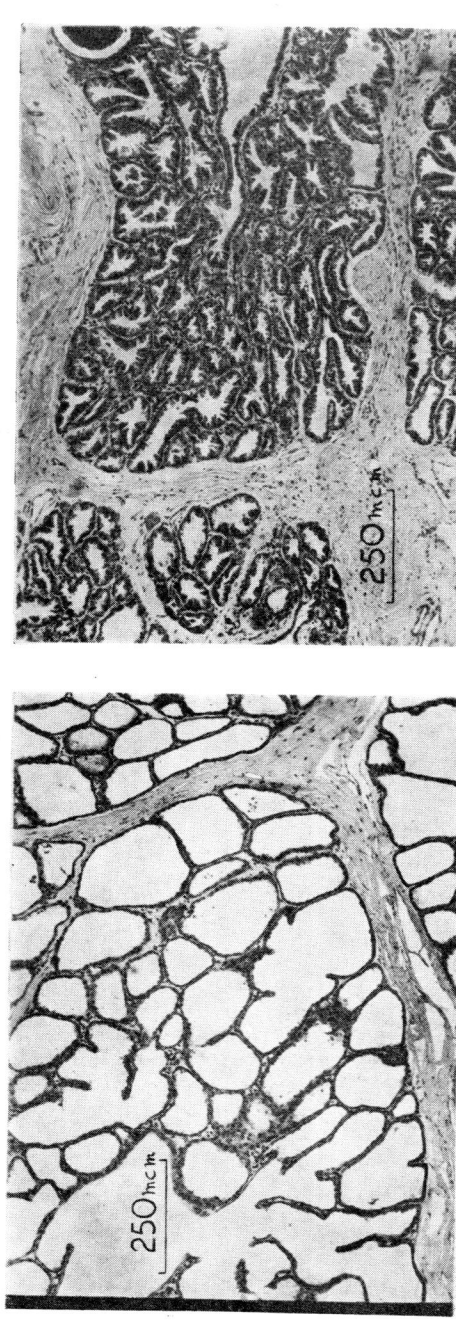
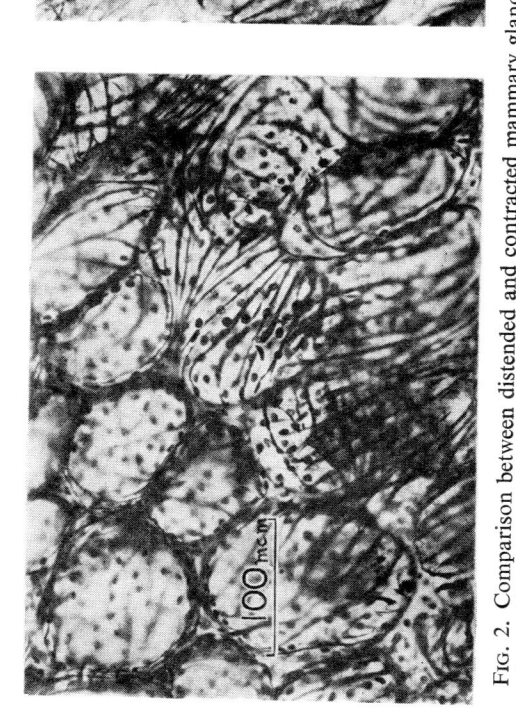

FIG. 2. Comparison between distended and contracted mammary glands of the goat. *Top left*: part of a lobule from the left half of an udder fixed while distended with milk. *Top right*: the right half of the udder from the same goat which was milked out as completely as possible before autopsy; note the contracted lobules with collapsed alveoli and ducts lined with a thick folded epithelium. *Bottom left*: myoepithelium on the surface of distended alveoli; section taken from the same left half as above. *Bottom right*: myoepithelium of contracted alveoli; section taken from the same right half as above. (From Richardson, 1949.)

The mesh-like arrangement of the stellate processes of the myoepithelial cells around the alveoli, their longitudinal orientation along the smaller milk ducts and their configuration before and after milking suggested (Richardson, 1949) that they were actively involved in milk ejection. Figure 2, which is reproduced by kind permission of Mr. K. C. Richardson, illustrates his studies carried out on goats belonging to the herd of this Institute. The morphology of the myoepithelial cells in the gland distended with milk is well shown, as is also the changed aspect of the latter after milking. An active role for the myoepithelium in alveolar contraction is supported by the work of Zaks (1951), Levitskaya (1955) and Linzell (1955), who observed that locally applied posterior pituitary hormones caused contraction of the alveoli in the mammary gland of the mouse *in situ* and also a shortening and widening of the milk ducts. It has also been shown recently that neurohypophysial hormones can induce milk ejection *in vitro* (van Dongen and Hays, 1966).

NEUROHYPOPHYSIAL HORMONES AND MAMMARY GLAND ACTION POTENTIALS

Forbes, Forbes and Neyland (1955) reported that the milk-ejection reflex in women was accompanied by a slow action potential discharge recorded from the areola of the breast. The electrical discharge began a few seconds before the patient signalled the tingling sensation often associated with the milk-ejection reflex. Similar electrical phenomena could be evoked by the intravenous administration of oxytocin into the same subjects before suckling. Later control experiments (Forbes, Neyland and Fox, 1960) were considered to eliminate the possibility that these electrical effects were due to sweat gland activity and it was believed (Deane and Forbes, 1956) that they were associated with contraction of the mammary gland myoepithelium in response to oxytocin. More recently Findlay (1966) has studied action potentials recorded from segmental nerves supplying the mammae of lactating rabbits subjected to various stimuli. Of interest in the present context is the finding that intravenous oxytocin evoked action potential discharges in the nerve coincident with the rise in intramammary pressure which, incidentally, considerably outlasted the electrical discharge.

CHANGES IN THE MILK-EJECTION RESPONSE TO NEUROHYPOPHYSIAL HORMONES DURING PREGNANCY AND LACTATION

Changes in the mammary response to oxytocin and vasopressin during various physiological states have only been studied to an appreciable extent in man (Sala, 1964). In the non-pregnant woman the mammary gland is unresponsive to the intravenous injection of doses as large as 1000 mU oxytocin. The sensitivity of the myoepithelium to oxytocin increases from the beginning of pregnancy and after the 14th–17th week 100 mU are sufficient to induce a threshold milk-ejection pressure response. By the 18th–20th week a response is obtained to 1 mU and the threshold remains at this level throughout the rest of gestation. The myoepithelial sensitivity to vasopressin follows a similar pattern except that the threshold doses needed are 40–50 times greater than those for oxytocin.

Conflicting results have been obtained in a number of species regarding the changes in the sensitivity of the mammary gland to oxytocin during lactation (for references see Denamur, 1965). The reason for these discrepancies is most probably to be sought in the wide variations in the amount of milk present in the mammary gland at different phases of the lactational cycle. Thus, it seems likely that the apparent response to oxytocin would be impaired during early lactation and involution when the gland is relatively empty. In the involuting rat mammary gland, filled intraductally with milk to overcome the problem of lack of secretion, 3–5 times more oxytocin is required to evoke a threshold response than during lactation (DeNuccio and Grosvenor, 1967), but a milk-ejection response is still obtainable even after an 11-day involutionary period.

SPECIES DIFFERENCES IN THE REQUIREMENT FOR OXYTOCIN IN MILK REMOVAL

In many of the species studied, e.g. rat (Eayrs and Baddeley, 1956; Grosvenor, 1964; Edwardson and Eayrs, 1967), rabbit (Mena and Beyer, 1963) and cat (Beyer et al., 1962) interruption of the neural pathways from the mammary gland to the brain results in a failure of lactation. If milk secretion is maintained by hormonal replacement therapy the young can only obtain milk if oxytocin is injected at suckling, showing that the integrity of the milk-ejection reflex is essential for emptying of the gland.

By contrast, in small ruminants the milk-ejection reflex does not appear to be essential for milk removal. This view arises from experiments involving complete deafferentation of the udder in sheep and goats (Tsakhaev, 1958; Tverskoï, 1958; Denamur and Martinet, 1959; Linzell, 1963) in which normal milk yields were obtained provided that the udders were carefully massaged at the end of the milking. The administration of oxytocin to these animals does not further increase the milk yield except when large amounts of milk are present in the gland (Denamur and Martinet, 1960). The studies of Yokoyama and Ôta (1965) on goats anesthetized during milking and of Folley and Knaggs (1966) who found oxytocin in the jugular blood of goats during only a minority of milkings, even though the milk yields were normal, also indicate that oxytocin release is not indispensable for obtaining a normal milk yield in this species. A conditioned reflex release of oxytocin was precluded in the experiments involving deafferentation of the udder since primiparous animals were used. As noted above, the milking routine in these experiments usually ended with a vigorous massage of the udder and it is therefore possible that milk removal might have been assisted by the local contraction of the myoepithelial cells surrounding the alveoli in response to the mechanical stimulation of the udder, as described for the rabbit (Cross, 1954; Yokoyama, 1956) and rat (Linzell, 1955; Grosvenor, 1965). Moreover, the goat udder contains a large proportion of cisternal tissue and milk sinuses which might be readily evacuated by a thorough milking procedure.

INHIBITION OF THE MILK-EJECTION ACTIVITY OF OXYTOCIN

Inhibition nvolving mammary vasoconstriction. A number of factors discussed below produce a constriction of the blood capillaries in the mammary gland which results in an inhibition of the milk-ejection response to injected oxytocin, since access of the hormone to the myoepithelial cells is prevented. Local cooling of the mammary gland or a lowering of the body temperature usually result in constriction of the mammary gland capillaries. In our experience the *in vivo* mammary gland preparations for the assay of milk-ejection activity are highly susceptible to reduction of the environmental or general body temperature (Knaggs, 1966). Another inhibitory phenomenon, not strictly vasoconstriction, but an occlusion of the mammary gland capillaries occurs when the glands are overdistended with milk (Cross and Silver, 1956).

A reflex nervous vasoconstriction may occur as a result of emotional e.g. fright, pain, worry, or other physiological factors which activate the sympathetic nervous system. The mammary blood vessels have been shown to be very sensitive to the action of sympathetic adrenergic vasoconstrictor nerve fibers (Hebb and Linzell, 1951; Linzell, 1953).

There are also a large number of vasoconstrictor substances, some of which occur naturally, which may cause a constriction of the mammary gland capillaries. The most important of these are adrenaline and noradrenaline which were shown by Hebb and Linzell (1951), Linzell (1953) and Cross and Silver (1962a) to have a powerful vasoconstrictor action on the mammary gland. These two substances are released during activation of the sympathetico-adrenal system or by various substances which cause their release by a direct action on the adrenal medulla. The injection of adrenaline has been shown to inhibit the milk-ejection normally evoked by endogenous or exogenous oxytocin in a variety of species, e.g. cow (Ely and Petersen, 1941; Bílek and Janovsky, 1958), sow (Braude and Mitchell, 1952; Whittlestone, 1954b), dog (Pickford, 1960), rabbit (Cross, 1953) and the perfused bovine udder preparation (Peeters, Sierens and Silver, 1952). The mechanism by which adrenaline prevents the milk-ejection response to oxytocin has not been clearly defined. Presumably mammary vasoconstriction plays a large part in inhibiting the mammary gland responses to oxytocin. There is also the possibility that adrenaline may act directly on the mammary myoepithelial cells making them refractory to oxytocin. The work of Linzell (1955) suggested that this is not so, as adrenaline applied directly to the mammary tissue did not prevent alveolar contraction in response to the topical application of oxytocin. However, more recently Chan (1965) has presented rather compelling evidence that the action of adrenaline in inhibiting the galactokinetic effect of oxytocin is exerted directly on the myoepithelial cells. From experiments on the mammary gland of the lactating rabbit involving the use of adrenergic blocking agents he concluded that the inhibitory effect of adrenaline was independent of the vasoconstrictor properties of the catecholamine and, moreover, adrenaline inhibited the contractile response of the rabbit mammary strip to oxytocin *in vitro*.

Synthetic angiotensin II possesses some milk-ejection activity when injected intra-arterially into the lactating guinea-pig at a dose of 1–2 μg. (Knaggs, 1966). This dose of angiotensin also temporarily inhibits the response to subsequent injections of oxytocin, possibly as a result of a vasoconstrictor action of angiotensin on the mammary gland, or alternatively because of the action of adrenaline released from the adrenal medulla under the stimulus of angiotensin (Feldberg and Lewis, 1964). Similarly, synthetic bradykinin which gives a threshold milk-ejection response after the intra-arterial injection of 1 μg into the guinea-pig mammary gland (Knaggs, 1966) temporarily inhibits the milk-ejection response to further oxytocin probably by causing a release of adrenaline from the adrenal medulla (Feldberg and Lewis, 1964). Histamine which may be present in blood after tissue injury produces a very marked tachyphylaxis of the mammary gland and inhibition of the response to subsequent oxytocin injections (Knaggs, 1966). This may be due to a direct inhibitory action of histamine on the mammary gland or to the fact that histamine induces the release of plasma kinins (Edery and Lewis, 1963) which in turn precipitate the release of adrenaline. 5-Hydroxytryptamine applied topically to mouse mammary tissue (Linzell, 1955) or injected intra-arterially into the mammary gland of the lactating guinea-pig (Knaggs, 1966) also causes a pronounced reduction in the mammary response to oxytocin.

Inhibition not necessarily involving mammary vasoconstriction. Vasopressin, although it has inherent milk-ejection activity has also been reported to inhibit the galactokinetic action of oxytocin. Kullander (1963) observed that when vasopressin and oxytocin were infused simultaneously into the lactating rabbit in ratios varying from 1:1 to 1:4 then the milk-ejection responses normally produced by oxytocin were greatly diminished or abolished. Lower ratios of vasopressin: oxytocin had no effect. The mechanism of this effect is obscure; it does not appear to be mediated by adrenaline release, and vasopressin does not potentiate the inhibitory action of adrenaline. Pressor effects are also eliminated since the amounts of vasopressin involved are too small to affect the blood pressure. This antagonism may be of importance in view of the reports that vasopressin and oxytocin are released simultaneously during suckling (Cross, 1950; Kalliala and Karvonen, 1951; Kalliala, Karvonen and Leppänen, 1952; Peeters and Coussens, 1950; Peeters, Stormorken and Vanschoubroek, 1960). However, the ratio of the amount of vasopressin: oxytocin released at suckling is of the order of 1:100 in the rabbit (Cross, 1951) and 1:30 in the dog (Pickford, 1960), ratios which would have no antagonistic effect according to Kullander (1963). By contrast Chaudhury, Chaudhury and Lu (1961) found that 10 mU vasopressin given intraperitoneally immediately before suckling had no effect on milk ejection in the lactating guinea-pig. We ourselves have observed no inhibitory effect of arginine or lysine vasopressin on the milk-ejection response to oxytocin when injected intra-arterially into the mammary gland of the lactating guinea-pig two minutes before the oxytocin. Moreover, Tindal, Knaggs and Turvey (1968) found that the intravenous injection of a solution containing equal amounts of oxytocin and vasopressin into the lactating guinea-pig gave the same milk-ejection response as the same amount of oxytocin injected alone. Similar results were obtained by Gaitan, Cobo and Mizrachi (1964) in lactating women.

The fact that thiol compounds such as thioglycollate irreversibly inactivate oxytocin and vasopressin by reducing their S-S bridges was first demonstrated by van Dyke et al. (1942). It has since been shown that thiols exert a second and distinct type of inhibitory effect on the biological actions of oxytocin (Martin and Schild, 1962). This antagonism occurs at the level of the target tissue and is believed to involve competition for the receptor sites. Since the chemical inactivation of oxytocin is a slow process (Martin and Schild, 1962) the latter effect is probably responsible for the inhibition by thioglycollate of the contraction of rat mammary strips in response to oxytocin reported by Smith (1961).

The effect of removing Ca^{++} from the bath fluid of preparations of rat and rabbit mammary strips is to render the strips nonreactive to oxytocin (Moore and Zarrow, 1965; Poláček, Krejčí and Rudinger, 1967). This effect may be reversed by returning the calcium concentration to normal. A fourfold increase in the calcium concentration augments the mammary response to oxytocin, but larger increases produce an irreversible loss of responsiveness of the rat mammary strip (Poláček et al., 1967). In these mammary strip preparations an increase in the potassium concentration has no effect on the response of the rat tissue (Poláček et al., 1967), but with rabbit tissue replacement of the sodium in Tyrode solution with potassium leads to a progressive but partially reversible decrease in the response to oxytocin (Moore and Zarrow, 1965).

In addition to those discussed above a number of other inhibitory factors have also been reported. In anesthetized preparations the milk-ejection response is considerably affected by variations in the depth of anesthesia. Immediately after injection of some anesthetic agents (e.g. pentobarbital sodium, urethane) the sensitivity of the response is temporarily depressed (Knaggs, 1966). The anesthetic may affect the central and peripheral mechanisms which control vasomotor tone in the body and cause mammary vasoconstriction, or it may exert its inhibitory effect directly on the myoepithelial cells. Satisfactory oxygenation of the blood and tissues is essential to maintain the response to injected oxytocin in the actively contracting mammary gland according to van Dyke et al. (1955). In contrast, Cross and Silver (1962a) found that a reduction in O_2 tension in the gland produced by breathing a mixture of O_2 and N_2 did not affect the milk-ejection response to exogenous oxytocin. However, marked hypoxia or hypercapnia caused inhibition of the milk-ejection response to oxytocin by activation of the sympathetico-adrenal system (Cross and Silver, 1962b). Electrical stimulation of the efferent nerves to the mammary glands results in an inhibition of the milk-ejection response to oxytocin in the guinea-pig, rabbit and goat mammary gland (Linzell, 1955; Cross, 1955b; see also references cited by Barȳshnikov, 1965). The Russian interpretation of this phenomenon is that the stimulation causes a spasm of the smooth muscle around the larger milk ducts which prevents the egress of milk. Finally, it may be noted here that several synthetic analogues of oxytocin have been prepared which exhibit an antagonism toward the mammary response to oxytocin. These inhibitory analogues are discussed in a later section (see p. 307).

BIOASSAY OF MILK-EJECTION ACTIVITY

Several mammary gland preparations are used for the detection and bioassay of the milk-ejection activity of oxytocin and its synthetic analogues. From a pharmacological standpoint the lactating mammary gland is most suitable for the bioassay of oxytocin, particularly in extracts of body fluids or tissues, since its response to the hormone is highly specific when compared with that of the uterine myometrium and spontaneous contractions are rarely encountered. Measurements of the milk-ejection responses of the lactating mammary gland *in situ* after the intravenous or close intra-arterial injection of oxytocin form the basis of a number of preparations; mouse (Vorherr, 1965); guinea-pig (Tindal and Yokoyama, 1960, 1962); rabbit (Turner and Cooper, 1941; Cross and van Dyke, 1953; van Dyke *et al.*, 1955; Berde and Cerletti, 1957; Fitzpatrick, 1961); sow (Whittlestone, 1952, 1953); woman (Friedman, 1960). Turner and Cooper (1941) observed the contractions of the mammary gland through the skin of the abdomen in the rabbit, whereas Whittlestone (1952, 1953) used the duration and volume of milk flow in the sow as criteria for the intensity of the response. Most of the *in vivo* methods, however, depend on measurements of the changes in intramammary pressure by techniques involving cannulation of the gland, or by use of external pressure recording systems such as that described for the human breast by Friedman (1960). The anesthetized lactating rabbit preparation is relatively insensitive by the intravenous route of injection, but the sensitivity is greatly increased (threshold 100 μU) when the close intra-arterial route (Fitzpatrick, 1961) is used. The lactating guinea-pig preparation (Tindal and Yokoyama, 1960, 1962) is essentially similar but considerably more sensitive than the rabbit method, especially when the close intra-arterial route is employed which has a threshold of 1–5 μU oxytocin, the intravenous threshold being 50 μU oxytocin. Higher thresholds (i.v., 500–2000 μU; i.a., 50–100 μU) have been given for a slightly modified version of this technique as used by Beránková-Ksandrová *et al.* (1966).

Several *in vitro* mammary gland preparations are also used for determining the milk-ejection activity of oxytocin. Narrow strips of tissue cut from lactating glands are suspended in an organ bath maintained at constant temperature, with a calculated resting tension applied to the strips. The isometric contractile force produced by the addition of oxytocin to the bath is measured. Smith (1961) described such a preparation using rat mammary tissue, which was later modified by Rydén and Sjöholm (1962) who obtained threshold responses from 2–50 μU oxytocin. Beránková-Ksandrová et al. (1966) using isolated mammary strips from the guinea-pig obtained threshold responses to 500 μU oxytocin. The mammary strip method was originated by Méndez-Bauer et al. (1960) who used rabbit mammary tissue and this preparation was more fully investigated by Moore and Zarrow (1965) who found a threshold of 100 μU. Since both myoepithelial and smooth muscle elements are present in the mammary gland (Richardson, 1949; Linzell, 1955) it is not clear to what extent the contraction of each of these two tissues contributes to the total mammary response to oxytocin. Recently a very sensitive technique has been developed utilizing small blocks of mammary tissue from lactating rats and observing the time taken for the ejection of milk to occur after the immersion of the blocks in a solution containing oxytocin (van Dongen and Hays, 1966). The threshold of this method is 1×10^{-6} μU oxytocin.

The *in vitro* techniques have the advantages that interference from anesthesia and homeostatic mechanisms is eliminated and the tissue retains its ability to react to oxytocin for several days and may be stored at low temperatures and used when required. However, a long interval of 5–10 min is needed between successive doses of oxytocin, whereas injections may be given every 2–3 min with the gland *in situ*. Statistically the *in vitro* methods show a lack of precision when compared with the *in vivo* techniques. A comprehensive study of the relative specificity of the various mammary gland assay preparations has not been made. However, the *in vitro* methods are in general the less specific and many respond to relatively small concentrations of acetylcholine, 5-hydroxytryptamine, histamine, adrenaline, and noradrenaline (Moore and Zarrow, 1965; van Dongen and Marshall, 1967). With the exception of acetylcholine, much higher concentrations of these substances than normally occur in the body fluids are necessary to increase the intramammary pressure *in vivo*. However, the threshold concentration of acetylcholine is approximately 1–2000 times that of oxytocin (Folley and Knaggs, 1966) in the non-atropinized animal; in the atropinized guinea-pig the threshold concentration of acetylcholine after intra-arterial injection is approximately 2,500,000 times that of oxytocin (Knaggs, 1966).

MILK-EJECTION ACTIVITY OF SYNTHETIC ANALOGUES OF OXYTOCIN

The synthesis of a large number of analogues of oxytocin and vasopressin and the study of their pharmacological properties has been undertaken in order to determine the relationship between chemical structure and biological activity with the ultimate object of finding compounds of clinical interest and also of elucidating the underlying mechanism of their various biological effects. Such investigations have been concerned principally with variations in the sequence, stereostructure, side chains, and chemical functional groups of the constituent amino-acid residues, alterations in the size of the disulfide ring and the effect of shortening the tripeptide side chain. Table 2 contains details of a number of analogues of oxytocin which are of particular interest in regard to their milk-ejecting ability.

Table 2a shows that of the naturally occurring neurohypophysial hormones oxytocin is the most active in respect of galactokinetic activity. Nevertheless, it is of interest that two other neurohypophysial hormones, isotocin ([Ser^4, Ile^8]-oxytocin) and mesotocin ([Ile^8]-oxytocin) which occur in the pituitaries of some teleosts and Amphibia respectively are almost as active. The substitution of leucine in position 8 by a basic amino acid, e.g. arginine vasotocin, arginine and lysine vasopressin, enhances the pressor and antidiuretic activities and diminishes the milk-ejection and oxytocic activities.

So far, only one compound, deamino-oxytocin, has been prepared which has a higher specific milk-ejection activity than oxytocin itself. Since this compound has a relatively low pressor activity and has been reported to be resistant to pregnancy oxytocinase in man (Golubow, Chan and du Vigneaud, 1963) it is of obvious clinical interest for possible use in certain types of lactational disorder. In this connection Althabe *et al.*, (1966) reported that deamino-oxytocin was about 1.5 times as active as oxytocin in causing milk ejection in women in early lactation, a result which is in good agreement with assay results obtained with mammary gland preparations *in vivo* (see Table 2b).

Numerous analogues have been prepared which exhibit a selective increase in milk-ejection activity relative to the other biological activities. Table 2c contains particulars of 19 of these analogues which include only those having at least one-tenth of the specific milk-ejection activity of oxytocin which is taken as 450 U/mg. It is evident from the data in Table 2 and from similar data pertaining to analogues not included in the table (see reviews by Sawyer, 1961; du Vigneaud, 1964; Berde and Boissonnas, 1966) that the milk-ejection activity is in general less susceptible

TABLE 2. MILK-EJECTION ACTIVITIES OF SYNTHETIC ANALOGUES OF OXYTOCIN

	Milk-ejection activity U./mg ± S.E.	Oxytocic activity (isolated rat uterus) U./mg	Pressor activity (rat) U./mg	Reference
a. Natural posterior pituitary hormones				
Oxytocin	450 ± 30	450	5	Boissonnas et al., 1961.
Mesotocin, [Ile^8]-oxytocin	328 ± 21	289	6.3	Boissonnas et al., 1961.
Isotocin, [Ser^4, Ile^8]-oxytocin	300 ± 15	150	0.06	Berde and Boissonnas, 1966.
Arginine vasotocin, [Arg^8]-oxytocin	~210;	115	245	Berde and Boissonnas, 1966.
Arginine vasopressin	65 ± 8	16	400	Berde and Boissonnas, 1966.
Lysine vasopressin	60 ± 10	5	270	Berde and Boissonnas, 1966.
Glumitocin, [Ser^4, Gln^8]-oxytocin	Not known	Not known	Not known	Acher et al., 1965.
b. Structural modifications increasing specific milk-ejection activity				
Deamino-oxytocin	541 ± 13; 677; 775	803	1.44	Ferrier et al., 1965; Knaggs, 1966; Althabe et al., 1966.
c. Structural modifications increasing milk-ejection activity relative to other biological activities (>45 U./mg milk-ejection activity)				
[3-β-diethylalanine]-oxytocin	398	305	1.4	Eisler et al., 1966.
[4-Asparagine]-oxytocin	300 ± 128	108	0.13	Berde and Boissonnas, 1966.
Deamino-4-decarboxamido-oxytocin	266 ± 2	93	0	Branda et al., 1966.
[4-Serine]-oxytocin	255 ± 45	195	0.1	Berde and Boissonnas, 1966.
[2-p-Methylphenylalanine]-oxytocin	243	19	0	Zhuze et. al, 1964,
[4-Alanine]-oxytocin	240 ± 55	36	0.01	Berde and Boissonnas, 1966.
4-Decarboxamido-oxytocin	225	72	0.	Branda et al., 1966.
[3-Valine]-oxytocin	207 ± 14	59	0.2	Berde and Boissonnas, 1966.

TABLE 2 (cont.)

	Milk-ejection activity U./mg ± S.E.	Oxytocic activity (isolated rat uterus) U./mg	Pressor activity (rat) U./mg	Reference
[2-Phenylalanine]-oxytocin (deoxy-oxytocin)	141 ± 21	32	0.4	Berde and Boissonnas, 1966.
[3-alloIsoleucine]-oxytocin	125	25	0.2	Berde and Boissonnas, 1966.
[3-Norvaline]-oxytocin	85	7	0.1	Berde and Boissonnas, 1966.
[2-Phenylalanine]-deamino-oxytocin	65.6; 60	25	0.04	Knaggs, 1966; du Vigneaud, 1964.
[3-O-Methylthreonine]-oxytocin	65	35	0.07	Eisler et al., 1966.
[2-p-Ethylphenylalanine]-oxytocin	60	6.5	0	Zhuze et al., 1964.
[9-Sarcosine]-oxytocin	55	36	0.01	Berde and Boissonnas, 1966.
[8-D-Leucine]-oxytocin	50	20	0.01	Berde and Boissonnas, 1966.
[1-Mercaptoacetic acid]-oxytocin	50	25	0.01	Jarvis and du Vigneaud, 1967.
[8-Glycine]-oxytocin	46 ± 7	16	0.6	Berde and Boissonnas, 1966.

d. *Structural modifications decreasing milk-ejection activity relative to other biological activities*

[8-Citrulline]-oxytocin	238	500	7	Berde and Boissonnas, 1966; van Dyke et al., 1963.

e. *Analogues with an inhibitory effect on the milk-ejection activity of oxytocin*

Prolyl oxytocin				Beránková-Ksandrová et al., 1966.
Glycyl oxytocin	Hormonogens			Beránková-Ksandrová et al., 1966.
Leucyl oxytocin				Beránková-Ksandrová et al., 1966.
Phenylalanyl oxytocin				Beránková-Ksandrová et al., 1966.
Glycylglycyl oxytocin				Beránková-Ksandrová et al., 1966.
Leucylleucyl oxytocin	Hormonogens			Beránková-Ksandrová et al., 1966.
Leucylglycylglycyl oxytocin				Beránková-Ksandrová et al., 1966.

to diminution by alterations in the structure of the molecule than the other biological activities of oxytocin. Of the 19 analogues shown, 6 may be of potential clinical interest for use in the treatment of lactational disorders related to the functioning of the milk-ejection reflex, because the ratio of milk-ejection: oxytocic activity is in all cases greater than 3 and the ratios of milk-ejection activity: pressor and antidiuretic activities respectively are greater than those of oxytocin. These six compounds are [Phe(pMe)^2]-oxytocin, [Ala^4]-oxytocin, 4-decarboxamido-oxytocin, [Val^3]-oxytocin, [Phe^2]-oxytocin and [aIle^3]-oxytocin. Of these analogues, the galactokinetic effect of [Val^3]-oxytocin in lactating women has been reported (Friedman, 1960). A preliminary clinical study of [aIle^3]-oxytocin has been briefly described by Jungmannova *et al.* (1964). It is interesting to note that [Val^3]-oxytocin is eliminated from the circulation of rats more slowly than oxytocin (Smith and Ginsburg, 1961).

An interesting exception to the above mentioned generalization that milk-ejection activity is on the whole the biological activity of oxytocin most resistant to the effects of changes in the molecular structure is the analogue formed by the substitution of leucine in position 8 by citrulline. [Cit^8]-oxytocin shows a decrease in milk-ejection activity relative to oxytocic and pressor activities (Table 2d).

Table 2e gives particulars of seven oxytocin analogues which inhibit the galactokinetic effect of oxytocin *in vivo*. All these compounds are characterized by an amino acid or short peptide chain attached to the terminal amino group of oxytocin (Beránková-Ksandrová *et al.*, 1966). One of these seven analogues, Leu-Gly-Gly-oxytocin exerts its inhibitory effect only after intravenous injection and not after close intra-arterial injection into the mammary gland or on the mammary strip *in vitro* (Bisset, 1964). Most of these compounds exert a prolonged effect on the mammary gland *in vivo* together with tachyphylaxis. The prolonged action is believed to be due to the slow liberation of oxytocin by the action of aminopeptidases and the inhibitory effects might be ascribed to saturation of receptor sites by the liberated hormone. Synthetic compounds showing this phenomenon have been called hormonogens (Beránková-Ksandrová *et al.*, 1966). Two observations are in accord with the hormonogen concept: first, Bisset (1964) and Beránková-Ksandrová *et al.* (1966) have reported that the galactokinetic effect of single injections of oxytocin can be inhibited by slow intravenous infusions of the hormone; second, compounds such as *N*-methyl-oxytocin, sarcosyl oxytocin and D-leucyl oxytocin which would probably not be attacked by aminopeptidases do not show the actions typical of hormonogens (Beránková-Ksandrová *et al.*, 1966).

ADDITIONAL MAMMARY EFFECTS OF OXYTOCIN

GALACTOPOIETIC EFFECT

In addition to its galactokinetic action by virtue of which the yield of milk at a given milking can be increased by a single injection of oxytocin at the expense of the yield at the next milking because of the expulsion of the residual milk from the alveoli, it has been reported by several workers (for references see Cowie and Folley, 1957; Benson and Fitzpatrick, 1966) that regular injections of oxytocin into lactating animals produce longterm increases in the yield of milk and butter fat. It seems unlikely that this apparent galactopoietic effect of oxytocin could be due to the action of the hormone in preventing the build up of pressure in the alveoli to an extent at which it might inhibit milk secretion, since there is much evidence (see Elliot, 1959a, b) that, at least in the cow, milk secretion continues at an undiminished rate for at least 20 hr after milking. In the experiments which we are considering the animals were milked more frequently than this. Alternative mechanisms for the possible galactopoietic effect of oxytocin which have been proposed are that it might stimulate the release from the anterior pituitary of hormones concerned in galactopoiesis, or that it may directly stimulate the metabolism of the mammary parenchymal cells.

STIMULATION OF CARBOHYDRATE METABOLISM OF MAMMARY PARENCHYMAL CELLS

Both synthetic oxytocin and synthetic vasopressin increase the oxidation of [1-^{14}C]-glucose and [6-^{14}C]-glucose in the parenchyma of slices taken from the mammary glands of lactating rats, rabbits and mice and of [1-^{14}C]-glucose in mammary slices taken from pregnant rats and rabbits (Goodfriend and Topper, 1961). Oxytocin exerted its maximal effect at concentrations of 10^{-8} to 10^{-6}M in which range the similar well-known action of insulin was additive which suggested that the mechanism of the oxytocin effect was different from that of insulin. On the other hand, glucose oxidation in rat liver slices is not affected by oxytocin or vasopressin. The effect on glucose oxidation in the mammary gland does not appear to be mediated by a facilitation of glucose entry into the cell, or to any action on the enzymes involved in phosphorylation or oxidation in the pentose phosphate cycle, but since the effect is inhibited by puromycin, Cohen, Brenneman and Topper (1962) suggested that it may be due to a specific effect on protein biosynthesis, perhaps involving the formation of an enzyme protein concerned in glucose oxidation.

RESORPTION OF MILK CONSTITUENTS

Studies by Azimov and his colleagues (Azimov, 1959; Azimov, Orlov and Belugina, 1962) using $Na_2H^{32}PO_4$, $^{45}CaCl_2$ and ^{35}S-methionine have indicated the possibility of a two-way transference of some milk constituents between the blood and the mammary secretion in lactating cows and goats. Azimov believes that this resorptive process plays an important role in milk secretion and he showed that the speed of resorption was increased during milking or by the injection of posterior pituitary extract. Azimov's ideas on the importance of reabsorption in mammary function have been supported by the electron microscope studies of Bargmann, Fleischhauer and Knoop (1961) who reported the presence of numerous microvilli on the luminar surface of the mammary parenchymal cells of the golden hamster forming a brush border, thus increasing the available surface area for the passage of solutes from the alveolar secretion into the cells.

RETARDATION OF MAMMARY INVOLUTION

It was shown by Benson and Folley (1956, 1957) that regular injections of oxytocin into rats after weaning markedly retarded the involution of the mammary gland and that this effect was abolished by hypophysectomy. A similar effect was exerted by vasopressin (Benson and Folley, 1957) and [Val^3]-oxytocin (Benson, Folley and Tindal, 1960). These results were subsequently confirmed by a number of authors (for review see Meites and Nicoll, 1966; Benson and Fitzpatrick, 1966), but the interpretation has given rise to a certain amount of controversy, for discussion of which the reader is referred to reviews by Benson and Fitzpatrick (1966) and Meites (1968). Although the oxytocin effect bears a resemblance to those which can be obtained by the application of the suckling stimulus without milk removal (Selye, 1934) or to injections of prolactin, which led Benson and Folley (1957) to consider the possibility that central mechanisms might be involved, more recent biochemical studies on the mammary gland lead to a different conclusion. Thus, Ôta, Shinde and Yokoyama (1965) found that in rats weaned between days 11–13 of lactation, oxytocin, like prolactin, tended to maintain the DNA content of the abdominal mammary glands in keeping with the maintenance of the alveolar structure; on the other hand, the functional integrity of the mammary tissue as indicated by the RNA and phosphoprotein content was supported by prolactin treatment but not by oxytocin. Similarly, in the rabbit weaned at the 5th day of lactation, Denamur (1962) found that oxytocin, unlike prolactin, did not prevent the decline in the RNA content of the mammary gland. In this case, however, the DNA was not maintained either. In general agreement with this is the fact that it has so far not proved possible to counteract the well-known fall in the respiratory metabolism of mammary slices after weaning by injections of oxytocin (Folley and McNaught, 1956, 1957; Ôta and Yokoyama, 1958; Yokoyama and Ôta, 1959).

MAMMARY UPTAKE OF OXYTOCIN

The possibility exists that the lactating mammary gland might play an important role in the inactivation of oxytocin in the blood or in its removal therefrom, since it has been shown (Ginsburg and Smith, 1959) that intravenously injected oxytocin disappears more rapidly from the circulation in the lactating than in the non-lactating rat. This indicates that in the lactating animal as compared with the non-lactating one an additional organ or mechanism exists in which preferential uptake of oxytocin takes place. The organ concerned is almost certainly the lactating mammary gland. It would appear that excretion of oxytocin into the milk is not an important route for the disposal of the hormone since Noddle (1962) failed to find significant amounts of oxytocin in the milk after intravenous injections of large doses of the hormone.

REFERENCES

BOOKS, REVIEWS AND MONOGRAPHS

BARȲSHNIKOV, I. A. (1959). Reflex regulation of lactation. *Dairy Sci. Abstr.*, 21: 47–53.
BARȲSHNIKOV, I. A. (1965). Nervous control of mammary function. The reflex regulation of lactation. *Proc. 2nd Int. Congr. Endocr.*, vol. 1, pp. 655–659. Excerpta Medica Foundation, Amsterdam.
BENSON, G. K. and FITZPATRICK, R. J. (1966). The neurohypophysis and the mammary gland. *The Pituitary Gland*, vol. 3, pp. 414–452. Harris, G. W. and Donovan, B. T. (eds.). Butterworths, London.
BERDE, B. (1963). *Pharmacologie des Hormones Neurohypophysaires et de leurs Analogues Synthétiques.* Masson & Cie, Paris.
BERDE, B. and BOISSONNAS, R. A. (1966). Synthetic analogues and homologues of the posterior pituitary hormones. *The Pituitary Gland*, vol. 3, pp. 624–661. Harris G. W. and Donovan, B. T. (eds.). Butterworths, London.
BOISSONNAS, R. A., GUTTMANN, ST., BERDE, B. and KONZETT, H. (1961). Relationships between the chemical structures and the biological properties of the posterior pituitary hormones and their synthetic analogues. *Experientia*, 17: 377–390.
CALDEYRO-BARCIA, R. (1961). Factors controlling the actions of the pregnant human uterus. *Physiology of Prematurity*, pp. 11–117. Kowlessar, M. (ed.). Josiah Macy Jr. Foundation Publications, New York.
COWIE, A. T. and FOLLEY, S. J. (1957). Neurohypophysial hormones and the mammary

gland. *The Neurohypophysis*, pp. 183–201. Heller, H. (ed.). Butterworths, London.

CROSS, B. A. (1955a). The posterior pituitary gland in relation to reproduction and lactation. *Br. med. Bull.*, **11**: 151–155.

CROSS, B. A. (1961). Neural control of lactation. *Milk: the Mammary Gland and its Secretion*, pp. 229–277. Kon, S. K. and Cowie, A. T. (eds.). Academic Press, New York.

CROSS, B. A. (1966). Neural control of oxytocin secretion. *Neuroendocrinology*, vol. 1, pp. 217–259. Martini, L. and Ganong, W. F. (eds.). Academic Press, New York.

DENAMUR, R. (1965). The hypothalamo-neurohypophysial system and the milk-ejection reflex. *Dairy Sci. Abstr.*, **27**: 193–224, 263–280.

DU VIGNEAUD, V. (1964). An organic chemical approach to the study of the significance of the chemical functional groups of oxytocin to its biological activities. *Proc. Robert A. Welch Foundation Conferences on Chemical Research*, VIII, pp. 133–163.

ELLIOT, G. M. (1959a). The direct effect of milk accumulation in the udder of the dairy cow upon milk secretion rate. *Dairy Sci. Abstr.*, **21**: 435–439.

ELLIOT, G. M. (1959b). The effect on milk yield of the length of milking intervals used in twice a day milking, twice and three times a day milking and incomplete milking. *Dairy Sci. Abstr.*, **21**: 481–490.

FITZPATRICK, R. J. (1961). The estimation of small amounts of oxytocin in blood. *Oxytocin*. pp. 358–379. Caldeyro-Barcia, R. and Heller, H. (eds.). Pergamon Press, Oxford.

FOLLEY, S. J. (1952). Aspects of pituitary-mammary gland relationships. *Recent Prog. Horm. Res.*, **7**: 107–137.

HAMMOND, J. (1936). The physiology of milk and butter fat secretion. I. Milk pressure in the udder. *Vet. Rec.*, **16**: 519–527.

HARRIS, G. W. (1958). The central nervous system, neurohypophysis and milk ejection. *Proc. R. Soc. B.*, **139**: 263–276.

KNAGGS, G. S. (1966). Blood oxytocin levels in relation to lactation and reproduction Ph. D. Thesis. University of Reading.

MEITES, J. (1968). Control of prolactin secretion. *La Physiologie de la Reproduction chez les Mammifères*. Colloq. int. C.N.R.S. Paris, 1966.

MEITES, J. and NICOLL, C. S. (1966). Adenohypophysis: Prolactin. *A. Rev. Physiol.*, **28**: 57–88.

SAWYER, W. H. (1961). Neurohypophysial hormones. *Pharmac. Rev.*, **13**: 225–277.

SCHÄFER, E. A. (1898). Mechanism of the secretion of milk. *Textbook of Physiology*, vol. 1, pp. 662–668. Schäfer, E. A. (ed.). Pentland, Edinburgh and London.

VAN DYKE, H. B., ADAMSON, K. JR. and ENGEL, S. L. (1955). Aspects of the biochemistry and physiology of the neurohypophyseal hormones. *Recent Prog. Horm. Res.*, **11**: 1–41.

ZAKS, M. G. (1962). *The Motor Apparatus of the Mammary Gland*. Oliver & Boyd, Edinburgh and London.

ORIGINAL PAPERS

ACHER, R., CHAUVET, J., CHAUVET, M. T. and CREPY, D. (1965). Phylogénie des peptides neurohypophysaires: isolement d'une nouvelle hormone, la glumitocine (Ser_4-Gln_8-ocytocine) présente chez un poisson cartilagineux, la raie *(Raia clavata)*. *Biochim. Biophys. Acta*, **107**: 393–396.

ALTHABE, O. JR., ARNT, I. C., BRANDA, L. A. and CALDEYRO-BARCIA, R. (1966). Comparison of the milk-ejecting potencies of oxytocin and deamino-oxytocin in lactating women. *J. Endocr.*, **36**: 7-14.
AZIMOV, G. I. (1959). Some processes accompanying the secretion of milk. *Proc. 15th Dairy Congr.* vol. 1, pp. 15-19.
AZIMOV, G. I., ORLOV, A. F. and BELUGINA, O. P. (1962). Milk secretion and re-absorption from the udder. *Nature, Lond.*, **193**: 985-986.
BARGMANN, W., FLEISCHHAUER, K. and KNOOP, A. (1961). Über die Morphologie der Milchsekretion. II. Zugleich eine Kritik am Schema der Sekretionsmorphologie. *Z. Zellforsch. mikrosk. Anat.*, **53**: 545-568.
BELLER, F. K., KRUMHOLZ, K. H. and ZEININGER, K. (1958). Vergleichende Oxytocin-Bestimmungen gemessen durch den lactagogen Effect der Milchdrüse. *Acta Endocr., Copenh.*, **29**: 1-8.
BENSON, G. K. and FOLLEY, S. J. (1956). Oxytocin as a stimulator for the release of prolactin from the anterior pituitary. *Nature, Lond.*, **177**: 700.
BENSON, G. K. and FOLLEY, S. J. (1957). The effect of oxytocin on mammary gland involution in the rat. *J. Endocr.*, **16**: 189-201.
BENSON, G. K., FOLLEY, S. J. and TINDAL, J. S. (1960). Effects of synthetic oxytocin and valyl oxytocin on mammary involution in the rat. *J. Endocr.*, **20**: 106-111.
BERÁNKOVÁ-KSANDROVÁ, Z., BISSET, G. W., JOŠT, K., KREJČÍ, I., PLIŠKA, V., RUDINGER, J., RYCHLÍK, I. and ŠORM, F. (1966). Synthetic analogues of oxytocin acting as hormonogens. *Brit. J. Pharmac. Chemother.*, **26**: 615-632.
BERDE, B. and CERLETTI, A. (1957). Démonstration expérimentale de l'action de l'ocytocine sur la glande mammaire. *Gynaecologia*, **144**: 275-278.
BERDE, B. and CERLETTI, A. (1960). Über die Wirkung pharmakologischer Oxytocindosen auf die Milchdrüse. *Acta Endocr., Copenh.*, **34**: 543-557.
BEYER C., MENA, F., PACHECO, P. and ALCARAZ, M. (1962). Blockage of lactation by brain stem lesions in the cat. *Amer. J. Physiol.*, **202**: 465-468.
BÍLEK, J. and JANOVSKÝ, M. (1958). Vliv adrenalinu na ejekci mléka vyvolanou oxytocinem. *Živočišná výroba*, **4**: 677-682.
BISSET, G. W. (1964). The effect on milk-ejecting activity of modifying two functional groups in oxytocin. *Proc. 2nd Int. Pharmacol. Meeting*, vol. 10, pp. 21-30. Rudinger, J. (ed.). Pergamon Press, Oxford.
BRANDA, L. A., DRABAREK, S. and DU VIGNEAUD, V. (1966). The synthesis and pharmacological properties of deamino-4-decarboxamido-oxytocin (1-β-mercaptopropionic acid-4-α-aminobutyric acid-oxytocin). *J. Biol. Chem.*, **241**: 2572-2575.
BRAUDE, R. and MITCHELL, K. G. (1952). Observations on the relationship between oxytocin and adrenaline in milk ejection in the sow. *J. Endocr.*, **8**: 238-241.
CHAN, W. Y. (1965). Mechanism of the epinephrine inhibition of the milk ejecting response to oxytocin. *J. Pharmac. Exp. Ther.*, **147**: 48-53.
CHAUDHURY, R. R., CHAUDHURY, M. R. and LU, F. C. (1961). Stress-induced block of milk ejection. *Brit. J. Pharmac. Chemother.*, **17**: 305-309.
CLEVERLEY, J. D. (1967). Unpublished results.
COHEN, J., BRENNEMAN, A. R. and TOPPER, Y. J. (1962). The stimulation by oxytocin and acetylcholine of glucose oxidation by lactating-rat mammary-gland slices: inhibition of the hormone effects by puromycin. *Biochim. Biophys. Acta*, **63**: 554-556.
COWIE, A. T., FOLLEY, S. J., CROSS, B. A., HARRIS, G. W., JACOBSOHN, D. and RICHARDSON, K. C. (1951). Terminology for use in lactational physiology. *Nature, Lond.*, **168**: 421.

CROSS, B. A. (1950). Suckling antidiuresis in rabbits. *Nature, Lond.*, **166**: 612–613.
CROSS, B. A. (1951). Suckling antidiuresis in rabbits. *J. Physiol., Lond.*, **114**: 447–453.
CROSS, B. A. (1953). Sympathetico-adrenal inhibition of the neurohypophysial milk-ejection mechanism. *J. Endocr.*, **9**: 7–18.
CROSS, B. A. (1954). Milk ejection resulting from mechanical stimulation of mammary myoepithelium in the rabbit. *Nature, Lond.*, **173**: 450–451.
CROSS, B. A. (1955b). The hypothalamus and the mechanism of sympathetico-adrenal inhibition of milk ejection. *J. Endocr.*, **12**: 15–28.
CROSS, B. A. and VAN DYKE, H. B. (1953). The effects of highly purified posterior pituitary principles on the lactating mammary gland of the rabbit. *J. Endocr.*, **9**: 232–235.
CROSS, B. A., GOODWIN, R. F. W. and SILVER, I. A. (1958). A histological and functional study of the mammary gland in normal and agalactic sows. *J. Endocr.*, **17**: 63–74.
CROSS, B. A. and SILVER, I. A. (1956). Milk ejection and mammary engorgement. *Proc. Roy. Soc. Med.*, **49**: 978–979.
CROSS, B. A. and SILVER, I. A. (1962a). Mammary oxygen tension and the milk-ejection mechanism. *J. Endocr.*, **23**: 375–384.
CROSS, B. A. and SILVER, I. A. (1962b). Central activation of the sympathetico-adrenal system by hypoxia and hypercapnia. *J. Endocr.*, **24**: 91–103.
DEANE, H. W. and FORBES, A. (1956). Myoepithelial cells and their function. *J. Appl. Physiol.*, **9**: 495–496.
DENAMUR, R. (1962). Effets chez la lapine de l'ocytocine et de la prolactine sur les acides nucléiques de la glande mammaire. *C. R. Hebd. Séanc. Acad. Sci., Paris*, **225**: 1786–1788.
DENAMUR, R. and MARTINET, J. (1953). Sensibilité de la glande mammaire de la chèvre aux hormones posthypophysaires. *C. R. Séanc. Soc. Biol.*, **147**: 1217–1220.
DENAMUR, R. and MARTINET, J. (1959). Le rôle du système nerveux de la glande mammaire dans l'entretien de la lactation. *Archs. Sci. Physiol.*, **13**: 271–352.
DENAMUR, R. and MARTINET, J. (1960). Physiological mechanisms concerned in the maintenance of lactation in the sheep and goat. *Nature, Lond.*, **185**: 252–253.
DENUCCIO, D. J. and GROSVENOR, C. E. (1967). Effect of suckling and hormones on contractility of involuting rat mammary gland. *Amer. J. Physiol.*, **212**: 149–156.
DONKER, J. D. (1958). Lactation studies. I. Effects upon milk ejection in the bovine of various injection treatments using oxytocin and relaxin. *J. Dairy Sci.*, **41**: 537–544.
EAYRS, J. T. and BADDELEY, R. M. (1956). Neural pathways in lactation. *J. Anat.*, **90**: 161–171.
EDERY, H. and LEWIS, G. P. (1963). Kinin-forming activity and histamine in lymph after tissue injury. *J. Physiol., Lond.*, **169**: 568–583.
EDWARDSON, J. A. and EAYRS, J. T. (1967). Neural factors in the maintenance of lactation in the rat. *J. Endocr.*, **38**: 51–59.
EISLER, K., RUDINGER, J. and ŠORM, F. (1966). Amino acids and peptides. LXV. Analogues of oxytocin with isoleucine replaced by L-diethylalanine, L-cyclopentylglycine, and L- and D-cyclohexylglycine. *Colln. Czech. Chem. Commun.*, **31**: 4563–4580.
ELY, F. and PETERSEN, W. E. (1941). Factors involved in the ejection of milk. *J. Dairy Sci.*, **24**: 211–223.
FELDBERG, W. and LEWIS, G. P. (1964). The action of peptides on the adrenal medulla. Release of adrenaline by bradykinin and angiotensin. *J. Physiol., Lond.*, **171**: 98–108.

Ferrier, B. M., Jarvis, D. and du Vigneaud, V. (1965). Deamino-oxytocin. *J. Biol. Chem.*, **240**: 4264–4266.

Findlay, A. L. R. (1966). Sensory discharges from lactating mammary glands. *Nature, Lond.*, **211**: 1183–1184.

Folley, S. J. and Knaggs, G. S. (1965). Levels of oxytocin in the jugular vein blood of goats during parturition. *J. Endocr.*, **33**: 301–315.

Folley, S. J. and Knaggs, G. S. (1966). Milk-ejection activity (oxytocin) in the external jugular vein blood of the cow, goat, and sow, in relation to the stimulus of suckling or milking. *J. Endocr.*, **34**: 197–214.

Folley, S. J. and McNaught, M. L. (1956). The rôle of the suckling stimulus in the maintenance of lactation. *Ann. Rep. Natn. Inst. Res. Dairying*, 59–60.

Folley, S. J. and McNaught, M. L. (1957). The rôle of the suckling stimulus in the maintenance of lactation. *Ann. Rep. Natn. Inst. Res. Dairying*, 58–59.

Forbes, A., Forbes, A. P. and Neyland, M. (1955). Action potentials in the human mammary gland. *J. Appl. Physiol.*, **7**: 675–682.

Forbes, A., Neyland, M. and Fox, S. (1960). Electric response in the mammary gland. *J. Appl. Physiol.*, **15**: 511–514.

Friedman, E. A. (1960). Direct measurement of milk ejection pressure in unanaesthetized lactating humans. *Amer. J. Obstet. Gynec.*, **80**: 119–123.

Fuchs, A. R. and Wagner, G. (1963). Quantitative aspects of release of oxytocin by suckling in unanaesthetised rabbits. *Acta Endocr., Copenh.*, **44**: 581–592.

Gaines, W. L. (1915). A contribution to the physiology of lactation. *Amer. J. Physiol.*, **38**: 285–312.

Gaitan, E., Cobo, E. and Mizrachi, M. (1964). Evidence for the differential secretion of oxytocin and vasopressin in man. *J. Clin. Invest.*, **43**: 2310–2322.

Ginsburg, M. and Smith, M. W. (1959). The fate of oxytocin in male and female rats. *Brit. J. Pharmac. Chemother.*, **14**: 327–333.

Golubow, J., Chan, W. Y. and du Vigneaud, V. (1963). Effect of human pregnancy serum on avian vasodepressor activities of oxytocin and desamino-oxytocin. *Proc. Soc. Exp. Biol. Med.*, **113**: 113–115.

Goodfriend, T. L. and Topper, Y. J. (1961). Effects of oxytocin, vasopressin and acetylcholine on glucose metabolism in mammary tissue *in vitro*. *J. Biol. Chem.*, **236**: 1241–1243.

Grosvenor, C. E. (1964). Lactation in the rat mammary glands after spinal cord section. *Endocrinology*, **74**: 548–553.

Grosvenor, C. E. (1965). Contraction of lactating rat mammary gland in response to direct mechanical stimulation. *Amer. J. Physiol.*, **208**, 214–218.

Hebb, C. O. and Linzell, J. L. (1951). Some conditions affecting the blood flow through the perfused mammary gland, with special reference to the action of adrenaline. *Quart. J. Exp. Physiol.*, **36**: 159–175.

Jarvis, D. and du Vigneaud, V. (1967). The effect of decreasing the size of the ring present in deamino-oxytocin by one methylene group on its biological properties. *J. Biol. Chem.*, **242**: 1768–1771.

Jungmannová, Č., Brotánek, V., Kazda, S. and Rudinger, J. (1964). Physiological and clinical effects of alloisoleucyl³-oxytocin. *Oxytocin and its Analogues*, pp. 106–108. Meeting of Polish Endocr. Soc. Kraków, 1964.

Kalliala, H. and Karvonen, M. J. (1951). Antidiuresis during suckling in lactating women. *Annls Med. Exp. Biol. Fenn.*, **29**: 233–241.

Kalliala, H., Karvonen, M. J. and Leppänen, V. (1952). Release of antidiuretic hormone during nursing in the dog. *Annls Med. Exp. Biol. Fenn.*, **30**: 96–107.

KULLANDER, S. (1963). Studies on the hormonal control of the milk-ejection activity in the lactating rabbit. *Acta Endocr., Copenh.*, **44**: 313–324.
LEVITSKAYA, E. S. (1955). Prizhiznennoe issledovanie raboty vyvodnogo apparata molochnoi zhelezy beloĭ myshi. *Trudȳ Inst. Fiziol. I. P. Pavlova*, **4**: 58–62.
LINZELL, J. L. (1952). The silver staining of myoepithelial cells, particularly in the mammary gland, and their relation to the ejection of milk. *J. Anat.*, **86**: 49–57.
LINZELL, J. L. (1953). The blood and nerve supply to the mammary glands of the cat, and other laboratory animals. *Brit. Vet. J.*, **109**: 427–433.
LINZELL, J. L. (1955). Some observations on the contractile tissue of the mammary glands. *J. Physiol., Lond.*, **130**: 257–267.
LINZELL, J. L. (1963). Some effects of denervating and transplanting mammary glands. *Quart. J. Exp. Physiol.*, **48**: 34–60.
MARTIN, P. J. and SCHILD, H. O. (1962). Effects of thiols on oxytocin and vasopressin receptors. *Nature, Lond.*, **196**: 382–383.
MARTINET, J. and DENAMUR, R. (1960). Étude préliminaire des mécanismes de l'évacuation du lait de la glande mammaire chez la chèvre et la brebis. *Archs Sci. physiol.*, **14**: 35–96.
MENA, F. and BEYER, C. (1963). Effect of high spinal section on established lactation in the rabbit. *Amer. J. Physiol.*, **205**: 313–316.
MÉNDEZ-BAUER, C. J., CABOT, H. M. and CALDEYRO-BARCIA, R. (1960). A new test for the biological assay of oxytocin. *Science, N. Y.*, **132**: 299–301.
MOORE, R. D. and ZARROW, M. X. (1965). Contraction of the rabbit mammary strip *in vitro* in response to oxytocin. *Acta Endocr., Copenh.*, **48**: 186–198.
NODDLE, B. A. (1962). Metabolism of oxytocin in the mammary gland. *Proc. Int. Union physiol. Sci.*, 22nd Int. Congr. Leiden, vol 2. Comm. No. 523.
ÔTA, K., SHINDE, Y. and YOKOYAMA, A. (1965). Relationship between oxytocin and prolactin secretion in maintenance of lactation in rats. *Endocrinology*, **76**: 1–8.
ÔTA, K. and YOKOYAMA, A. (1958). Effect of oxytocin administration on respiration of lactating mammary gland tissues in rats. *Nature, Lond.*, **182**: 1509–1510.
PEETERS, G. and COUSSENS, R. (1950). The influence of the milking act on the diuresis of the lactating cow. *Archs. Int. Pharmacodyn. Thér.*, **84**: 209–220.
PEETERS, G., SIERENS, G. and SILVER, M. (1952). Expulsion of milk in the isolated perfused udder of the cow. *Archs. Int. Pharmacodyn. Thér.*, **88**: 413–423.
PEETERS, G., STORMORKEN, H. and VANSCHOUBROEK, F. (1960). The effect of different stimuli on milk ejection and diuresis in the lactating cow. *J. Endocr.*, **20**: 163–172.
PICKFORD, M. (1960). Factors affecting milk release in the dog and the quantity of oxytocin liberated. *J. Physiol., Lond.*, **152**: 515–526.
POLÁČEK, I., KREJČÍ, I. and RUDINGER, J. (1967). The action of oxytocin and synthetic analogues on the isolated mammary-gland myoepithelium of the lactating rat: effect of some ions. *J. Endocr.*, **38**: 13–24.
RICHARDSON, K. C. (1949). Contractile tissues in the mammary gland, with special reference to myoepithelium in the goat. *Proc. Roy. Soc., B*, **136**: 30–45.
RICHARDSON, K. C. (1951). Structural investigation of the contractile tissues in the mammary gland. *Colloques Int. Cent. Natn. Rech. Scient.*, **32**: 167–170b.
RYDÉN, G. and SJÖHOLM, I. (1962). Assay of oxytocin by rat mammary gland *in vitro*. *Brit. J. Pharmac. Chemother.*, **19**: 136–141.
SALA, N. L. (1964). The milk-ejecting effect induced by oxytocin and vasopressin during human pregnancy. *Amer. J. Obstet. Gynec.*, **89**: 626–634.
SALA, N. L. (1965). Milk ejecting effect induced by various octapeptides in human beings. *Acta Physiol. Latinoam.*, **15**: 191–199.

SELYE, H. (1934). On the nervous control of lactation. *Amer. J. Physiol.*, **107**: 535–538.
SILVER, I. A. (1954). Myoepithelial cells in the mammary and parotid glands. *J. Physiol., Lond.*, **125**: 8P–9P.
SMITH, M. W. (1961). Some properties of rat mammary tissue. *Nature, Lond.*, **190**: 541–542.
SMITH, M. W. and GINSBURG, M. (1961). Fate of synthetic oxytocin analogues in the rat. *Brit. J. Pharmac. Chemother.*, **16**: 244–252.
THEOBALD, G. W. (1959). Separate release of oxytocin and antidiuretic hormone. *J. Physiol., Lond.*, **149**: 443–461.
TINDAL, J. S., KNAGGS, G. S. and TURVEY, A. (1968). Preferential release of oxytocin from the neurohypophysis after electrical stimulation of the afferent path of the milk-ejection reflex in the brain of the guinea-pig. *J. Endocr.*, **40**: 205–214.
TINDAL, J. S. and YOKOYAMA, A. (1960). Bioassay of milk ejection hormone (oxytocin) in body fluids in relation to the milk-ejection reflex. *Ann. Rep. Natn. Inst. Res. Dairying*, 52–53.
TINDAL, J. S. and YOKOYAMA, A. (1962). Assay of oxytocin by the milk-ejection response in the anaesthetized lactating guinea pig. *Endocrinology*, **71**: 196–202.
TSAKHAEV, G. A. (1958). O sekretornoĭ funktsii molochnoĭ zhelezy v usloviyakh ee izolyatsii ot tsentral'noĭ nervoi sistemy. *Liet TSR Mokslu. Akad. Biol. Inst. Darb.*, **3**: 229–245.
TURNER, C. W. and COOPER, W. D. (1941). Assay of posterior pituitary factors which contract the lactating mammary gland. *Endocrinology*, **29**: 320–323.
TVERSKOĬ, G. B. (1958). Sekretsiya moloka v koz posle polnoĭ pererezki spinnogo mozga. *Dokl. Akad. Nauk. SSSR*, **123**: 1137–1139.
VAN DONGEN, C. G. and HAYS, R. L. (1966). A sensitive *in vitro* assay for oxytocin. *Endocrinology*, **78**: 1–6.
VAN DONGEN, C. G. and MARSHALL, J. M. (1967). Effect of various hormones on the milk ejection response of tissue isolated from the rat mammary gland. *Nature, Lond.*, **213**: 632–633.
VAN DYKE, H. B., CHOW, B. F., GREEP, R. O. and ROTHEN, A. (1942). The isolation of a protein from the pars neuralis of the ox pituitary with constant oxytocic, pressor and diuresis-inhibiting activites. *J. Pharmac. Exp. Ther.*, **74**: 190–209.
VAN DYKE, H. B., SAWYER, W. H. and OVERWEG, N. I. A. (1963). Pharmacologic activities of the 8-citrulline analogues of oxytocin and vasopressin. *Endocrinology*, **73**: 637–639.
VORHERR, H. (1965). Eine neue Methode sum Oxytocin-Nachweis an der lactierenden Maus. *Arch. Exp. Path. Pharmak.*, **251**: 123.
WIEDERMAN, J. and STONE, M. L. (1962). Effect of oxytocin on myoepithelium of the breast. *J. Appl. Physiol.*, **17**: 539–542.
WHITTLESTONE, W. G. (1952). The milk-ejecting activity of extracts of the posterior pituitary gland. *J. Endocr.*, **8**: 89–95.
WHITTLESTONE, W. G. (1953). The milk-ejection response of the sow to standard doses of oxytocic hormone. *J. Dairy Res.* **20**: 13–15.
WHITTLESTONE, W. G. (1954a). Intramammary pressure changes in the lactating sow. I. The effect of oxytocin. *J. Dairy Res.*, **21**: 19–30.
WHITTLESTONE, W. G. (1954b). The effect of adrenaline on the milk-ejection response of the sow. *J. Endocr.*, **10**: 167–172.
YOKOYAMA, A. (1956). Milk-ejection responses following administration of "tap" stimuli and posterior pituitary extracts. *Endocr. Jap.*, **3**: 32–38.

YOKOYAMA, A. and ÔTA, K. (1959). Effects of administration of oxytocin and prolactin on lactating activity of mammary glands in rats. *Endocr. Jap.*, **6**: 259–267.
YOKOYAMA, A. and ÔTA, K. (1965). The effect of anaesthesia on milk yield and maintenance of lactation in the goat and rat. *J. Endocr.*, **33**: 341–351.
ZAKS, M. G. (1951). Novye dannye o funktsii motornogo apparata vymeni. *Sbornik dokladov vtoroĭ vsesoyuznoĭ konferentsii po molochnomu delu*, pp. 150–163. Davidov, R. B. (ed.). Sel'khozgiz, Moscow.
ZHUZE, A. L., JOŠT, K., KASAFÍREK, E. and RUDINGER, J. (1964). Amino acids and peptides. XLV. Analogues of oxytocin with O-ethyltyrosine, p-methylphenylalanine, and p-ethylphenylalanine replacing tyrosine. *Colln. Czech. Chem. Commun.*, **29**: 2648–2662.

CHAPTER 9

EFFECTS OF NEUROHYPOPHYSIAL HORMONES AND THEIR SYNTHETIC ANALOGUES ON LOWER VERTEBRATES

B. K. Follett

Department of Zoology,
The University,
Leeds 2, England

INTRODUCTION

Until recently, research into the functions of the neurohypophysial peptides has been largely confined to a few mammalian species; studies in lower vertebrates have been and still are comparatively rare. Moreover, these investigations often appear to have been greatly, if not unduly, influenced by the discoveries that in the mammals the hormones act primarily on the kidney and the uterus. However, it is now realized that other target organs for the neurohypophysial hormones exist; thus these peptides alter water and electrolyte metabolism at sites other than the kidney and may also play a significant role in controlling the adenohypophysis. Nevertheless the major responses at the cellular level appear to be consistent throughout the vertebrate series in that the peptides accelerate the osmotic flow of water and increase ion transport across cell membranes. They also appear to have an action on muscular tissues of the reproductive tract and to induce hyperglycaemia in most groups of vertebrates. It is perhaps these fundamental actions that have attracted many physiologists to place more emphasis on the lower vertebrates as a source of material for their investigations. For example, the relatively simple structure of the anuran bladder has led to considerable advances in understanding the biochemical events associated with hormonally induced water and electrolyte transfer. These findings may well have relevance to the mechanisms whereby the neurohypophysial hormones increase water absorption in the distal tubule of the mammalian kidney.

It should perhaps be emphasized that in a review concerning the effects of the neurohypophysial peptides on lower vertebrates, many responses will be described which are more likely to be of pharmacological than of physiological significance. Judgements as to the exact functions of the hormones must remain subjective as long as little is known of either the normal levels of the peptides in the circulation or of their half-lives in the blood. Wherever possible, indirect evidence such as changes in the histological appearance or the hormone content of the neurosecretory system after a specific treatment will be presented to support a truly physiological function of the peptides.

The reader's attention is drawn to other reviews concerned with the functions of the hormones in lower vertebrates, in particular two monographs edited by Heller (1957, 1963) and the recent papers by Dodd, Perks and Dodd (1966) and Bentley (1966a).

THE CYCLOSTOMES

Neurohypophysial peptides do not affect the overall water balance of the fresh water lamprey, *Lampetra fluviatilis* (Heller and Bentley, 1963, 1965). Moreover, in contrast with higher fishes, the peptides have no action on glomerular filtration rate and urine volume (Table 1). However, in large doses they increase sodium loss through the kidney (Bentley and Follett, 1963); oxytocin was the most effective peptide tested although arginine vasotocin, vasopressin and [3-valine]-oxytocin were also active (Bentley and Follett, 1962). The physiological significance of these results is difficult to assess since the amounts of hormone used were much greater than the quantity stored in the lamprey's neurohypophysis. Furthermore, adaptation of lampreys to media of increasing salinity did not alter the concentration of arginine vasotocin in the pars nervosa (Bentley and Follett, 1963).

Evidence for a possible function of the neurohypophysial hormones in controlling the secretion of the pars intermedia is provided by Oztan and Gorbman (1960). They showed that the neurosecretory system of larval lampreys *(Petromyzon marinus)* responds to light; continuous illumination depleted the system of stainable neurosecretory material while the converse was true in larvae kept in the dark. Bentley and Follett (1965) found that the peptides had a metabolic action in inducing hyperglycaemia in the lamprey. Further studies are required to establish this response as a true endocrine function but it is an effect which occurs in other vertebrate groups (Mirsky, 1963; Bentley, 1965, 1966b).

TABLE 1. EFFECTS OF NEUROHYPOPHYSIAL HORMONES ON WATER LOSS IN FISH

Species	Medium	Peptide used	Effect on GFR	Effect on Urine volume	Effect on Water reabsorption
Lampetra fluviatilis	F-W	AVT	0^1	0^1	0^1
Ameiurus	F-W	AVP		0^2	
Carassius auratus	F-W	AVP		$+^3$	
		AVT	$+^{4,5}$	$+^{4,5}$	$0^{4,5}$
		O	$+^{4,5}$	$+^{4,5}$	$0^{4,5}$
		SIO	$-^4$	$-^4$	0^4
		LVP	0^5	0^5	0^5
Salmo gairdneri	Salt-loaded	AVP		$-(?)^6$	
	F-W	AVP	$+^7$		
Salmo irideus	F-W	AVP		0^8	
	Spawning in S-W	AVP		$-^8$	
Anguilla anguilla	F-W	SIO	$+^9$		$-^9$
Protopterus aethiopicus	F-W	AVT	$+^{10}$	$+^{10}$	0^{10}
		O	$0,+^{10}$	$0,+^{10}$	0^{10}
		IO	0^{10}	0^{10}	0^{10}

The abbreviations for the peptides are: AVT, arginine vasotocin; AVP, arginine vasopressin; LVP, lysine vasopressin; O, oxytocin; SIO, [4-serine, 8-isoleucine]-oxytocin and IO, [8-isoleucine]-oxytocin. F-W refers to fresh water, S-W to sea water.

The effects are summarized as 0, no change; +, increase and −, decrease.

References:

1. Bentley and Follett (1963).
2. Burgess *et al.* (1933).
3. Sexton (1955).
4. Maetz *et al.* (1964).
5. Maetz (1963).
6. Holmes, W. N. (1959).
7. Holmes, W. N. and McBean (1963).
8. Holmes, R. L. (1961).
9. Rankin *et al.* (1967).
10. Sawyer (1966).

THE ELASMOBRANCHS

Evidence for an action of the peptides in this group is extremely sparse (see Dodd *et al.*, 1966). Water retention was not produced in the Nurse shark *(Gingylostoma cirratum)* by an extract of skate neural lobes (Heller and Bentley, 1965). The isolated oviduct of *Scyliorhinus caniculus* and *Squalus acanthias* show strong spontaneous contractions *in vitro* (Dodd *et al.*, 1966) but oxytocin, even in large doses, did not alter the contractions. Mackay (1931) reported a sustained rise in blood pressure in the dogfish *(Squalus acanthias)* after large doses of extracts from the whole mammalian neurohypophysis. The active peptide appears to have been oxytocin since vasopressin is without effect in this species (Waring and Landgrebe, 1950).

In elasmobranchs the neurosecretory axons of the hypothalamo-neurohypophysial system do not form a discrete pars nervosa but interdigitate freely with the pars intermedia (Dodd, 1963; Dodd *et al.*, 1966). This suggests a possible functional relationship and is supported by the observations of Knowles (1965) who found apparent synaptic contacts between the neurosecretory fibers (Types A and B) and the intrinsic endocrine cells of the pars intermedia in the dogfish, *Scyliorhinus*. Transplantation of the pars neurointermedia of the skate to a distal site results in a high secretion rate of MSH (Chevins and Dodd, personal communication). If a functional relationship exists therefore, it would appear to be inhibitory.

THE TELEOST FISHES

The teleost fishes form the largest single group of vertebrates with over 20,000 species. They are found throughout the entire range of aquatic habitats, the majority of species are limited to either fresh water or to sea water but many are euryhaline and several show a well-marked migration during their life cycle. It is not surprising, therefore, that the possible control of their water and electrolyte balance by neurohypophysial hormones has received attention. Earlier studies have been summarized by Fontaine (1956) and Pickford and Atz (1957); the results were inconclusive and led to the widely held view, expressed by Sawyer (1961a), that the hormones might never reach the systemic circulation but affect only the adenohypophysis. More recently, however, the studies of Maetz and his collaborators in France have provided evidence for systemic effects on both water and electrolyte metabolism.

EFFECTS ON WATER METABOLISM

Burgess, Harvey and Marshall (1933) failed to obtain an antidiuresis in *Ameiurus* after the injection of vasopressin. The lack of a water balance effect was also shown in a range of Teleost species (Boyd and Dingwall, 1939; Fontaine and Raffy, 1950; Callamand *et al.*, 1951; Heller and Bentley, 1965).

More detailed studies have included direct estimations of urine loss under the influence of neurohypophysial hormones and in a few the glomerular filtration rate has been estimated. Table 1 summarizes the most pertinent results. The diuresis obtained with vasopressin by Sexton (1955) in the goldfish was analyzed in detail by Maetz and his co-workers (Maetz, et al., 1964; Bourguet, Lahlouh and Maetz, 1964) and reviewed by Maetz (1963). They showed that arginine vasotocin (0.04–0.2 µg, i.e. 6–30 mU pressor activity) and oxytocin (20–200 mU) caused a rapid increase in urine flow which lasted 1 to 2 hr. The diuresis was caused solely by an increase in the glomerular filtration rate, no change in tubular water reabsorption was found. In contrast, one of the endogenous teleost principles, [4-serine, 8-isoleucine]-oxytocin, had no diuretic effect and two to three hours after injection caused a mild antidiuresis. Increases in filtration rate caused by neurohypophysial peptides have also been reported by W. N. Holmes and McBean (1963) in *Salmo gairdneri* and by Rankin, Chan and Chester Jones (1967) in the eel *(Anguilla anguilla)*. In contrast, R. L. Holmes (1961) found that the urine volume of spawning trout failed to decrease when they were placed in sea water but vasopressin caused an immediate antidiuresis. This response was not observed in non-spawning trout.

The diuretic action of the neurohypophysial peptides could have physiological value to a fish in fresh water since it is continuously subject to hydration and requires mechanisms to excrete the excess water. However, direct evidence that the hormones play a physiological role in controlling the glomerular filtration rate is still lacking, although it is perhaps significant that the injection of a hypotonic saline solution (30 mM) into *Carassius* caused a pronounced diuresis and a re-establishment of the normal equilibrium condition (Bourguet et al., 1964).

EFFECTS ON SODIUM BALANCE

Neurohypophysial peptides affect sodium balance at both renal and extrarenal sites. Thus Maetz et al. (1964) found that arginine vasotocin and oxytocin increased the sodium influx across the gills of the goldfish. However, arginine vasotocin and oxytocin increased sodium as well as water loss through the kidney, although the peptides did not affect tubular sodium absorption. Taken overall, therefore, the hormones caused a net loss of sodium from the animal. In contrast, [4-serine, 8-isoleucine]-oxytocin caused a net uptake of sodium since it increased sodium influx and yet had no action on the kidney. These experiments illustrate well the problems of investigating electrolyte balance in fishes and perhaps explain why so few studies can be described as adequate.

The demonstration of effects on sodium fluxes across the gill suggested a function for the peptides in a euryhaline teleost, where the adaptation from fresh water to sea water requires a reversal in the overall direction of net sodium movement (see Maetz, 1963). Motais (Motais and Maetz, 1964; Motais, 1967) has investigated sodium fluxes in the euryhaline flounder *(Platichthys flesus)*. In fresh water the sodium exchange across the gills is very low and only about 1% of the body sodium is exchanged per hour. On placing flounders in sea water the gills become progressively more permeable to sodium until about 25% of body sodium is exchanged each hour, this process is reversed if flounders are placed again in fresh water (Motais and Maetz, 1964; Motais, Garcia Romeu and Maetz, 1966). It now appears that virtually all the change in sodium influx across the gill and a very large proportion of the efflux, about 90%, in the flounder, occurs instantaneously on placing a euryhaline fish in a medium of different salinity. These rapid alterations could be explained by a mechanism of exchange diffusion (Ussing, 1960) across the gill membranes (Motais *et al.*, 1966). Although such a mechanism may have advantages to the fish it would not alter the *net* movement of sodium. However, in all the euryhaline species examined, which include the eel *(Anguilla)*, the mullet *(Mugil)*, the killifish *(Fundulus)* and the flounder, there is an additional mechanism for regulating sodium outflux, and thus net sodium flux, across the gill (Motais *et al.*, 1966). This additional mechanism which is absent in stenohaline species, is distinguishable from exchange diffusion since it adapts more slowly to a change in external salinity. Motais *et al.* (1966) consider that this is the mechanism which might possibly be influenced by endocrine secretions. Thus prolactin is extremely effective in depressing the remaining sodium outflux after transference of hypophysectomized *Fundulus* from sea water to fresh water (Maetz *et al.*, 1967), and a similar though less pronounced effect is seen in *Anguilla* (Maetz, Mayer and Chartier-Baraduc, 1967). In contrast the transfer from fresh water to sea water would require an increased and maximal outflux of sodium from the gill. Neurohypophysial peptides appear to have an action here for Motais and Maetz (1964) found that oxytocin increased gill permeability to sodium. Oxytocin also accelerated the sodium outflux associated with the change from fresh to sea water. Recently, Motais and Maetz (1967) confirmed these results with low doses of arginine vasotocin (50 mU pressor activity); the efflux in vasotocin-treated flounders transferred to sea water was 910 ± 140 μEq/hr/kg b.w. after 1 hr compared with 350 ± 20 μEq/hr/kg in the controls ($P < 0.01$). The efflux of the vasotocin-treated animals remained greater even after 7 hr in sea water. Aldosterone appears to slow down the readjustment of the sodium outflux in sea water (Motais, 1967).

The transference of trout from fresh to sea water causes a depletion of hormone from the neural lobe (Carlson and Holmes, 1962), differential assays showed the fall to be restricted to arginine vasotocin (Lederis, 1964).

MISCELLANEOUS EFFECTS

Vasopressor effects of neurohypophysial peptides in the eel *(Anguilla)* have been reported recently by Chan and Chester Jones (1967). Arginine vasotocin, oxytocin and [4-serine, 8-isoleucine]-oxytocin caused a pronounced elevation in blood pressure in the ventral aorta and a smaller rise in the dorsal aorta. The effect is discernible for a long period of time, up to 6 hr after the injection of [4-serine, 8-isoleucine]-oxytocin. However, adrenergic blocking agents, e.g. phentolamine, abolish the pressor effects suggesting that the responses may not be a direct effect. Nevertheless, further studies are required, for an action of hormones on the hemodynamics of the gill and kidney could indirectly affect salt and water balance.

Viviparity and ovoviviparity occur in many species of fish and the observation in some live-bearers, such as guppies *(Lebistes* spp.), that the young are expelled with force is suggestive of a mechanism not dissimilar from oviposition and parturition. Indeed the injection of neurohypophysial hormones can induce spawning behavior and the delivery of the young in several species (Houssay, 1931; Haempel, 1950; Ishii, 1961). Extracts of frog or fish neural lobes were more effective than mammalian extracts (Ishii, 1961). Oviposition in the rice fish, *Oryzias latipes*, has been studied by Egami and Ishii (1962). Egg-laying only takes place in the presence of a male and is believed to operate by way of a neurohormonal reflex arc involving tactile stimuli on various areas of the skin (Egami and Nambu, 1961) and the release of an ovipositioning hormone from the pars nervosa. The only evidence for the latter is that mammalian neurohypophysial extracts will cause oviposition in isolated females (Egami, 1959); nevertheless these observations are of interest and require further study. Sawyer and Pickford (1963) have reported a striking depletion of [4-serine, 8-isoleucine]-oxytocin from the pituitaries of female *Fundulus* during the spawning season. The reason is unknown although large doses of oxytocin induce a spawning reaction in this species (Wilhelmi, Pickford and Sawyer, 1955).

The structure of the neurosecretory system in the Teleostei (Dodd and Kerr, 1963) suggests that the neurohypophysial peptides might cause the release of adenohypophysial hormones, in particular from the pars intermedia. However, no direct evidence is available although Knowles and Vollrath (1966) found changes in type A_2 neurosecretory fibers of the eel after changing the background illumination. Leatherland (1967) could not correlate changes in the stainability of the eel neurosecretory system with specific stimuli: he found that a variety of 'stress' reactions caused a rapid depletion of neurosecretory material followed by a compensatory increase in stainability, usually within 24 hr. Jasinski, Gorbman and Hara (1966) found that electrical stimulation of the olfactory tract in goldfish depletes completely the stainable neurosecretory material in cells of the preoptic nucleus as well as in the axons. No precise function for such a release has been suggested but the experiments are unique in demonstrating the highly labile state of the system. The discharge of material is very rapid and granules appear to move towards the pars nervosa at a rate of about 2 mm/min. Restitution of stainability throughout the whole system requires about $1-1\frac{1}{2}$ hr only.

THE DIPNOI

Arginine vasotocin did not have an effect on water retention in the African lungfish *(Protopterus aethiopicus)*, although arginine vasotocin and oxytocin increased net sodium loss significantly (Heller and Bentley, 1965). More recently these responses have been studied in detail by Sawyer (1966). The i.p. injection of small doses of arginine vasotocin (55–900 mU pressor activity/kg) caused a rapid diuresis resulting from an increase in glomerular filtration rate. There was no effect on tubular water reabsorption. Oxytocin caused diuresis in only three of six animals while a few experiments with [8-isoleucine]-oxytocin gave inconsistent results.

A more striking response to vasotocin was the great increase in sodium excretion through the kidney. The rate of loss was increased several hundred-fold in some experiments. The explanation of this effect is not altogether clear although, as Sawyer (1966) emphasizes, arginine vasotocin may not depress tubular sodium reabsorption. The increase in sodium loss might have been due to the fact that sodium reabsorption had not increased in proportion to the filtered load which had risen from the effect on the filtration rate.

The responses in the lungfish therefore, resemble those found in the teleost fishes and cyclostomes rather than those in the Amphibia in which the peptides depress the glomerular filtration rate and increase tubular sodium reabsorption (Jard and Morel, 1963).

THE AMPHIBIANS

In contrast with the groups already discussed, the actions of neurohypophysial hormones in the Amphibia have been extensively investigated. However, the emphasis has again been placed on effects on water and electrolyte metabolism and until recently, research has been confined largely to the anuran amphibians (frogs and toads).

EFFECTS OF THE HORMONES IN ANURA

A clear-cut effect was first described by Brunn (1921) who showed that mammalian neurohypophysial extracts increased the body weight of frogs sitting in water. This phenomenon has been shown to be a composite response caused by a renal antidiuresis (Houssay and Potick, 1929), an increase in water uptake through the skin (Novelli, 1936) and a promotion of water reabsorption from the urinary bladder (Ewer, 1952a). The magnitude of the overall effect depends not only on the dose and peptide but also on the habitat of the species (Steggerda, 1937; Ewer, 1952b; Bentley, et al., 1958). Heller and Bentley (1965) in a study of the water balance effect throughout the Amphibia, showed that the maximal water retention under the influence of neurohypophysial hormones varied from 1–2 ml/100 cm^2 body surface/hr in *Pelobates cultripes* and *Discoglossus pictus*, representatives of the more primitive Anura, to 17 ml/100 cm^2/hr in the Hylidae *(Hyla hyla)*, an advanced and ecologically more successful group of frogs. A fully aquatic toad, *Xenopus laevis*, gave no water balance response to neurohypophysial hormones, a result similar to that obtained in the fishes. The effects in terrestrial amphibians appear to represent a physiological function for Levinsky and Sawyer (1953) and Jancsó (1955) reported that the pituitary of dehydrated frogs contained less antidiuretic principle than that of well-hydrated controls. The use of highly purified preparations of the hormones has shown that species vary in their sensitivity to individual peptides (Heller and Bentley, 1965). In general arginine vasotocin was most effective although in *Bufo bufo* the mammalian hormone arginine vasopressin was almost as effective. Oxytocin, which is probably present in many anurans, was invariably much less active. In addition to effects on water metabolism neurohypophysial hormones can also act on the overall sodium balance to cause a net uptake of the ion although the effect does not occur in all anurans (Heller and Bentley, 1965).

The effects of the peptides on the three separate target organs, namely the kidney, the skin and the bladder have been analyzed.

The kidney. The antidiuretic effect of neurohypophysial peptides is due to both a decrease in the glomerular filtration rate and an increase in tubular water reabsorption (Pasqualini, 1938; Jancsó, 1955; Sawyer, 1957; Jard and Morel, 1963). In *Rana esculenta* Jard and Morel (1963) showed that very small doses (0.03 μg) of arginine vasotocin or lysine vasotocin ([8-lysine]-oxytocin), which were estimated to yield a plasma concentration of 10^{-10}M, were effective in causing an antidiuresis. The observed response resulted largely from an increased tubular water reabsorption while the fall in the glomerular filtration rate was relatively slight. In addition the vasotocins induced an increase in tubular sodium reabsorption with no effect on potassium absorption. The effects of the vasotocins in the tubule are highly specific for much larger doses of oxytocin and lysine vasopressin had no effects on the tubule although they caused a slight decrease in the glomerular filtration rate. Moreover, oxytocin and [8-isoleucine]-oxytocin completely inhibit the tubular actions of the vasotocins when administered in large quantities, lysine vasopressin had no inhibitory action (Morel and Jard, 1963a). In discussing these results, Morel and Jard (1963b) suggest that the inhibition is competitive at the site of attachment of the vasotocins in the kidney, and that the attachment is made by some component of the ring structure. However, the results of Morel and Jard may not apply generally to all anurans. Thus Uranga and Sawyer (1960) obtained an antidiuresis in *Rana catesbeiana* with large doses of oxytocin (up to 10 U/kg) and vasopressin, smaller doses (1 U/kg) resulted in a diuresis which was associated with an increase in filtration rate. In this case an apparent inhibition of the antidiuretic properties of vasotocin might be due to a simple antagonism. Sawyer (1963a) also reports an antidiuretic action of oxytocin and vasopressin in the grass frog *(Rana pipiens)* and two further species of toads *(Bufo arenarum* and *B. marinus)*.

It appears, therefore, that the anuran kidney has at least two sites where hormones affect its function. The tubular site is highly specific to arginine vasotocin and its action is similar to that of vasopressin in the kidney of mammals. There is a second and perhaps less specific site of action where neurohypophysial hormones alter glomerular filtration, presumably by a variation of blood pressure and flow.

The skin. An increase in water uptake through the skin was first suggested by the results of Brunn (1921) but was first demonstrated unequivocally by Novelli (1936). The dependence of the response on an osmotic flow of water was shown by Stewart (1949) and Sawyer (1951) who abolished the water balance effect by placing frogs in iso- or hyper-osmotic solutions.

However, studies in intact animals were complicated by the presence of the kidney and most recent work has concentrated on permeability studies of a piece of skin *in vitro*. Koefoed-Johnsen and Ussing (1953) showed an increased net transfer of water from the outer to the inner surface of the skin *in vitro* after the application of neurohypophysial hormones to the inner surface. The osmotic permeability ("filtration permeability") to water was several times greater than the diffusion permeability through the skin as measured by the deuterium flux. This difference has been interpreted (Koefoed-Johnsen and Ussing, 1953) as indicating that under the influence of an osmotic gradient water moves not by diffusion but as a continuous "bulk" flow through minute pores in the skin. Neurohypophysial hormones would dilate such pores and increase the net transfer of water. Although most attractive the theory cannot be regarded as proven since the essential element, the difference between the osmotic and diffusion permeabilities, was based on experiments using labelled molecules. Such molecules would require more successful collisions to traverse a pore than the unlabelled water molecules and thus the diffusion permeability might give a falsely low value (see Bentley, 1966a).

Considerable species differences exist between the rate of water transfer across the skin and its response to neurohypophysial hormones (Maetz, 1963). Thus the net water flux, without hormone and under the influence of an osmotic difference of 205 mOsm, was 21.4 $\mu l/cm^2/hr$ in *Bufo bufo*, 9.3 $\mu l/cm^2/hr$ in *Rana esculenta* and 5.0 $\mu l/cm^2/hr$ in the fully aquatic *Xenopus laevis*. The addition of neurohypophysial peptides raised the net water transfer to 45.7 $\mu l/cm^2/hr$ in *B. bufo* and to 17.1 $\mu l/cm^2/hr$ in *R. esculenta*; however, no change was observed in *Xenopus laevis*. These results support the suggestion that the response to the hormones is of ecological importance. Bourguet and Maetz (1961) have shown that arginine vasotocin is the most potent hormone on the water transfer process and that this peptide affects the skin at a concentration in the order of 10^{-10} M.

Ionic fluxes through the amphibian skin are also affected by neurohypophysial peptides (Jørgensen, Levi and Ussing, 1946). Maetz (1963) has shown in intact *Bufo regularis*, that oxytocin, lysine vasopressin and an extract of pituitaries from *B. bufo* cause a net uptake of sodium resulting from a sharp increase of the influx without any consistent change in the efflux. As with the effect on water transfer the peptides stimulate sodium transport across the isolated skin (Fuhrman and Ussing, 1951). The net flux of sodium as measured by a double-isotope technique (^{23}Na and ^{24}Na) is equal to the short-circuit current (Ussing, 1954), i.e. that current which must be applied across the skin as a counter-potential to nullify the spontaneous potential. This preparation has proved to be a most elegant tool for analysing the effects of the hormones on sodium transport across both the amphibian skin (e.g. Maetz, 1963) and urinary bladder (Bentley, 1966a). The peptides act only on the inner surface of the skin (Maetz, 1963). Arginine vasotocin is the most active peptide (Jard, Maetz and Morel, 1960; Bourguet and Maetz, 1961) and has an effect at a concentration of 10^{-10} M.

Since neurohypophysial hormones produce a simultaneous increase in passive osmotic permeability to water and in active sodium transport, it is of interest to enquire whether they act at a single receptor site. Recent evidence suggests the presence of two receptors. Thus Bourguet and Maetz (1961) were able to demonstrate in the frog bladder and skin that various peptides may produce a similar increase in water permeability while stimulating sodium transport to a quite different degree. Moreover, Maetz (1963) and Bentley and Heller (1964) were able to stimulate sodium transport across the skin without any effect on water transfer in the toad, *Xenopus laevis* and the newts *Triturus alpestris* and *T. cristatus*.

The actions of the hormones in increasing water uptake would seem to be of physiological value but the significance of accelerating sodium uptake is more difficult to assess. Frogs will certainly take up sodium from the medium in which they are placed (Krogh, 1939) even at a concentration of 10^{-5} M (pond water is normally less than 10^{-3} M) but whether the neurohypophysial hormones are actually responsible is not clear. An additional function of the peptides on skin sodium transport might also be the conservation of sodium that diffuses across the membranes. The increased flux of sodium also helps to increase the net transfer of water although it plays a minor role (Maetz, 1960).

The bladder. The storage of urine in the anuran bladder and its possible significance as a reservoir has been realized for a long time (Darwin, 1839). Indeed, in certain arid living species of Australian frogs the capacity of the bladder may exceed 50% of the body weight (Main and Bentley, 1964). Neurohypophysial peptides increase water reabsorption from the bladder in the intact frog (Ewer, 1952a) and cause a net osmotic transfer *in vitro* across the bladder wall (Bentley, 1958). The isolated bladder also transports sodium against an electrochemical gradient from its mucosal to serosal surface. This transport is increased by neurohypophysial hormones (Leaf, Anderson and Page, 1958; Bentley, 1960). The rate of sodium transport is sufficient to account for the short-circuit current across the bladder. In all these respects, therefore, the bladder has properties similar to the anuran skin. However, the skin is a complex structure compared with the urinary bladder and consists of several layers of cells and numerous glands. The isolated bladder has thus proved to be a better preparation for studying the action of hormones. The technique described by Bentley (1958) now appears to be in general usage. A comprehensive review of the physiology of the amphibian bladder has recently been published by Bentley (1966a). The reader is referred to this account for a more detailed description of the effects of neurohypophysial hormones.

The water-transfer activity across either the toad or frog bladder has been determined for a large number of both synthetic and naturally occurring analogues of oxytocin (see Jard, Maetz and Morel, 1960; Sawyer, 1963b; Rasmussen *et al.*, 1963; Schwartz and Livingstone, 1964); in contrast, few determinations of the sodium transporting activity (natriferic) have been made (Bentley, 1963; Follett and Heller, 1964; Ferguson, 1964). The presence of a highly basic residue at position eight greatly contributes to either water-transfer or natriferic activity. As the basicity is decreased from arginine through citrulline to leucine activity declines. It is also clear that an oxytocic ring confers more biological activity than a vasopressor ring. Within the oxytocic ring, position three is essential for activity. The mere removal of a methyl group to produce [3-valine]-oxytocin virtually abolishes the activity. Of further interest is deamino-oxytocin: this analogue which lacks the free amino group on the first cysteine residue, has a much reduced water transfer activity compared with oxytocin. In contrast deamino-oxytocin has enhanced oxytocic, fowl vasodepressor and rat antidiuretic activities (Chan and du Vigneaud, 1962). Differences between activity in *Rana* and *Bufo* are relatively minor when the error of the assay is taken into consideration. However, the substitution of glutamine by serine at position four greatly reduced biological activity in *Rana* but was less effective in *Bufo*. The [4-asparagine]-oxytocin analogue also has considerable potency in *Bufo*. The mammalian antidiuretic response has also been tested with many analogues, the conclusions reached have been similar in that a basic residue at position eight enhances potency (Sawyer, 1961b).

The mechanism of action of the neurohypophysial peptides on the bladder has been extensively investigated during the past five years. As in the skin there appear to be at least two receptor elements, one altering sodium and the other water transfer. This was suggested by the results of Bourguet and Maetz (1961) and confirmed recently by Lichtenstein and Leaf (1965), who abolished the vasopressin-induced sodium transport by the application of amphotericin B to the mucosal surface of the bladder. The increased water transfer was unaffected. The exact sites of action are still unclear although the peptides will only act on the serosal surface (Leaf and Hays, 1961). This suggests that the receptor sites might be located at this point although it is perfectly possible that the peptides may only enter through the serosal surface and then have a direct action at some point in the cell (Bentley, 1966a).

The discovery in 1962 by Orloff and Handler that adenosine-3', 5'-monophosphate (cyclic AMP) in low doses accelerates both water transfer and sodium transport across the toad bladder suggested that the peptides may not act directly. They might function through an intermediate in a similar manner to that described for other hormones such as catecholamines and glucagon (see Sutherland, Øye and Butcher, 1965). Bentley (1966a) has drawn up a hypothetical scheme which involves the neurohypophysial peptides activating adenyl cyclase, the latter increasing the entry of sodium into the bladder cells. The elevated sodium content could then activate an ATP-ase which results in the liberation of phosphate-bond energy and the transfer of sodium out of the cell. The cyclic-AMP formed may also activate a phosphorylase which could alter the permeability of the mucosal barrier to water.

EFFECTS OF THE HORMONES IN URODELA

Bentley and Heller (1964, 1965) have recently investigated the effects on water and sodium balance in the urodele amphibians. In all species they obtained an increase in weight after neurohypophysial hormones, although the intensity of the effect was related to the habitat of the species. Thus the maximal increase in body weight in the wholly aquatic mud puppy *(Necturus)* and larval axolotl *(Ambystoma)* was only 2–6% whereas a rise of 14–20% was found in terrestrial newts *(Triturus alpestris, T. cristatus)* and the fire salamander *(Salamandra maculosa)*. Similar small water balance effects after the injection of arginine vasotocin have been reported by Alvarado and Johnson (1965) in larval and adult *Ambystoma*. The most effective neurohypophysial peptide was invariably arginine vasotocin (Bentley and Heller, 1964) followed by arginine and lysine vasopressin and by oxytocin, a similar grading in activity was found in the Anura (Heller and Bentley, 1965).

As discussed previously the overall water balance response in Anura is a composite effect caused by actions on three effector sites, namely the kidney, skin and bladder. In a typical toad *(Bufo marinus)* neurohypophysial hormones increase body weight by 15–22%, nearly half of the water retained was reabsorbed from the bladder, the antidiuresis and skin uptake contributing the remainder (Bentley and Ferguson, 1967).

It is of interest, therefore, that in the urodeles the relative significance of these effector sites is completely different (Bentley and Heller, 1964, 1965). In *Triturus, Necturus* and *Ambystoma* the effect of the peptides was caused solely by a renal action. For example, in *Triturus* arginine vasotocin decreased urine flow from 261 to 109g/kg b.w./day while the concentration of sodium in the urine was unaltered. This infers that the hormone acts primarily by decreasing the glomerular filtration rate. In support of these results *in vivo*, Bentley and Heller (1964) showed that neurohypophysial peptides failed to alter the net water flux across the isolated skin or bladder of these species. Alvarado and Johnson (1965) report a sixfold fall in the filtration rate after vasotocin in *Ambystoma*. In contrast the weight gain in *Salamandra* is due entirely to reabsorption of water from the urinary bladder: arginine vasotocin had no effect on water transfer across the isolated skin and also failed to alter kidney function. (Bentley and Heller, 1965).

A net sodium uptake resulted from the injection of arginine vasotocin into *Triturus* (Bentley and Heller, 1964) and into larval and adult *Ambystoma* (Alvarado and Johnson, 1965). Part of this effect was due to a decreased urinary loss of sodium but a net influx was also measurable. The results in *Ambystoma* suggested an accelerated sodium uptake across the skin, a response well characterized in the anurans. Bentley and Heller (1964) were unable to confirm this with *Ambystoma* skin *in vitro* although this may have been a reflection of the inability of the skin to survive in such conditions. However, arginine vasotocin increased clearly the short-circuit current across the skin of *Triturus*.

MISCELLANEOUS EFFECTS OF THE HORMONES

The hypothalamic neurosecretory system of both Anura and Urodela ends primarily in the pars nervosa although fine neurosecretory axons are also present in the pars eminens (Dodd and Kerr, 1963). It is possible that secretions from these axons could influence the release of adenohypophysial hormones. Jørgensen and Larsen (1963) have presented evidence that arginine vasopressin accelerates the release of ACTH from the transplanted pars distalis of *Bufo bufo*. However, lesions experiments (Jørgensen, 1965) do not appear to implicate the neurosecretory system in the control mechanism. The strict criteria necessary to establish unequivocally the identity of a hypothalamic releasing factor (see Guillemin, 1963) have not yet been presented for any compound in the amphibian hypothalamus and more work is urgently required in this field.

Woolley (1959) obtained alterations in systemic blood pressure with oxytocin and vasopressin in both frogs and toads. The doses used were very large, however, and the response would appear to be pharmacological rather than physiological. Arginine vasotocin in small doses induces hyperglycemia in toads (Bentley, 1965). Again the significance of this response is unknown although it occurs in all vertebrate groups. Another response which may have a physiological role was discovered by Heller, Ferreri and Leathers (1967): neurohypophysial hormones cause contraction of the oviduct in both anurans and urodeles. Considerable differences in sensitivity were found but in all species used arginine vasotocin was the most active peptide tested.

THE REPTILES

An action of neurohypophysial hormones on the reptilian kidney was first shown by Burgess *et al.* (1933) who induced an antidiuresis in the alligator with Pitressin. The effect was caused by a fall in the glomerular filtration rate with no change in tubular water reabsorption. This was confirmed by Sawyer and Sawyer (1952). Bentley (1959) obtained an antidiuresis with Pitressin in the lizard, *Trachysaurus rugosus*. Indirect evidence suggested that the effect was primarily on the glomerulus. More recently, the underlying physiology of the reptilian kidney has been further analysed in snakes (LeBrie and Sutherland, 1962; Dantzler, 1967), crocodiles (Coulson and Hernandez, 1964; Schmidt-Nielsen and Skadhauge, 1967) and chelonids (Dantzler and Schmidt-Nielsen, 1966). Experiments in which reptiles were dehydrated and in which an action of neurohypophysial hormones is most likely, have shown that the relative importance of the glomerular filtration rate, tubular reabsorption and absorption through the bladder or cloaca differs markedly between species. Thus in the fresh-water turtle, *Pseudemys scripta* (Dantzler and Schmidt-Nielsen, 1966) and in water snakes of the genus *Natrix* (LeBrie and Sutherland, 1962), dehydration results in large changes in the filtration rate and alterations in tubular permeability. However, in desert-living forms such as the tortoise *Gopherus agassizii* (Dantzler and Schmidt-Nielsen, 1966), geckos *(Hemodactylus* sp.) and the lizard *Phrynosoma cornutum* (Roberts and Schmidt-Nielsen, 1966) dehydration had little effect on filtration rate or on the renal tubules. The ureteral urine was hypo- or iso-osmotic and the final volume of voided urine was determined by bladder or cloacal absorption. Schmidt-Nielsen and Skadhauge (1967) have demonstrated a similar mechanism of control over water excretion in the crocodile *(Crocodylus acutus)*.

These results suggest actions of neurohypophysial hormones and are supported by direct experiments in water snakes (LeBrie and Sutherland, 1962; Dantzler, 1967) and in the fresh-water turtle (Dantzler and Schmidt-Nielsen, 1966). Dantzler (1967) found that very low doses of arginine vasotocin depressed the glomerular filtration rate and increased tubular water reabsorption in *Natrix*. However, the greater magnitude and duration of the effect on the tubules suggests that tubular permeability to water is more sensitive to vasotocin than is the filtration rate. These findings differ from those of LeBrie and Sutherland (1962) who found the primary site of action of vasopressin to be the glomerulus, while increased tubular permeability to water occurred only at low filtration rates. It is likely, however, that differences between these workers are merely a reflection of experimental technique. In fresh-water turtles (Dantzler and Schmidt-Nielsen, 1966) low doses of an extract of turtle pituitaries (2–9 mU pressor activity) elicited a clear cut tubular effect, whereas larger doses (72 mU activity) had an almost wholly glomerular action. These data support Dantzler (1967) in considering the tubule as the primary site of action. Measurements of Tm for para-amino-hippuric acid in *Natrix* indicated that vasotocin depresses the filtration rate by altering the number of functional glomeruli rather than changing the filtration rate at each glomerulus (Dantzler, 1967). The actions of neurohypophysial peptides in the other reptiles in which water excretion is apparently dependent on bladder or cloacal function requires analysis, especially since Bentley (1962) found no effect of arginine vasotocin on water or sodium transport in the bladder of the tortoise *Testudo graeca*. Indirect evidence which implicates the neurohypophysis in water conservation comes from Hirano (1966) who found that an injection of 10% sodium chloride solution or deprivation of water caused a fall in the hormone content of the pars nervosa in the turtle, *Clemmys japonica*.

Dantzler (1967) showed that oxytocin and 8-isoleucine oxytocin in small doses caused a relatively transient antidiuresis in *Natrix*. The effect appeared to result from a vasodepression caused by these peptides which lowered the filtration rate. Arginine vasotocin had no effect on blood pressure. The systemic vascular effects of the peptides in reptiles appear to be highly variable (e.g. Woolley, 1959) and as in other vertebrate groups a physiological function is not yet apparent.

Arginine vasotocin induced increased tubular reabsorption of sodium in *Natrix* (Dantzler, 1967) similar to that found by Jard and Morel (1963) in frogs. In contrast, however, with the amphibians there was also an increased tubular absorption of potassium.

The oviduct also appears to be a site of action of the peptides. Sawyer, Munsick and van Dyke (1961) found that arginine vasotocin and vasopressin contracted the turtle oviduct strongly implying a possible action in egg-laying. Clausen (1940) has reported that in several groups of viviparous snakes (*Natrix* spp., *Storeria* spp., *Thamnophis* spp.) mammalian posterior pituitary extract precipitated parturition when gestation was at an advanced stage. Oxytocin induced oviposition within one hour in the ovoviviparous lizard *(Zootoca vivipara)*; this effect was obtained in mid-gestation as well as late in pregnancy (Panigel, 1956).

THE BIRDS

Particular interest has again centred upon possible effects on the avian kidney, especially because birds are the first group to possess a loop of Henle and to produce a hypertonic urine. However, the nature of avian excreta, in particular the insolubility of uric acid, has made the problem difficult experimentally. Nevertheless, commercial posterior pituitary preparations have been shown to be antidiuretic in chickens (Burgess *et al.*, 1933; Korr, 1939); the effect appeared to result from actions on both the tubule and filtration rate. Arginine vasotocin is approximately six times as potent as vasopressin in inducing antidiuresis; oxytocin is almost invariably diuretic and usually raises the filtration rate (Sawyer, 1963b). However, more recent studies in the domestic fowl (Skadhauge, 1964; Dantzler, 1966) suggest that vasotocin has no effect on the filtration rate but only on tubular reabsorption of water. The restriction of the response to the renal tubules would be similar to the renal action of neurohypophysial peptides in the mammals.

There is a considerable amount of indirect evidence implicating the peptides in avian water exchanges. Thus neurohypophysectomy results in diabetes insipidus (Shirley and Nalbandov, 1956) and hypothalamic lesions induce polyuria and polydipsia (e.g. Ralph, 1960). Depletion of stainable neurosecretory material from the pars nervosa and activation of the supraoptic and paraventricular nuclei following dehydration has been reported in many species of birds (e.g. Follett and Farner, 1966). Moreover, dehydration in the Japanese Quail *(Coturnix coturnix japonica)* is accompanied by a fall in the hormone content of the hypothalamohypophysial system (Follett and Farner, 1966). The reduction in arginine vasotocin content of the pars nervosa (82.1%) was greater than that of oxytocin (57.9%), the difference between the means was statistically significant ($P < 0.02$). The mean loss of vasotocin from the pars eminens (36.0%) was much less ($P < 0.001$) than the loss from the pars nervosa. These results suggest arginine vasotocin to be the active antidiuretic principle.

The cloaca of birds has long been considered as a possible site of water and electrolyte absorption. It is not known if neurohypophysial hormones act at this site although water transfer from the cloaca is unlikely since the urine is hypertonic to the plasma.

The vasodepressor activity of oxytocin in the domestic fowl is well known and forms the basis of an assay for the peptide (Coon, 1939). The potency of many analogues of oxytocin has been tested on this preparation (Sawyer 1961b; Berde and Boissonnas, 1966). In contrast with the requirements for biological activity on the frog bladder, the fowl vasodepressor response is not very specific. Nevertheless modifications of the ring size, shortening of the lateral peptide chain, lengthening of the N-terminal position and alterations in position 2 abolish activity. Position eight does not appear to be critical for activity, e.g. the replacement of leucine (oxytocin) by isoleucine, valine, citrulline or lysine only affects the activity slightly. Positions within the ring are more important but [4-serine, 8-isoleucine]-oxytocin and [3-valine]-oxytocin still retain considerable potency. Deamino-oxytocin is even more potent than oxytocin: the explanation is not clear although the analogue is less susceptible to plasma peptidases (Golubow, Chan and du Vigneaud, 1963). The effect of the neurohypophysial peptides on the blood pressure of other birds has also been investigated (e.g. Woolley, 1959). Oxytocin is vasodepressive in most species although it causes a rise in blood pressure in the pigeon (Waring, Morris and Stephens, 1956). It should perhaps be emphasized that no physiological function for the vasodepressor response has yet been forthcoming.

Neurohypophysial hormones also have a strong contractile action on the isolated fowl oviduct and the response has been used as a bioassay (Sawyer, 1961b). Arginine vasotocin was the most active peptide tested (640 U/mg) followed by arginine vasopressin (240 U/mg), lysine vasotocin (75 U/mg) and oxytocin (29 U/mg). A physiological function for the response appears likely. Thus Munsick, Sawyer and van Dyke (1960) showed that an intravenous injection of arginine vasotocin (30 mU) induced oviposition within 90 sec. Tanaka and Nakajo (1962) found a considerable depletion of arginine vasotocin from the chicken neural lobe after oviposition with only a small decrease in oxytocin content. More direct evidence is the fact that the plasma concentration of vasotocin rises during egg-laying from 167 μU/ml just prior to oviposition to 7059 μU/ml at oviposition ($P < 0.01$). Within 20 min of egg-laying the level had fallen again to 1216 μU/ml (Sturkie and Lin, 1966). Stimulation of the preoptic area in chickens, which is associated with release of vasotocin, also induces premature oviposition (Opel, 1964). However, the neurohypophysis and its hormones do not appear essential for oviposition (Shirley and Nalbandov, 1956; Opel, 1965). This resembles the situation in mammals where oxytocin may aid in parturition but may not be essential (Fitzpatrick, 1966).

Hyperglycemia may be induced in chickens by oxytocin (Kook, Cho and Yun, 1964). A similar response is found to arginine vasotocin (Bentley, 1966a). The significance of this effect is obscure but it occurs in all vertebrate groups (Mirsky, 1963; Bentley and Follett, 1965; Bentley, 1965).

HYPOTHALAMIC CONTROL OF THE PARS DISTALIS

The avian hypothalamus has a conspicuously well developed median aminence which often contains large amounts of neurosecretory material derived from the hypothalamo-neurohypophysial tract (Farner and Oksche, 1962). The axons ending in this region appear to contain arginine vasotocin and oxytocin (Ishii, Hirano and Kobayashi, 1962; Hirano, 1966; Follett and Farner, 1966) and form a separate store which is physiologically independent from the pars nervosa. Thus dehydration depletes the pars nervosa without affecting stainability in the median eminence (Farner and Oksche, 1962). On the other hand, photoperiodically induced testicular growth in highly sensitive white-crowned sparrows *(Zonotrichia leucophrys gambelii)* caused a depletion of material from the median eminence without affecting the pars nervosa (Oksche et al., 1959; Farner and Oksche, 1962). These results led to the hypothesis that the neurosecretory material might affect gonadotrophin release and it assigned a primary role to the supraoptico-hypophysial tract in this mechanism. This theory gained support from the results of Benoit and Assenmacher in the domestic mallard in which hypothalamic lesions severing the neurosecretory tract caused an abolition of the release of gonadotrophin (e.g. Assenmacher, 1958; Gogan, Kordon and Benoit, 1963). However, consistent changes in the neurosecretory material of the median eminence and its hormones were not found in other species of birds undergoing photoperiodic stimulation (e.g. Wolfson and Kobayashi, 1962; Graber and Nalbandov, 1965; Follett and Farner, 1966). Moreover, Wilson and Farner (1965) showed in white-crowned sparrows that lesions of the neurosecretory tract did not abolish gonadal development. At this time therefore, the original hypothesis must be drastically revised if not abandoned altogether (see review by Farner and Follett, 1966). Nevertheless, the original findings of Oksche et al. (1959) still hold true and it is perfectly possible that the neurohypophysial peptides stored in the avian median eminence influence another function of the adenohypophysis.

CONCLUSIONS

It is evident that one of the major functions of the neurohypophysial hormones throughout the vertebrates is to control their water exchanges. The peptides invariably act to stabilize the internal milieu although this may require essentially opposite effects in fresh water fish and terrestrial vertebrates. Developmentally the kidney of the teleost fishes would appear to be the first definitive target organ, a range of neurohypophysial hormones having no effect on renal water excretion in the lamprey. In both the teleosts and the lungfishes the hormones cause a diuresis resulting from an increase in the glomerular filtration rate, while tubular water reabsorption remains unaffected. The mechanisms whereby the filtration rate is increased remains unknown although glomerular recruitment is likely. Alternatively, an increase in the filtration rate at each glomerulus is a possibility especially since Chan and Chester Jones (1967) demonstrated a vasopressor response to neurohypophysial peptides in the eel.

The evolution of terrestrial vertebrates imposed a very different problem in that the conservation of body water became of paramount importance. The studies of Bentley and Heller (1964) indicate that the primitive urodele amphibians have acquired an antidiuretic response to the neurohypophysial peptides. This action appears to be due to a decrease of glomerular filtration rate. One of the most intriguing problems which remains is the mechanism of this reversed effect on the filtration rate. A renal antidiuresis alone does not appear to be adequate for terrestrial life and the Anura have added further target organs for neurohypophysial hormones, namely the skin and bladder. In addition the peptides not only decrease filtration rate at the kidney but also increase tubular water reabsorption. The combined action on all these target organs has allowed the Anura to be ecologically more successful and even to inhabit arid areas (Bentley, Lee and Main, 1958). The effects on the bladder, and to a lesser extent on the skin, have also proved useful in understanding the biochemical events associated with water absorption and electrolyte transport. The urinary bladder preparation mimics *in vitro* many of the properties of the renal tubules of the mammalian kidney and has revealed actions at the cellular level not only of the neurohypophysial hormones but also of the mineralocorticoids.

Vertebrates above the level of the Amphibia no longer have a highly permeable skin and the effects of the peptides on water balance are restricted to the kidney. The action on the glomerular filtration rate becomes progressively less important and the tubular responses dominate (Dantzler, 1966, 1967), until in the mammals the glomerular effects have largely disappeared.

Neurohypophysial hormones have relatively minor effects on electrolyte balance in mammals although they may aid in the counter-current concentrating mechanism by increasing sodium transport from the ascending limb of the loop of Henle (Pickford, 1966), or by some other effect (see Chapter 8a). However, in lower vertebrates the peptides increase sodium transport against an electrochemical gradient in a variety of tissues including the renal tubule, the teleost gill and the amphibian skin and bladder. The physiological significance of these responses is not always clear, for example in fresh water cyclostomes and teleosts, but the matter requires further analysis. This is especially so in marine teleosts in which the peptides may have an essential role in removing excess sodium from the body derived from intestinal absorption. It is of interest that in all the lower vertebrates, the receptor site of the target organ is exquisitely sensitive to arginine vasotocin, the mammalian antidiuretic principles being relatively very much less active.

The muscular tissue of the reproductive tract may be responsive to neurohypophysial peptides in all vertebrate groups. It is tempting to infer that the hormones play a normal role in oviposition but definitive evidence in the lower vertebrates is only available in the domestic fowl where assays show a rise in the plasma arginine vasotocin level during egg-laying (Sturkie and Lin, 1966). The most effective peptide in contracting the oviduct is again arginine vasotocin. A role for the "oxytocin-like" hormones has not yet been discovered.

Finally the neurohypophysial peptides may influence the release of adenohypophysial hormones in the lower vertebrates. However, direct experimental evidence is lacking and recent studies on the hypothalamic releasing mechanisms in mammals do not invoke the neurohypophysial peptides. Nevertheless, the high concentration of stainable neurosecretory material in the avian median eminence argues for an action on the pars distalis, and the anatomical interdigitation of the pars nervosa and pars intermedia in elasmobranchs and teleosts strongly suggests a functional relationship.

REFERENCES

BOOKS, REVIEWS AND MONOGRAPHS

BENTLEY, P. J. (1966a). The physiology of the urinary bladder of Amphibia. *Biol. Rev.*, **41**: 275–316.

BERDE, B. and BOISSONNAS, R. A. (1966). Synthetic analogues and homologues of the posterior pituitary hormones. *The Pituitary Gland*, vol. 3, pp. 624–661. Harris G. W. and Donovan B. T. (eds.). Butterworths, London.

COULSON, R. A. and HERNANDEZ, T. (1964). *Biochemistry of the Alligator*, pp. 138 Louisiana State University Press, Baton Rouge.
DARWIN, C. (1839). *Journal of researches into the natural history and geology of the countries visited during the voyage of H.M.S. Beagle around the world*.
DODD, J. M. (1963). The pituitary complex. *Techniques in Endocrine Research*, pp. 161–185. Eckstein, P. and Knowles, F. G. W. (eds.). Academic Press, London.
DODD, J. M. and KERR, T. (1963). Comparative morphology and histology of the hypothalamo-neurohypophysial system. *Symp. Zool. Soc. Lond.*, 9: 5–27.
DODD, J. M., PERKS, A. M. and DODD, M. H. I. (1966). Physiological functions of neurohypophysial hormones in sub-mammalian vertebrates. *The Pituitary Gland*, vol. 3, pp. 578–623. Harris, G. W. and Donovan, B. T. (eds.). Butterworths, London.
FARNER, D. S. and FOLLETT, B. K. (1966). Light and other environmental factors affecting avian reproduction. *J. Anim. Sci.*, 25: 90–118.
FARNER, D. S. and OKSCHE, A. (1962). Neurosecretion in birds. *Gen. Comp. Endocr.*, 2: 113–147.
FITZPATRICK, R. J. (1966). The posterior pituitary gland and the female reproductive tract. *The Pituitary Gland*, vol. 3, pp. 453–505. Harris, G. W. and Donovan B. T. (eds.). Butterworths, London.
FONTAINE, M. (1956). The hormonal control of water and salt-electrolyte metabolism in fish. *Mem. Soc. Endocr.*, 5: 69–82.
GUILLEMIN, R. (1963). Sur la nature des substances hypothalamiques qui controlent la sécrétion des hormones antéhypophysaires. *J. Physiol., Paris*, 55: 7–44.
HELLER, H. (ed.). (1957). *The Neurohypophysis*. Butterworths, London.
HELLER, H. (ed.). (1963). Comparative aspects of neurohypophysial morphology and function. *Symp. Zool. Soc. Lond.*, 9.
HELLER, H. and BENTLEY, P. J. (1963). Comparative aspects of the actions of neuro, hypophysial hormones on water and sodium metabolism. *Mem. Soc. Endocr.-* 13: 59–65.
JANCSÓ, N. (1955). *Speicherung*. Akadémiai Kiadó, Budapest.
JØRGENSEN, C. B. (1965). Brain-pituitary relationships in amphibians, birds and mammals: on the origin and nature of the neurons by which hypothalamic control of pars distalis functions are mediated. *Archs Anat. microsc. Morph. exp.*, 54: 261–276.
JØRGENSEN, C. B. and LARSEN, L. O. (1963). Neuro-adenohypophysial relationships. *Symp. Zool. Soc. Lond.*, 9: 59–82.
KROGH, A. (1939). *Osmotic Regulation in Aquatic Animals*. Cambridge University Press.
LEAF, A. and HAYS, R. M. (1961). The effects of neurohypophysial hormones on permeability and transport in a living membrane. *Recent Prog. Horm. Res.*, 17: 467–492.
MAETZ, J. (1963). Physiological aspects of neurohypophysial function in fishes with some reference to the Amphibia. *Symp. Zool. Soc., Lond.*, 9: 107–140.
MOREL, F. and JARD, S. (1963b). Experiments concerning the first steps of the mechanism of action of neurohypophysial hormones on the kidney. *Mem. Soc. Endocr.*, 13: 67–75.
MOTAIS, R. (1967). Les mécanismes d'échanges ioniques branchiaux chez les Téléostéens. Leur rôle dans l'osmoregulation. *Ann. Inst. Océanog., Monaco*, 45: 1–83.
PICKFORD, G. E. and ATZ, J. W. (1957). *The Physiology of the Pituitary Gland in Fishes*, New York Zoological Society, New York.
PICKFORD, M. (1966). Neurohypophysis and kidney function. *The Pituitary Gland*, vol. 3, pp. 374–399. Harris, G. W. and Donovan, B. T. (eds.). Butterworths, London.

SAWYER, W. H. (1957). The antidiuretic action of neurohypophysial hormones in Amphibia. *The Neurohypophysis*, pp. 171–182. Heller, H. (ed.). Butterworths, London.
SAWYER, W. H. (1961a). Comparative physiology and pharmacology of the neurohypophysis. *Recent Prog. Horm. Res.*, **17**: 437–465.
SAWYER, W. H. (1961b). Neurohypophysial hormones. *Pharmac. Rev.*, **13**: 225–277.
SAWYER, W. H. (1963a). In discussion. *Mem. Soc. Endocrinol.*, **13**: 97.
SAWYER, W. H. (1963b). Neurohypophysial peptides and water excretion in the vertebrates. *Mem. Soc. Endocrinol.*, **13**: 45–59.
SCHWARTZ, I. L. and LIVINGSTONE, L. (1964). Cellular and antidiuretic aspects of the antidiuretic action of vasopressins and related peptides. *Vitams Horm.*, **22**: 261–358.
SUTHERLAND, E. W., ØYE, I. and BUTCHER, R. W. (1965). The action of epinephrine and the role of the adenyl cyclase system in hormone action. *Recent. Prog. Horm. Res.*, **21**: 623–647.
USSING, H. H. (1954). Active transport of inorganic ions. *Symp. Soc. Exp. Biol.*, **8**: 407–422.
USSING, H. H. (1960). The alkali metal ions in isolated systems and tissues. In *Handbuch der Experimentellen Pharmakologie*, vol. 13, pp. 1–195. Springer, Berlin.
WARING, H. and LANDGREBE, F. W. (1950). Hormones of the posterior pituitary. *The Hormones*, vol. 2, pp. 427–514. Pincus, G. and Thimann, K. V. (eds.). Academic Press, New York.

ORIGINAL PAPERS

ALVARADO, R. H. and JOHNSON, S. R. (1965). The effects of arginine vasotocin and oxytocin on sodium and water balance in *Ambystoma*. *Comp. Biochem. Physiol.*, **16**: 531–546.
ASSENMACHER, I. (1958). Recherches sur le contrôl hypothalamique de la fonction gonadotrope préhypophysaire chez le canard. *Archs Anat. Microsc. Morph. Exp.*, **47**: 447–572.
BENTLEY, P. J. (1958). The effects of neurohypophysial extracts on water transfer across the wall of the isolated urinary bladder of the toad, *Bufo marinus*. *J. Endocr.*, **17**: 201–209.
BENTLEY, P. J. (1959). Studies on the water and electrolyte metabolism of the lizard *Trachysaurus rufosus* (Gray). *J. Physiol., Lond.*, **145**: 37–47.
BENTLEY, P. J. (1960). The effects of vasopressin on the short-circuit current across the wall of the isolated bladder of the toad, *Bufo marinus*. *J. Endocr.*, **21**: 161–170.
BENTLEY, P. J. (1962). Studies on the permeability of the large intestine and urinary bladder of the tortoise (*Testudo graeca*) with special reference to the effects of neuro-hypophysial and adrenocortical hormones. *Gen. Comp. Endocr.*, **2**: 323–328.
BENTLEY, P. J. (1963). A method for the detection and estimation of small amounts of arginine vasotocin. *J. Endocr.*, **24**: 295–296.
BENTLEY, P. J. (1965). Hyperglycaemic effects of vasotocin in toads. *Nature, Lond.*, **206**: 1053–1054.
BENTLEY, P. J. (1966b). Hyperglycaemic effect of neurohypophysial hormones in the chicken, *Gallus domesticus*. *J. Endocr.*, **34**: 527–528.

BENTLEY, P. J. and FERGUSON, D. R. (1967). The role of the toad urinary bladder in the amphibian "water balance effect" of neurohypophysial hormones. *J. Endocr.*, **37**: 349–350.

BENTLEY, P. J. and FOLLETT, B. K. (1962). The action of neurohypophysial and adrenocortical hormones on sodium balance in the cyclostome, *Lampetra fluviatilis*. *Gen. Comp. Endocr.*, **2**: 329–335.

BENTLEY, P. J. and FOLLETT, B. K. (1963). Kidney function in a primitive vertebrate, *Lampetra fluviatilis*. *J. Physiol., Lond.*, **169**: 902–918.

BENTLEY, P. J. and FOLLETT, B. K. (1965). The effects of hormones on the carbohydrate metabolism of the lamprey *(Lampetra fluviatilis)*. *J. Endocr.*, **31**: 127–137.

BENTLEY, P. J. and HELLER, H. (1964). The action of neurohypophysial hormones on the water and sodium metabolism of urodele amphibians. *J. Physiol., Lond.*, **171**: 434–453.

BENTLEY, P. J. and HELLER, H. (1965). The water-retaining action of vasotocin on the fire salamander *(Salamandra maculosa)*: the role of the urinary bladder. *J. Physiol., Lond.*, **181**: 124–129.

BENTLEY, P. J., LEE, A. K. and MAIN, A. R. (1958). Comparison of dehydration and hydration of two genera of frogs *(Heleioporus* and *Neobatrachus)* that live in areas of varying aridity. *J. Exp. Biol.*, **35**: 677–684.

BOURGUET, J. and MAETZ, J. (1961). Arguments en faveur de l'indépendance des mécanismes d'action de divers peptides neurohypophysaires sur le flux osmotique d'eau et sur le transport actif de sodium au sein d'un même récepteur: études sur la vessie et la peau de *Rana esculenta* L. *Biochim. Biophys. Acta*, **52**: 552–565.

BOURGUET, J., LAHLOUH, B. and MAETZ, J. (1964). Modifications expérimentales de l'équilibre hydrominéral et osmorégulation chez *Carassius auratus*. *Gen. Comp. Endocr.*, **4**: 563–576.

BOYD E. M. and DINGWALL, M. (1939). The effect of pituitary (posterior lobe) extract on the body water of fish and reptiles. *J. Physiol., Lond.*, **95**: 501–507.

BRUNN, F. (1921). Beitrag zur Kenntnis der Wirkung von Hypophysenextrakten auf den Wasserhaushalt des Frosches. *Z. ges. exp. Med.*, **25**: 170–175.

BURGESS, W. W., HARVEY, A. M. and MARSHALL, E. K. (1933). The site of the antidiuretic action of pituitary extract. *J. Pharmac. Exp. Ther.*, **49**: 237–249.

CALLAMAND, D., FONTAINE, M., OLIVEREAU, M. and RAFFY, A. (1951). Hypophyse et osmoregulation chez les poissons. *Bull Inst. Océanogr. Monaco*, No. 984.

CARLSON, I. H. and HOLMES, W. N. (1962). Changes in the hormone content of the hypothalamo-hypophysial system of the rainbow trout *(Salmo gairdneri)*. *J. Endocr.*, **24**: 23–32.

CHAN, D. K. O. and CHESTER JONES, I. (1967). The regulation of blood pressure in the European eel, *Anguilla anguilla* L. *Gen. Comp. Endocr.*, **9**: 439.

CHAN, W. Y. and DU VIGNEAUD, V. (1962). Comparison of the pharmacologic properties of oxytocin and its highly potent analogue, desamino-oxytocin. *Endocrinology*, **71**: 977–982.

CLAUSEN, H. J. (1940). Studies on the effect of ovariotomy and hypophysectomy on gestation in snakes. *Endocrinology*, **27**: 700–704.

COON, J. M. (1939). A new method for the assay of posterior pituitary extracts. *Archs Int. Pharmacoldyn. Thér.*, **62**: 79–99.

DANTZLER, W. H. (1966). Renal response of chickens to infusion of hypertonic sodium chloride solution. *Amer. J. Physiol.*, **210**: 640–646.

DANTZLER, W. H. (1967). Glomerular and tubular effects of arginine vasotocin in water snakes *(Natrix sipedon)*. *Amer. J. Physiol.*, **212**: 83–91.

DANTZLER, W. H. and SCHMIDT-NIELSEN, B. (1966). Excretion in freshwater turtle *(Pseudemys scripta)* and desert tortoise *(Gopherus agassizii)*. *Amer. J. Physiol.*, **210**: 198–210.

EGAMI, N. (1959). Preliminary note on induction of spawning reflex and oviposition in *Oryzias latipes* by the administration of neurohypophysial substances. *Annotnes Zool. Jap.*, **32**: 13–17.

EGAMI, N. and ISHII, S. (1962). Hypophysial control of reproductive functions in teleost fishes. *Gen. Comp. Endocr.*, Suppl. 1: 248–253.

EGAMI, N. and NAMBU, M. (1961). Factors initiating mating behaviour and oviposition in the fish *Oryzias latipes*. *J. Fac. Sci. Tokyo Univ.*, Sec. IV, **9**: 263–278.

EWER, R. F. (1952a). The effect of pituitrin on fluid distribution in *Bufo regularis* Reuss. *J. Exp. Biol.*, **29**: 173–177.

EWER, R. F. (1952b). The effects of posterior pituitary extracts on water balance in *Bufo carens* and *Xenopus laevis* together with some general considerations on anuran water economy. *J. Exp. Biol.*, **29**: 429–439.

FERGUSON, D. R. (1964). Neurohypophysial hormones in mammals. M. D. Thesis. University of Bristol.

FOLLETT, B. K. and FARNER, D. S. (1966). The effects of the daily photoperiod on gonadal growth, neurohypophysial hormone content, and neurosecretion in the hypothalamo-hypophysial system of the Japanese Quail *(Coturnix coturnix japonica)*. *Gen. Comp. Endocr.*, **7**: 111–124.

FOLLETT, B. K. and HELLER, H. (1964). The neurohypophysial hormones of bony fishes and cyclostomes. *J. Physiol., Lond.*, **172**: 74–91.

FONTAINE, M. and RAFFY, A. (1950). Le facteur hypophysaire de retention d'eau chez les Téléostéens. *C. R. Séanc. Soc. Biol.*, **144**: 617–618.

FUHRMAN, F. A. and USSING, H. H. (1951). A characteristic response of the isolated frog skin potential to neurohypophysial principles and its relation to the transport of sodium and water. *J. Cell. Comp. Physiol.*, **38**: 109–130.

GOGAN, F., KORDON, C. and BENOIT, J. (1963). Retentissement de lésions de l'éminence médians sur la gonadostimulation du Canard. *C. R. Séanc. Soc. Biol.* **157**: 2133–2136.

GOLUBOW, J., CHAN, W. Y. and DU VIGNEAUD, V. (1963). Effect of human pregnancy serum on avian depressor activities of oxytocin and desamino-oxytocin. *Proc. Soc. Exp. Biol. Med.*, **113**: 113–115.

GRABER, J. W. and NALBANDOV, A. V. (1965). Neurosecretion in the White Leghorn Cockerel. *Gen. Comp. Endocr.*, **5**: 485–492.

HAEMPEL, O. (1950). Untersuchungen über den Einfluss von Hormonen auf den Geschlechtszyklus von *Lebistes reticulatus* (Pet). *Z. Vitamin-Hormon-Ferment Forsch.* **3**: 261–277.

HELLER, H. and BENTLEY, P. J. (1965). Phylogenetic distribution of the effects of neurohypophysial hormones on water and sodium metabolism. *Gen. Comp. Endocr.*, **5**: 96–108.

HELLER, H., FERRERI, E. and LEATHERS, D. H. G. (1967). The effect of neurohypophysial hormones on the amphibian oviduct. *J. Endocr.*, **37**: xxxix.

HIRANO, T. (1966). Neurohypophysial hormones in the median eminence of the bullfrog, turtle and duck. *Endocr. Jap.*, **13**: 59–74.

HOLMES, R. L. (1961). Kidney function in migrating salmonids. *Rep. Challenger Soc.*, **3**: 23.

HOLMES, W. N. (1959). Studies on the hormonal control of sodium metabolism in the rainbow trout *(Salmo gairdneri)*. *Acta Endocr. Copnh.*, **31**: 587–602.

Holmes, W. N. and McBean, R. L. (1963). Studies on the glomerular filtration rate of rainbow trout *(Salmo gairdneri)*. *J. Exp. Biol.*, **40**: 335–341.
Houssay, B. A. (1931). Action sexuelle de l'hypophyse sur les poissons et des reptiles. *C. R. Séanc. Soc. Biol.*, **106**: 377–378.
Houssay, B. A. and Potick, D. (1929). Cited in Heller, H. (1950). The comparative physiology of the neurohypophysis. *Experientia*, **6**: 368–376.
Ishii, S. (1961). Artificial parturition in the top minnow. *Zool. Mag., Tokyo*, **70**: 3–4.
Ishii, S., Hirano, T. and Kobayashi, H. (1962). Neurohypophysial hormones in the avian median eminence and pars nervosa. *Gen. Comp. Endocr.*, **2**: 433–440.
Jard, S. and Morel, F. (1963). Actions of vasotocin and some of its analogues on salt and water excretion by the frog. *Amer. J. Physiol.*, **204**: 222–226.
Jard, S., Maetz, J. and Morel, F. (1960). Action de quelques analogues de l'ocytocine sur différents récepteurs de l'osmorégulation chez *Rana esculenta*. *C. R. hebd. Séanc. Acad. Sci., Paris*, **251**: 788–790.
Jasinski, A., Gorbman, A. and Hara, T. J. (1966). Rate of movement and redistribution of stainable neurosecretory granules in hypothalamic neurons. *Science, N.Y.*, **154**: 776–778.
Jørgensen, C. B., Levi, H. and Ussing, H. H. (1946). On the influence of the neurohypophyseal principles on the sodium metabolism in the axolotl *(Ambystoma mexicanum)*. *Acta Physiol. Scand.*, **12**: 350–371.
Knowles, F. G. W. (1965). Evidence for a dual control, by neurosecretion, of hormone synthesis and hormone release in the pituitary of the dogfish, *Scylliorhinus stellaris*. *Phil. Trans. Roy. Soc. Ser. B*, **249**: 435–455.
Knowles, F. G. W. and Vollrath, L. (1966). Neurosecretory innervation of the pituitary of the eels *Anguilla* and *Conger*. I. The structure and ultrastructure of the neuro-intermediate lobe under normal and experimental conditions. *Phil. Trans. Roy. Soc. Ser. B*, **250**: 311–327.
Koefoed-Johnsen, V. and Ussing, H. H. (1953). The contributions of diffusion and flow. The effect of neurohypophysial hormone on isolated anuran skin to the passage of D_2O through living membranes. *Acta Physiol. Scand.*, **28**: 60–76.
Kook, Y., Cho, K. B. and Yun, K. O. (1964). Metabolic effects of oxytocin in the chicken. *Nature, Lond.*, **204**: 385–386.
Korr, I. (1939). The osmotic function of the chicken kidney. *J. Cell. Comp. Physiol.*, **13**: 175–193.
Leaf, A., Anderson, J. and Page, L. B. (1958). Active sodium transport by the isolated toad bladder. *J. Gen. Physiol.*, **41**: 657–68.
Leatherland, J. F. (1967). Structure and function of the hypothalamo-neurohypophysial complex and associated ependymal structures in the fresh water eel *(Anguilla anguilla* L.). Ph. D. Thesis, University of Leeds.
LeBrie, S. J. and Sutherland, I. D. W. (1962). Renal function in water snakes. *Amer. J. Physiol.*, **203**: 995–1000.
Lederis, K. (1964). Fine structure and hormone content of the hypothalamo-neurohypophysial system of the rainbow trout *(Salmo irideus)* exposed to sea water. *Gen. Comp. Endocr.*, **4**: 638–661.
Levinsky, N. G. and Sawyer, W. H. (1953). Significance of the neurohypophysis in the regulation of fluid balance in the frog. *Proc. Soc. Exp. Biol. Med.*, **82**: 272–274.
Lichtenstein, N. S. and Leaf, A. (1965). Effect of amphotericin B on the permeability of the toad bladder. *J. Clin. Invest.*, **44**: 1328–42.

MACKAY, M. E. (1931). The action of some hormones and hormone-like substances on the circulation in the skate. *Contr. Can. Biol. Fish.*, Ser. B, **7**: 17–29.
MAETZ, J. (1960). Corrélation entre les actions des hormones neurohypophysaires sur le transport actif de sodium et le flux osmotique d'eau à travers la peau des amphibiens. *Acta Endocr. Copnh.*, **35**, Suppl. 51.
MAETZ, J., MAYER, N. and CHARTIÈR-BARADUC, M. M. (1967). La balance minérale du sodium chez *Anguilla anguilla* en eau de mer, en eau douce et au cours de transfert d'un milieu à l'autre: Effects de l'hypophysectomie et de la prolactine. *Gen. Comp. Endocr.*, **8**: 177–188.
MAETZ, J., BOURGUET, J., LAHLOUH, B. and HOURDRY, J. (1964). Peptides neurohypophysaires et osmoregulation chez *Carassius auratus*. *Gen. Comp. Endocr.*, **4**: 508–523.
MAETZ, J., SAWYER, W. H., PICKFORD, G. E. and MAYER, N. (1967). Evolution de la balance minérale du sodium chez *Fundulus heteroclitus* au cours de transfert d'eau de mer en eau douce: Effects de l'hypophysectomie et de la prolactine. *Gen. Comp. Endocr.*, **8**: 163–176.
MAIN, A. R. and BENTLEY, P. J. (1964). Water relations of Australian burrowing frogs and tree frogs. *Ecology*, **45**: 379–82.
MIRSKY, I. A. (1963). Relative effects of insulin, oxytocin and vasopressin on the free fatty acid concentration of the plasma of non-diabetic and diabetic dogs. *Endocrinology*, **73**: 613–618.
MOREL, F. and JARD, S. (1963a). Inhibition of frog *(Rana esculenta)* antidiuretic action of vasotocin by some analogues. *Amer. J. Physiol.*, **204**: 227–232.
MOTAIS, R. and MAETZ, J. (1964). Action des hormones neurohypophysaires sur les échanges de sodium (mesurés à l'aide du radio-sodium Na^{24}) chez un téléostéen euryhalin, *Platichthys flesus* L. *Gen. Comp. Endocr.*, **4**: 210–224.
MOTAIS, R. and MAETZ, J. (1967). Arginine vasotocine et évolution de la perméabilité branchiale au sodium au cours du passage d'eau douce en eau de mer chez le Flet. *J. Physiol.*, Paris, **59**: 271.
MOTAIS, R., GARCIA ROMEU, F. and MAETZ, J. (1966). Exchange diffusion effect and euryhalinity in teleosts. *J. Gen. Physiol.*, **50**: 391–423.
MUNSICK, R. A., SAWYER, W. H. and VAN DYKE, H. B. (1960). Avian neurohypophysial hormones: pharmacological properties and tentative identification. *Endocrinology*, **66**: 860–871.
NOVELLI, A. (1936). Lóbulo posterior de las hipofisis e imbición de los batrachios II. Mecanesmo de su acción. *Revta Soc. Argent. Biol.*, **12**: 163.
OKSCHE, A., LAWS, D. F., KAMEMOTO, F. I. and FARNER, D. S. (1959). The hypothalamo-hypophysial neurosecretory system of the White-crowned Sparrow, *Zonotrichia leucophrys gambelii*. *Z. Zellforsch. mikrosk. Anat.*, **51**: 1–42.
OPEL, H. (1964). Premature oviposition following operative interference with the brain of the chicken. *Endocrinology*, **74**: 193–200.
OPEL, H. (1965). Oviposition in chickens after removal of the posterior lobe of the pituitary by an improved method. *Endocrinology*, **76**: 673–677.
ORLOFF, J. and HANDLER, J. S. (1962). The similarity of effects of vasopressin, adenosine-3',5'-phosphate (cyclic AMP) and theophylline on the toad bladder. *J. Clin. Invest.*, **41**: 702–709.
OZTAN, N. and GORBMAN, A. (1960). Responsiveness of the neurosecretory system of larval lampreys *(Petromyzon marinus)* to light. *Nature, Lond.*, **185**: 167–168.
PANIGEL, M. (1956). Contribution à l'étude de l'ovoviviparité chez les reptiles. Gesta-

tion et parturition chez le lézard vivipare *Zootoca vivipara*. *Ann. Sci. Nat. (Zool.)*, **18**: 569–668.

PASQUALINI, R. Q. (1938). Action des extraits pituitaires sur la diurèse du crapaud. *C. R. Séanc. Soc. Biol.*, **129**: 1240–1241.

RALPH, C. L. (1960). Polydipsia in the hen following lesions in the supraoptic hypothalamus. *Amer. J. Physiol.*, **199**: 528–530.

RANKIN, J. C., CHAN, D. K. O. and CHESTER JONES, I. (1967). Kidney function in the European eel, *Anguilla anguilla* L. *Gen. Comp. Endocr.*, **9**: 484–485.

RASMUSSEN, H., SCHWARTZ, I. L, YOUNG, R. and MARC-AURELE, J. (1963). Structural requirements for the action of neurohypophysial hormones upon the isolated amphibian urinary bladder. *J. Gen. Physiol.*, **46**: 1171–89.

ROBERTS, G. S. and SCHMIDT-NIELSEN, B. (1966). Renal ultrastructure and the excretion of salt and water by three terrestrial lizards. *Amer. J. Physiol.*, **211**: 476–486.

SAWYER, W. H. (1951). Effect of posterior pituitary extract on permeability of frog skin to water. *Amer. J. Physiol.*, **164**: 44–48.

SAWYER, W. H. (1966). Diuretic and natriuretic responses of lungfish *(Protopterus aethiopicus)* to arginine vasotocin. *Amer. J. Physiol.*, **210**: 191–197.

SAWYER, W. H. and PICKFORD, G. E. (1963). Neurohypophysial principles of *Fundulus heteroclitus*: characteristics and seasonal changes. *Gen. Comp. Endocr.*, **3**: 439–445.

SAWYER, W. H. and SAWYER, M. K. (1952). Adaptive responses to neurohypophysial fractions in vertebrates. *Physiol. Zool.*, **25**: 84–98.

SAWYER, W. H., MUNSICK, R. A. and VAN DYKE, H. B. (1961). Evidence for the presence of arginine vasotocin (8-arginine oxytocin) and oxytocin in neurohypophyseal extracts from amphibians and reptiles. *Gen. Comp. Endocr.*, **1**: 30–36.

SCHMIDT-NIELSEN, B. and SKADHAUGE, E. (1967). Function of the excretory system of the crocodile *(Crocodylus acutus)*. *Amer. J. Physiol.*, **212**: 973–980.

SEXTON, A. W. (1955). Factors influencing the uptake of sodium against a diffusion gradient in the goldfish gill. *Diss. Abstr.*, **15**: 2270–2271.

SHIRLEY, H. V. and NALBANDOV, A. V. (1956). Effects of neurohypophysectomy in domestic chickens. *Endocrinology*, **58**: 477–483.

SKADHAUGE, E. (1964). Effects of unilateral infusion of arginine-vasotocin into the portal circulation of the avian kidney. *Acta Endocr. Copnh.*, **47**: 321–330.

STEGGERDA, F. R. (1937). Comparative study of water metabolism in amphibians ininjected with Pituitrin. *Proc. Soc. Exp. Biol. Med.* **36**: 103–106.

STEWART, W. C. (1949). Effect of mammalian (posterior lobe) pituitary extract on water balance of frogs when placed in different osmotic environments. *Amer. J. Physiol.*, **157**: 412–417.

STURKIE, P. D. and LIN, Y. (1966). Release of vasotocin and oviposition in the hen. *J. Endocrinol.*, **35**: 325–326.

TANAKA, K. and NAKAJO, S. (1962). Participation of neurohypophysial hormone in oviposition in the hen. *Endocrinology*, **70**: 453–458.

URANGA, J. and SAWYER, W. H. (1960). Renal responses of the bullfrog to oxytocin, arginine vasotocin and frog neurohypophysial extract. *Amer. J. Physiol.*, **198**: 1287–1290.

WARING, H., MORRIS, L. and STEPHENS, G. (1956). The effect of pituitary posterior lobe extracts on the blood pressure of the pigeon. *Aust. J. Exp. Biol. Med. Sci.*, **34**: 235–238.

WILHELMI, A. E., PICKFORD, G. E. and SAWYER, W. H. (1955). Initiation of the spawning reflex in *Fundulus* by the administration of fish and mammalian neurohypophysial preparations and synthetic oxytocin. *Endocrinology*, **57**: 243–252.

WILSON, F. E. and FARNER, D. S. (1965). Effects of hypothalamic lesions on testicular growth. *Fedn Proc. Fedn Am. Socs Exp. Biol.*, **24**: 129.

WOLFSON, A. and KOBAYASHI, H. (1962). Phosphatase activity and neurosecretion in the hypothalamo-hypophysial system in relation to the photoperiodic gonadal response in *Zonotrichia albicollis*. *Gen. Comp. Endocr.*, **1**: 168–179.

WOOLLEY, P. (1959). The effect of posterior lobe pituitary extracts on blood pressure in several vertebrate classes. *J. Exp. Biol.*, **36**: 453–458.

CHAPTER 10

CELLULAR MODE OF ACTION OF VASOPRESSIN*

Alexander Leaf and Geoffrey W. G. Sharp

Departments of Medicine, Massachusetts General Hospital and Harvard Medical School, Boston, Massachusetts

THE primary action of vasopressin in mammals is to regulate the renal tubular reabsorption of water. This action, on the epithelium of distal portions of the nephron, occurs at concentrations of the hormone far lower than those required to elicit its known extrarenal effects such as milk ejection, stimulation of the uterus or vasoconstriction. Vasopressin, or antidiuretic hormone (ADH), is lacking in the circulation of the hydrated animal and under these conditions a dilute urine flows from the collecting ducts. In the dehydrated animal ADH is secreted and increases the permeability of the distal portions of the nephron to water. Water is reabsorbed along the osmotic gradient which exists between the dilute urine, of the distal portion of the nephron and collecting duct, and the medullary interstitium. A small volume of concentrated urine is finally excreted.

The nature of the permeability change involved has been the subject of active investigation in recent years. Because of the difficulties of studying permeability properties in renal tubular epithelium the effects of vasopressin on more accessible tissues, the skin and urinary bladder of frogs and toads, have been studied. These tissues, which respond to ADH with a permeability change probably analogous to that in the kidney, have contributed much to our current knowledge. The studies of Koefoed-Johnsen and Ussing (1953) on frog skin provided the first major conceptual advance in our understanding of the mode of action of vasopressin.

The work to be summarized here is drawn largely from investigations on the urinary bladder of the toad because of its ability to perform func-

---

*Supported in part by grants from the John. A. Hartford Foundation, Inc. and the U.S. Public Health Service (No. HE-06664 from the National Heart Institute, and AM-04501 from the National Institute of Arthritis and Metabolic Diseases).

tions which are carried out in mammals by the epithelium of the distal portions of the renal tubule, its accessibility for studies *in vitro*, and its relatively simple structure.

Ewer (1952) observed that the urinary bladder of the toad served as a reservoir of water which can be reabsorbed during periods of water deprivation or rapidly in response to injections of antidiuretic hormone. In the hydrated toad the transparently thin bilobed bladder with its content of hypotonic urine may occupy one-third to one-half of the entire abdominal cavity. Histologically this tissue consists of a single layer of specialized epithelial cells lining the mucosal or urinary surface of the bladder. This functional epithelium is supported on a loose stroma of connective tissue in which are occasional bundles of smooth muscle and capillaries. The contramucosal surface is a serosa. The total solute concentration of such urine may be as low as 50 mOsm per kg water, as dilute as the human kidney can excrete during maximal water diuresis. Such dilute urine may remain in the bladder for hours without apparent decrease in volume or increase in solute concentration.

WATER TRANSPORT

Although in the absence of antidiuretic hormone the bladder acts like a tight vessel for the contained urine, Table 1 (Hays and Leaf, 1962) shows that the unidirectional permeability to water measured isotopically with deuterated or tritiated water is quite high. Measurements were made

TABLE 1. EFFECT OF VASOPRESSIN ON DIFFUSION PERMEABILITY (UNIDIRECTIONAL WATER FLUX) OF ISOLATED TOAD BLADDER TO WATER MEASURED WITH DHO OR THO IN THE ABSENCE OF AN OSMOTIC GRADIENT (HAYS AND LEAF, 1962; LEAF, 1965).

	Periods (30 min)			Mean difference (Period 2–1)	S.E. of mean difference	P
	1	2	3			
	μl cm^{-2} hr^{-1}					
Control	343	338	339	−5	±9	>0.5
With hormone*	338	543	599	+205	±35	<0.001

* Hormone added at end of first period (2 units commercial vasopressin to medium bathing serosal surface). Control includes ten experiments; seven measured from mucosal-to-serosal surface and three in opposite direction.

Hormone-treated group includes thirteen experiments; nine were mucosal-to-serosal fluxes and four were measured in reverse direction.

15 ml frog Ringer's solution bathing each surface; area of chambers, 3.14 cm^2.

in vitro with the bladder wall separating two halves of a lucite chamber. Isotopically labeled water was added to the medium bathing one side of the bladder and its rate of appearance on the opposite side was determined. Results are expressed as microliters of water crossing one square centimeter of bladder wall per hour. It is seen that the rate of transport remains quite constant over three successive 30-min periods. Furthermore, addition of vasopressin (mammalian antidiuretic hormone) to the medium bathing the serosal surface of the half-bladder after the first 30-min control period produced a significant increase in the unidirectional diffusion permeability to water by some 70%.

Quite a different impression of the permeability of the bladder to water is obtained if one measures the net transfers of water across this tissue. This may be done either gravimetrically by weighing the volume of solutions placed on either side of the bladder initially and again at the termination of an experiment, or volumetrically by having one-half of the chamber sealed and connected to a horizontal calibrated pipette in which the volume flow per unit time may be continuously monitored. Because of the distensibility of the bladder wall it is necessary to support it against a nylon or dacron mesh during these observations so that the volume of the half chamber does not change due to billowing of the bladder to one side or the other. The results of a large number of measurements of net transport of water made in the absence and presence of antidiuretic hormone are shown in Fig. 1 (Hays and Leaf, 1962). The abscissa is the osmotic gradient across the bladder wall obtained by diluting the medium bathing the mucosal surface to the desired concentration, but keeping constant that at the opposite serosal surface. The ordinate is the net water transport or flux.

In the absence of an osmotic gradient, with or without antidiuretic hormone, essentially no net transfer of water occurs. We conclude, therefore, that the high isotopic permeability presented in Table 1 represents an equal permeability to water in the two directions across the tissue, from mucosal-to-serosal and serosal-to-mucosal surfaces. The lower line of Fig. 1 indicates the very small net transfers of water across the bladder which occur in the absence of the hormone, despite large osmotic gradients (160 mOsm per kg water on the abscissa is equivalent to some 4 atm of hydrostatic pressure). This is consistent with the findings mentioned of dilute urine remaining in the bladder for long periods of time with little or no detectable change in concentration. The upper line shows the large net transfer of water which may occur in the presence of vasopressin. At the higher osmotic gradients studied, the volume of water crossing unit area of bladder per minute is equal to the total water content of the same

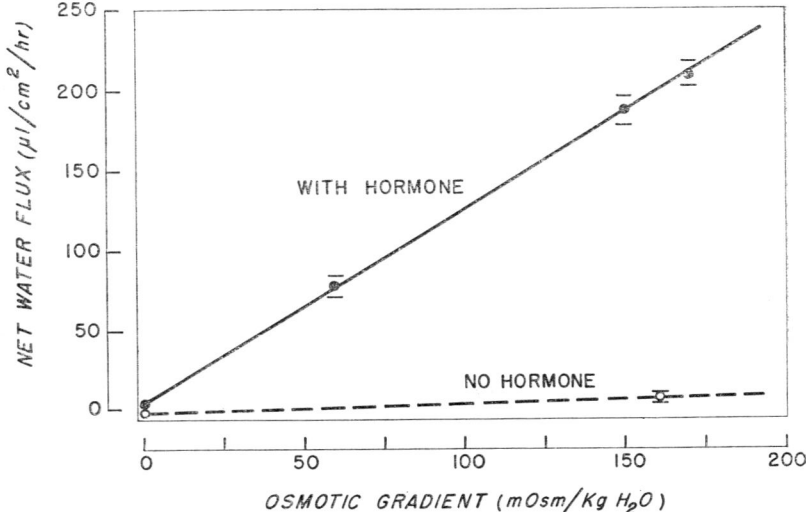

FIG. 1. Dependence of net water flux on osmotic gradient in presence or absence of neurohypophysial hormone. With hormone the points at osmotic gradients of 59, 150, and 170 represent six, eight and fifteen experiments, respectively, and their mean values and S. E. of means are 77.2 ± 6.9, 186 ± 8.8, and 209 ± 7.9 μl per cm² per hour, respectively. The regression equation relating water movement to osmotic gradient is $y = 1.22x+4.22$. Twelve experiments without hormone but with an osmotic gradient of 160 mOsm per kg water gave a mean net flux of $+4.3\pm1.3$ μl per cm² per hour (Hays and Leaf, 1962; Leaf, 1965).

area of tissue and attains a magnitude of more than one-third the simultaneously determined unidirectional permeability to water.

The finding that net movement of water is proportional to the transepithelial osmotic gradient and that no net water transfer occurs in the absence of such an external driving force indicates that water moves passively across the bladder. Furthermore, the hormonal effects on net water transport can be demonstrated in the complete absence of sodium ions (Hays and Leaf, 1962) and, therefore, the active transport of sodium by this tissue contributes very little directly to net water transport. The osmotic gradients *in vivo* arise from the active reabsorption of sodium, and this is the energy-requiring step in water reabsorption.

The findings thus indicate that water moves passively across the toad bladder and that, in spite of a high isotopic permeability to water, very little net movement occurs in the absence of the hormone. Vasopressin has the ability to induce large net transfers of water with only a moderate further increase in the unidirectional diffusion permeability. Before asking in what way the hormone modifies the bladder to produce these effects on the transport of water, it may be useful to digress briefly and to consider some current views regarding water itself which make these effects possible.

The uniqueness and suitability of water as a substrate for life has long been appreciated (Henderson, 1913). The structure of water which accounts for its unusual properties is the subject of extensive study at present. Although many questions about liquid water remain unsolved, it is a fact that water is a highly associated liquid which is pertinent to the present discussion. The crystallographic study of ice indicates it to consist of regular tetrahedrally placed molecules of water (Pauling, 1960). Each molecule of water is surrounded by the four nearest neighbor molecules and the resulting tetrahedral configuration is stabilized by hydrogen bonding of the water molecules. Each molecule is maximally bonded by two hydrogen bonds to its nearest neighbors. Pauling (1960) has pointed out that when ice melts at zero degrees, the heat of melting is sufficient to break only some 15% of the hydrogen bonds present in the fully co-ordinated structure of ice. The residual hydrogen bonds in liquid water account for many of its unique properties.

Obviously the physical properties of ice and water are so different that the latter cannot contain in a static state 85% of the structure of the former. The association between a molecule and its neighbors can be only temporary, as the structure is continually broken down by thermal agitation. Such associations need persist over small regions or clusters for times long enough that the order be "seen" by X-ray or even infra-red radiation and longer than the relaxation time for rotation of a single water molecule, about 10^{-12} sec. Thus water is continuously and rapidly making, breaking and reforming clusters. Frank (1958) has picturesquely referred to the "flickering cluster" structure of water. From their statistical mechanical theory of water, Némethy and Scheraga (1962) have estimated the average size of clusters of water molecules in liquid water at 20° C to be approximately 57 molecules. Below this temperature the size of the aggregates will be larger and at higher temperatures, smaller. Only in the vapor phase, however, does water behave like a monomer.

Various factors are known to increase or stabilize the structure of water and others to break down its structure. It has long been appreciated that individual water molecules are permanent electrical dipoles because of the asymmetrical arrangement of the negative oxygen and positive hydrogen atoms in the V-shaped molecule of water. The interaction of these dipoles with the strong electrical fields of ions results in ionic hydration shells. More recently it has been appreciated (Frank, 1958) that water exists in an increased state of order in apposition to non-polar molecules or surfaces. Since the physical properties of bulk water and bulk ice are so different we may expect the properties of water to vary between these extremes at local sites. Since the coefficient of self diffusion of water is 2.4×10^{-5} cm^2 sec^{-1} at 25°C (Wang, Robinson and Edelman, 1953) and that of water in ice is 1.0×10^{-10} cm^2 sec^{-1} at -1.5 to -2.0°C (Kuhn and Thürkauf, 1958), the transport properties of water may be expected to be strongly dependent upon the degree to which it is structured.

In the measurements of the diffusion permeability of the bladder presented in Table 1, labeled water was added to the medium bathing one surface of the bladder and its rate of appearance in the medium bathing the opposite surface determined in the absence of net transfers of water across the tissue to prevent effects from solvent drag. The individual tagged water molecule penetrates the barrier by diffusion, a process of isotopic exchange, in which the gradient of chemical potential of the isotopic species or a gradient of specific activity is the driving force and is equal to the entropy of mixing multiplied by the absolute temperature. As the isotopic water molecule penetrates the barrier it will be subject to the frictional forces between water and water, f_{ww}, and between water and membrane, f_{wm}, as it randomly jumps from one position to the next in response to thermal agitation. It may at one moment be associated with one cluster of water molecules and the next moment be part of another cluster. In the absence of net transfers of water across the bladder, the clusters will have no overall direction and the progress of the labeled water molecules will depend upon the molecular friction between it and its neighboring water, f_{ww}, or membrane molecules, f_{wm}. In a very finely porous membrane $f_{wm} > f_{ww}$ but in coarse, porous membranes, since they are mole friction terms, f_{wm} diminishes and f_{ww} becomes the determining factor, as in self-diffusion. From the self-diffusion coefficient, $D°$, of water in water a "molecular radius" of the diffusing species may be computed from the Einstein-Stokes relation (Einstein, 1905):

$$D° = \frac{kT}{6\pi\eta\alpha} = \frac{RT}{f_{ww}}$$

where k is Boltzmann's constant, R is the gas constant, T is absolute temperature, α is the radius of the diffusing species, and η is the viscosity of bulk water.

The resultant value of α is constant for measurements made over a considerable temperature range indicating that in the process of diffusion we are dealing with the transport of a single moving particle. Furthermore, the magnitude of α (~ 0.1 nm) indicates that the moving unit in diffusion is a single water molecule. The low value for α as compared with the known molecular radius of water of 0.138 nm from X-ray crystallography is probably due to the limitations of Stokes' law when applied to the movement of particles which approximate in size those of the suspending medium.

When the transport process involves movement of single water molecules as in diffusion or movement through channels so small that dimensions approach that of a water molecule, then the ratio of the two unidirectional fluxes, J_{12} and J_{21}, across the barrier are proportional only to the ratio of the chemical activity of the water on the two sides of the barrier, a_1 and a_2. Thus:

$$\frac{J_{12}}{J_{21}} = \frac{a_1}{a_2}$$

This condition is not favorable for net transport of water as can be quickly appreciated by substituting concentrations of water for activities in the experiments shown in Fig. 1. In these experiments the medium bathing the serosal surface was kept isotonic at 220 mOsm per kg of water and the mucosal medium was diluted. With 160 mOsm per kg of water as the difference in the concentration of water across the bladder,

$$\frac{J_{12}}{J_{21}} = \frac{55.56 - 0.06}{55.56 - 0.22} = 1.003$$

If J_{12} is taken from Table 1 as 340 μl cm^{-2} gr^{-1}, then J_{21} will be 339 μl cm^{-2} hr^{-1}, whereas the observed net flux averaged some 200 μl cm^{-2} hr^{-1}. Diffusion is thus an ineffectual means of producing net transfer of water and can account for only a small fraction of the observed water transport across the bladder in the presence of vasopressin.

In contrast to the process of diffusion, net water movement across a barrier in response to a gradient of hydrostatic or osmotic pressure will depend on the movement of individual water molecules only when the dimensions of the channels through which the water moves approximate the dimensions of individual water molecules. Through all pores of larger dimensions the associated nature of water will result in the movement of clusters of water molecules which thereby reduces the friction per molecule and allows larger net transfers of water for a given pressure difference than could occur by diffusion alone. To account for the observed net transfers of water across the bladder in the absence of vasopressin and again with the hormone the mean pore radius (Koefoed-Johnsen and Ussing, 1953; Pappeinhemer, Renkin and Borrero, 1951; Solomon, 1960; Robbins and Mauro, 1960) must be some 0.8 nm and 4.0 nm respectively.

It may now be asked in what way neurohypophysial hormones modify the bladder to produce the effects on water transport. Koefoed-Johnsen and Ussing (1953) have proposed the most satisfactory explanation at the present time on the basis of the "pore hypothesis". According to their hypothesis, net water movement occurs predominantly by bulk flow in aqueous pores through the bladder rather than by diffusion, and vasopressin increases the net transfer of water by enlarging the radius of individual pores. Since diffusion is dependent on the area (or pore radius squared) available for penetration by the diffusing species while laminar flow, according to the Poiseuille equation, is a function of the fourth power of the radius of the individual pores, a small increase in radius of individual pores, Δr, will affect diffusion only by $(r+\Delta r)^2 - r^2$ while bulk flow will be increased by $(r+\Delta r)^4 - r^4$. They picture neurohypophysial hormones as altering the responsive membrane from one containing many small pores to one containing fewer larger pores. Little change in area or diffusion permeability would be consistent with large increases in bulk transfer of water with vasopressin according to this hypothesis of hormonal action. Examination of the permeability of the bladder to small solutes, however, shows the inapplicability of any explanation for the hormonal action on the transport of water which requires the presence of large pores only.

SOLUTE TRANSPORT

That neurohypophysial hormones may affect permeability to solute molecules as well as to water was first indicated by Andersen and Ussing (1957) who found that vasopressin produced an increase in permeability of the isolated toad skin to thiourea and acetamide.

The striking feature of this effect on the permeability of the toad bladder to small molecules is its specificity. Figure 2 (Leaf and Hays, 1962) contrasts the large increase in permeability to urea and acetamide that followed addition of vasopressin with the absence of an effect on thiourea. Of some 40 compounds whose rate of penetration has been tested, only in the case of certain small uncharged amides and certain low molecular weight alcohols listed in Table 2 was the permeability of the toad bladder increased by vasopressin (Maffly et al., 1960).

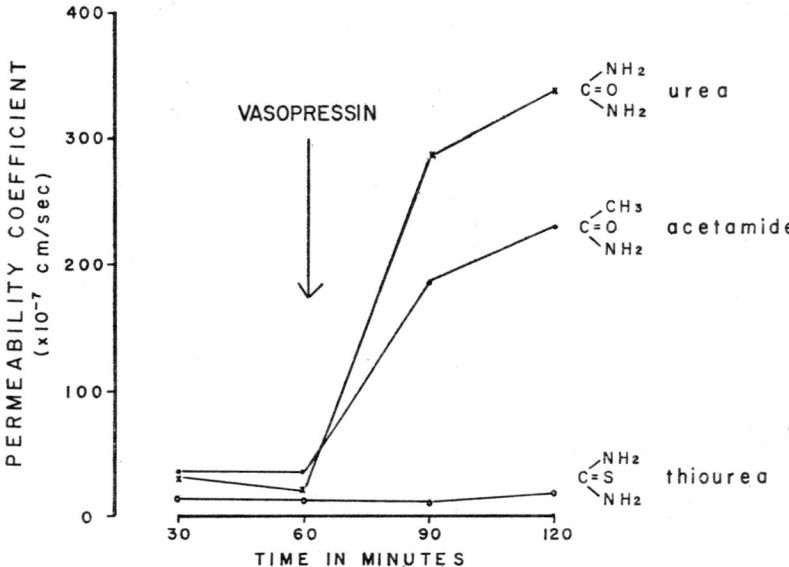

FIG. 2. Effect of vasopressin on the permeability of the toad bladder to urea, acetamide and thiourea. The appropriately labeled molecule was added to the medium bathing one surface of the membrane and its rate of appearance on the opposite side was determined. After two periods of 30 min each, vasopressin was added to the serosal medium and an additional two periods determined. In every instance the permeability to urea and acetamide was enhanced by the hormone, while permeability to thiourea was unaffected (Maffly et al., 1960; Leaf, 1965).

The mode of penetration of the toad bladder by urea and the few similar small molecules appears to be passive, as was demonstrated for water. They penetrate the bladder at equal rates in both directions as shown in Table 3 for urea (Maffly et al., 1960). The permeabilities from mucosal-to-serosal surface and from serosal-to-mucosal surface were simultaneously determined using ^{14}C-urea and ^{15}N-urea to measure the two unidirectional permeability coefficients. Although vasopressin produced approximately a ten-fold average increase in the permeability coefficients, the values in the two directions remained equal. Furthermore, no evidence for carrier-mediated or facilitated diffusion by either self-depression or competition studies was obtained (Leaf and Hays, 1962). Thus these compounds appear to pass through the rate-limiting permeability barrier of the bladder by a process of free diffusion without interaction with the

TABLE 2. COMPOUNDS PENETRATING THE TOAD BLADDER MORE RAPIDLY WITH VASOPRESSIN (LEAF, 1965; LEAF AND HAYS, 1962).

	Molecular weight	Permeability coefficients K_{trans} (10^{-7} cm sec^{-1})		S.E. of mean difference	n
		Vasopressin			
		Before	After		
Amides					
Urea (NH$_2$CONH$_2$)	60	26	274	±5	37
Acetamide (CH$_3$CONH$_2$)	29	44	196	±26	9
Propionamide (CH$_3$CH$_2$CONH$_2$)	73	97	215		2
Butyramide (CH$_3$CH$_2$CH$_2$CONH$_2$)	87	132	180		4
Cyanamide (NH$_2$C≡N)	42	127	282	±31	6
Urethane (NH$_2$COOCH$_2$CH$_3$)	89	581	639	±18	6
Dimethylformamide HCON(CH$_3$)$_2$	73	174	259	±10	6
Nicotinamide (C$_5$H$_4$NCONH$_2$)	122	26	40	±2	6
Methylacetamide (CH$_3$CONHCH$_3$)	73	87	242	±16	6
Water and alcohols					
Water (HOH)	18	944	1580	±35	8
Methanol (CH$_3$OH)	32	825	913	±19	9
Ethanol (CH$_3$CH$_2$OH)	46	575	678	±20	8
Ethylene glycol (CH$_2$OHCH$_2$OH)	62	16	35	±6	6
Inorganic ions					
Sodium	23	36	52	±2.7	14

TABLE 3. SIMULTANEOUS PERMEABILITY COEFFICIENTS FOR UREA IN THE TWO DIRECTIONS THROUGH THE TOAD BLADDER (MAFFLY et al., 1960; LEAF, 1965).

Hormone	No. of periods	Permeability coefficients			S.E. of Δ
		M−S*	S−M*	Δ	
		$\times 10^{-7}$ cm sec^{-1}			
Absent	17	26.0	26.8	0.8	±2.3
Present	13	251.3	261.2	9.9	±7.9

* Mucosal-to-serosal and serosal-to-mucosal permeabilities measured simultaneously with ^{15}N− and ^{14}C-labeled urea.

bladder. However, since the very fact of specificity necessitates interaction with the barrier, one suspects the presence of hydrogen bonding which is the form of interaction most likely to escape detection by the criteria of self-depression or competition.

An effect of solvent flow through the bladder on the penetration of the bladder by urea has been demonstrated (Leaf and Hays, 1962). Imposing net transport of water across the bladder during simultaneous measurements of the two unidirectional fluxes of urea distorted the flux ratio from a value of unity by accelerating the urea flux in the direction of water movement and retarding the flux upstream. This finding indicates that urea and water probably occupy some common channel during a portion, at least, of their course across the bladder. Sidel and Hoffman (1963) have observed solvent drag on urea using a synthetic liquid "membrane" of well stirred mesityl oxide separating two aqueous solutions in which transport of water probably occurs in droplets, certainly not in continuous aqueous channels. These considerations make one interpret the evidence of a solvent drag effect on urea with some caution.

Another means of testing the interaction of solute and solvent as they cross a permeability barrier is to evaluate the reflection coefficient, σ. This expression has been introduced by Staverman (1951) to indicate the penetration of membranes by solute relative to solvent. A truly semipermeable membrane will act as a perfect sieve, the concentration of impermeant solute in the filtrate will be zero, and $\sigma = 1.0$. On the other hand, the concentration of solute in the filtrate from a nonselective barrier will be the same as in the original medium, and $\sigma = 0$.

Table 4 (Leaf and Hays, 1962) shows the reflection coefficients obtained for thiourea, chloride and urea in the presence of large net transfers of water averaging some 200 μl cm^{-2}hr^{-1}. The reflection coefficient for

TABLE 4. REFLECTION COEFFICIENTS FOR THIOUREA, CHLORIDE, AND UREA THROUGH TOAD BLADDER (LEAF, 1965; LEAF AND HAYS, 1962).

	No. of experiments	Mean Δ_w	Mean σ	Range of σ
		$\mu l\ cm^{-2}hr^{-1}$		
Thiourea	6	200	0.995	0.988 – 1.000
Chloride	3	207	0.993	0.990 – 0.994
Urea	29	200	0.79	

Reflection coefficient, $\sigma = 1 - \dfrac{\overline{\text{Net solute flux}}}{\text{Net water flux} \cdot \text{Medium concentration}}$

thiourea and chloride were essentially 1.0, indicating that even in the presence of large net movements of water the membrane retains a high degree of impermeability to thiourea and chloride. Even urea is retarded some 80% in its rate of penetration relative to that of water. Thus thiourea and chloride are excluded from access to the channels in which bulk flow of water occurs and the results, even with respect to urea, are not ambiguous in indicating that water and urea move in the same channels (Kedem and Katchalsky, 1958).

SODIUM TRANSPORT

In contrast to water and the urea-like compounds which move passively, the toad bladder—like the renal tubular epithelium—actively transports sodium ions from urine to body fluids (Leaf, Anderson and Page, 1958). Energy derived from metabolism is used to pump sodium ions uphill thermodynamically from luminal fluid to body fluids. This transport is highly specific for sodium ions. It is of interest that this transport activity of the bladder can be stimulated by mammalian neurohypophysial hormones. This is shown in Fig 3. Even a very large amount of vasopressin added to the medium bathing the mucosal or urinary surface has no effect on sodium transport. The same amount of hormone added to the serosal medium produces a prompt and large stimulation of the current. It has been shown by simultaneous measurements of sodium flux across the bladder using two different radioactive isotopes of sodium that all the increase in short-circuit current after vasopressin results from an increase in the transport of sodium from mucosal-to-serosal surfaces (Leaf and Dempsey, 1960).

The increase in sodium transport associated with exposure of the bladder to vasopressin is accompanied, as expected, by an increase in

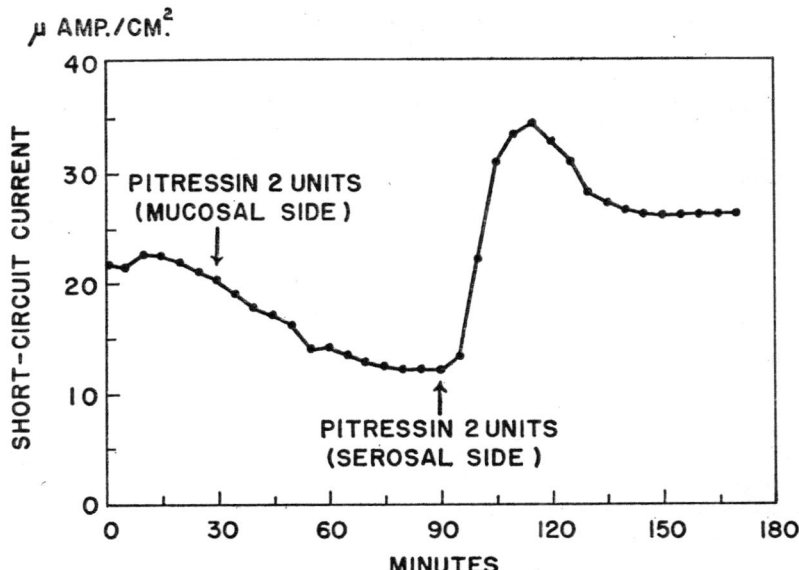

FIG. 3. Demonstration of the unilateral stimulatory effect of neurohypophysial hormone. When Pitressin was added to the Ringer's solution bathing the mucosal surface no effect on short-circuit current was noted. The same amount of hormonal preparation added to the solution bathing the serosal side resulted in a prompt and large stimulation (Leaf et al., 1958; Leaf, 1965).

metabolism (Leaf and Dempsey, 1960). Part A, Table 5, shows the increase in oxygen consumption stimulated by vasopressin. The metabolic effects are, however, not a direct effect of the hormone but only secondary to its action on sodium transport. Thus, when sodium is removed from the bathing medium so that there is no sodium to be transported, the stimulation of oxygen consumption by the hormone is abolished as shown in Part B, Table 5. In the absence of sodium, however, neurohypophysial hormones still exert their usual effects on the permeability of the bladder to water and urea (Hays and Leaf, 1962).

A recent study by Civan, Kedem and Leaf (1966) further indicates that the action of vasopressin with respect to the permeability of the bladder to sodium involves a passive process. Under conditions of zero net transport of sodium is achieved by reducing the electrochemical gradient for chloride ions across the tissue to zero, the driving force for sodium would vanish across any "passive" permeability barrier. The addition of

TABLE 5. EFFECT OF NEUROHYPOPHYSIAL HORMONES ON QO_2 OF TOAD BLADDER (LEAF, 1965).

Measurements of oxygen consumption were made for three consecutive hours on paired bladder halves in Warburg vessels by classical manometric techniques. Hormone was added at the end of one hour to one bladder half while the other served as control. Measurements were made in sodium Ringer's solution (A) and in sodium-free Ringer's solution (B) in which all the sodium had been replaced by magnesium or choline.

	Hours			Mean difference (hours 2–1)	S.E. of mean difference	P
	1	2	3			
A. Sodium Ringer's solution	(10 paired experiments)					
Control	1.20	1.22	1.06	+0.02	±0.03	0.6
With hormone*	1.23	1.72	1.76	+0.49	±0.05	<0.001
B. Sodium-free Ringer's solution	(19 paired experiments)					
Control	1.01	0.97	0.93	−0.04		
With hormone*	1.12	1.12	1.10	0		

* Hormone added at end of first hour

vasopressin in this special situation did not regularly increase the transepithelial electrical potential although it caused the usual drop in its electrical resistance. The results suggest an action of vasopressin only on permeability barriers to sodium and not directly upon the active energy-requiring transport processes affecting this ion.

Thus far, there is no direct evidence that vasopressin affects sodium transport in the mammalian nephron but the evidence with respect to an effect on the transport of urea is definite.

SITE OF ACTION OF VASOPRESSIN

Having considered the penetration of the bladder wall by water, by solutes generally, by a special group of solutes typified by urea, and by sodium ions, one may try to draw these separate phenomena together into a unified concept of the permeability properties of this tissue and of the action of vasopressin on it. Some unity can be achieved by examining the site at which the hormonal effect is mediated. Since such a site of action must coincide with a rate-limiting permeability barrier the identification of such sites will aid in the localization of the important permeability barriers within the tissue.

The most direct approach to the site of the hormonal effect on permeability was that of Peachey and Rasmussen (1961) whose work has been confirmed by Jard (personal communication). These workers exposed the mucosal surfaces of bladders to hypotonic fluid in the presence and absence of vasopressin. Following appropriate preparation they then examined the tissue histologically. In the absence of hormone there was no swelling of the epithelial layer of cells in spite of the hypotonic fluid bathing the mucosal surface. In the presence of vasopressin these cells were markedly swollen. When the same hypotonic solution was applied to the serosal surface of the tissue the cells were observed to swell promptly in the absence of the hormone. These observations, taken together with the knowledge that vasopressin induces large net transfers of water across the bladder when the mucosal bathing medium is hypotonic, clearly indicate that a permeability barrier at or near the mucosal surface normally excludes water from the cells. Neurohypophysial hormones affect this mucosal barrier to allow water to cross the tissue; during this process osmotic swelling of the epithelial layer cells occurs.

MacRobbie and Ussing (1961) came to similar conclusions from direct measurements of the thickness of the epithelial layer of frog skin. This tissue swells only when its outside surface is bathed with hypotonic fluid in the presence of vasopressin. This finding implies that a barrier to penetration by water near the outside surface of the skin had been reduced allowing net transport of water, as occurs in the toad bladder and renal tubule, with concomitant swelling of the epithelial cells.

Recently Civan and Frazier (1967) have reported another kind of observation which supports a mucosal site of action of vasopressin with respect to permeability of the bladder to ions. They impaled the mucosal cells with micropipets and measured the electrical resistance from mucosal medium to micropipet tip within the mucosal layer of cells. Simultaneously the electrical resistance across the bladder was measured. Vasopressin caused a decrease in resistance across the bladder which was entirely or mostly accounted for by the drop in resistance across the mucosal surface of the epithelial layer of cells.

Though not so direct, similar evidence may be obtained from radioisotope experiments. Table 6 (Leaf, 1965) shows the effect of vasopressin on the permeability of the bladder to labeled water (THO), urea and thiourea and to the accumulation of the isotopic species within the tissue (% labeling) in the steady state following addition of the isotopic species to the medium bathing the mucosal surface. In the case of THO and C^{14}-

TABLE 6. EFFECT OF VASOPRESSIN ON PERMEABILITY AND LABELING OF TOAD BLADDER BY THO ^{14}C-UREA, AND ^{14}C-THIOUREA ADDED TO THE MUCOSAL MEDIUM (LEAF, 1965).

	No. of paired experiments	Permeability coefficients ($K_{trans} \times 10^{-7}$ cm sec^{-1}) vasopressin		% labeling* vasopressin		Δ	S.E. of mean difference	P
		absent	present	absent	present			
THO	10	940	1600	20.8	27.2	6.4	±2.3	0.02
C^{14}-urea	8	18	329	11	38	27	±3.9	<0.001
C^{14}-thiourea	7	13	13	2.6	3.5	0.9	±0.4	0.1

* % labeling = $\dfrac{\text{average concentration in tissue water}}{\text{concentration in mucosal medium}}$ (×100).

Since vasopressin increased the transepithelial permeability coefficient, K_{trans}, and the tissue labeling for water, urea, and thiourea, its site of action must be at or near the mucosal surface of the bladder.

urea the increase in transport across the bladder is associated with an increased content of the radioactive species within the tissue. This finding is again consistent with an action of vasopressin to increase the permeability of a barrier in or near the apical surface of the mucosal layer of cells with respect to each species. By contrast, vasopressin has no significant effect on the low permeability of the bladder to thiourea and the tissue labeling was also not significantly affected by the hormone. Furthermore, the very low tissue labeling averaging 2.6 and 3.5% in seven paired experiments in the absence and the presence of vasopressin set an upper limit for tissue labeling since they include ^{14}C-thiourea adherent to the mucosal surface which was not removed by blotting, as well as molecules in transit across the tissue. This indicates that the selective barrier which effectively screens out most solute molecules must also be located very near the mucosal surface.

If the relatively simple histology of the tissue is considered, the apical surface of the mucosal cells is bounded by a unit plasma membrane and it seems likely that the hormonal effect is exerted upon this membrane. The only structure regularly present outside the unit plasma membrane is the fuzzy deposit seen by electron microscopy (Peachey and Rasmussen, 1961), but this appears to be much too porous a structure to constitute the permeability barriers we are discussing, unless in life this layer is much more homogeneous and only in the process of fixation and histological preparation becomes fibrillar and porous. In either case one is dealing with a superficial barrier at the mucosal surface of the tissue. Such a location for the major permeability barrier in these tissues is advantageous as it protects the epithelial cells from being buffeted by the vicissitudes of urinary composition with respect to tonicity, pH, ammonium ions and other noxious factors which must be excreted in the urine at concentrations which would be toxic, if not lethal, to most cells.

An interesting feature of the functional orientation of the mucosal cells in this tissue is that the response to neurohypophysial hormones occurs only when these are added to the medium bathing the serosal surface despite the effect of the hormone at the mucosal or apical surface of the cells. We have been unable to detect any hormonal effects with even very large amounts of the hormones added to the mucosal medium. This may simply mean that the polypeptide hormones cannot gain access to their site of action from the mucosal medium because of the general impermeability of the apical barrier to most solutes. The actual receptor sites for the hormones may be located at the basal surface of the mucosal layer of cells and this would be consistent with the evidence presented elsewhere that the action of vasopressin is mediated through a series of chemical events induced by the hormone in this responsive tissue which includes the synthesis of adenosine 3', 5'-phosphate.

THE COMPLEX NATURE OF THE RESPONSIVE PERMEABILITY BARRIER

Ascribing the locus of action of vasopressin with respect to its effect on water, urea and sodium transport to a site in or near the apical surface of the mucosal layer of cells does not circumvent the apparent paradox that the tissue can remain selective to solute molecules of small dimensions at a time when large channels seem necessary to accommodate the net transport of water across the tissue. This apparent difficulty is readily overcome theoretically by assuming that the permeability barrier is not a simple homogeneous structure but a complex system of at least two barriers with different properties in series (Kedem and Katchalsky, 1963). Thus a dense diffusion barrier in series with an underlying porous barrier could theoretically account for the permeability properties of the bladder. The dense barrier might screen out most solutes but allow water, urea and sodium to pass. Modification of the porosity of the deeper barrier by vasopressin could then provide the specific changes in permeability induced by the hormone.

It seemed that such a dual barrier hypothesis was likely to remain in the realm of purely speculative probability until Lichtenstein and Leaf (1965) made the observation that amphotericin B added to the mucosal medium bathing the toad bladder separates the two barriers functionally. Amphotericin B is a polyene antibiotic known to react with sterols (Kinsky, Luse and van Deenen, 1966). For this reason it is toxic to fungi but not to bacteria which do not synthesize sterols and, therefore, contain none in their cell walls. By carefully adjusting the amounts of amphotericin B in experiments with the toad bladder, it was possible to remove the selective permeability barrier functionally, leaving the second barrier relatively intact. Figure 4 (Lichtenstein and Leaf, 1965) shows that amphotericin B added to the mucosal bathing medium resulted in a stimulation of sodium transport (short-circuit current) which was not further augmented by vasopressin. By contrast net transport of water across the tissue

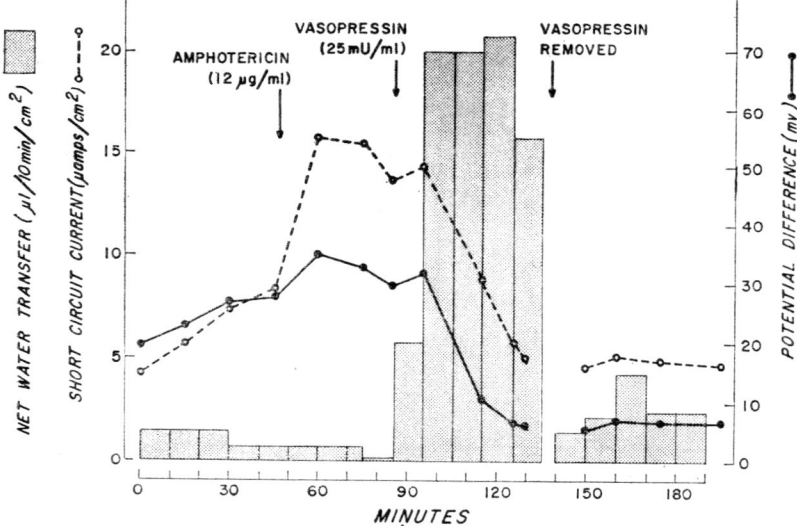

FIG. 4. Comparison of the effects of amphotericin B and vasopressin on short-circuit current, potential difference and net water movement across the toad bladder. Addition of amphotericin B to the mucosal medium produced a large increase in short-circuit current without affecting net movement of water. Subsequent addition of vasopressin failed to augment the short-circuit current, but produced its usual large effect on transport of water. When vasopressin was removed, the net transport of water was reduced. In this experiment sodium Ringer's solution was used as the serosal bathing medium and sodium Ringer's solution (diluted 1 : 4) as the mucosal bathing medium (Lichtenstein and Leaf, 1965).

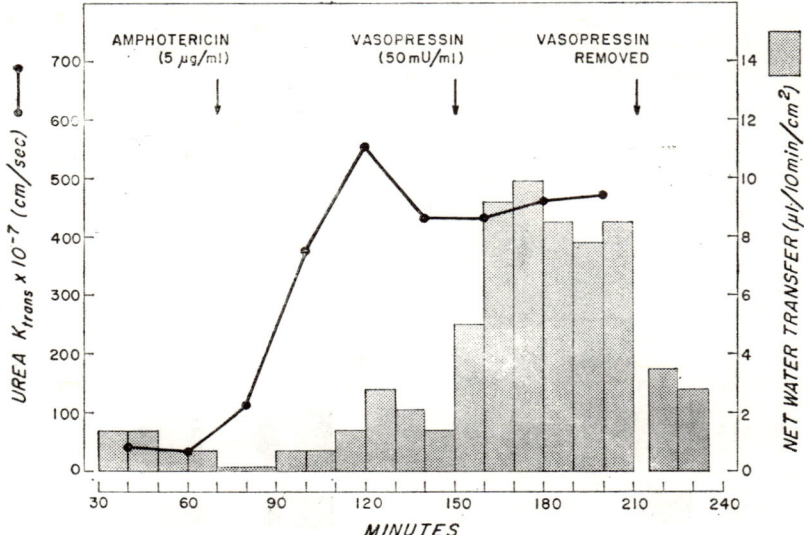

Fig. 5. Effect of amphotericin B and vasopressin on net water transfer and permeability to urea. Amphotericin B added to the mucosal bathing medium produced a large increase in the permeability of the bladder to urea and a slight increase in net water movement. Subsequently vasopressin had no further effect on the tissue permeability to urea but did cause the usual large increase in net water transfer. Removal of vasopressin reduced net water transfer to lower levels. In this experiment the initial short-circuit current was 56 μamp, the potential difference was 6 mv; the final values were 58 μamp, and 6 mv, respectively. Sodium Ringer's solution (diluted 1 : 1) on the mucosal side provided the osmotic gradient. K_{trans} = permeability coefficient (Lichtenstein and Leaf, 1965).

was not significantly affected by the concentration of amphotericin B used in this experiment but increased in typical fashion in response to vasopressin. A similar dissociation of the effects of amphotericin B and of vasopressin on the permeability of the bladder to urea and to net transfer of water could also be made, as shown in Fig. 5 (Lichtenstein and Leaf, 1965). After application of amphotericin B to the mucosal surface of the bladder the permeability of the tissue to all small solute molecules is markedly increased and cellular constituents leak out into the medium as has been shown in relation to the toxic effect of this antibiotic on molds (Kinsky, 1961a, b). Thus amphotericin functionally removes the selective permeability barrier in the bladder.

By quantitative comparisons of the changes in permeability induced by vasopressin and amphotericin B, it was possible to ascribe the hormonal effects discussed to either of the two series barriers as summarized in Fig. 6. Note that it is still necessary for the hormone to exert separate effects on each of the two hypothetical barriers.

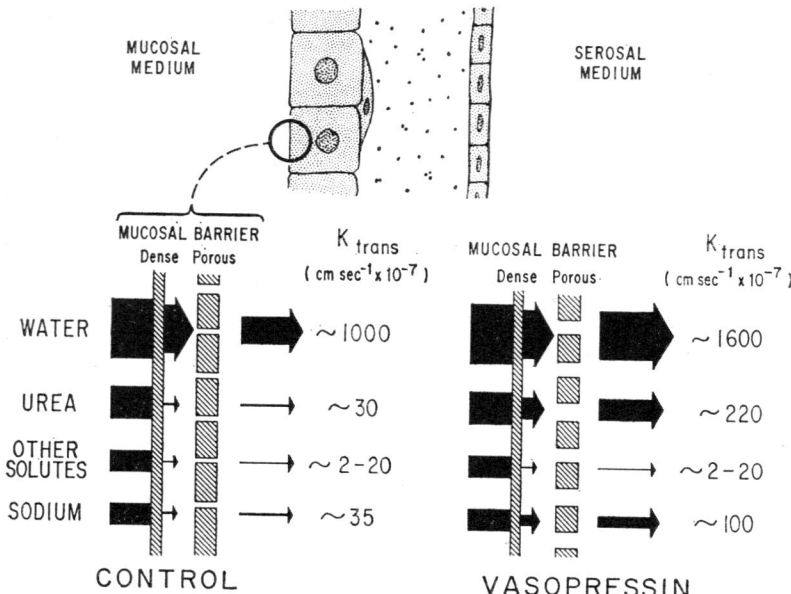

FIG. 6. Schematic representation of the mucosal permeability barrier. The urinary surface of the mucosal cells is represented as a dual barrier, a dense diffusion and a porous barrier, in series. All substances including water are retarded at the diffusion barrier. Vasopressin enhances the permeability of this tissue to urea and sodium by an effect on the dense diffusion barrier and to water by an effect on the porous barrier (Lichtenstein and Leaf, 1965).

Further investigations of the structure of cell membranes and the molecular changes induced in responsive membranes by neurohypophysial hormones will be necessary before it can be said whether it will ever be possible to account for the hormonal effects by a single action exerted at a single site.

PROPOSED MECHANISMS OF THE HORMONAL EFFECT

One attempt at a biochemical explanation for the observed effects of vasopressin on the permeability of membranes was that of Ginetzinsky and coworkers (Ginetzinsky, 1958, 1961; Ginetzinsky et al., 1960). They examined the mucopolysaccharide complexes in the intercellular cement of the basement membrane in distal portions of the nephron using histochemical techniques. They also estimated hyaluronidase activity in the urine. From their finding that the mucopolysaccharide complexes in the distal nephron disappeared and hyaluronidase activity increased in the urine during antidiuresis, they proposed that hyaluronidase was secreted by the renal epithelium in response to antidiuretic hormone. This enzyme then digested the intercellular cement and basement membrane making the renal tubule permeable to water by providing a pathway for water to move between the epithelial cells.

Dicker and Eggleton (1960) provided additional support for this hypothesis by confirming the presence of increased hyaluronidase in the urine after the injection of vasopressin in three normal subjects and in a patient with diabetes insipidus but found no hyaluronidase in the urine of two patients with nephrogenic diabetes insipidus. Thorn, Knudsen and Koefoed (1961) obtained antidiuresis in ethanol-anesthetized rats in water diuresis with bovine hyaluronidase injected in large amounts.

In spite of this supportive evidence an action of the hormone to create such pathways between cells seems unlikely to account for the very specific effects of the hormone on the transport of water and solutes. The effects of hyaluronidase injections were shown by Rosenfeld, Hirata and Brest (1963) to result from hemodynamic changes in the kidney. The assay method for hyaluronidase was criticized by Berlyne (1960) who showed that the assay was sensitive to the urinary electrolyte composition. With suitable controls for electrolyte composition, Berlyne found no relationship of urinary hyaluronidase activity and urine volume. Furthermore, bovine hyaluronidase even when added in large amounts to the medium bathing the isolated anuran bladders had no effects on the permeability of that tissue (Leaf, 1960; Bentley, 1962).

Another hypothesis was that vasopressin interacted with receptor sites in the kidney with formation of covalent bonds through thiol-disulfide exchange reactions which in turn effected the porosity of the responsive membrane (Fong et al., 1960; Rasmussen et al., 1960; Schwartz et al., 1960). The cystine in the ring structure of the hormone was thought to provide the essential disulfide group for these exchange reactions. When a synthetic polypeptide lacking a disulfide group was subsequently tested and found to be active, this hypothesis of the hormonal action was retracted (Schwartz, Rasmussen and Rudinger 1964).

A more fruitful current hypothesis of the hormonal action is that it stimulates production of adenosine 3′, 5′-phosphate (cyclic 3′, 5′-AMP) and that this compound is the intracellular mediator of the hormonal effect (Orloff and Handler, 1961, 1962). 3′, 5′-AMP appears similarly to serve as an intracellular mediator of the action of several other nonsteroidal hormones (Haynes and Berthet, 1957; Haynes, 1958; Sutherland and Rall, 1960). The major evidence in support of this hypothesis is the finding of Orloff and Handler that cyclic 3′, 5′-AMP added in high concentrations to the medium bathing the toad bladder will mimic the known actions of vasopressin on permeability of this tissue to water and to sodium. They also found that theophylline which inhibits the hydrolysis of cyclic 3′, 5′-AMP by the cyclic 3′, 5′-nucleotide phosphodiesterase has the same effect as vasopressin on the toad bladder *in vitro* and enhances the effects of cyclic 3′, 5′-AMP. Handler, Butcher, Sutherland and Orloff (1965) have shown, furthermore, that vasopressin increases the concentration of cyclic 3′, 5′-AMP in urinary bladder. This finding is in agreement with the report by Brown *et al.* (1963) that vasopressin increases the accumulation of cyclic 3′, 5′-AMP by the particulate fraction of a homogenate of dog kidney.

The evidence that cyclic 3′, 5′-AMP mimics the actions of vasopressin and that its concentration is increased in tissue exposed to vasopressin constitutes persuasive evidence that it is in fact an intermediary in the action of this hormone. Thus far known biochemical effects of cyclic 3′, 5′-AMP include activation of phosphorylase (Handler and Orloff, 1963) and of phosphofructokinase (Passonneau and Lowry, 1962; Mansour, 1963). How the activation of enzymes might be involved in the permeability changes produced by the hormone is not at present understood. The manner in which it acts to produce permeability changes is entirely unknown.

REFERENCES

BOOKS, REVIEWS, AND MONOGRAPHS

EINSTEIN, A. (1905). Über die von der molekularkinetischen Theorie der Wärme geförderte Bewegung von in ruhenden Flüssigkeiten suspendierten Teilchen. *Annalen der Physik*, **17**: 549. English trans., *Investigations on the Theory of the Brownian Movement*, pp. 9–12. Furth, R. (ed.). Methuen, London, 1926. Dover Publications, New York, 1956.

HENDERSON, L. J. (1913). *The fitness of the environment: An Inquiry into the Biological Significance of the Properties of Matter*. Macmillan, New York.

LEAF, A. (1965). Transepithelial transport and its hormonal control in the toad bladder. *Ergebn. Physiol.*, **56**: 216–263.

PAULING, L. (1960). *The Nature of the Chemical Bond*, 3rd ed., pp. 464–469. Cornell University Press, Ithaca, New York.

SOLOMON, A. K. (1960). Pores in the cell membrane. *Scient. Amer.*, **203**: 146–156.
SUTHERLAND, E. W. and RALL, T. W. (1960). The relation of adenosine-3',5'-phosphate and phosphorylase to the action of catecholamines and other hormones. *Pharmac. Rev.*, **12**: 265–299.

ORIGINAL PAPERS

ANDERSEN, B. and USSING, H. H. (1957). Solvent drag on non-electrolytes during osmotic flow through isolated toad skin and its response to antidiuretic hormone. *Acta Physiol. Scand.*, **39**: 228–239.
BENTLEY, P. J. (1962). Hyaluronidase, corticosteroids and the action of neurohypophysial hormones on the urinary bladder of the frog. *J. Endocr.*, **24**: 407–413.
BERLYNE, G. M. (1960). Urinary hyaluronidase, a method of assay and investigation of its relationship to the urinary concentrating mechanism. *Clin. Sci.*, **19**: 619–629.
BROWN, E., CLARKE, D. L., ROUX, V. and SHERMAN, G. H. (1963). The stimulation of adenosine 3', 5'-monophosphate production by antidiuretic factors. *J. Biol. Chem.*, **238**: PC 852–853.
CIVAN, M. M. and FRAZIER, H. S. (1967). Demonstration of an apical site of action of vasopressin in toad bladder epithelium. *J. Clin. Invest.*, **46**: 1045.
CIVAN, M. M., KEDEM, O. and LEAF, A. (1966). Effect of vasopressin on toad bladder under conditions of zero net sodium transport. *Am. J. Physiol.*, **211**: 569–575.
DICKER, S. E. and EGGLETON, M. G. (1960). Hyaluronidase and antidiuretic activity in urine of man. *J. Physiol., Lond.*, **154**: 378–384.
EWER, R. F. (1952). The effect of pituitrin on fluid distribution in *Bufo regularis* Reuss. *J. Exp. Biol.*, **29**: 173–177.
FONG, C. T. O., SILVER, L., CHRISTMAN, D. R. and SCHWARTZ, I. L. (1960). On the mechanism of action of the anti-diuretic hormone (vasopressin). *Proc. Natn. Acad. Sci., U.S.A.*, **46**: 1273–1277.
FRANK, H. S. (1958). Covalency in the hydrogen bond and the properties of water and ice. *Proc. Roy. Soc. Med.*, **247**: 481–492.
GINETZINSKY, A. G. (1958). Role of hyaluronidase in the reabsorption of water in renal tubules: the mechanism of action of the antidiuretic hormone. *Nature, Lond.*, **182**: 1218–1219.
GINETZINSKY, A. G. (1961). Relationship between urinary hyaluronidase and diuresis. *Nature, Lond.*, **189**: 235–236.
GINETZINSKY, A. G., KRESTINSKAYA, T. V., NATOCHIN, JU. V., SAX, M. G. and TITOVA, L. K. (1960). Evolution of the substrate acted upon by antidiuretic hormone. *Physiologia Bohemoslov.*, **9**: 166–171.
HANDLER, J. S., BUTCHER, R. W., SUTHERLAND, E. W. and ORLOFF, J. (1965). The effect of vasopressin and of theophylline on the concentration of adenosine 3',5', phosphate in the urinary bladder of the toad. *J. Biol. Chem.*, **240**: 4524–4526.
HANDLER, J. S. and ORLOFF, J. (1963). Activation of phosphorylase in toad bladder and mammalian kidney by antidiuretic hormone. *Amer. J. Physiol.*, **205**: 298–302.
HAYNES, R. C. (1958). The activation of adrenal phosphorylase by the adrenocorticotropic hormone. *J. Biol. Chem.*, **233**: 1220–1222.
HAYNES, R. C. and BERTHET, L. (1957). Studies on the mechanism of action of the adrenocorticotropic hormone. *J. Biol. Chem.*, **225**: 115–124.

HAYS, R. M. and LEAF, A. (1962). Studies on the movement of water through the isolated toad bladder and its modification by vasopressin. *J. Gen. Physiol.*, **45**: 905–919.
KEDEM, O. and KATCHALSKY, A. (1958). Thermodynamic analysis of the permeability of biological membranes to non-electrolytes. *Biochim. Biophys. Acta*, **27**: 229–246.
KEDEM, O. and KATCHALSKY, A. (1963). Permeability of composite membranes Part 3. Series array of elements. *Trans. Faraday Soc.*, **59**: 1941–1953.
KINSKY, S. C. (1961a). The effect of polyene antibiotics on permeability in Neurospora crassa. *Biochem, Biophys. Res. Commun.*, **4**: 353–357.
KINSKY, S. C. (1961b). Alterations in the permeability of Neurospora crassa due to polyene antibiotics. *J. Bacteriol.*, **82**: 889–897.
KINSKY, S. C., LUSE, S. A. and VAN DEENEN, L. L. M. (1966). Interaction of polyene antibiotics and artificial membrane systems. *Fedn Proc. Fedn Am. Socs exp. Biol.*, **25**: 1503–1510.
KOEFOED-JOHNSEN, V. and USSING, H. H. (1953). The contributions of diffusion and flow to the passage of D_2O through living membranes. *Acta Physiol. Scand.*, **28**: 60–76.
KUHN, W. and THÜRKAUF, M. (1958). Isotopentrennung beim Gefrieren von Wasser and Diffusionskonstanten von D und ^{18}O im Eis. *Helv. Chimica Acta*, **41**: 938–971.
LEAF, A. (1960). Some actions of neurohypophyseal hormones on a living membrane. *J. Gen. Physiol.*, **43**: 175–189.
LEAF, A., ANDERSON, J. and PAGE, L. B. (1958). Active sodium transport by the isolated toad bladder. *J. Gen. Physiol.*, **41**: 657–668.
LEAF, A. and DEMPSEY, E. F. (1960). Some effects of mammalian neurohypophyseal hormones on metabolism and active transport of sodium by the isolated toad bladder. *J. Biol. Chem.*, **235**: 2160–2163.
LEAF, A. and HAYS, R. M. (1962). Permeability of the isolated toad bladder to solutes and its modification by vasopressin. *J. Gen. Physiol.*, **45**: 921–932.
LICHTENSTEIN, N. S. and LEAF, A. (1965). Effect of amphotericin B on the permeability of the toad bladder. *J. Clin. Invest.*, **44**: 1328–1342.
MACROBBIE, E. A. C. and USSING, H. H. (1961). Osmotic behavior of the epithelial cells of frog skin. *Acta Physiol. Scand.*, **53**: 348–365.
MAFFLY, R. H., HAYS, R. M., LAMDIN, E. and LEAF, A. (1960). The effect of neurohypophyseal hormones on the permeability of the toad bladder to urea. *J. Clin. Invest.*, **39**: 630–641.
MANSOUR, T. E. (1963). Studies on heart phosphofructokinase: purification, inhibition and activation. *J. Biol. Chem.*, **238**: 2285–2292.
NÉMETHY, G. and SCHERAGA, H. A. (1962). Structure of water and hydrophobic bonding in proteins. I. A model for the thermodynamic properties of liquid water. *J. Chem. Phys.*, **36**: 3382–3400.
ORLOFF, J. and HANDLER, J. S. (1961). Vasopressin-like effects of adenosine 3′,5′-phosphate (cyclic 3′,5′-AMP) and theophylline in the toad bladder. *Biochem. Biophys. Res. Commun.*, **5**: 63–66.
ORLOFF, J. and HANDLER, J. S. (1962). The similarity of effects of vasopressin, adenosine-3′,5′-phosphate (cyclic AMP) and theophylline on the toad bladder. *J. Clin. Invest.*, **41**: 702–709.
PAPPENHEIMER, J. R., RENKIN, E. M. and BORRERO, L. M. (1951). Filtration, diffusion and molecular sieving through peripheral capillary membranes. *Amer. J. Physiol.*, **167**: 13–46.
PASSONNEAU, J. V., and LOWRY, O. H. (1962). Phosphofructokinase and the Pasteur effect. *Biochem. Biophys. Res. Commun.*, **7**: 10–15.

PEACHEY, L. D. and RASMUSSEN, H. (1961). Structure of the toad's urinary bladder as related to its physiology. *J. Biophys. Biochem. Cytol.*, **10**: 529–553.

RASMUSSEN, H., SCHWARTZ, I. L., SCHOESSLER, M. A. and HOCHSTER, G. (1960). Studies on the mechanism of action of vasopressin. *Proc. Nat. Acad. Sci., U.S.A.*, **46**: 1278–1287.

ROBBINS, E. and MAURO, A. (1960). Experimental study of the independence of diffusion and hydrodynamic permeability coefficients in collodion membranes. *J. Gen. Physiol.*, **43**: 523–532.

ROSENFELD, J. B., HIRATA, K. and BREST, A. (1963). The effect of hyaluronidase on the renal concentrating mechanism in the dog. *Amer. J. Med. Sci.*, **245**: 760.

SCHWARTZ, I. L., RASMUSSEN, H. and RUDINGER, J. (1964). Activity of neurohypophysial hormone analogues lacking a disulfide bridge. *Proc. Nat. Acad. Sci., U.S.A.*, **52**: 1044–1045.

SCHWARTZ, I. L., RASMUSSEN, H., SCHOESSLER, M. A., SILVER, L. and FONG, C. T. O. (1960). Relation of chemical attachment to physiological action of vasopressin. *Proc. Nat. Acad. Sci., U.S.A.*, **46**: 1288–1298.

SIDEL, V. W. and HOFFMAN, J. F. (1963). Apparent "solvent-drag" across a liquid membrane. *Biophysical Society Abstracts, Chicago Mtg.*

STAVERMAN, A. J. (1951). The theory of measurement of osmotic pressure. *Rec. Trav. chim. Pays-Bas Belg.*, **70**: 344–352.

THORN, N. A., KNUDSEN, P. J., and KOEFOED, J. (1961). Antidiuretic effect of large doses of bovine testicular hyaluronidase in rats. *Acta Endocr., Copnh.*, **38**: 571–576.

WANG, J. W., ROBINSON, C. V. and EDELMAN, I. S. (1953). Self-diffusion and structure of liquid water. III. Measurements of the self-diffusion of liquid water with H^2, H^3 and O^{18} as tracers. *J. Amer. Chem. Soc.*, **75**: 466–470.

CHAPTER 11

FATE OF THE NEUROHYPOPHYSIAL HORMONES*

Henry D. Lauson

*Department of Physiology,
Albert Einstein College of Medicine of Yeshiva University,
New York, New York, U.S.A.*

It is convenient to describe the irreversible removal of vasopressin and oxytocin from the blood in terms of the clearance concept. The quantity removed per minute at a specific site is a direct function of the concentration of the hormone in the plasma and, for a first approximation, may be taken to be simply proportional to the plasma concentration over a given limited range. The total (or organ) irreversible removal rate (microunits/min) divided by the arterial plasma concentration (microunits/ml) is the total (or organ) plasma clearance (ml/min). In the steady state, the quantity of hormone removed by an organ per unit time is the product of the plasma flow through the organ and the quantity removed from each unit volume of perfusing plasma (Fick principle). Clearance is also the ratio of this product to the concentration in the incoming plasma—that is, plasma flow multiplied by extraction ratio. The total plasma clearance is the sum of all organ clearances.

CLEARANCE IN THE STEADY STATE

Under steady-state conditions, in which the plasma concentration of the hormone is unchanging, the rate of irreversible removal is equal to the rate of its secretion (or, during suppression of secretion, to the rate of a constant intravenous infusion of exogenous hormone). Total clearance

---

* Investigations by the author and his associates cited in this chapter were supported in part by a grant (AM-01588) from the National Institute of Arthritis and Metabolic Diseases, National Institutes of Health, United States Public Health Service.

is equal to the rate of secretion (or infusion) divided by the arterial plasma concentration. No assumptions are needed concerning binding to plasma or tissue proteins, diffusion into extravascular fluids, or uniformity of concentration in these fluids.

The steady state method has been used in only a few studies of the total clearance of exogenous vasopressin in rats (Ginsburg, 1957; Sawyer, 1963; Czaczkes and Kleeman, 1964) and in dogs (Lauson and Bocanegra, 1961; Share, 1962; Czaczkes and Kleeman, 1964). Clearance of exogenous oxytocin has been measured in this way apparently only in the human female late in pregnancy and in the postpartum period (González-Panizza *et al.*, 1961). The method has not yet been applied to estimation of total clearance of endogenous neurohypophysial hormones, although this seems theoretically possible. However, the steady-state clearance of endogenous vasopressin in the dog has been measured in one organ, the liver, as the product of the hepatic plasma flow and the arterial-hepatic venous difference of concentration of vasopressin in the plasma (Usami and Chien, 1963).

Measurement of the total clearance of exogenous hormone requires constant intravenous infusion during a long enough interval to assure stabilization of the plasma concentration. Concurrent endogenous secretion would lead to under-estimation of the true clearance. Ways of minimizing this error are (a) to infuse the peptide at very high rates, (b) to suppress endogenous secretion by overhydration, ethanol administration or both, or (c) to use an animal or patient with severe diabetes insipidus as the subject.

TOTAL CLEARANCE IN THE TRANSIENT STATE

In most investigations the clearances of vasopressin and oxytocin have been estimated from analysis of the curve of disappearance of the peptide from the plasma following a single intravenous injection. Interpretation is much more difficult than in the case of steady-state analysis.

The transient approach was examined in some detail in a recent review (Lauson, 1967), and it was concluded that at present a two-compartment model is needed "in which (a) total clearance represents the rate constant of the process of irreversible removal from the plasma and in which (b) some, most or all of the hormone is free to diffuse (reversibly) out of the plasma into the interstitial fluid at least." Disappearance of the hormone from the plasma in the first few minutes after intravenous injection will often seem to follow a single exponential course even though both processes occur simultaneously. Total (irreversible) clearance, calculated as the product of the slope and the apparent volume of distribution, will be erroneously large because of the outward diffusion component. The magnitude of the error is inversely related to the magnitude of the clearance. In the intact rat, in which clearances of vasopressin and oxytocin are relatively large (Ginsburg and Heller, 1953; Ginsburg and Smith, 1959), the disappearance from plasma in the early minutes is predominantly due to irreversible clearance; net outward diffusion is severely curtailed. However, in the nephrectomized rat with complete exclusion of the splanchnic circulation, in which irreversible clearance is essentially zero, the early disappearance of oxytocin is entirely due to (reversible) diffusion out of the plasma (Ginsburg and Smith, 1959). Yet, in both cases, the plasma concentration of oxytocin appears to decline semilogarithmically in the first minutes after injection, the zero-time intercepts are approximately equal to the quotient of the injected dose divided by the plasma volume, and the slopes differ by less than a ratio of 2 to 1.

Nevertheless, the single injection method seems to be appropriate for the study of the kinetics of removal of oxytocin from the plasma, because in its two most studied physiological roles—expulsion of the fetus and ejection of milk (see reviews by Fitzpatrick and Walmsley, 1965; Folley and Knaggs, 1965a; Fitzpatrick, 1966; Benson and Fitzpatrick, 1966)—oxytocin appears to be secreted in "slugs" or "spurts" (Lauson, 1960; Fitzpatrick, 1961), which are reasonably well simulated by single injections. But in this "slope analysis", the relative contributions of diffusion and irreversible clearance cannot be readily distinguished. For the estimation of the plasma clearance of vasopressin, the steady-state method is the more appropriate one, because normally this hormone is secreted continuously to maintain relatively steady physiological antidiuresis.

Because most of the available data on the removal of vasopressin and oxytocin from the plasma were obtained by means of the single injection method, the question of possible binding to plasma proteins must be considered.

PHYSICAL STATE OF VASOPRESSIN AND OXYTOCIN IN THE BLOOD

BINDING BY ERYTHROCYTES

There is no evidence to suggest that vasopressin or oxytocin is carried in or on red blood cells. Studies in the rat (Heller and Zaidi, 1957), dog (Bocanegra and Lauson, 1961) and man (Ginsburg, unpublished experiments, cited by Heller and Ginsburg, 1966) show that vasopressin added to whole blood can be entirely accounted for in assays of the plasma. The same is true for endogenous vasopressin in blood from dogs after hemorrhage (Bocanegra and Lauson, 1961) and for oxytocin added to the blood of rats (Ginsburg and Smith, 1959) and of man and sheep (Fitzpatrick, 1961).

BINDING BY PROTEINS IN THE PLASMA

It is possible that vasopressin and oxytocin are secreted into the blood attached to or accompanied by the neurohypophysial carrier protein, neurophysin, but according to Ginsburg and Ireland (1964) and Heller and Ginsburg (1966), it is unlikely that more than a very small fraction of the hormone could remain bound to neurophysin in the circulating blood.

Estimates of the extent to which the peptides are bound to plasma proteins vary widely within and among species (Lauson, 1967). There seems to be general agreement that such binding is probably relatively weak and rapidly reversible. This is suggested by the fact that under some conditions the extraction of vasopressin from plasma passing through the liver and kidneys of rats must approach 100% (Ginsburg and Heller, 1953; Ginsburg, 1957; Sawyer, 1963). In this circumstance, practically all of the vasopressin, protein-bound as well as free, would have to cross the endothelium of the capillaries during a single passage of blood through these organs.

Data on the binding of vasopressin by serum or plasma proteins are most discordant in the case of the rat. Thorn and Silver (1957) found that virtually all of the endogenous vasopressin (present in very high concentrations) in serum migrated with β-globulins during starch electrophoresis (4° C and pH 8.6) and was also retained in the impermeate during ultrafiltration of the serum through collodion. Thorn (1959a) then showed that an undetermined fraction of arginine vasopressin added to rat serum migrated "in a fairly broad zone in the globulin region" during similar starch electrophoresis. Smith and Thorn (1965), using Sephadex gel filtration, found that a very large fraction of exogenous arginine vasopressin was bound to the proteins of rat plasma; addition of calcium ions in high concentration abolished the binding. However, Czaczkes and Kleeman (1964) were unable, by dialysis and ultrafiltration through cellophane, to demonstrate any binding of the endogenous vasopressin present in physiological concentrations in rat serum. Moreover, endogenous vasopressin in plasma of hemorrhaged rats was mostly ultrafilterable (Beuzeville and Lauson, 1967).

In cats, the presence of endogenous and exogenous vasopressin in thoracic duct lymph in relatively high lymph/plasma concentration ratios, despite the considerable capacity of lymph to inactivate *in vitro*, suggests that the fraction of the hormone bound to plasma proteins is not very large (Tata et al., 1965).

In dogs, Brook and Share (1966) definitively established that all of the endogenous vasopressin in plasma circulates in the free peptide form. Bocanegra and Lauson (1961) found that about three-fourths of endogenous vasopressin in plasma from hemorrhaged dogs was ultrafilterable through cellophane. Physiological amounts of endogenous vasopressin are entirely free in dog serum according to Czaczkes and Kleeman (1964).

Exogenous vasopressin (Parke-Davis Pituitrin) dialyzed more slowly from human plasma than from 0.9% sodium chloride solution (unpublished observations of Heller and Lederis, cited by Heller, 1957). Endogenous vasopressin in plasma from children with nephrogenic diabetes insipidus is essentially all ultrafilterable (Holliday et al., 1963). Endogenous vasopressin in physiological concentrations in plasma of normal men is entirely free (Czaczkes et al., 1964).

Relatively few data are available on the binding of oxytocin to plasma proteins. Heller (1957) cited the earlier studies which suggested that the ultrafilterability of oxytocin (as well as vasopressin) was decreased when posterior pituitary extracts were mixed with blood or plasma. In the experiment of Heller and Lederis (unpublished observations) illustrated in fig. 1 of Heller (1957), synthetic oxytocin in one volume of either human plasma or buffer solution was dialyzed to equilibrium against four volumes of the buffer; approximately 25% of the original oxytocin remained bound to plasma proteins at equilibrium. Thorn (1959a) added synthetic oxytocin to rat serum; an undetermined fraction migrated with a broad zone of globulins during starch electrophoresis (4° C, pH 8.6). Oxytocin in nephrectomized rats without splanchnic circulation distributes into a volume equivalent to 431 ml/kg (Ginsburg and Smith, 1959). Radioactive oxytocin penetrates deeply into many body tissues (Aroskar et al. 1964).

In brief, the extent to which endogenous and exogenous vasopressin and oxytocin are bound to plasma proteins in various mammals is uncertain. The weight of the evidence suggests that relatively large fractions circulate in the free peptide form. Even if binding should be extensive, it seems likely that it is sufficiently weak and reversible to affect the kinetics of removal of the hormones from the plasma in only a minor way.

TOTAL CLEARANCE OF VASOPRESSIN AND OXYTOCIN

STEADY-STATE DATA

Ginsburg (1957) found that the total plasma clearance of Pitressin (probably a mixture of arginine and lysine vasopressins) averaged 34 ml/min kg in conscious hydrated rats in which constant intravenous infusion produced high plasma concentrations. This is equivalent to 100% of the plasma volume per minute. Sawyer (1963) reported values of 52 ml/min kg (1.5 times plasma volume per minute) for arginine vasopressin and 21 ml/min kg for lysine vasopressin in rats with high plasma concentrations. Czaczkes and Kleeman (1964) infused four overhydrated, ethanol-anesthetized rats with arginine vasopressin at physiological rates. With a steady-state plasma concentration of 2 microunits/ml, the total clearance averaged only 8.5 ml/min kg. It is therefore possible that the clearance of vasopressin is a function of its concentration in plasma.

In non-overhydrated dogs anesthetized with pentobarbital, the total clearance of arginine vasopressin averaged about 9–11 ml/min kg when plasma concentrations were high (Lauson and Bocanegra, 1961; Share, 1962; Lauson *et al.*, 1965). With physiological plasma concentrations of 4 and 8 microunits/ml in two experiments on one dog, Czaczkes and Kleeman (1964) found total clearances of arginine vasopressin to be only 3.7 ml/min kg; steady-state plasma concentrations of 19 and 40 microunits/ml were associated with clearances of 5.8 and 5.3 ml/min kg.

Blood concentrations of oxytocin were measured by González-Panizza *et al.* (1961) in women in late pregnancy or in the postpartum period during constant intravenous "macroinfusions". In one woman with a dead fetus, given 16,000,000 microunits/min for 30 min, the total plasma clearance was about 740 ml/min. The time from the beginning of the infusion at which the concentration reached one-half the steady-state value was 6.5 min; the half-time of the disappearance of the hormone after cessation of the infusion was only 2.7 min. As was suggested by the authors, this large difference between these two half-times is compatible with diffusion of oxytocin out of the plasma through a perceptible barrier during the infusion. Upon cessation of the infusion, diffusional re-entry must have occurred, but in the face of the large clearance there was probably too little time for it to have appreciably retarded the decrease in concentration. The slope of the disappearance curve through the fifth post-infusion minute was ln $2/2.7$ min, or 0.256 min^{-1}; its dimensions are clearance/apparent volume of distribution (Lauson, 1960). Dividing the steady-state clearance of 740 ml/min by 0.256 min^{-1} yields an estimate of the apparent volume of distribution of 2900 ml, which is close to the value for plasma volume in an adult woman. (This situation resembles that in dogs infused with vasopressin in which apparent volume of distribution, calculated in this way, averaged only 1.14 times the plasma volume (Lauson and Bocanegra, 1961)). The rate constant of the exponentially increasing plasma concentration during the infusion of oxytocin is equivalent to ln 2/6.5 min, or 0.106 min^{-1}. Dividing this into the steady-state clearance, yields an estimate of the apparent volume of distribution of 7000 ml, which is equivalent to a major fraction of the extra-cellular fluid volume. These considerations suggest that extensive diffusion occurred.

In two women studied in the postpartum period by this group infusions of 8,000,000 microunits/min were given. Total plasma clearances were approximately 1700 and 1850 ml/min. Post-infusion half-lives were 4.0 and 2.5 min, and the apparent volumes of distribution (calculated from these half-lives) were about 9900 and 6650 ml. If, in these non-pregnant women, only the liver and kidneys (and mammary glands) cleared oxytocin irreversibly from the plasma, the extraction ratios in these organs must have been very large. In a pregnant woman near term, who also received 8,000,000 microunits/min, the clearance was 1333 ml/min, the post-infusion half-life was 1.8 min, and the apparent volume of distribution was about 3450 ml. In a second pregnant woman, the same infusion rate produced a steady-state plasma concentration of only about 1670 microunits/ml, indicating a total plasma clearance of about 4800 ml/min. This is more than an average resting cardiac output of plasma per minute; possibly the plasma oxytocinase was unusually potent in this woman.

DATA BASED ON SINGLE INJECTIONS

In rats, the disappearance of antidiuretic activity of vasopressin from the plasma follows a rapid semilogarithmic course after single injections, and the apparent volume of distribution is roughly equal to the plasma volume (see reviews by Heller and Ginsburg (1966) and Lauson (1967)). The clearance can therefore be characterized reasonably well in terms of the half-life in plasma. The early values of about 0.86 min (Ginsburg and Heller, 1953, Ginsburg, 1954) were obtained in ether-anesthetized rats injected with Pitressin in doses of 1,000,000 microunits/kg. A half-life of 1.5 min can be calculated from the data of Crawford and Pinkham (1954) who used the same dosage of Pitressin. Unpublished observations of Ginsburg (1960) (cited by Heller and Ginsburg, 1966) showed a half-life of 1.1 min for arginine vasopressin and 1.7 min for lysine vasopressin. In the control rats of Smith and Thorn (1965) the half-life of arginine vasopressin was 1.1 min. All of these results were obtained with injections of very large doses. Czaczkes and Kleeman (1964) injected much smaller amounts into overhydrated, ethanol-anesthetized rats. As the plasma concentration of arginine vasopressin decreased from 50 to 8 to 1.6 microunits/ml, the half-life increased from 1.5 to 1.9 to 3.5 min, suggesting that clearance is some direct function of plasma concentration.

Oxytocin clearance in rats after single injections of 2,000,000 microunits/kg was studied by Ginsburg and Smith (1959). The half-lives in intact males, females in estrus, pregnant females and lactating females were 1.65, 1.73, 2.01 and 1.19 min, respectively. The half-lives of oxytocin and two of its analogues, [3-phenylalanine]-oxytocin and [3-valine]-oxytocin, measured under similar conditions in intact males by Smith and Ginsburg (1961), were 1.75, 1.44 and 3.86 min, respectively. In lactating females, the corresponding values were 1.26, 1.25 and 3.70 min.

In rabbits, Chaudhury and Walker (1959) found a half-life of 3.3 min for oxytocin after injection of 2,000,000 microunits/kg. Their more limited data on vasopressin (Pitressin) are better fitted with a double exponential curve; the half-life of the second component is about 4 min.

Half-lives of about 5 min can be calculated for the pressor and oxytocic activities in the blood of decapitated cats injected intravenously with large doses of beef posterior pituitary extract (Jones and Schlapp, 1936).

The half-life of arginine vasopressin in the plasma of anesthetized dogs following cessation of constant infusions averaged 5.4 and 4.9 min, respectively, in the studies of Lauson and Bocanegra (1961) and of Share (1962). The half-life after single injections was 6.8 min in Share's experiments. Silver et al. (1961) found a half-life of 5.0 min for tritiated arginine vasopressin. Initial plasma concentrations in these studies were well above the physiological range. With initial plasma concentrations of 4–6 microunits/ml, the half-life of exogenous arginine vasopressin and of endogenous antidiuretic hormone in over-hydrated, conscious dogs was 7.5 min (Czaczkes and Kleeman, 1964).

In one conscious, lactating goat, Folley and Knaggs (1965b) followed the semilogarithmic decrease in plasma oxytocin concentration at close intervals for 7 min after a single intravenous injection of oxytocin. The half-life was 1.37 min, and the apparent volume of distribution was 87 ml/kg, which is roughly 1.6 times the plasma volume.

Knaggs (1967) injected 1,000,000 microunits intravenously into a conscious 102 kg sow which had recently lost a premature litter. The decrease of plasma concentration followed a semi-logarithmic course during the 4 min in which concentrations were measurable. The half-life was only 0.62 min, the zero-time intercept was 437 microunits/ml, and the apparent volume of distribution was 2290 ml, or 22.4 ml/kg, a value somewhat less than the expected plasma volume. Total clearance, calculated from this volume and the slope, was 25 ml/min kg, of which diffusional loss must have represented a substantial fraction.

The disappearance of vasopressin from the plasma of two normal men (70, 71 kg) who were injected intravenously on two occasions each with 4 units of Pitressin or Tonephin (Hoechst) (*ca.* 57,000 microunits/kg) followed a double exponential course (Schröder and Rott, 1959). The half-life of the second component (observed during the 10–30 min interval after the injection) was about 7.7 min. The apparent volume of distribution, calculated as dose divided by the zero-time intercept of the second component, was 135 ml/kg. Total plasma clearance, estimated as the product of the slope and volume of distribution, was about 850 ml/min, or 12 ml/min kg. In 3 human subjects studied by Silver *et al.* (1961), the half-life during the first 10–12 min after intravenous injection of very large doses of tritiated arginine vasopressin ranged from 2.3–5.5 (average, 3.9) min. This short half-life is similar to that observed by Schröder and Rott (1959) in the corresponding period. These data are strikingly different from those obtained by Czaczkes *et al.* (1964) who injected physiological doses of arginine-vasopressin into overhydrated normal men. With initial plasma concentrations of 5.9–14.5 microunits/ml, the half-life of the disappearance curve (which was semilogarithmic throughout the 40–50 min period of observation) averaged 21 min; the apparent volume of distribution (27 ml/kg) was less than plasma volume. These authors also showed that 72 hr of dehydration shortened the half-life to 10 min, while 72 hr of overhydration prolonged it to 42 min.

RENAL, HEPATIC AND MAMMARY CLEARANCE OF VASOPRESSIN AND OXYTOCIN

That the kidneys clear vasopressin from the blood has been known since Dale (1909) first showed that pressor material was excreted after injection of posterior pituitary extracts. Excretion of exogenous antidiuretic material was first demonstrated by Heller and Urban (1935) and of oxytocic material by Larson (1935). The possible participation of other organs in the clearance process was suggested by the fact that homogenates of various tissues, in addition to those of kidneys, could inactivate vasopressin and oxytocin (Heller and Urban, 1935; Jones and

Schlapp, 1936; Larson, 1938, 1939). Subsequent studies in the whole animal, isolated perfused organs and isolated tissues indicate that the kidneys and liver are the only organs which irreversibly remove the neurohypophysial hormones from the blood to any measurable extent; however, in the lactating female rat the mammary glands also participate significantly.

STUDIES IN THE WHOLE ANIMAL

Ginsburg and Heller (1953) observed a decrease in the rate of disappearance of intravenously injected Pitressin (a) in nephrectomized rats, (b) in rats with most of the splanchnic circulation excluded, and (c) in rats with a combination of both. The kidneys accounted for something over half and the liver for the balance of the total clearance. In Crawford and Pinkham's experiments (1954), the renal fraction was about two-thirds of the total clearance of Pitressin in the rats which were injected with the same dose as was used by Ginsburg and Heller (1953). Ether anesthesia was used in both of these studies, and plasma concentrations of Pitressin were very high. The renal and hepatic extraction ratios must have been close to 100%. Much smaller extraction ratios (hepatic, about 10%; renal, 24%) were found in overhydrated, ethanol-anesthetized rats with physiological plasma concentrations of arginine vasopressin (Beuzeville and Lauson, 1964, 1966). From these extraction ratios and estimates of the organ blood flows (which were relatively large under these conditions), renal and hepatic fractions were estimated to represent 60 and 40% of the total vasopressin clearance, respectively (Lauson, 1967).

Oxytocin clearance by the kidneys and liver (and mammary glands in the lactating female) was studied in rats by Ginsburg and Smith (1959). In nephrectomized males with the splanchnic circulation completely excluded, total (irreversible) clearance was essentially zero, but the rapid decline of plasma concentration during the first 7 min after injection of the oxytocin revealed the importance of diffusion out of the plasma in the interpretation of curves of disappearance of these peptides. As in the case of vasopressin, something over half of the total clearance could be attributed to renal clearance. In the intact lactating female rat, total clearance was some 40% greater than in the estrous female or intact male. After nephrectomy plus complete exclusion of the splanchnic circulation in lactating rats, the slope of the disappearance curve was still about one-third that in the intact lactating rat, and the plasma continued to be cleared of oxytocin by a single exponential process until the concentration could no longer be measured. For the most part, qualitatively similar results were obtained by Smith and Ginsburg (1961) with the analogues, [3-

phenylalanine]-oxytocin and [3-valine]-oxytocin. The half-lives of [3-phenylalanine]-oxytocin were indistinguishable from those of oxytocin in lactating females, intact males, males without splanchnic circulation, nephrectomized males and males deprived of both kidneys and splanchnic circulation. The corresponding half-lives for [3-valine]-oxytocin were 2–3 times longer. In the males without kidneys and splanchnic circulation the very slow disappearance of [3-valine]-oxytocin suggested the existence of a "permeability barrier".

In the rabbit, the half-life of oxytocin in the circulation after large single injections was prolonged from a control value of 3.3 min to 7.9 min after nephrectomy and to 5.5 min after exclusion of the splanchnic circulation (Chaudhury and Walker, 1959).

In overhydrated, conscious dogs, the hepatic extraction ratio for vasopressin is so small that Mathé and Altman (1954) were unable to show any differences in the antidiuretic response to physiological doses of Pitressin when these were alternately infused into a peripheral vein and into a catheter previously inserted into a splenic vein. Using the same approach, Lauson et al. (1965) re-investigated the problem more extensively and demonstrated that the extraction ratio is about 12%. In analogous experiments they found that the renal extraction was about 25%. From these extraction ratios and plasma flow data, it was estimated that the hepatic and renal clearances represented about one-third and two-thirds, respectively, of the total clearance. Usami and Chien (1963) provided clear proof in anesthetized, non-overhydrated dogs that the liver clears endogenous vasopressin. The extraction ratio remained constant at about 21–24% as graded hemorrhage progressively reduced the liver blood flow. These data suggest that in the dog the hepatic extraction ratio may not be able to increase much above 25%, whereas in the rat it apparently can approach 100% (Ginsburg and Heller, 1953).

In lactating sheep, Manunta and Marongiu (1961) injected oxytocin alternately into a peripheral vein and into the portal vein (via a previously inserted catheter) while continuously recording mammary duct pressure. The much smaller pressure response to the intraportal injection suggests that a large fraction of the hormone had been removed in its first passage through the liver.

EXCRETION IN THE URINE

A major fraction of endogenous vasopressin appears to be bound to large molecules in the urine of kangaroo rats (Ames and van Dyke, 1950), rats (Gilman and Goodman, 1937; Ames and van Dyke, 1950; Thorn, 1959b), dogs (Ames et al., 1950) and man (Bercu et al., 1950). The nature and source of the macromolecules is unknown. The fact that high recoveries of the total antidiuretic activity in urine are possible with the zinc ferrocyanide method of Noble *et al.* (1939) suggests that both free and bound vasopressin are precipitated in this procedure. The endogenous antidiuretic material in human urine is identical with arginine vasopressin on paper chromatography (Mayer, 1960) and paper electrophoresis (Kuroda, 1963). In rat urine, Thorn (1959b) showed that the activity was destroyed by trypsin and chymotrypsin but not by carboxypeptidase; this is the pattern exhibited by vasopressin. Friedberg and Vorherr (1960) inactivated urinary antidiuretic substance with plasma from pregnant women.

The oxytocic substance in the urine of rats was not dialyzable in the studies of Aujard *et al.* (1955), but the substance was not definitely identified as oxytocin. In the recent important study of Aroskar *et al.* (1964), 3 radioactive products were found on paper chromatograms of urine excreted by rats after intravenous injection of oxytocin labeled with tritium in the leucine residue. One was identified as probably unchanged oxytocin. This biologically active oxytocin accounted for two-thirds of the excreted radioactivity and represented 12% of the original 15,000,000 microunit dose per rat. The other two radioactive urinary substances, not further characterized in this study, were assumed to be metabolic products of oxytocin which had retained the label.

The urinary clearance of Pitressin in conscious, overhydrated rats represented 21% of the concurrent total clearance (constant infusion method) and was 1.24 times as large as the inulin clearance (Ginsburg, 1957). Sawyer (1963) showed that the urinary clearances of lysine and arginine vasopressins were similar in rats even though the total clearance of the latter was 2.5 times as large as that of lysine vasopressin. Thus, the urinary clearances of lysine vasopressin and of arginine vasopressin represented 27 and 12% of the respective total clearances. The ratios of these urinary clearances to the concurrent inulin clearances were 0.75 and 0.79, respectively. Lauson *et al.* (1965) reported that the urinary clearance of arginine vasopressin in anesthetized dogs was roughly equal to the glomerular filtration rate and, furthermore, could account for about all of the vasopressin extracted from the plasma flowing through the kidneys. Towbin and Ferrell (1963) found in stop-flow studies in dogs that tritiated arginine vasopressin was excreted by glomerular filtration alone, but the ratio of vasopressin clearance/glomerular filtration rate averaged only 0.6 (range, 0.2–0.8), suggesting variable binding to plasma proteins. Plasma concentrations in all of these urinary clearance studies were unphysiologically high.

There have been no comparable studies on the urinary clearance of oxytocin.

Data on the fraction of injected vasopressin excreted into the urine were recently reviewed (Lauson, 1967). This fraction, which is roughly equivalent to the ratio of urinary clearance to total clearance, ranged from about 5–30%. Among these reports, two are especially interesting. Smith and Thorn (1965) showed that acutely induced hypercalcemia in rats increased the fraction of arginine vasopressin excreted from a control value of 7% to 24% of the injected dose. Dicker and Eggleton (1960) compared the urinary excretion of intramuscularly injected lysine-vasopressin in 2 patients with nephrogenic diabetes insipidus with that in control subjects. The 2 patients excreted 47 and 79% of the dose; the controls excreted 5–11%. Thus a correlation was established between the inability of the kidneys to respond to the hormone and a possible inability of the kidneys to inactivate it.

Little has been published on the urinary excretion of oxytocin. Larson (1939) reported that anesthetized cats and dogs excreted about 24–28% of the oxytocic content of a large dose of posterior pituitary extract. In one non-pregnant woman, given oxytocin intravenously at the rate of 8,000,000 microunits/min for 27 min, urinary excretion of oxytocin increased to a rate of about 1,050,000 microunits/min during the last 7 min of the infusion; urinary clearance was therefore about 13% of the total clearance (González-Panizza et al., 1961). If the total clearance had been similar to that in the two postpartum women studied by this group (1700–1850 ml/min), this urinary clearance would have been of the order of 230 ml/min.

In the absence of data on simultaneously measured urinary excretion and plasma concentration of endogenous vasopressin in man, separate selected data from the literature were used to make an estimate of roughly 4–10 ml/min for the urinary clearance (Lauson, 1967). This is equivalent to about 3–8% of the glomerular filtration rate. These estimates are consistent with a total endogenous vasopressin clearance of about 150 ml/min for physiological conditions in normal man (Czaczkes et al., 1964).

STUDIES IN ISOLATED ORGANS

The first study of vasopressin clearance in an isolated perfused organ was that of Eser and Tüzünkam (1950) who found that vasopressin recirculating through a guinea pig liver in Tyrode's solution for three hours was almost completely inactivated. Little et al. (1966) studied the clearance of arginine vasopressin in blood-perfused isolated rat livers.

In single passage experiments, the extraction ratio increased from 24% at low plasma concentrations to 63% at very high concentrations. When vasopressin was allowed to recirculate, the disappearance followed an approximately semilogarithmic course (while the plasma concentration exceeded 100 microunits/ml). Non-viable livers (perfused with cyanide or left either unperfused or unoxygenated for 1–2 hr) extracted vasopressin as effectively as did normal livers. In the classical heart–lung–kidney experiments of Starling and Verney (1925) and Verney (1926), it is likely that the kidney inactivated antidiuretic hormone (Lauson, 1967).

STUDIES IN ISOLATED TISSUES

Heller and Zaidi (1957) were able to extract less than 0.2% of an injected dose of Pitressin from kidneys of rats removed 3 min after the injection. They estimated that during this time 25% of the dose should have been cleared by the kidneys; nearly all of this therefore must have been rapidly inactivated. Smith and Sachs (1961) and Smith (1962) emphasized the importance of studying inactivation in slices under conditions in which inactivating enzymes are not released into the medium; kidney slices under such conditions unquestionably convert vasopressin into inactive molecules. Slices from the papillary zone are most effective (Thorn and Willumsen, 1963a). Smith (1962, 1963) found that hyaluronidase increased and calcium decreased the rate of inactivation (the latter was also demonstrated by Thorn and Willumsen, 1963b); these effects were attributed to changes in cell permeability to vasopressin. The rate of inactivation of vasopressin in kidney slices was not affected by addition of dinitrophenol, diisopropyl-phosphofluoridate, trypsin inhibitor, ethylenediamine tetraacetate and phosphate, but oxytocin in excess amounts and p-chloromercuribenzoate decreased the rate (Smith and Sachs, 1961). When glomeruli are separated from the tubular elements in rat kidney homogenates, only the latter are able to inactivate vasopressin (Heller and Zaidi, 1957). Glomerular elements from rabbit kidneys were less effective in destroying oxytocin than were the tubular elements (Chaudhury and Walker, 1959).

A partially purified fraction of the supernatant fluid separated from kidney homogenates apparently is capable of reducing the S–S bond of vasopressin (Dicker and Greenbaum, 1958), and may also contain enzymes which attack the three amide groups on the molecule (Dicker, 1960). In the rat kidney, the supernatant was the most effective of the subcellular fractions in inactivating vasopressin (Dicker and Greenbaum, 1956), but in the rabbit kidney, the mitochondrial fraction was most active in destroying oxytocin (Chaudhury and Walker, 1959).

A possible early step in the *inactivation* of vasopressin by the kidney may involve the same kind of disulfide binding-mechanism (thiol-disulfide exchange reaction) that was described by Fong et al. (1960) and by Schwartz et al. (1960, 1964) in relation to *activation* of the antidiuretic response to vasopressin. However, it is significant that in analogous experiments, the extent of binding of oxytocin, which is inactivated by the rat kidney *in vivo* almost as effectively as is vasopressin (Ginsburg and Smith, 1959), was apparently related to its antidiuretic potency. That is, only when large enough doses were given to produce near-maximal antidiuresis was oxytocin found to be bound in appreciable amounts (Schwartz et al., 1964). It is possible, therefore, that binding of this kind may be an early step in the initiation of both action and inactivation of these hormones. These observations and ideas probably have a bearing on questions arising from data of other experiments: (a) The antidiuresis in a rat due to an intravenous injection of lysine vasopressin has a shorter duration than that resulting from a dose of arginine vasopressin which causes an equally intense effect (Sawyer, 1958), but (b) the half-life of lysine vasopressin in plasma is more than twice that of arginine vasopressin (Sawyer, 1963). (c) Other analogues differ from arginine vasopressin in the persistence of their effects after intravenous injection of doses producing equally intense antidiuresis (Sawyer et al., 1962; van Dyke et al., 1963; Chan, 1965).

The early literature on inactivation of oxytocin and vasopressin by liver homogenates and extracts has been reviewed by Heller (1957) and Heller and Ginsburg (1966). Rychlík (1964), in an interesting summary of recent experiments of his group, formulated the inactivation of oxytocin by liver extracts as a two-stage reaction: (a) reversible reduction of the disulfide bond and (b) irreversible degradation of the linear peptide, dihydro-oxytocin, from the amino end by an aminopeptidase which does not attack the active hormone itself. The first step requires glutathione, and the enzyme has tentatively been called "glutathione-oxytocin transhydrogenase".

INACTIVATION OF OXYTOCIN AND VASOPRESSIN BY SERUM FROM PREGNANT WOMEN

Inactivation of oxytocin by serum from pregnant women was first described by Fekete (1930), and Dieckmann et al. (1950) were the first to show, by valid methods, the inactivation of the antidiuretic activity of vasopressin by blood from pregnant women. The extensive investigations in this field have been reviewed by Tuppy (1960), Tuppy and Wintersberger (1964) and Heller and Ginsburg (1966). It now seems established that the same enzyme(s) attacks both oxytocin and vasopressin in the same manner. Tuppy and Nesvadba (1957) showed that the site of attack on oxytocin is the peptide bond between the amino-terminal half of cystine (position 1) and tyrosine (position 2). Riad (1967) demonstrated that the same bond in lysine vasopressin is cleaved by pregnancy serum. This confirmed the conclusion reached by Stoklasa and Wintersberger (1959), who found that the purified enzyme inactivated both hormones at the same rate.

Oxytocinase activity has been localized in two bands by vertical gel electrophoresis (Glendening *et al.* 1965). Golubow *et al.* (1963) showed that deamino-oxytocin is not inactivated by pregnancy serum, which suggests that the free amino group is essential for attachment of the hormone to the enzyme. Interestingly, this amino group is also required for the binding of oxytocin to neurophysin (Hope, 1964).

That this serum enzyme is not of major importance in vasopressin metabolism during pregnancy was shown by Roth and Slater (1962). The difference in duration of antidiuresis in response to the same dose of vasopressin during late pregnancy and again, in the same patients, in the postpartum period suggests that vasopressinase activity accounts for about 20% of the total clearance of vasopressin during late pregnancy (Lauson, 1967).

REFERENCES

BOOKS. REVIEWS, AND MONOGRAPHS

BENSON, G. K. and FITZPATRICK, R. J. (1966). The neurohypophysis and mammary glands. *The Pituitary Gland*, Vol. 3, pp. 414–452. Harris, G. W. and Donovan, B. T. (eds.). University of California Press, Berkeley and Los Angeles.

DICKER, S. E. (1960). The inactivation of oxytocin *in vitro*. *Polypeptides which Affect Smooth Muscles and Blood Vessels*, pp. 79–82. Schachter, M. (ed.). Pergamon Press, Oxford.

FITZPATRICK, R. J. (1961). The estimation of small amounts of oxytocin in blood. *Oxytocin*, pp. 358–379. Caldeyro-Barcia, R. and Heller, H. (eds.). Pergamon Press, Oxford.

FITZPATRCK, R. J. (1966). The posterior pituitary gland and the female reproductive tract *The Pituitary Gland*, Vol. 3, pp. 453–504. Harris, G. W. and Donovan, B. T. (eds..). University of California Press, Berkeley and Los Angeles.

FITZPATRICK, R. J. and WALMSLEY, C. F. (1965). The release of oxytocin during parturition. *Advances in Oxytocin Research*, pp. 51–73. Pinkerton, J. H. M. (ed.). Pergamon Press, Oxford.

FOLLEY, S. J. and KNAGGS, G. S. (1965a). Oxytocin levels in the blood of ruminants with special reference to the milking stimulus. *Advances in Oxytocin Research*, pp. 37–49. Pinkerton, J. H. M. (ed.). Pergamon Press, Oxford.

GONZÁLEZ-PANIZZA, V. H., SICA-BLANCO, Y. and MÉNDEZ-BAUER, C. (1961). The fate of injected oxytocin in the pregnant woman near term. *Oxytocin*, pp. 347–357. Caldeyro-Barcia, R. and Heller, H. (eds.). Pergamon Press, Oxford.

HELLER, H. (1957). The state and concentration of the neurohypophysial hormones in the blood. *Ciba Fdn Collog. Endocr.*, **11**: 3–14.

HELLER, H. and GINSBURG, M. (1966). Secretion, metabolism and fate of the posterior pituitary hormones. *The Pituitary Gland*, vol. 3, pp. 330–373. Harris, G. W. and Donovan, B. T. (eds.). University of California Press, Berkeley.

HOPE, D. B. (1964). On the nature of the hormone-protein binding in van Dyke protein. *Oxytocin, Vasopressin and their Structural Analogues*, pp. 99–107. Rudinger, J. (ed.). Macmillan, New York.

LAUSON, H. D. (1967). Metabolism of antidiuretic hormones. *Amer. J. Med.*, **42**: 713–744.

LAUSON, H. D. (1960). Vasopressin and oxytocin in the plasma of man and other mammals. *Hormones in Human Plasma*, pp. 225–293. Antoniades, H. N. (ed.). Little, Brown, Boston.

RYCHLÍK, I. (1964). Inactivation of oxytocin and vasopressin by tissue enzymes: a basis for the design of analogues. *Oxytocin, Vasopressin and their Structural Analogues*, pp. 153–162. Rudinger, J. (ed.). Macmillan, New York.

SAWYER, W. H. (1963). Neurohypophysial peptides and water excretion in the vertebrates. *Mem. Soc. Endocr.*, **13**: 45–58.

SCHWARTZ, I. L., RASMUSSEN, H., LIVINGSTON, L. M. and MARC-AURELE, J. (1964). Neurohypophyseal hormone-receptor interactions, *Oxytocin, Vasopressin and their Structural Analogues*, pp. 125–131. Rudinger, J. (ed.). Macmillan, New York.

TUPPY, H. (1960). Enzymic inactivation and degradation of oxytocin and vasopressin, *Polypeptides which Affect Smooth Muscles and Blood Vessels*, pp. 49–58. Schachter, M. (ed.). Pergamon Press, Oxford.

TUPPY, H. and WINTERSBERGER, E. (1964). Investigations of pregnancy serum oxytocinase. *Oxytocin, Vasopressin and their Structural Analogues*, pp. 143–151. Rudinger, J. (ed.). Macmillan, New York.

ORIGINAL PAPERS

AMES, R. G., MOORE, D. H. and VAN DYKE, H. B. (1950). The excretion of posterior pituitary antidiuretic hormone in the urine and its detection in the blood. *Endocrinology*, **46**: 215–227.

AMES, R. G. and VAN DYKE, H. B. (1950). Antidiuretic hormone in the urine and pituitary of the kangaroo rat. *Proc. Soc. Exp. Biol. Med.*, **75**: 417–420.

AROSKAR, J. P., CHAN, W. Y., STOUFFER, J. E., SCHNEIDER, C. H., MURTI, V. V. S. and DU VIGNEAUD, V. (1964). Renal excretion and tissue distribution of radioactive oxytocin in rats. *Endocrinology*, **74**: 226–232.

AUJARD, C., CSÁNYI, E. and LE BRETON, E. (1955). Recherches sur l'activité oxytocique des urines. *Archs Sci. Physiol.*, **9**: 71–82.

BERCU, B. A., ROKAW, S. N. and MASSIE, E. (1950). Antidiuretic action of the urine of patients in cardiac failure. *Circulation*, **2**: 409–413.

BEUZEVILLE, C. F. and LAUSON, H. D. (1964). The question of vasopressin removal by the liver in rats. *Fedn Proc. Fedn Amer. Socs Exp. Biol.*, **23**: 150.

BEUZEVILLE, C. F. and LAUSON, H. D. (1966). Removal of vasopressin by the kidney in rats. *Fedn Proc. Fedn Amer. Socs Exp. Biol.*, **25**: 254.
BEUZEVILLE, C. F. and LAUSON, H. D. (1967). Unpublished preliminary observations.
BOCANEGRA, M. and LAUSON, H. D. (1961). Ultrafilterability of endogenous antidiuretic hormone from plasma of dogs. *Amer. J. Physiol.*, **220**: 486–492.
BROOK, A. H. and SHARE, L. (1966). On the question of protein-binding and the diffusibility of circulating antidiuretic hormone in the dog. *Endocrinology*, **78**: 779–785.
CHAN, W. Y. (1965). Effects of neurohypophysial hormones and their deamino analogues on renal excretion of Na, K and water in rats. *Endocrinology*, **77**: 1097–1104.
CHAUDHURY, R. R. and WALKER, J. M. (1959). The fate of injected oxytocin in the rabbit. *J. Endocr.*, **19**: 189–192.
CRAWFORD, J. D. and PINKHAM, B. (1954). The removal of circulating antidiuretic hormone by the kidney. *Endocrinology*, **55**: 699–700.
CZACZKES, J. W. and KLEEMAN, C. R. (1964). The effect of various states of hydration and the plasma concentration on the turnover of antidiuretic hormone in mammals. *J. Clin. Invest.*, **43**: 1649–1658.
CZACZKES, J. W., KLEEMAN, C. R. and KOENIG, M. (1964). Physiologic studies of antidiuretic hormone by its direct measurement in human plasma. *J. Clin. Invest.*, **43**: 1625–1640.
DALE, H. H. (1909). The action of extracts of the pituitary body. *Biochem. J.*, **4**: 427–447.
DICKER, S. E. and EGGLETON, M. G. (1960). Hyaluronidase and antidiuretic activity in urine of man. *J. Physiol., Lond.*, **154**: 378–384.
DICKER, S. E. and GREENBAUM, A. L. (1956). Inactivation of the antidiuretic activity of vasopressin by tissue homogenates. *J. Physiol., Lond.*, **132**: 199–212.
DICKER, S. E. and GREENBAUM, A. L. (1958). The destruction of the antidiuretic activity of vasopressin by -SH active compounds. *J. Physiol., Lond.*, **141**: 107–116.
DIECKMANN, W. J., EGENOLF, G. F., MORLEY, B. and POTTINGER, R. E. (1950). The inactivation of the antidiuretic hormone of the posterior pituitary gland by blood from pregnant patients. *Amer. J. Obstet. Gynec.*, **60**: 1043–1049.
ESER, S. and TÜZÜNKAM, P. (1950). La foie et l'hormone antidiurétique. *Ann. Endocr.*, **11**: 124–130.
FEKETE, K. (1930). Beiträge zur Physiologie der Gravidität. *Endokrinologie*, **7**: 364–369.
FOLLEY, S. J. and KNAGGS, G. S. (1965b). Levels of oxytocin in the jugular vein blood of goats during parturition. *J. Endocr.*, **33**: 301–315.
FONG, C. T. O., SILVER, L., CHRISTMAN, D. R. and SCHWARTZ, I. L. (1960). On the mechanisms of action of the antidiuretic hormone (vasopressin). *Proc. Nat. Acad. Sci., U.S.A.*, **46**: 1273–1277.
FRIEDBERG, V. and VORHERR, H. (1960). Adiuretinuntersuchungen im Blut und Urin während und nach Operationen. *Klin. Wschr.*, **38**: 1155–1158.
GILMAN, A. and GOODMAN, L. (1937). The secretory response of the posterior pituitary to the need for water conservation. *J. Physiol., Lond.*, **90**: 113–124.
GINSBURG, M. (1954). The secretion of antidiuretic hormone in response to haemorrhage and the fate of vasopressin in adrenalectomized rats. *J. Endocr.*, **11**: 165–176.
GINSBURG, M. (1957). The clearance of vasopressin from the splanchnic vascular area and the kidneys. *J. Endocr.*, **16**: 217–226.
GINSBURG, M. and HELLER, H. (1953). The clearance of injected vasopressin from the circulation and its fate in the body. *J. Endocr.*, **9**: 283–291.
GINSBURG, M. and IRELAND, M. (1964). Binding of vasopressin and oxytocin to protein in extracts of bovine and rabbit neurohypophyses. *J. Endocr.*, **30**: 131–145.

Ginsburg, M. and Smith, M. W. (1959). The fate of oxytocin in male and female rats. *Brit. J. Pharmacol. Chemother.*, **14**: 327–333.

Glendening, M. B., Titus, M. I., Schroeder, S. A., Mohun, G. and Page, E. W. (1965) The destruction of oxytocin and vasopressin by the aminopeptidases in sera from pregnant women. *Amer. J. Obstet. Gynec.*, **92**: 815–820.

Golubow, J., Chan, W. Y. and du Vigneaud, V. (1963). The effect of human pregnancy serum on avian depressor activities of oxytocin and desamino-oxytocin. *Proc. Soc. Exp. Biol. Med.*, **113**: 113–115.

Heller, H. and Urban, F. F. (1935). The fate of antidiuretic principle of post-pituitary extracts. *J. Physiol., Lond.*, **85**: 502–518.

Heller, H. and Zaidi, S. M. (1957). The metabolism of exogenous and endogenous antidiuretic hormone in the kidney and liver *in vivo*. *Brit. J. Pharmacol Chemother.*, **12**: 284–292.

Holliday, M. A., Burstin, C. and Harrah, J. (1963). Evidence that the antidiuretic substance in the plasma of children with nephrogenic diabetes insipidus is antidiuretic hormone. *Pediatrics, Springfield*, **32**: 384–388.

Jones, A. M. and Schlapp, W. (1936). The action and fate of injected posterior pituitary extracts in the decapitated cat. *J. Physiol., Lond.*, **87**: 144–157.

Knaggs, G. S. (1967). Biological half-life of intravenously injected oxytocin in the circulation of the sow. *J. Endocr.*, **37**: 229–230.

Kuroda, R. (1963). The antidiuretic hormone (ADH) and heart insufficiency. 1. Comparative evaluation of methods of extracting ADH from human urine and isolation of antidiuretic hormones by paper electrophoresis. *Folia Endocr. Jap.*, **38**: 1069–1078. (In Japanese.)

Larson, E. (1935). Tolerance and fate of posterior lobe pituitary extract. *J. Pharmac. Exp. Ther.*, **54**: 151.

Larson, E. (1938). Tolerance and fate of the pressor principle of posterior pituitary extracts in anesthetized animals. *J. Pharmac. Exp. Ther.*, **62**: 346–361.

Larson, E. (1939). Fate of the injected oxytocic principle of posterior pituitary in anesthetized cats and dogs. *J. Pharmac. Exp. Ther.*, **67**: 175–186.

Lauson, H. D. and Bocanegra, M. (1961). Clearance of exogenous vasopressin from plasma of dogs. *Amer. J. Physiol.*, **200**: 493–497.

Lauson, H. D., Bocanegra, M. and Beuzeville, C. F. (1965). Hepatic and renal clearance of vasopressin from plasma of dogs. *Amer. J. Physiol.*, **209**: 199–214.

Little, J. B., Klevay, L. M., Radford, E. P., Jr. and McGandy, R. B. (1966). Antidiuretic hormone inactivation by isolated perfused rat liver. *Amer. J. Physiol.*, **211**: 786–792.

Manunta, G. and Marongiu, A. (1961). Inattivazione dell'oxytocina *in vivo* negli ovini. *Boll. Soc. ital. Biol. sper.*, **37**: 510–512.

Máthé, G. and Altman, J. (1954). Contribution experimentale a l'étude de l'inactivation hépatique de la pitressine. *Presse Méd.* **62**: 983–985.

Mayer, F. S. (1960). Identification of the antidiuretic substance in human urine. *Acta Endocr., Copnh.*, **35**: 568–574.

Noble, R. L., Rinderknecht, H. and Williams, P. C. (1939). The apparent augmentation of pituitary antidiuretic action by various retarding substances. *J. Physiol., Lond.*, **96**: 293–301.

Riad, A. M. (1967). Studies on the enzymatic degradation of oxytocin and vasopressin by human pregnancy serum. *Acta Endocr., Copnh.*, **54**: 618–628.

Roth, K. and Slater, S. (1962). Inactivation of vasopressin during pregnancy. *Amer. J. Obstet. Gynec.*, **83**: 1325–1336.

SAWYER, W. H. (1958). Differences in antidiuretic responses of rats to the intravenous administration of lysine and arginine vasopressin. *Endocrinology*, **63**: 694–698.

SAWYER, W. H., CHAN, W. Y. and VAN DYKE, H. B. (1962). Antidiuretic responses to neurohypophysial hormones and some of their synthetic analogues in dogs and rats. *Endocrinology*, **71**: 536–540.

SCHRÖDER, R. and ROTT, D. (1959). Über die Bestimmung und das Verhalten von ADH im menschlichen Plasma. *Klin. Wschr.*, **37**: 1175–1181.

SCHWARTZ, I. L., RASMUSSEN, H., SCHOESSLER, M. A., SILVER, L. and FONG, C. T. O. (1960). Relation of chemical attachment to physiological action of vasopressin. *Proc. Nat. Acad. Sci., U.S.A.*, **46**: 1288–1298.

SHARE, L. (1962). Rate of disappearance of arginine vasopressin from circulating blood in the dog. *Amer. J. Physiol.*, **203**: 1179–1181.

SILVER, L., SCHWARTZ, I. L., FONG, C. T. O., DEBONS, A. F. and DAHL, L. K. (1961). Disappearance of plasma radioactivity after injection of H^3- or I^{131}-labeled arginine vasopressin. *J. Appl. Physiol.*, **16**: 1097–1099.

SMITH, M. W. (1962). The effect of hyaluronidase and cortisol on the inactivation of vasopressin by rat kidney slices. *J. Endocr.*, **24**: 415–424.

SMITH, M. W. (1963). The effect of calcium on the inactivation of vasopressin by rat kidney slices. *J. Physiol., Lond.*, **166**: 22–23P.

SMITH, M. W. and GINSBURG, M. (1961). Fate of synthetic oxytocin analogues in the rat. *Brit. J. Pharmacol., Chemother.*, **16**: 244–252.

SMITH, M. W. and SACHS, H. (1961). Inactivation of arginine vasopressin by rat kidney slices. *Biochem. J.*, **79**: 663–669.

SMITH, M. W. and THORN, N. A. (1965). The effects of calcium on protein-binding and metabolism of arginine vasopressin in rats. *J. Endocr.*, **32**: 141–151.

STARLING, E. H. and VERNEY, E. B. (1925). The secretion of urine as studied on the isolated kidney. *Proc. Roy. Soc., Lond.*, B, **97**: 321–363.

STOKLASA, E. and WINTERSBERGER, E. (1959). Zum Mechanismus des Oxytocin- und Vasopressin-Abbaues durch Schwangerenserum. *Arch. Exp. Path. Pharmak.*, **236**: 358–364.

TATA, P., HELLER, J. and GAUER, O. H. (1965). Über die antidiuretische Aktivität in der Lymphe von Katzen. *Pflügers Arch. ges. Physiol.*, **283**: 222–229.

THORN, N. A. (1959a). Binding *in vitro* of highly-purified arginine-vasopressin and synthetic oxytocin to rat serum globulin. *Acta Endocr., Copnh.*, **30**: 472–476.

THORN, N. A. (1959b). Some chemical properties of antidiuretic material in the urine of rats. *Acta Endocr., Copnh.*, **32**: 128–133.

THORN, N. A. and SILVER, L. (1957). Chemical form of circulating antidiuretic hormone in rats. *J. Exp. Med.*, **105**: 575–583.

THORN, N. A. and WILLUMSEN, N. B. S. (1963a). Inactivation of arginine-and lysine-vasopressin by slices from different zones of the rat kidney and by rat liver slices. *Acta Endocr., Copnh.*, **44**: 545–562.

THORN, N. A. and WILLUMSEN, N. B. S. (1963b). Inhibitory action of calcium on the inactivation of antidiuretic hormone by rat kidney slices. *Acta Endocr., Copnh.*, **44**: 563–569.

TOWBIN, E. J. and FERRELL, C. B. (1963). Stop flow study renal excretion of tritiated vasopressin. *J. Clin. Invest.*, **42**: 987.

TUPPY, H. and NESVADBA, H. (1957). Über die Aminopeptidaseaktivität des Schwangerenserum und ihre Beziehung zu dessen Vermögen, Oxytocin zu inaktivieren. *Mh. Chem.*, **88**: 977–988.

USAMI, S. and CHIEN, S. (1963). Role of hepatic blood flow in regulating plasma concentration of antidiuretic hormone after hemorrhage. *Proc. Soc. Exp. Biol. Med.*, **113**: 606–609.

VAN DYKE, H. B., SAWYER, W. H. and OVERWEG, N. I. A. (1963). Pharmacologic activities of the 8-citrulline analogues of oxytocin and vasopressin. *Endocrinology*, **73**: 637–639.

VERNEY, E. B. (1926). The secretion of pituitrin in mammals, as shown by perfusion of the isolated kidney of the dog. *Proc. Roy. Soc., Lond.*, B, **99**: 487–517.

CHAPTER 12(a)

CLINICAL PHARMACOLOGY: OXYTOCIN

G. W. Theobald

Obstetric Unit, University College Hospital, London

It was originally thought that posterior pituitary extract had a diuretic effect and it is a matter of interest that the first clinical application of this extract was in the form of "diuretic tablets" given by mouth (Blair Bell, 1909). The earliest use of posterior pituitary extract in obstetrics was in the treatment of "shock, uterine atony and intestinal paresis" (Blair Bell, 1909). Two years later Hofbauer (1911) injected the extract both intramuscularly and intravenously to augment the pains of labor. As a result of the observations of Knaus (1926) that posterior pituitary extract could be absorbed both sublingually and *per rectum*, Hofbauer and Hoerner (1927) tried the sublingual route clinically but discarded it in favor of its intra-nasal application.

The induction of premature labor was first done in London in 1756 and remained for a long time a peculiarly English procedure because continental obstetricians preferred to do symphysiotomy recommended by Sigault in 1777. For a century and a half the main ground for inducing premature labor was cephalo-pelvic disproportion and the reason it was done was because the maternal mortality from Caesarean section was then so high. The method used was low amniotomy and its main defects were (1) the induction-delivery time was often prolonged, and (2) the infant often failed to survive the ordeal. Watson (1914, 1922) was the first in modern times to institute a routine method of medical induction of labor, without amniotomy, which included giving castor oil, quinine, an enema, and if necessary intramuscular injections of posterior pituitary extract in heavy dosage. It may be observed that the Editor of *Practical Medicine*, Series 1921, believed "it more than possible that a man could receive damages at law for the loss of a wife or child, if it were shown that Pituitrin was administered before delivery".

The whole picture of induction of labor was changed by the introduction of the physiological intravenous oxytocin drip (Theobald *et al.*, 1948) and of the sulfonamides, together with the antibiotics. The latter have made Caesarean section safe and the treatment of choice in cases of significant cephalo-pelvic disproportion, whereas the former completely changed and widened the scope of the operation. It is now so safe and satisfactory that it is widely performed during the last two weeks of pregnancy in the treatment of a raised blood pressure and proteinuria and also to limit postmaturity. Some there are who look forward to the time when the last two weeks of pregnancy can be dispensed with.

Oxytocin is also used in pharmacological amounts, either by itself or in combination with ergometrine (Ergonovine), to prevent or treat postpartum hemorrhage, and also by some in the treatment of breast engorgement in the early puerperium.

This section will therefore concern itself with: (a) the standardization of oxytocin, (b) its actions other than on the uterus or mammary gland, (c) its effect on the mammary gland, (d) its use in postpartum hemorrhage, and (e) its use in the induction of labor and in enhancing uterine activity during labor.

STANDARDIZATION OF OXYTOCIN

In 1925 a Committee of the League of Nations adopted the U. S. P. Standard Reference Powder as the international standard for posterior pituitary extracts, 0.5 mg of this powder being equivalent to one international unit. The standard powder was made from the whole posterior lobes of cattle, collected immediately after death and ground in acetone to remove water and fat. Until 1928 posterior pituitary extracts were standardized only for their oxytocic activity. A standard powder, obtained in the same manner and similar to the international standard powder, is kept in most countries concerned with such problems and the unit is the specific oxytocic, vasopressor or antidiuretic activity present in it. Syntocinon (=synthetic oxytocin) is standardized by the rat uterus method and stabilized by buffering to an acid pH of between 3.0 and 4.0. Small quantities of chlorbutol and of ethanol are added as preservatives. One mg Syntocinon has an oxytocic activity of about 450 I.U.

An increased concentration of oxytocin in the blood of the order of 70 nU/ml may greatly increase uterine activity in man at the time of the onset of labor. Such figures must be borne in mind when studying reports of the pharmacological effects of oxytocin on the vascular system, for when calculated on the basis of molecular weight it is from 2.5 to 5 times more active than isoprenaline (Pickford, 1961, 1964). It is further noteworthy that hormones given in monumental amounts may have different and even opposite effects from those when given in physiological amounts. Vasopressin given in massive dosage may cause a temporary rise in the blood pressure in man and less antidiuretic effect than when given in physiological dosage (Theobald, 1955), whereas estrogen given in excessive amounts may block rather than expedite motility and conductivity in the pregnant uterus (Jung, 1965).

ACTION OF OXYTOCIN ON STRUCTURES OTHER THAN THE UTERUS

The amount of glucose in the blood rises during normal spontaneous labor in man, but the expected rise is prevented by an intravenous oxytocin infusion (Fairweather, 1965). The underlying mechanism is not understood.

Pharmacological amounts of oxytocin given to dogs have been shown to modify urinary excretion and renal clearances. Provided the rate of urine secretion was slow it induced an increase in the excretion of sodium and chloride, and occasionally in that of potassium. Whereas ADH exerts a strong antidiuretic action without affecting renal clearances, oxytocin increases renal plasma flow (RPF) without affecting glomerular filtration rate (GFR) or the systemic blood pressure (Dicker and Heller, 1946; Berde, 1959; Pickford, 1961).

It was shown in rats (van Dyke et al., 1955) and in man (Theobald, 1955) that pharmacological amounts of oxytocin have an antidiuretic effect. The effect of intravenous oxytocin on water diuresis in the woman varies during the different phases of the menstrual cycle and causes responses at the end of pregnancy which differ markedly from those obtained during the puerperium (Howarth et al., 1963).

The intravenous injection of oxytocin usually causes vascular dilatation in man, dog and cat, but this action can be reversed by the previous administration of estrogen (Haigh et al., 1963; Deis and Pickford, 1964).

In the rat, kidneys perfused with blood from headless donors respond to aldosterone by diuresis which, in spite of reduced sodium concentration in the urine, often causes net sodium loss. An intravenous injection of oxytocin converts this abnormal action of aldosterone to the normal one of salt and water retention (Davy and Lockett, 1960).

Demunbrun et al. (1954) reported that the GFR, RPF, and tubular maxima were markedly reduced in dogs after neurohypophysectomy, and that the normal renal hemodynamics were restored by giving oxytocin but not by vasopressin.

Sacks (1924) stated that posterior pituitary extract conspicuously decreased the rate of edema formation in man, and further evidence has accumulated to suggest that this action is due to the oxytocin fraction (Ferguson, 1962).

It is established that the stimulus of coitus in the estrous rabbit excites a reflex activation of the adenohypophysis with consequent release of gonadotrophin. It has also been reported that the mere sight of the bull causes increased uterine activity in the cow (van Demark and Hays, 1952). Considering that the ascent of the spermatozoa *in utero* is far more rapid than can be accounted for by their inherent motility, it has been conjectured that their progress may be aided by reverse uterine peristalsis caused by oxytocin. There appears to be no experimental evidence in support of this supposition. The "pharmacological" actions of oxytocin may be of more significance than is often conceded provided the observations of Demunbrun et al. (1954) are confirmed.

MILK EJECTION

By means of a nervous reflex, suckling causes oxytocin release which acts on the contractile myoepithelial cells, causing milk ejection. Plain muscle is also present in the ducts but there is no evidence that oxytocin affects it. It was first proved by Cross and van Dyke (1953) that oxytocin was more effective than ADH in causing milk ejection in the rabbit. Theobald (1961) confirmed this observation in man and demonstrated that on the fourth day of the puerperium the intravenous infusion of 0.2 mU Syntocinon/min often sufficed to cause both milk ejection and mammary contractions. The composite trace made by Dr C.N. Smyth during a visit to Bradford in March, 1957, compares the effect of the intravenous infusion of 0.2 mU Syntocinon/min with that of suckling the other breast both on uterine activity, mammary contractions and milk ejection which was photographically recorded during the same time period (Fig. 1).

The vast literature on this subject has been reviewed by Petersen (1944), Folley (1956), and Denamur (1965). It will be noted that in man similar amounts of oxytocin when infused intravenously are equally effective in causing both uterine activity and milk ejection on the fourth day of the puerperium and that the effective amount corresponds closely with the minimum effective amount of ADH on water diuresis. The only further observations which will be made here concern (1) mammary contractions during pregnancy, labor and the puerperium, and (2) the use of oxytocin in pharmacological amounts to relieve breast engorgement and to improve poor lactation in man.

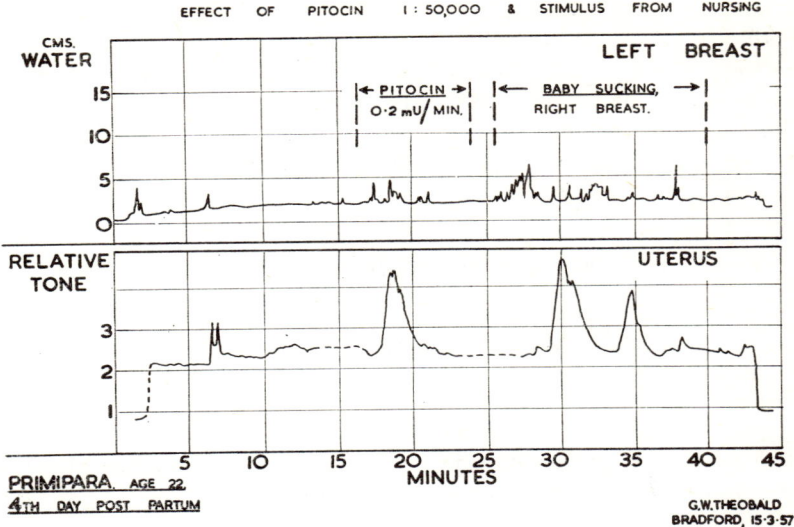

Fig. 1. Composite trace, external recording, comparing effects of the intravenous infusion of 0.2 mU Pitocin/min on mammary pressure and uterine tension compared with those caused by suckling the right breast (Theobald, 1961).

PRESSURE IN THE MAMMARY GLAND DURING
PREGNANCY, LABOR AND PARTURITION

Members of the Montevideo School (Caldeyro-Barcia, 1965) have introduced a polyethylene catheter into a mammary duct and by means of a pressure transducer have recorded intramammary pressures during pregnancy, parturition and the puerperium. The pressures recorded were probably caused by contraction of plain muscle as well as of the myoepithelial cells and it may well be that the pressure that suffices to cause adequate milk ejection is much less than that which is recorded by higher than threshold amounts of oxytocin. Further, the irritant effects of the catheter cannot be overlooked.

These highly interesting studies showed three points clearly. The first was that the rhythm of mammary contractions was not identical with those of the uterus. The same independence in rhythm of contractions was noted between those of the round ligaments and the uterus (Hendricks and Moawad, 1965). The second was that the average intramammary pressure rose from 1 mm Hg during pregnancy to 20 mm Hg between the 5th and 8th days of the puerperium. The third was that the threshold amount of oxytocin which produced a detectable response in intramammary pressure early in pregnancy was 100 mU whereas by mid-pregnancy the figure had dropped to 1 mU and thereafter showed no further change. The latter two figures might to no little extent be dependent on the amount of "milk" in the ducts.

RELIEF OF MAMMARY ENGORGEMENT

The fact that in normal puerperal women a nasal oxytocin spray causes milk ejection is easily demonstrated. It occurred to Haeger and Jacobsohn (1953) that this hormone might prove useful in the treatment of mammary engorgement and of poor lactation, and they claimed promising results. Subsequent trials have proved on the whole disappointing probably because mammary engorgement and poor lactation are not often primarily due to unsatisfactory milk ejection (Berde, 1959).

THE TREATMENT OF POSTPARTUM HEMORRHAGE

Seeing that the rest of this chapter will deal with physiological and paraphysiological amounts of oxytocin, it will be convenient to consider here its use in pharmacological amounts in the prevention and treatment of postpartum hemorrhage. This occurs much more frequently than is realized even in well-run maternity units. It is not known why this bleeding occurs, for although the intra-uterine pressure may exceed 400 mm Hg during the early puerperium, it is equally true that there may be no postpartum bleeding even when both the intra-uterine and the intramyometrial pressures are little above that of the atmosphere (Hendricks, 1966). For more than a century and a half ergot has been used in the treatment of postpartum hemorrhage and it is almost certain that midwives have used it for this purpose for many hundreds of years.

This is not the place to discuss the pharmacology of ergot, but it is of interest to record that whereas the intravenous injection of ergometrine (Ergonovine) causes an effect within 3 min, the old liquid extract of ergot acts almost as quickly when given by mouth as ergometrine injected intramuscularly. The two disadvantages of ergot are (1) that it may kill an unsuspected twin, and (2) that it may cause a steep rise in the blood pressure, but neither disadvantage is very real. Nevertheless, oxytocin has been used in some centers until the third stage is completed, when ergot is allowed if necessary. The intravenous use of posterior pituitary extract to prevent postpartum hemorrhage was advocated more than 40 years ago by Crichton (1920), and in recent years Syntometrine (0.5 mg ergometrine maleate plus 5 U oxytocin) has been introduced and used with success. This preparation, when injected intramuscularly, acts more quickly than ergometrine alone and combines the advantages of both substances. It does not obviate the danger to the second twin but neither does it appear to affect the blood pressure (Fliegner and Hibbard, 1966). It may be warned that the use of any of these preparations is not without danger if given before the birth of the anterior shoulder.

THE ACTION OF OXYTOCIN ON THE UTERUS

The first "modern" standardized bio-assay procedure was probably the isolated guinea-pig uterus preparation for testing posterior pituitary extracts (Dale and Laidlaw, 1912). Oxytocin causes the isolated uterus of most laboratory animals to contract, provided the hormonal state of the animal was satisfactory when the organ was removed and the ionic composition of the solution in which it is suspended is physiological. It was noted by Knaus (1925–1926) that the pregnant rabbit uterus does not respond to oxytocin except at the very end of pregnancy and this fact has been used as a method for quantitative comparison of the activities of oxytocin and related polypeptides (Berde and Cerletti, 1958).

The following three facts are pertinent. The first is that no bio-assay method gives any reliable guide as to the oxytocic effect of a synthetic peptide of the neurohypophysial type on the human uterus *in vivo* (Saameli, 1964). The second is that oxytocin has no demonstrable effect on the human myocardium or ureter (Caldeyro-Barcia, 1965) and actually exerts an inhibiting effect on intestinal motility in the anesthetized dog, on the guinea-pig tracheal chain and isolated ileum, and also on rabbit ileum. The inhibitory responses in the dog are not reduced by adrenergic blockade, ganglionic blockade or adrenergic neurone blockade. They are, however, reduced by atropine, without affecting the inhibitory responses to either epinephrine or papaverine (Levy, 1963).

Thirdly, it is generally agreed that oxytocin has little or no effect on the non-pregnant human uterus, whether *in vivo* or *in vitro*. Nevertheless, the uterine contractions which occur at the extreme ends of the menstrual cycle are almost indistinguishable from those occurring at the beginning of labor (Hendricks, 1965). The human uterus contracts without ceasing throughout the reproductive life of a woman and it is clear that all such contractions are "spontaneous" and are but modified by hormones, by the ionic concentrations in and around the myometrial cells, and by nervous impulses, both afferent and efferent. The astonishing fact is that pregnancy sensitizes the human myometrium to oxytocin and that this sensitivity increases pari passu with the growth of the placenta. It is therefore apparent that endogenous oxytocin cannot put a woman into labor but rather that physico-chemical changes in and around the myometrial cells sensitize the myometrium to the hormone.

MODE OF ACTION OF OXYTOCIN

Oxytocin acts by lowering the membrane potential of the uterine muscle. It causes an increase in the frequency of the trains of impulses and in the frequency of the discharges composing each train. It may also mobilize calcium ions. There are, however, odd facts about the behavior of oxytocin which are not explained by these observations. A rapid intravenous injection of 500 or 1000 mU oxytocin into a woman at term may fail to cause a single uterine contraction, but it may nevertheless cause a subsequent rise in myometrial sensitivity to oxytocin. An intravenous infusion of 2 mU oxytocin/min for 30 min may have no apparent effect on uterine activity, but contractions may begin some minutes after the infusion has been stopped. Lastly "oxytocin contractions" may persist for an hour or longer after the intravenous infusion has been stopped, and then gradually die away. It has been shown that oxytocin can still cause contraction of strips of myometrium after the membrane has been completely depolarized by immersion in potassium–Ringer's solution (Evans et al., 1958). It therefore seems likely that it can activate the contractile elements of plain muscle without the mediation of membrane depolarization. This may be a very relevant observation, but it would be interesting to speculate that oxytocin in some at present unknown way facilitates spread of conduction from muscle bundle to muscle bundle.

OXYTOCINASE

Fekete (1930) discovered that the serum of pregnant women inactivates oxytocin and it was later shown that the substance concerned is the enzyme oxytocinase. It is an aminopeptidase and acts equally well on both oxytocin and vasopressin (Tuppy, 1961). So far as is known it only occurs in the blood of pregnant women and of anthropoid apes. In women it can be detected shortly after the 16th day and increases 60-fold during pregnancy, reaching its maximum at term (Semm, 1961). Plasma obtained from 18 women at term was found to inactivate 50% of added Syntocinon in 4.54 ± 1.13 (S.D.) min (Mendez-Bauer et al., 1961).

Seeing that vasopressin inhibits water diuresis as effectively in pregnant as in non-pregnant women (Theobald, 1934), and that an intravenous infusion of 0.5 mU oxytocin/min may start labor at a time when the concentration of oxytocinase is at its highest, it is difficult to envisage the significance of this enzyme. The half-life of oxytocin in the non-pregnant woman has so far not been determined and it is possible that without this enzyme the half-life of oxytocin at term might be unduly extended. It is also possible that oxytocinase may be mainly concerned in protecting the placenta from overactivity of oxytocin (Tuppy, 1961).

MYOMETRIAL CHANGES DURING THE MENSTRUAL CYCLE COMPARED WITH THOSE WHICH OCCUR DURING PREGNANCY

The onset of labor in women is preceded by profound changes both in the cervix and in the myometrium, and these include alteration in electrolyte and water content both within and without the cells (Hawkins and Nixon, 1961), increase in the myometrium both of actomyosin and of high energy phosphates (Csapo, 1961; Kumar et al., 1962), marked increase in extensibility and in length-tension relation in myometrial strips (Schofield, 1966; Schofield and Wood, 1964) and changes in the physico-chemical structure of the cervix (Cullen and Harkness, 1964; Harkness and Harkness, 1961). It is interesting to conjecture that such changes precede the Braxton Hicks contractions and are in no way caused by them. Similar changes have been provoked in spayed animals by giving them estrogen, progesterone and relaxin, but on no occasion could the maximum changes in any of these parameters, such as are found at the end of pregnancy, be provoked; nor could the sensitivity *in vivo* of the myometrium to oxytocin be significantly altered. Giving large amounts of estradiol and medoxyprogesterone acetate (Provera) to women from the fourth to the ninth days of the cycle did not change the pattern of uterine activity which consisted of rapid contractions of low amplitude. After both hormones had been stopped for three to four days prelabor-like contractions were recorded. By this means it was found possible to provoke on the 8th day of the cycle the type of uterine activity normally limited to the period from the 27th day of one cycle to the 3rd of the next (Fig. 2). Further, marked uterine activity was recorded from the uterus of a woman of 52, who had had both ovaries removed two years previously, notwithstanding the fact that she had taken large doses of Provera for the previous seven days (Bengtsson and Theobald, 1966).

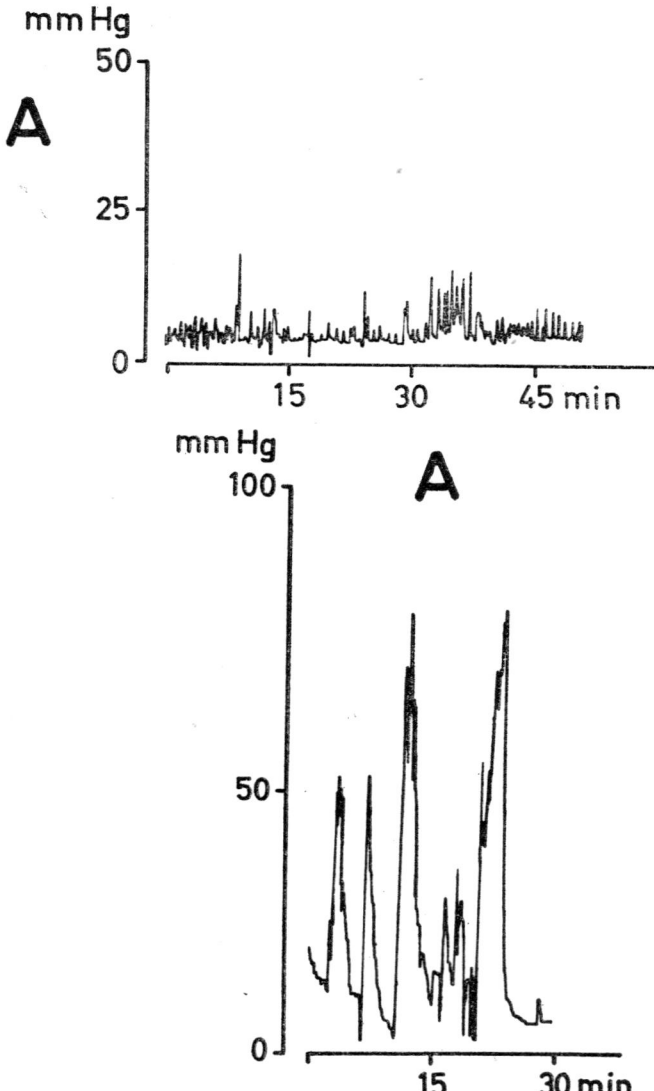

Fig. 2. Top trace from non-pregnant human uterus taken on third day of cycle. Lower trace from same patient on eighth day of cycle after she had taken 2 mg Linoral (ethinylestradiol, Schering) and 400 mg Provera (medoxyprogesterone acetate, Upjohn) daily from the third to the sixth day of the cycle and then stopped both for two days. (Modified from Bengtsson and Theobald, 1966.)

Estrogens given to a spayed animal cause an increase in all the mechanisms of uterine activity unless excessive amounts are given when the opposite effect is achieved (Jung, 1964). Many steroids have a blocking effect on the mechanical and electrical activity of the isolated parturient rat uterus, including testosterone, aldosterone and progesterone, the last being the most effective (Marshall, 1965). Progesterone also inhibits the activity of isolated strips from pregnant human myometrium (Barnes, 1965). The fact that large amounts of progesterone, or of one of its analogues, whether given directly into the myometrium or parenterally, have no consistent effect in preventing premature labor and that there is no fall in the blood level of progesterone in man before the onset of labor, have led Csapo (1961, 1965) to make the suggestion that the myometrium underlying the placenta receives a rich and immediate supply of progesterone from the placenta so that its conductivity is decreased.

This concept is difficult to entertain. In the first place a more rapid and pronounced effect on the uterus is caused if either posterior pituitary extract or ergometrine is injected directly into the muscle rather than intravenously. It is consequently not easy to believe that the twin effects of diffusion and absorption into the blood stream would not result in relative equilibrium of distribution throughout the organ. Secondly it would be difficult to understand how a woman with true placenta previa could go into labor if this were so. Thirdly, contractions of an order of 60 mm Hg can and do occur from 36 weeks onwards. A more fundamental objection to this concept is that there is no convincing evidence that progesterone *in vivo* is not as much concerned with causing as with inhibiting effective uterine activity. The change in the pattern of uterine activity characteristic of the ovulatory menstrual cycle is for frequent contractions of low amplitude to change to one of less frequent contractions of an amplitude exceeding 100 mm Hg. Such contractions, indistinguishable from pre-labor contractions, begin to occur at the very time that the amount of progesterone in the blood is increasing (Hendricks, 1965). Further, large amounts of Provera given for seven days to a woman aged 52 two years after both ovaries had been removed, failed to prevent marked uterine activity (Bengtsson and Theobald, 1966).

OXYTOCIN DURING PREGNANCY AND PARTURITION IN MAN

Theobald (1934) found that a single intravenous injection of 5 to 10 mU posterior pituitary extract caused minimum inhibition of water diuresis in the dog, man and the pregnant woman at term. Seeing that the results were so consistent, that the preparation used (Infundin) was standardized for its oxytocic content and that bovine glands are thought to contain roughly equal amounts of vasopressin and of oxytocin, he postulated that if oxytocin played any significant part in parturition its effective concentration in the blood would match that of vasopressin and be equivalent to that produced by an intravenous infusion of 0.2 to 1 mU oxytocin/min added to the pre-existing concentration of endogenous oxytocin (Theobald, 1936). The first "physiological" oxytocin drip was calculated on this basis and delivered 2.5 mU/min, and subsequently the optimum range was thought to lie between 2.5 and 5 mU/min. Everything above this range was regarded as pharmacological (Theobald *et al.*, 1948, 1956), potentially dangerous and no more effective. The implications of this view are that oxytocin only acts physiologically during labor and lactation. The fact that males secrete both oxytocin and lactogenic hormone affords no reason for supposing that the one is more useful to them than the other.

MEASUREMENT OF OXYTOCIN IN THE BLOOD

The problem just outlined could be solved immediately if the amount of oxytocin circulating in the blood could be measured. It has been shown (Fig. 1) that an increase in concentration of oxytocin in the blood of the order of 70 nano-units(nU)/ml suffices to cause both milk ejection and uterine activity and it seems improbable that a method will ever be discovered which could detect such a change in the concentration of oxytocin.

Rat mammary tissue *in vitro* at 5° C is equally sensitive to a number of polypeptides and to acetylcholine (Van Dongen and Marshall, 1967), but the method of Folley and Knaggs (1965) for measuring blood oxytocin has a claim to high specificity for oxytocin. Bisset's (1961) estimate of 4100 μU/ml in the internal jugular blood of a man is still quoted. Folley and Knaggs (1964, 1965a) found between 90 and 300 μU oxytocin/ml in the jugular blood of a goat while the kid was being expelled, and Fitzpatrick (1961), 3000 μU/ml in the jugular blood of the ewe while the lamb was being ejected. It would be desirable to establish whether such differences relate to species or to methods.

The surprising fact is that all workers in this field agree that the greatest amount of oxytocin in the blood is found just as the fetus is being ejected. Indeed, Folley and Knaggs (1965a) question whether oxytocin plays any part in initiating or controlling labor, and consider that its sole function may be to help in expelling the fetus. This is difficult to understand because both in man and in the sheep (Hindson *et al.*, 1965) contraction of the abdominal musculature is the chief factor concerned in ejecting the fetus. Seeing that stretching the vagina causes reflex milk ejection in the sheep and goat it may be that the large amounts of oxytocin said to be released at the end of the second stage of labor are *due* to the delivery and not the cause of it. In any case, unless species difference comes into play, it has still to be shown that small amounts of endogenous oxytocin do not play a part in initiating labor both in the sheep and the goat.

Coch *et al.* (1965) found up to 900 μU oxytocin in each ml plasma of external jugular vein blood of a woman in the second stage of labor. Further they found in *peripheral* blood plasma nearly 300 μU oxytocin/ml on the second day of the puerperium and 100 μU/ml on the eighth day. The amount of oxytocin in the jugular blood of the cow, mare, ewe and goat falls rapidly after delivery (Fitzpatrick and Walmsley, 1965; Folley and Knaggs, 1965) and yet it is maintained that about 750 mU oxytocin circulate in the peripheral blood of a puerperal woman at a time when the intravenous infusion of 0.5 mU/min may cause both milk ejection and a marked rise in uterine activity. This must be regarded as a serious criticism of the technique used, particularly as Caldeyro-Barcia (1961) has stated that the release of some 4 mU/min of oxytocin would suffice to cause both the uterine and mammary activity associated with normal spontaneous labor.

Saameli (1963) concluded that an average concentration of 3 μU oxytocin/ml in the blood sufficed to cause uterine activity during the last three weeks before the spontaneous onset of active labor in man. As oxytocin is either eliminated or inactivated in the body in an exponential manner (see also Chapter 11) he postulated that the blood level of the pre-existing endogenous oxytocin lay within wide limits in the same range as the injected hormone preparation. It has already been stated that the intravenous infusion of 0.2 mU oxytocin/min may initiate labor in a woman at term. Using the same formula as he did and likewise assuming the weight of the woman to be 70 kg, this infusion would result in a concentration of 70 nU exogenous oxytocin in each ml blood. This would indicate a fortyfold increase in myometrial sensitivity to oxytocin during the last few days or even hours of pregnancy, a figure obtained by dividing the 3000 nU oxytocin/ml found by Saameli by 70.

THE INDUCTION OF LABOR

"When the child is grown big and the mother cannot continue to provide him with enough nourishment, he becomes agitated, breaks through the membranes and incontinently passes into the external world." (HIPPOCRATES).

The genesis of the physiological oxytocin drip has been adumbrated (Theobald *et al.*, 1948), and from 1950 onwards an extensive literature on this subject has accumulated. The Bradford method was to do amniotomy and follow it the next day, if necessary, with an intravenous oxytocin infusion limited to 10 mU/min and rarely exceeding 5 mU/min. Some start with the intravenous oxytocin infusion and defer amniotomy until after labor has become established. The Montevideo School and Hendricks rarely give more than 8 mU oxytocin/min, but others increase the amount given until contractions occur, and then either keep it at that level or decrease it to the level that will maintain them.

It is worth determining at this stage whether there is any evidence that exogenous oxytocin makes any significant overall difference to the induction of labor. Tennent and Black (1954) induced labor over a period of three years by amniotomy alone in 1585 patients, or 18.3% of all their hospital deliveries. It can be assumed that at least 70% of these women went into labor within 24 hr, and it follows that some 475 did not. Of these 131 (28%) took between 3 and 7 days, and 35 (7%) took more than 7 days.

In the strictly comparable Bradford series of 3131 women over a period of four years (Theobald, 1963), 80% went into labor within 24 hr as the result of amniotomy alone, and of the 20% who did not 90% were in labor within 48 hr of the start of the oxytocin drip, or 97% of all those induced. The incidence of Caesarian section in both series was almost identical (about 3%). The simple fact which emerges is that the main function of exogenous oxytocin is to shorten the induction-delivery time and that it thus saves a few babies. These figures are shown in Table 1. The results during the years 1959–1960, when infusions delivering more than 5 mU/min were virtually forbidden, were as good as those in previous years, when this rule was less rigidly observed.

Some obstetricians seem to think that the sole value of the oxytocin infusion is to cause strong uterine contractions with the subconscious idea that they will suffice to deliver the infant. Barnes (1965), for example, holds that there is "no God-given dosage; the proper dosage of oxytocin per minute is that dosage which produces a term-type uterine contraction. ... We often can't tell when we are overdosing unless we have an intra-

TABLE 1. INDUCTION OF LABOR IN WOMEN THIRTYEIGHT OR MORE WEEKS PREGNANT. METHODS OF DELIVERY, 1957–60 (INCLUSIVE).

Out of 3331 cases of induction of labor, 21% required an oxytocin drip, the highest incidence being in Gravidae 4 and 4 +. Seventy-nine per cent of these women went into labor within 24 hr after amniotomy (Theobald, 1963).

	Total Numbers	Number of cases of			
		Oxytocin Drip	Spontaneous Delivery	Cæsarean Section	Forceps Extraction
Primigravidæ	1,187	273 (23)	928 (78)	48 (4)	211 (18)
Gravidæ 2 and 3	1,260	210 (17)	1,183 (94)	36 (3)	41 (3)
Gravidæ 4 and 4+	684	180 (26)	658 (96)	13 (2)	13 (2)
Totals	3,131	663 (21.0)	2,769 (89)	97 (3.1)	265 (8.5)

Percentage figures in brackets.

amniotic catheter present and a pressure tracing available. Under such circumstances, this medication is safe..."

In the United States labor is induced in two main categories of patients and usually not until the cervix is so ripe that European obstetricians would regard them as being in early labor. The first category includes the private patient, preferably a multigravida, by whose bedside the obstetrician sits until labor is completed. The second and smaller group consists of patients in whom labor is monitored by electronic equipment and in which the patient is not left alone for a single minute.

In this country, and in many centers in Europe, the patient is left largely in the care of the midwife without the help of any monitoring device. Under such circumstances a rate of infusion not exceeding 5 mU/min has been proved to be both effective and safe.

BUCCAL OXYTOCIN

The reintroduction of the method of giving oxytocin via the alimentary canal is a retrograde and dangerous step. Buccal oxytocin is given in heroic doses amounting to 4400 I.U. daily for two or more days. Its rate of absorption is problematical, but probably varies from patient to patient and in the same patient from hour to hour. It takes some time after the tablet has been placed before any effect on uterine activity is noticed, and it therefore follows that the removal of the tablet cannot prevent the continuing activity of the amount already absorbed. The advantage of the method, if successful, is that it involves no operative interference. It does limit conversation for two days and the tablet must be removed during meals. Further, an unknown percentage of those who have sucked the tablet for two days will have to submit to operative procedures. On the other hand, only 20% of the women who have amniotomy done will have to have an oxytocin infusion. Buccal oxytocin has been followed on not a few occasions by rupture of the uterus. Intravenous infusions of excessive doses of oxytocin can also kill, but the danger can be greatly minimized by careful monitoring whereas no such care can completely overcome the risks of buccal oxytocin.

EVIDENCE IN SUPPORT OF THE VIEW THAT A CHANGE IN SENSITIVITY OF THE MYOMETRIUM TO OXYTOCIN PRECEDES THE ONSET OF LABOR

In the first place it must be stressed that the only means of determining whether any change in myometrial sensitivity takes place between the 36th week and the onset of labor is to follow the uterine activity of the same woman over periods of hours, days and weeks. For this purpose the elegant technique of Alvarez and Caldeyro-Barcia (1950) is useless, and some form of external tocography is essential, such as that devised by Smyth (1957). The pattern of stylized regular contractions increasing stepwise during the last trimester of pregnancy matches biological reality less by similarity than by contrast, for the uterus at term often resembles the non-pregnant uterus (Hendricks, 1965) by showing phases of inactivity interspersed with those of marked activity.

The myometrium of a woman at term may fail to show any response to the repeated rapid injection of 1000 mU oxytocin. The trace in Fig. 3 shows fairly clearly a response to the rapid injection of 200 mU oxytocin.

Of the 3131 women in whom amniotomy was done in Bradford during

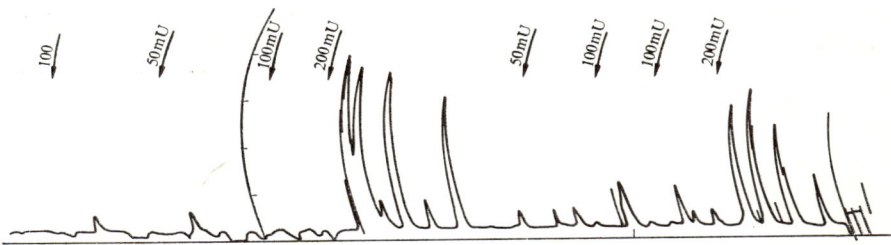

FIG. 3. Sensitivity test. External recording made with Smyth's guard-ring tocograph. A glucose-water drip was started and about an hour later various amounts of Syntocinon were injected rapidly into the rubber tubing close to the needle in the vein, at not less than 5-min intervals, while the drip tubing was temporarily clamped. The uterus responded to 200 mU and the patient was regarded as being sensitive to this amount (Theobald, 1968).

the years 1957–60 inclusive, only 663 required an oxytocin drip. Of these 463 needed it only for one day, and a further 129 for two days. Some women remained relatively insensitive to oxytocin for 4 days and then on the fifth morning proved sensitive to 2 mU oxytocin/min and delivered themselves rapidly (Theobald, 1963). Amniotomy by itself increases the sensitivity of the myometrium to oxytocin (Theobald and Lundborg, 1962). The significant point is that over 3000 women, selected for the operation by a large number of obstetricians according to definite criteria, were safely delivered with a Caesarean section rate of 3%, without any controlling apparatus, without any supervision other than that of the midwives, and without the oxytocin drip ever delivering more than 10 mU oxytocin/min and usually not more, and often less than 5mU/min. It may well be that part of the reason for the divergence of views on this matter between Caldeyro-Barcia and Theobald (1961), is due to the fact that the patients of the former were preselected for him by an obstetrician (Hendricks and Brenner, 1964). It is clearly important to explain why 10% of these women did not go into labor after amniotomy and an intravenous oxytocin infusion on two days, and why they did so during the next 48 hr. It is because most obstetricians will not allow the extended time limit between amniotomy and the onset of labour that the Caesarean section rate associated with induction of labor varies between 5 and 8% in many hospitals.

It has already been shown in Fig. 1 that the intravenous infusion of 0.2 mU Pitocin/min on the 4th day of the puerperium caused contractions both of the uterus and of the mammary gland and milk ejection. Increase in myometrial sensitivity to oxytocin before the onset of labor is well illustrated in Fig. 4. The patient was a Gravida 2 at term with intact membranes. In the upper trace the effect of the intravenous infusion of 2 mU oxytocin/min for 30 min is shown and can be compared with the lower trace similarly obtained two days later. The contractions died away after

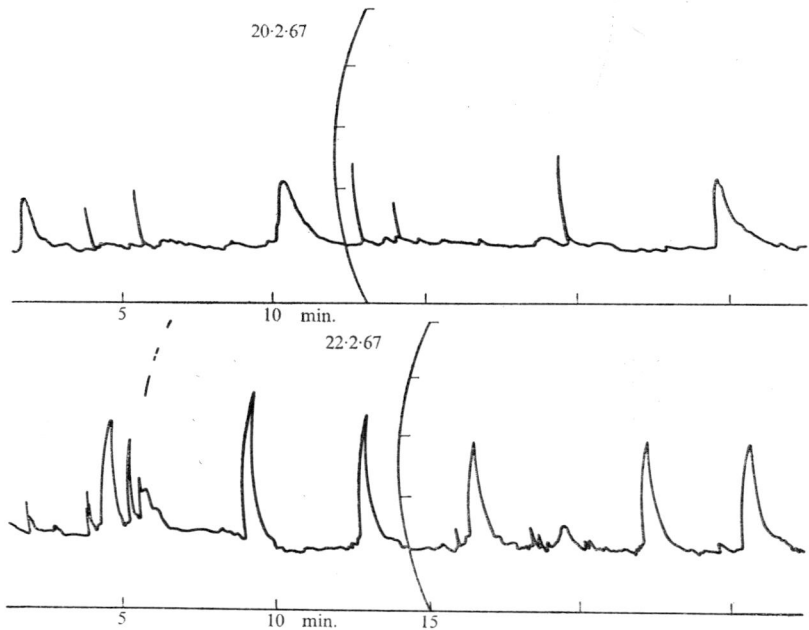

FIG. 4. External recording made with Smyth's tocograph. The patient was a Gravida 2, at term and with intact membranes. The top trace shows the effect of the intravenous infusion of 2 mU Syntocinon/min for 30 min after which it was discontinued. Three contractions of about 25 mm Hg occurred in 25 min. The five upward strokes are of no significance and were due either to fetal movements or to coughs. The lower trace was made in the same way 48 hr later and shows a different pattern of activity. Some of the six contractions were about 60 mm Hg. They died away after the infusion was stopped, but she went into labor the same night and was delivered early the next morning. The time marks are at 5-min intervals (Theobald, unpublished).

the infusion was stopped, but she went into labor the same night and was delivered early the next morning.

The great difference between initiating labor and its subsequent course is well illustrated by Gravidae 4 and 4 plus. They provide the highest percentage of those who are delivered within 6 hr of amniotomy, and also the highest percentage of those who fail to go into labor within 48 hours of the start of an oxytocin infusion. Once they start labor, its course is usually short. At 12 weeks the human pregnant uterus may fail to evacuate its contents notwithstanding the intravenous infusion of 10,000 mU oxytocin/min. Should the woman threaten abortion, however, the intravenous infusion of 5 mU/min may complete the process. Human myometrial strips removed at term are very much more sensitive to oxytocin than those removed at 21 weeks (Fuchs and Fuchs, 1963).

All this evidence is compatible with the view that the human myometrium acquires a sensitivity to oxytocin during pregnancy which usually reaches a high level between the 30th and 36th weeks and does not thereafter normally change much until just before labor starts. The matter is of consummate physiological interest and of profound clinical importance. Disaster threatens when the obstetrician increases the amount of oxytocin given at the very moment when the sensitivity of the myometrium increases.

The fact that forces are being exerted both to preserve and to terminate pregnancy are manifested in the recordings of intra-uterine activity before the onset of true labor. In their studies at Newcastle, Fairweather, Smart and Smart (1966) have noted systematic modulation in the peak pressures attained during contractions which could not be regarded as random, for some filled a Poisson distribution. Further, they were found to be repetitive. The guess of Hippocrates that the maturity of the fetus determined the length of pregnancy is not supported by the fact that "pregnancy" can continue in the monkey for more than 80 days after the fetus has been removed (van Wagenen and Newton, 1943).

CONCLUSIONS

Thanks to the introduction of the oxytocin drip, of the antibiotics, and the technique introduced by Alvarez and Caldeyro-Barcia (1950), by far the most accurate and scientific work on the uterus *in vivo* has been done in man. This is due to the fact that women can cooperate willingly, and the investigation can be made without any anesthetic. Much of what we know about uterine activity in man was learned in primitive hospital wards by means of very simple tocographic devices and the obstetrician's hand.

It has not been proved that oxytocin is essential to labor, but neither is there convincing evidence that normal labor can occur without it. Hypophysectomy does not exclude the possibility that sufficient oxytocin is available to institute labor. The fact that in man an intravenous infusion of oxytocin of the order of 2 mU/min suffices to cause both effective uterine activity and milk ejection at the appropriate times, affords presumptive evidence that oxytocin was devised by nature for these twin purposes. Perhaps oxytocin should be regarded as a fine regulator of parturition just as vasopressin may be thought of as a fine regulator of renal water excretion.

All uterine activity is "spontaneous" and is but modified by sodium, potassium, magnesium and calcium ions, by nervous impulses and by various hormones. The real problem is why the uterus tolerates the fetus and not why labor starts. Once these "tolerating" factors are removed it might be expected that the uterus would revert to its normal behavior and try to expel anything in its cavity. It is interesting to speculate that at the auspicious moment, oxytocin in some at present unknown manner facilitates conductivity from muscle bundle to muscle bundle, so that the whole uterus acts almost as if it were one single cell. Present concepts concerning its mode of action are inadequate and certainly do not explain how and why oxytocin contractions may persist for an hour or more after the infusion is stopped before they die away. Oxytocin is potent and must be treated with respect whether in preventing postpartum hemorrhage, inducing labor or given to increase uterine activity during labor.

More than 2000 years after Hippocrates, Michael Foster (1888) wrote; "We may be said to be in the dark as to why the uterus, after remaining for months subject only to futile contractions, is suddenly thrown into powerful and efficient action and, within maybe a few hours or even less, can get rid of the burden which it has borne with such tolerance for so long a time". Eighty years later we are able to induce labor with confidence and can be reasonably sure that both the onset and end of pregnancy are determined by the Biological Clock about which we know nothing.

REFERENCES

BOOKS, REVIEWS AND MONOGRAPHS

BARNES, A. C. (1965). *Initiation of Labor*, pp. 68, 214. Marshall, J. M. and Burnet, W. M. (eds.). U.S. Public Health Service Publication No. 1390, Washington.

BERDE, B. (1959). Some observations on the circulatory effects of oxytocin, vasopressin and similar polypeptides. *Recent Progress in Oxytocin Research.*, pp. 73–84. Pinkerton, J. H. M. (ed.). Charles C. Thomas, Springfield, Ill.

BISSET, G. W. (1961). Assay of oxytocin and vasopressin. *Oxytocin*, pp. 380–398. Caldeyro-Barcia, R. and Heller, H. (eds.). Pergamon Press, Oxford.

CALDEYRO-BARCIA, R. (1961). Factors controlling the actions of the pregnant uterus. *Physiology of Prematurity*, pp. 73–84. Kowlessar, M. (ed.). John Macy Jr. Foundation, New York.

CALDEYRO-BARCIA, R. (1965). *Initiation of Labor*, pp. 29–34, 63. Marshall, J. M. and Burnet, W. M. (eds.). U. S. Public Health Service Publication No. 1390, Washington.

CALDEYRO-BARCIA, R. and SERENO, J. A. (1961). The response of the human uterus to oxytocin throughout pregnancy. *Oxytocin*, pp. 177–202. Caldeyro-Barcia, R. and Heller, H. (eds.). Pergamon Press, Oxford.
CSAPO, A. (1961). Defence mechanism of pregnancy. *Progesterone and the Defence Mechanism of Pregnancy*, 1st ed., pp. 3–27. Wolstenholme, G. E. W. and Cameron, M. P. (eds.). Churchill, London.
CSAPO, A. (1965). Effects of progesterone on uterine activity. *Initiation of Labor*, pp. 75–93. Marshall, J. M. and Burnet, W. M. (eds.). U.S. Public Health Service Publication, No. 1390, Washington.
DENAMUR, R. (1965). The hypothalamic-neurohypophysial system and the milk ejection reflex. *Dairy Sci. Abstr.* 27 (5): 193–224; (6): 263–280.
FITZPATRICK, R. J. (1961). The estimation of small amounts of oxytocin in blood. *Oxytocin*, pp. 358–377. Caldeyro-Barcia, R. and Heller, H. (eds.). Pergamon Press, Oxford
FITZPATRICK, R. J. and WALMSLEY, C. F. (1965). The release of oxytocin during parturition. *Advances in Oxytocin Research*, pp. 51–71. Pinkerton, J. H. M. (ed.). Pergamon Press, Oxford.
FOLLEY, S. J. (1956). *The Physiology and Biochemistry of Lactation*. Oliver & Boyd, Edinburgh.
FOLLEY, S. J. and KNAGGS, G. S. (1965b). Oxytocin levels in the blood of ruminants with special reference to the milking stimulus. *Advances in Oxytocin Research*, pp. 37–44. Pinkerton, J. H. M. (ed.). Pergamon Press, Oxford.
HENDRICKS, C. H. (1965). Regulation of smooth muscle activity in vivo. *Muscle*, pp. 349–362. Paul, W. M., Daniel, E. E., Kay, C. M. and Monckton, G. (eds.). Pergamon Press, Oxford.
JUNG, H. (1965). Effects of progesterone on uterine activity. *Initiation of Labor*, pp. 75–93. Marshall, J. M. and Burnet, W. M. (eds.). U. S. Public Health Service Publication No. 1390, Washington.
MARSHALL, J. M. (1965). *Initiation of labor*, pp. 16–25, 57–66. Marshall, J. M. and Burnet, W. M. (eds.). U.S. Public Health Service Publication, No. 1390, Washington.
MÉNDEZ-BAUER, C. J., CARBALLO, M. A., CABOT, H. M., NEGREIROS DE PAIVA, C. E. and GONZÁLEZ-PANIZZA, V. H. (1961). Studies on plasma oxytocinase. *Oxytocin*, pp. 325–335. Caldeyro-Barcia, R. and Heller, H. (eds.). Pergamon Press, Oxford.
PETERSEN, W. E. (1944). Lactation. *Physiol. Rev.*, 24: 340–371.
PICKFORD, M. (1961). Some extra-uterine actions of oxytocin. *Oxytocin*, pp. 68–79. Caldeyro-Barcia, R. and Heller, H. (eds.). Pergamon Press, Oxford.
PICKFORD, M. (1964). Effects of neurohypophysial hormones on the vascular system. *Proc. 2nd Int. Pharmac. Meeting*, pp. 31–35. Pergamon Press, Oxford.
SEMM, K. (1961). The significance of oxytocinase in pregnancy and labour. *Oxytocin*, pp. 336–340. Caldeyro-Barcia, R. and Heller, H. (eds.). Pergamon Press, Oxford.
THEOBALD, G. W. (1955). *The Pregnancy Toxaemias: or the Encymonic Atelositeses*, p. 80. Kimpton, London.
THEOBALD, G. W. (1961). The synthesis of divergent observations concerning oxytocin. *Oxytocin*, pp. 212–225. Caldeyro-Barcia, R. and Heller, H. (eds.). Pergamon Press, Oxford.
THEOBALD, G. W. (1963). Induction of labour and of premature labour. *British Obstetric Practice*, 3rd ed., pp. 1055–1088. Claye, A. (ed.). Heinemann, London.
THEOBALD, G. W. (1968). Oxytocin reassessed. *Obstet. Gynec. Survey*, 23: 109–131.
TUPPY, H. (1961). Biochemical studies of oxytocinase. *Oxytocin*, pp. 315–324. Caldeyro-Barcia, R. and Heller, H. (eds.). Pergamon Press, Oxford.

VAN DYKE, H. B., ADAMSON, K. JR. and ENGEL, S. L. (1955). Aspects of the biochemistry and physiology of the neurohypophysial hormones. *Recent Prog. Horm. Res.* **11**: 1-35.

WATSON, B. P. (1914). Development of obstetrics. *Can. Med. Ass. J.* **4**: 469-480.

ORIGINAL PAPERS

ALVAREZ, H. and CALDEYRO-BARCIA, R. (1950). Contractility of the human uterus recorded by new methods. *Surg. Gynec. Obstet.*, **91**: 1-13.

BELL, W. BLAIR (1909). Therapeutic value of the infundibular extract in shock, uterine atony and intestinal paresis. *Brit. Med. J.* **ii**: 1609-1613.

BENGTSSON, L. PH. and THEOBALD, G. W. (1966). The effects of oestrogen and gestagen on the non-pregnant human uterus. *J. Obstet. Gynaec. Brit. Cwlth.*, **73**: 273-281.

BERDE, B. and CERLETTI, A. (1958). Quantitative comparison of substances related to oxytocin: a new test. *Acta Endocr., Copnh.*, **27**: 314-324.

COCH, J. A., BROVETTO, J., CABOT, H. M., FIELITZ, C. A. and CALDEYRO-BARCIA, R. (1965). Oxytocin-equivalent activity in the plasma of women in labor and during the puerperium. *Amer. J. Obstet. Gynec.*, **91**: 10-17.

CRICHTON, E. C. (1920). Personal communication.

CROSS, B. A. and VAN DYKE, H. B. (1953). The effects of highly purified posterior pituitary principles on the lactating mammary gland of the rabbit. *J. Endocr.*, **9**: 232-235.

CULLEN, B. M. and HARKNESS, R. D. (1964). Effects of ovariectomy and of hormones on collagenous framework of the uterus. *Amer. J. Obstet. Gynec.*, **206**: 621-627.

DALE, H. H. and LAIDLAW, P. P. (1912). A method of standardizing pituitary (infundibular) extracts. *J. Pharmacol. Exp. Ther.*, **4**: 75-95.

DAVY, M. J. and LOCKETT, M. F. (1960). Actions and interactions of aldosterone monoacetate and neurohypophysial hormones on the isolated cat kidney. *J. Physiol., Lond.*, **152**: 206-219.

DEIS, R. P. and PICKFORD, M. (1964). The effect of autonomic blocking agents on uterine contractions of the rat and guinea-pig. *J. Physiol., Lond.*, **173**: 215-225.

DEMUNBRUN, T. W., KELLER, A. D., LEVKOFF, A. H. and PURSER, R. M. (Jr.). (1954). Pitocin restoration of renal hemodynamics to pre-neurohypophysectomy levels. *Amer. J. Physiol.*, **179**: 429-434.

DICKER, S. E. and HELLER, H. (1946). The renal action of posterior pituitary extract and its fractions as analysed by clearance experiments in rats. *J. Physiol., Lond.*, **104**: 353-360.

EVANS, D. H. L., SCHILD, H. O. and THESLEFF, S. (1958). Effects of drugs on depolarized plain muscle. *J. Physiol., Lond.*, **143**: 474-485.

FAIRWEATHER, D. V. I. (1965). Changes in serum non-esterified fatty acid levels in spontaneous and in oxytocin induced labour. *J. Obstet. Gynaec. Brit. Cwlth.*, **72**: 408-415.

FAIRWEATHER, D. V. I., SMART, D. and SMART, E. (1966). Personal communication.

VON FEKETE, K. (1930). Beiträge zur Physiologie der Gravidität. *Endokrinologie*, **7**: 364-369.

FERGUSON, J. K. W. (1962). Personal communication.

FLIEGNER, J. R. and HIBBARD, B. M. (1966). Active management of the third stage of labour. *Brit. Med. J.*, **ii**: 622-623.

FOLLEY, S. J. and KNAGGS, G. S. (1964). Observations on oxytocin release in ruminants. *J. Reprod. Fertil.*, **8**: 265–266.
FOLLEY, S. J. and KNAGGS, G. S. (1965a). Levels of oxytocin in the jugular vein blood of goats during parturition. *J. Endocr.*, **33**: 301–315.
FUCHS, A.-R. (1964). Oxytocin and the onset of labour in rabbits. *J. Endocr.*, **30**: 217–224.
FUCHS, A.-R. and FUCHS, F. (1963). Spontaneous motility and oxytocin response of the pregnant and non-pregnant human uterine muscle *in vitro*. *J. Obstet. Gynaec. Brit. Cwlth.*, **70**: 658–664.
HAEGER, K. and JACOBSOHN, D. (1953). A contribution to the study of milk ejection in women. *Acta Physiol. Scand.*, **30**: Suppl. 3., 152–160.
HAIGH, A. L., KITCHIN, A. H. and PICKFORD, M. (1963). The effect of oxytocin on handblood flow in man following the administration of an oestrogen and isoprenaline. *J. Physiol., Lond.*, **169**: 161–166.
HARKNESS, M. L. R. and HARKNESS, R. D. (1961). The mechanical properties of the uterine cervix of the rat during involution and after parturition. *J. Physiol., Lond.* **156**: 112–120.
HAWKINS, D. F. and NIXON, W. C. W. (1961). The influence of oestrogen and progesterone on the electrolytes of the human uterus. *J. Obstet. Gynaec. Brit.Cwlth.*, **68**: 62–67.
HENDRICKS, C. H. (1964). A new technique for the study of motility in the non-pregnant human uterus. *J. Obstet. Gynaec. Brit. Cwlth.*, **71**: 712–715.
HENDRICKS, C. H. (1966). Inherent motility patterns and response characteristics of the non-pregnant human uterus. *Amer. J. Obstet. Gynec.*, **96**: 824–843.
HENDRICKS, C. H. and BRENNER, W. E. (1964). Patterns of increasing uterine activity in late pregnancy and the development of uterine responsiveness to oxytocin. *Amer. J. Obstet. Gynec.*, **90**: 485–492.
HENDRICKS, C. H. and MOAWAD, A. H. (1965). Round ligament motility *in vivo* studies in man. *J. Obstet. Gynaec. Brit. Cwlth.*, **72**: 618–625.
HINDSON, J. C., SCHOFIELD, B. M., TURNER, C. B. and WOLFF, H. S. (1965). Parturition in the sheep. *J. Physiol., Lond.*, **181**: 560–567.
HOFBAUER, J. (1911). Hypophysenextrakt als Wehemittel. *Zentbl. Gynäk.*, **35**: 137–141.
HOFBAUER, J. and HOERNER, J. K. (1927). The nasal application of pituitary extract for the induction of labor. *Amer. J. Obstet. Gynec.*, **14**: 137–148.
HOWARTH, A. T., LUNDBORG, R. A. and THEOBALD, G. W. (1963). The antidiuretic effect of oxytocin in man. *J. Physiol., Lond.*, **168**: 16–17P.
KNAUS, H. H. (1925–26). On the active principles of the pituitary extract. *J. Pharm. Exp. Ther.*, **26**: 337–346.
KNAUS, H. H. (1926). The action of pituitary extract administered by the alimentary canal. *Brit. Med. J.*, **i**: 337–346.
KUMAR, D., RUSSELL, J. J. and BARNES, A. C. (1962). Studies in human myometrium during pregnancy. *Amer. J. Obstet. Gynec.*, **84**: 586–590.
LEVY, B. (1963). The intestinal inhibiting response to oxytocin, vasopressin and bradykinin. *J. Pharmacol. Exp. Ther.*, **140**: 356–366.
SACKS, B. (1924). Observations upon the vascular reactions in man in response to Infundin, with special reference to the behaviour of the capillaries and venules. *Heart*, **11**: 353–370.
SAAMELI, K. (1963). An indirect method for the estimation of oxytocin blood concentration and half-life in pregnant women near term. *Amer. J. Obstet. Gynec.*, **85**: 186–192.

SAAMELI, K. (1964). Quantitative comparison between oxytocin and four related neurohypophysial peptides on the human uterus in situ. Brit. J. Pharmacol. Chemother., **23**: 176–183.
SCHOFIELD, B. M. (1966). The increased extensibility of pregnant myometrium. J. Physiol., Lond., **182**: 690–694.
SCHOFIELD, B. M. and WOOD, C. (1964). Length-tension relation in rabbit and human myometrium. J. Physiol., Lond., **175**: 125–133.
SMYTH, C. N. (1957). The guard-ring tocodynamometer. J. Obstet. Gynaec. Brit. Cwlth., **64**: 59–66.
TENNENT, R. A. and BLACK, M. D. (1954). Surgical induction of labour in modern obstetric practice. Brit. Med. J., **ii**: 833–837.
THEOBALD, G. W. (1934). The alleged relation of hyperfunction of the posterior lobe of the hypophysis to eclampsia and the nephropathy of pregnancy. Clin. Sci., **1**: 225–239.
THEOBALD, G. W. (1936). A centre, or centres, in the hypothalamus controlling menstruation, ovulation, pregnancy and parturition. Brit. Med. J., **i**: 1038–1041.
THEOBALD, G. W. (1959). The separate release of oxytocin and antidiuretic hormone. J. Physiol., Lond., **149**: 443–461.
THEOBALD, G. W., GRAHAM, A., CAMPBELL, J., GANGE, P. D. and DRISCOLL, W. J. (1948). The use of post-pituitary extract in physiological amounts in obstetrics. Brit. Med. J., **2**: 123–127.
THEOBALD, G. W., KELSEY, H. A. and MUIRHEAD, J. M. B. (1956). The pitocin drip. J. Obstet. Gynaec. Brit. Cwlth., **63**: 641–662.
THEOBALD, G. W. and LUNDBORG, R. A. (1962). Changes in myometrial sensitivity to oxytocin provoked in different ways. J. Obstet. Gynaec. Brit. Cwlth., **69**: 417–427.
TUPPY, H. (1960). Personal communication.
VAN DEMARK, N. L. and HAYS, R. L. (1952). Uterine motility responses to mating. Amer. J. Physiol., **170**: 518–521.
VAN DONGEN, C. G. and MARSHALL, J. M. (1967). Effect of various hormones on the milk ejection response of tissue isolated from the rat mammary gland. Nature, Lond., **213**: No. 5076, 632–633.
VAN WAGENEN, G. S. and NEWTON, W. H. (1943). Pregnancy in the monkey after removal of the fetus. Surg. Gynec. Obstet., **77**: 539–543.
WATSON, B. P. (1922). Further experience with pituitary extract in the induction of labor. Amer. J. Obstet. Gynec., **4**: 603–608.

CHAPTER 12(b)

CLINICAL PHARMACOLOGY: VASOPRESSIN

Reginald Hall

Royal Victoria Infirmary, Newcastle upon Tyne
and
Department of Medicine
University of Newcastle upon Tyne

ARGININE vasopressin is the human antidiuretic hormone and this is its main role in man. The designation vasopressin is unfortunate, since vasopressin does not alter the blood pressure in physiological doses and in man its action on the cardiovascular system can only be demonstrated in pharmacological doses.

Three main topics will be considered in this section.

A. Vasopressin deficiency causing the syndrome of diabetes insipidus.
B. Inappropriate secretion of vasopressin.
C. The use of lysine vasopressin to test pituitary–adrenal function.

VASOPRESSIN DEFICIENCY (DIABETES INSIPIDUS)

Deficient production of vasopressin or failure of the renal tubules to respond to the hormone results in the passage of large volumes of dilute urine. As a consequence of the polyuria the patient is thirsty and drinks more.

HYPOTHALAMO-NEUROHYPOPHYSIAL DIABETES INSIPIDUS

About one-third of such cases are caused by primary and secondary tumors in the region of the pituitary though tumors do not usually cause diabetes insipidus unless there is suprasellar extension or surgical interference. Craniopharyngioma is the commonest suprasellar tumor causing diabetes insipidus which is also a feature of tumors of the pineal gland.

Metastatic carcinoma in the region may abolish the response to hyperosmolality without interfering with that to nicotine suggesting a different site of action of the two stimuli (see below).

In another third of the cases there is no apparent cause for the diabetes insipidus. Although viral or "degenerative" causes have been suggested, it seems likely that some such cases will eventually be shown to result from metabolic disturbances in the neurosecretory system.

A further third of cases result from a variety of lesions including trauma, the Hand–Schüller–Christian syndrome, sarcoidosis and other granulomata, syphilis, basal meningitis and encephalitis. After head injury, usually when there has been a fracture of the base of the skull, the polyuria may not be apparent for several days and may be followed by an interval of apparent improvement lasting a further few days. The diabetes insipidus which then follows is of variable severity and often remits by the end of a year.

A rare hereditary form of diabetes insipidus has been described transmitted as a Mendelian dominant and causing symptoms early in life (Rodeck, 1955).

NEPHROGENIC DIABETES INSIPIDUS

The renal tubules may fail to respond to vasopressin because of a genetic defect, transmitted as a sex-linked recessive, the polyuria occurring in males soon after birth. If untreated, the severe dehydration results in mental retardation. Family studies have revealed asymptomatic heterozygous female carriers who show slight impairment of maximum concentrating capacity. Potassium depletion, hypercalcemia and amyloidosis may also cause polyuria unresponsive to vasopressin.

Clinical features of diabetes insipidus. Polyuria is the main complaint, and sleep is very often disturbed. Attempts to limit the volume of urine by fluid restriction lead to intolerable thirst and dehydration. The daily urine output varies, often being in the region of 5 liters but occasionally as much as 20–30 liters. There may be evidence of a local lesion in the region of the pituitary

Diagnosis. This is often obvious from the clinical context, e.g. the polyuria which follows head injury or pituitary operations. There are many causes of polyuria which must be distinguished from diabetes insipidus. If there is polyuria with a urine volume less than 4 liters per day accompanied by a raised blood urea the diagnosis is likely to be chronic renal failure, hypercalciuria, potassium deficiency or Fanconi's syndrome. If the urine volume is greater than 5 liters per day with a normal blood urea, the diagnosis is more likely to be diabetes insipidus, compulsive water drinking, hypercalciuria or familial nephrogenic diabetes insipidus. Chronic renal failure often causes polyuria, possibly due to an osmotic diuresis induced by the load of urea presented to a limited number of nephrons. A salt diuresis may follow relief of urinary obstruction. Chronic pyelonephritis causes renal tubular defects and polyuria in some cases. Examination of the urine for albumin, casts, pus cells and organisms, and plasma urea and electrolyte estimations will indicate renal disease. In chronic renal disease the urine specific gravity is fixed at 1.010, whereas in most instances of diabetes insipidus the urinary specific gravity is about 1.001. In diabetes mellitus, polyuria with a high urine specific gravity results from the osmotic diuresis produced by glucose. Serum potassium and calcium estimations will usually indicate polyuria caused by hypokalemia and hypercalcemia. When these diseases have been excluded and the polyuria confirmed the diagnosis usually lies between diabetes insipidus and compulsive water drinking (psychogenic polydipsia). The primary defect in the latter is an increased water intake with secondary polyuria. Compulsive water drinkers are usually middle-aged women with some psychological abnormality. Normal or only marginally impaired vasopressin output or action can be demonstrated by the tests outlined below. Administration of vasopressin does not improve the symptoms in these patients and continued drinking may cause water intoxication, whereas in patients with impaired vasopressin secretion correction of the deficiency is always beneficial. The very rare hereditary nephrogenic diabetes insipidus is easily excluded by the lack of response to vasopressin.

Since vasopressin cannot be routinely assayed in the blood, its presence or absence is demonstrated by tests which normally stimulate its release. Vasopressin administration may be used to determine the efficiency of the kidney in concentrating urine.

Stimulation of endogenous vasopressin release. Vasopressin output from the pituitary may be increased by a rise in plasma osmolality and by a fall in plasma volume. The precise sites of the volume and osmoreceptors has not yet been determined. Since emotion and various drugs such as nicotine, morphine and ether stimulate vasopressin release they should be avoided during the period of investigation. Ethanol causes a diuresis by interfering with vasopressin release.

Plasma osmolality may be increased by restriction of fluid intake or by administration of hypertonic saline.

24-hour fluid deprivation test. The intake of fluids, ice-cream and fruit is prohibited for 24 hr. Plasma electrolytes and osmolality and urinary specific gravity or osmolality are measured at the beginning and periodically during the test. In normal subjects there is little change in plasma electrolytes or osmolality, there is a rise in urinary osmolality up to 1800 mOsm/kg H_2O and specific gravity usually up to 1.030. In severe diabetes insipidus there is evidence of hemoconcentration and failure of urinary concentration, the specific gravity of the urine seldom exceeding 1.010. The patient must be weighed at the beginning of the test and the procedure terminated if weight loss exceeds 3% of the original weight. The test can be dangerous if these precautions are not strictly adhered to and it should only be carried out in hospital. In some patients with compulsive water drinking, renal concentrating power is impaired and a clear distinction is occasionally difficult.

Six-and-a-half hour fluid deprivation test (Dashe et al., 1963). This is a most satisfactory test for routine use, being safe and simple to carry out. In *normal subjects* the initial serum osmolality reported was 285 ± 4.4 mOsm/kg water and the final value after $6\frac{1}{2}$ hr fluid deprivation was 286 ± 5.5 mOsm/kg. The urinary concentration rose to 756–1496 mOsm/kg and the urine/serum osmolality ratio for the last hour of the test was 3.8 ± 0.9 (1.9–5.2). In *diabetes insipidus* all 13 cases studied showed a plasma osmolality of 300 mOsm/kg or more by the end of the test, the final concentration exceeding the initial by an average of 12 mOsm/kg. Less concentrated urine was secreted, and the mean urine:serum ratio over the last hour was 0.93 ± 0.45. In patients with *pituitary damage not requiring vasopressin* variable results were obtained but usually there was a rise in serum osmolality during the test averaging 3.7 ± 4.7 mOsm/kg. In three cases of psychogenic polydipsia the initial serum osmolality ranged from 270–288 mOsm/kg and remained constant during the test. The urine/serum ratio was within the normal range.

Plasma osmolality. Isolated observations of plasma osmolality can help in the diagnosis of diabetes insipidus where the level is usually raised if the patient is not receiving treatment. Low values may be found if the patient with diabetes insipidus is being overtreated with vasopressin and in most cases of psychogenic polydipsia.

Infusion of hypertonic saline (Hickey and Hare, 1944). This test is not recommended for routine use. The large salt load may precipitate cardiac failure and may itself cause an osmotic diuresis preventing a fall in urine flow. Catheterization of the patient may be necessary to ensure accurate urine collections and this carries its own risk of introducing infection. The patient is hydrated initially by drinking 20 ml of water per kg body weight in three equal drinks at 20-min intervals over the first hour. Two and a half per cent sodium chloride solution is infused intravenously to give 0.25 ml per kg body weight over 45 min. Urine is collected, by catheter if necessary, at 15-min intervals during the hour before the infusion, during the infusion, and for 30 min afterwards. Urinary output is recorded as ml per minute at the end of each 15 min period. The diuresis initially established should exceed 5 ml/min before the saline infusion is started. In normal subjects hypertonic saline stimulates vasopressin output and there is a considerable reduction in urine flow both during and after the infusion. Failure of vasopressin release or action is indicated by a continued diuresis.

Oral sodium chloride test (Jadresic and Maira, 1962). This test depends on the rise of plasma osmolality produced by orally administered saline. A 1% sodium chloride solution by mouth increases the osmotic pressure of the plasma of the fasting patient by about the same amount as an intravenous injection of 2.5% sodium chloride after heavy hydration. The test is easily applied, is safe and can be carried out without elaborate equipment in outpatients. Intravenous infusion and catheterization are avoided. The procedure is as follows:

Day 1—fluids are withheld from midnight. The patient empties his bladder in the morning and drinks one liter of water in 15 min. Urine is passed at half-hourly intervals for 2 hr and the total volume passed is expressed as a percentage of 1 liter.

Day 2—as for Day 1 except that 1 liter of 1% sodium chloride is drunk instead of water.

In all subjects tested after the water load very nearly, or more than 70% of the volume ingested, was excreted in 2 hr.

With the saline solution normal subjects (20 were tested) excreted less than 25% of the load, and a similar result was obtained in one patient with psychogenic polydipsia. In two cases of polyuria with hypercalciuria the excretion was 46% and 34%. All seven patients with diabetes insipidus had a urinary excretion of over 65% and usually the value was similar to that obtained after the water load.

Nicotine test (Walker, 1949). Nicotine can be used to stimulate vasopressin output but enough must be given by inhalation or injection to cause nausea, sweating and dizziness. The fall in blood pressure which results may affect the glomerular filtration rate. Nicotine should not be given by injection to patients with coronary artery disease. The test is usually carried out without prior restriction of fluids. Nicotine acid tartrate is given cautiously intravenously over 3–5 min in a dose of 3–6 mg, the larger dose being given to smokers, or the smoke from two cigarettes is vigorously inhaled and the urine output is measured over the following 3 hr at hourly intervals. In normal subjects there is an 80% decrease in urine flow and a rise in urine concentration most marked in the first hour. Persistence of polyuria is seen in severe cases of diabetes insipidus but there is considerable overlap in partial cases. In some cases of diabetes insipidus polyuria cannot be reduced by hyperosmolality but is affected by nicotine. These findings suggest that the osmoreceptor center is separate from that responding to nicotine.

Administration of vasopressin. Administration of vasopressin to test the kidney's ability to respond to the hormone should theoretically precede the other tests outlined above. Vasopressin is given without any alteration in the patient's fluid intake, measurements of plasma osmolality and urine volume and osmolality should be recorded at $\frac{1}{2}$ –1 hr intervals for several hours. Fluid intake should also be measured and the patient's clinical condition assessed. Vasopressin may be administered intravenously (0.5–1.0 I. U. of aqueous Pitressin solution with caution (see p. 29)) or by intramuscular injection, e.g. vasopressin tannate in oil, 5 units. In normal persons the urine volume falls and a concentrated urine is produced. Depending on the fluid intake the plasma osmolality often falls. In patients with diabetes insipidus a normal response is usually obtained but occasionally subnormal responses are seen possibly as a result of tubular damage caused by the high fluid output. In patients with psychogenic polydipsia, unlike those with diabetes insipidus, fluid intake is unabated and signs of water intoxication may develop. Plasma osmolality falls and usually there is a fall in urine output and a variable rise in urine concentration depending on the degree of impaired tubular function which has resulted from the polyuria. In patients with nephrogenic diabetes insipidus urine concentration remains low and output high.

Treatment. Whenever possible the underlying cause should be treated, though diabetes insipidus may be aggravated or even induced by surgical interference in the pituitary-hypothalamic region.

Hydration. If fluid intake is inadequate because of admission to hospital, investigations, mental abnormality, damage to the adjacent thirst center or other reasons, dehydration rapidly occurs and adequate fluid should always be given.

Hormonal replacement therapy. There are four types of vasopressin preparation available differing in routes of administration, effectiveness and duration of action.

(a) *Pitressin tannate in oil.* Chronic diabetes insipidus can be treated with intramuscular or subcutaneous injections of Pitressin tannate in oil. The duration of action varies in different patients but usually daily or alternate day injections will be needed. Treatment should be started with 0.5 ml (ampoules are of 1 ml containing 5 I. U.) on alternate days and the dose varied according to response. The vial needs warming in water for several minutes prior to thorough shaking, otherwise the Pitressin tannate will not be suspended in the oil base. Injections should be given in the evening to ensure good control during the night and the site of injection should be varied. Allergic reactions are rare.

(b) *Aqueous Pitressin solution* (available in ampoules of 0.5 and 1.0 ml containing 20 I. U. per ml) is useful for diagnostic purposes and for treatment of acute diabetes insipidus, e.g. after pituitary surgery. Injections of 0.5–1.0 I.U. cause maximal antidiuresis; after intravenous injections the effect only lasts 1–2 hr. Pallor, elevation of blood pressure, angina, intestinal colic and uterine cramps may result if the dose is too large. Because of its brief action and the side effects mentioned this preparation has no place in the routine therapy of diabetes insipidus. Intravenous infusion of 20 units of aqueous Pitressin solution in 200 ml of 5% dextrose over 15–20 min may reduce portal venous pressure by reducing splanchnic arterial inflow and thereby reduce bleeding from esophageal varices (Edmunds and West, 1962). It has a somewhat limited value, but is worth trying.

(c) *Posterior pituitary powder* is a crude posterior pituitary extract containing vasopressin and oxytocin in equal amounts. It is usually available in 40 mg capsules equivalent to 40 units of vasopressin. Ten to fifty mg of the powder can be taken as snuff or insufflated into the nostril several times daily, after each micturition. Chronic rhinitis and ulceration can prove troublesome and bronchospasm or other allergic manifestations are not infrequent. Antibodies cross-reacting with human posterior pituitary can develop but these may not be clinically significant (Pepys *et al.*, 1966).

(d) *Lysine vasopressin nasal spray* (Sandoz) is available in spray containers of 5 ml containing 50 I.U. of synthetic lysine vasopressin, (Lypressin) in 1 ml. The patient should be advised to hold the container upright and spray the inside of one or both nostrils by squeezing the container. The dose of the spray can be adjusted to the patient's response by advising him to use it after each act of micturition. Five to 20 I.U. may be required 3-7 times daily or more. Side effects are uncommon, but nasal congestion with ulceration of nasal mucosa has been reported. There may be scope for an improved method of delivering the spray possibly at a fixed dose rate. Some patients find it difficult to use the spray effectively in its present form. Trial of the spray is recommended in patients who prefer to avoid intramuscular injections, who exhibit allergic reactions to other preparations and in those with mild to moderate diabetes insipidus. It may be a useful supplement to treatment with intramuscular long-acting vasopressin in severe cases. The spray is more expensive to use than alternative preparations (Dashe et al., 1964; Barltrop, 1963).

Diuretic agents. Chlorothiazide and benzothiadiazide (thiazide) diuretics cause a reduction in urine flow in patients with diabetes insipidus (Crawford and Kennedy, 1959). Other diuretics also have this effect which is maximal for the thiazide diuretics and diminishes progressively with mercurial compounds, spirolactones and triamterene in that order and is not exerted by acetazolamide (Migone and Ambrosoli, 1965). The diuretics are also effective in nephrogenic diabetes insipidus where vasopressin is ineffective.

Their mechanism of action is not fully understood and several factors may be involved. As a result of sodium loss and a reduction in plasma volume there is a fall in glomerular filtration rate. More complete reabsorption of glomerular filtrate at the proximal tubule causes reduction in the amount of salt and water presented to the distal tubule (Earley and Orloff, 1964) from which less sodium is reabsorbed because of the action of the thiazide. Hence a smaller volume of urine with a higher concentration of solute is produced. Other causes of a reduced filtration rate, e.g. dehydration and hypotension also cause a reduction in urine flow suggesting that this hypothesis is tenable, though not all patients show a fall in glomerular filtration rate after thiazides. The thiazides may also increase the permeability of the collecting ducts to water, an action suppressed by cortisone (Migone and Ambrosoli, 1965). The mechanism of action may also include a central thirst-reducing factor as well as the renal component (Skadhauge, 1963). These drugs are useful in patients who experience side effects with vasopressin and also in nephrogenic diabetes insipidus. They rarely reduce the urine volume to normal but a reduction to 50% of the urine output before treatment can usually be achieved. Doses similar to those used for the treatment of edema are necessary, e.g. 1.0–1.5 g chlorothiazide daily. Potassium depletion should be looked for and supplements of potassium may be necessary.

Chlorpropamide. Chlorpropamide, a sulfonylurea compound used in the treatment of diabetes mellitus has recently been reported to reduce urine flow in diabetes insipidus (Arduino *et al.*, 1966). In three patients with diabetes insipidus there was a reduction in free water clearance and urine output though no effect was obtained in two cases of nephrogenic diabetes insipidus. Even with doses of 500 mg per day there was no clinical manifestation of hypoglycemia. The action of the drug appears similar to that of vasopressin and further investigations are required to determine its usefulness and its mode of action.

INAPPROPRIATE SECRETION OF VASOPRESSIN

In 1938 Winkler and Crankshaw reported a patient with a carcinoma of the bronchus who had hyponatremia and a high rate of excretion of sodium in the urine. Schwartz *et al.* (1957) described two similar patients who excreted hypertonic urine despite having hypotonic plasma and an expanded extracellular fluid volume. They pointed out that the only known cause for secretion of hypertonic urine in the presence of hypotonic plasma is excess of vasopressin. They showed that the hyponatremia in these patients was largely dilutional and suggested that it was due to overproduction of vasopressin, which was inappropriate because under normal circumstances the low plasma osmolality should have reduced vasopressin output. Since then more than 25 patients have been described with this syndrome, all except one associated with oat cell carcinoma of the bronchus. The exception was a case of carcinoma of the duodenum (Lebacq and Delaere, 1965).

This dilutional hyponatremia may also occur in a wide variety of non-malignant conditions, e.g. after head injury (Epstein and Levitin, 1959; Carter, Rector and Seldin, 1961), in cerebrovascular disease (Goldberg and Handler, 1960), in pituitary tumors (Goldberg and Handler, 1960; van't Hoff and Zilva, 1961), in encephalitis, poliomyelitis and cerebral hemorrhage (Peters *et al.*, 1950), in tuberculous meningitis (Rapoport *et al.*, 1951), in a variety of non-malignant chest conditions, staphylococcal pneumonia (Stormont and Waterhouse, 1962) and pulmonary tuberculosis (Sims *et al.*, 1950), and in myxedema and acute intermittent porphyria (Goldberg, 1963).

Clinical features. The clinical features specific to dilutional hyponatremia are largely those of water intoxication with depression, lethargy, mental confusion, anorexia and generalized muscular weakness. They can easily be attributed to the underlying disease but usually respond promptly to correction of the hyponatremic state. There may also be hypothermia and prolongation of duration of the tendon reflexes such as occurs in hypothyroidism. Hyponatremia may be found before there is any other clinical evidence of bronchial carcinoma and should always alert the clinician to this diagnosis.

Investigations. The abnormalities found are the result of the inappropriate secretion of vasopressin causing overhydration. Plasma sodium is low, usually less than 120 mEq/l and occasionally as low as 100 mEq/l. Plasma chloride and urea are also low and plasma potassium is low or normal. Despite the low plasma sodium concentration there is no evidence of hemoconcentration and the hematocrit is normal or low. The plasma volume is normal or increased, the extracellular volume and the total body water are increased. Plasma osmolality is low, almost always less than 270 mOsm/kg and the urinary osmolality is higher than that of the plasma. The glomerular filtration rate, measured by inulin or creatinine clearance, is normal. There is excessive urinary loss of sodium despite the low plasma sodium level. This is probably due to reduction of aldosterone secretion consequent upon the expanded plasma volume. In a patient described by Barraclough *et al.* (1966) the rate of aldosterone secretion was measured and found to be low (9 μg/day compared with the normal range of 44–160 μg/day on a 96 mEq sodium intake). A majority of patients show an additional proximal renal tubular defect of reabsorption of glucose, amino acids, potassium and sodium, so that their hyponatremia is due to depletion as well as dilution. There may also be an acidification defect demonstrable when these patients are loaded with ammonium chloride. The aminoaciduria is of generalized distribution. It is possible that these proximal tubular defects are, at least in part, the result of potassium depletion. Patients with dilutional hyponatremia are unable to excrete a water load and this test can provide additional confirmation of the diagnosis. After a control collection of urine and serum, 20 ml of water per kg body weight is drunk in 1 hr and urine and serum collected at hourly intervals for a further 3 hr. Normal subjects showed a prompt fall in urine osmolality, an increase in free water clearance and prompt excretion of 52–98% of the water load in 3 hr (Lee *et al.*, 1961). By contrast patients with hyponatremia showed only a slight fall in urine osmolality, there was no significant free water clearance and less than 69% of the water load was excreted.

Differential diagnosis. Hyponatremia *per se* gives little information as to the sodium balance of an individual patient. It may be present when the total body sodium is high, low or normal. In various diseases associated with edema such as cirrhosis of the liver, congestive heart failure and the nephrotic syndrome, total body sodium may be increased in the presence of hyponatremia. Edema is not usually present in the syndrome under consideration. Depletion of total body sodium due to gastrointestinal loss, adrenocortical insufficiency and "salt-losing nephritis" may also be associated with hyponatremia. These conditions usually result in hemoconcentration, extrarenal uremia and hypotension. A raised blood urea concentration and hematocrit and a lowered plasma volume suggests sodium depletion. Patients with dilutional hyponatremia are not usually hypotensive.

Adrenocortical insufficiency causes most problems in diagnosis since it may also be the result of spread from a bronchogenic carcinoma. Skin pigmentation may occur in either condition. Tests of adrenocortical function easily differentiate the two disorders, plasma cortisol or 11-hydroxycorticosteroids showing a prompt rise after ACTH (or the synthetic ACTH preparation Synacthen) in patients with dilutional hyponatremia.

Pathogenesis. The cause of the hyponatremia and renal salt loss in patients with malfunction of the central nervous system is not fully understood. By inference they are likely to have inappropriate secretion of vasopressin probably of hypothalamic-pituitary origin but the nature of the stimulus causing this overproduction is unknown. Histological lesions were not found in the areas normally involved in vasopressin synthesis (Goldberg and Handler, 1960). It is possible that decreased blood flow to the volume receptor area, whose site is not yet precisely localized, might be responsible for increased vasopressin production in the presence of an expanded plasma volume. Patients with cerebrally-determined hyponatremia are usually in the older age group where cerebrovascular disease is common.

In hyponatremia of non-malignant pulmonary origin it is possible that displacement or stimulation of some receptor situated in the mediastinum may be involved. Receptors influencing urine volume are thought to be located in the right atrium but the mechanism involved is uncertain. Afferent stimuli from mediastinal receptors to the hypothalamus may run in the vagus nerve and constitute a further theoretical source of stimuli.

In hyponatremia associated with bronchogenic carcinoma there is now little doubt that the responsible agent is vasopressin produced in the tumor. In two such patients increased plasma levels of an antidiuretic compound have been demonstrated (Lee *et al.*, 1964; Bower *et al.*, 1964).

In both cases large amounts of antidiuretic material were extracted from the tumor. This finding makes it unlikely that reflex stimulation of hypothalamic-pituitary vasopressin production by the tumor was responsible, unless the tumor also had an increased avidity for the hormone. Unger *et al.* (1964) have suggested that certain malignant tumors act as hormonal sponges, accumulating various circulating hormones and releasing them intermittently as a result of breakdown of malignant cells. Strong evidence against the trapping hypothesis was provided by Bower *et al.* (1964) who reported a patient with the syndrome in whom there was complete destruction of the posterior pituitary and in whom no neurosecretory material could be demonstrated by specific staining in either the supraoptic or the paraventricular nuclei. Again the concentration of vasopressin found in tumors is often 100 times greater than that in the plasma even after the inevitable losses involved in processing and extracting the material. This level would imply a concentrating ability greater than that of any tissue apart from the neurohypophysis.

Further evidence that vasopressin is produced by the tumor is the improvement in the syndrome after radiotherapy (Ivy, 1961) or nitrogen mustard and radiotherapy (Schwartz *et al.*, 1960). After irradiation of a primary tumor it was found to contain lower levels of vasopressin than the non-irradiated secondaries (Bower *et al.*, 1964). It seems very likely therefore that the source of the vasopressin-like material is the tumor itself. The nature of the antidiuretic compound must next be considered. Final proof that the material is arginine vasopressin awaits chemical analysis of tumor tissue. Circumstantial evidence is strong that the material is indeed arginine vasopressin. Methods used for identification have so far been bioassay (Barraclough *et al.* 1966) and radioimmunoassay (Utiger, 1966). Barraclough *et al.* (1966) assayed plasma, urine and primary and secondary tumor material in the water loaded rat against synthetic arginine vasopressin as described by Lee *et al.* (1964). They concluded that the antidiuretic activity in the tumor and urine extracts could be ascribed to arginine vasopressin since the following requirements were fulfilled:

(1) The onset and duration of the antidiuresis and increase in urine conductivity were essentially similar for extracts and for arginine vasopressin. (2) There was no change in arterial pressure. (3) Assays measuring change in urine volume and change of urine conductivity gave virtually identical results. (4) The slopes of the log dose–response curves of arginine vasopressin and extracts were essentially parallel. (5) Treatment with 0.01 M sodium thioglycollate for 30 min abolished the activity. (6) During a mannitol diuresis in a rat the extract did not change the urine volume.

These criteria are adequate to distinguish arginine vasopressin from lysine vasopressin but do not themselves exclude the possibility that the material is some closely related peptide. Berde (1965) also found that tumor extract vasopressin had a potency ratio for antidiuretic, pressor and galactokinetic activity very similar to arginine vasopressin.

Utiger (1966) has described a patient with carcinoma of the lung and hyponatremia in whom tumor extracts contained large amounts of arginine vasopressin or some very closely related peptide when determined by radioimmunoassay. The active material was extracted from tissue by acetic acid. Gel filtration and alkali inactivation studies confirmed the similarity of the material to arginine vasopressin but the assay did not distinguish between arginine and lysine vasopressin. Bioassay and radio-immunoassay results agree that the material obtained from tumor extracts is likely to be arginine vasopressin but, as mentioned previously, final proof depends on complete chemical analysis.

Many different hormones can be secreted by tumors or tissues unlike those which are normally responsible for their synthesis. What then is the explanation for the synthesis of these hormones by tumors? Two explanations have been put forward. The first suggests that hormones are synthesized by chance as a result of the "chaotic protein synthesis characteristic of neoplastic growth" (Bower and Gordan, 1965). Mutations of the DNA of malignant cells would allow coding of peptides with endocrine activity. Only part of the hormone molecule is usually required for the full hormonal activity, e.g. 24 of the 39 aminoacids of the ACTH molecule. Identification of tumor extracts with the natural hormone by bioassay and radioimmunoassay procedures suggests that both biologically and immunologically active parts of the hormone molecule are being synthesized. Again the production of more than one hormone by a tumor is not uncommon and this also makes the theory of random synthesis less likely. Overproduction of vasopressin has been associated with overproduction of ACTH in cases reported by Liddle et al. (1965), Rees et al. (1960) and Daly et al. (1963).

A more likely possibility is that tumor cells, like all other cells (except the sex cells) inherit an identical complement of DNA and therefore all the coded information requisite for synthesis of all normal proteins. Differentiation of cells involves reversible repression of specific segments of the DNA molecule possibly by combination of DNA with histones. Much of the DNA of a normal cell is masked. The malignant cell could revert to synthesis of various peptides by inactivation of the histone repressor or by deletion of a regulator gene which normally is postulated to produce a repressor which combines with the operator slowing the manufacture of messenger RNAs (Hobbs and Miller, 1966; *Lancet*, 1967). If "de-repression" is involved in tumor hormone synthesis the hormone produced by the tumor should be identical with the natural hormone. Bioassay and radioimmunoassay procedure suggest that this is likely in the case of vasopressin, ACTH, insulin and gastrin but final proof awaits chemical analysis.

Although relatively few cases of hyponatremia associated with bronchogenic carcinoma have been reported, the syndrome is probably often overlooked. Ross (1964) reported that in 100 consecutive admissions of patients with bronchogenic carcinoma, two were found to have dilutional hyponatremia and two overproduction of ACTH.

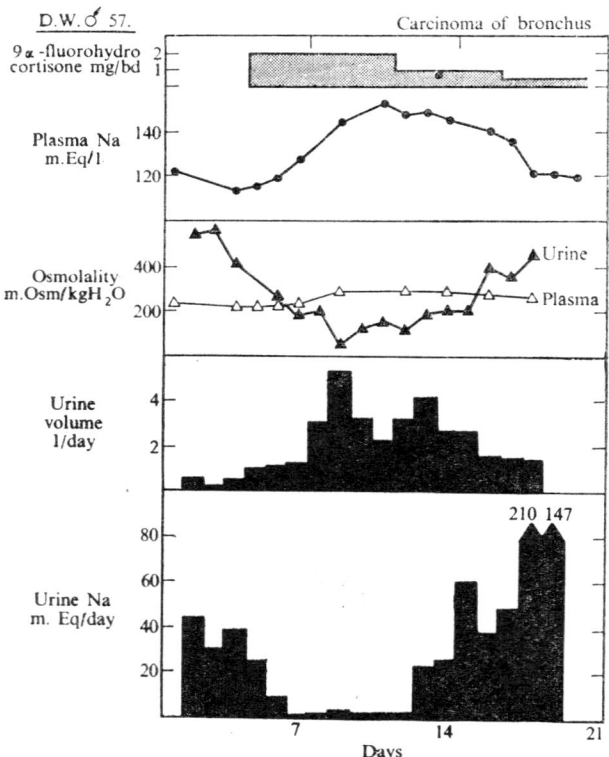

FIG. 1. Dilutional hyponatremia complicating carcinoma of the bronchus. Response to the administration of 9α-fluorohydrocortisone, 2 mg twice daily. (From Ross, E., 1964, by permission of Pitman Medical Publishing Co. Ltd.)

Therapy. Patients with dilutional hyponatremia respond well to limitation of fluid intake to about 1 liter per day and administration of 9α-fluorohydrocortisone in a dose of 2 mg twice daily if they do not have a proximal tubular defect (Fig. 1). There is a rapid rise in plasma sodium and the patient's mental state returns to normal. Hypokalemia may be caused

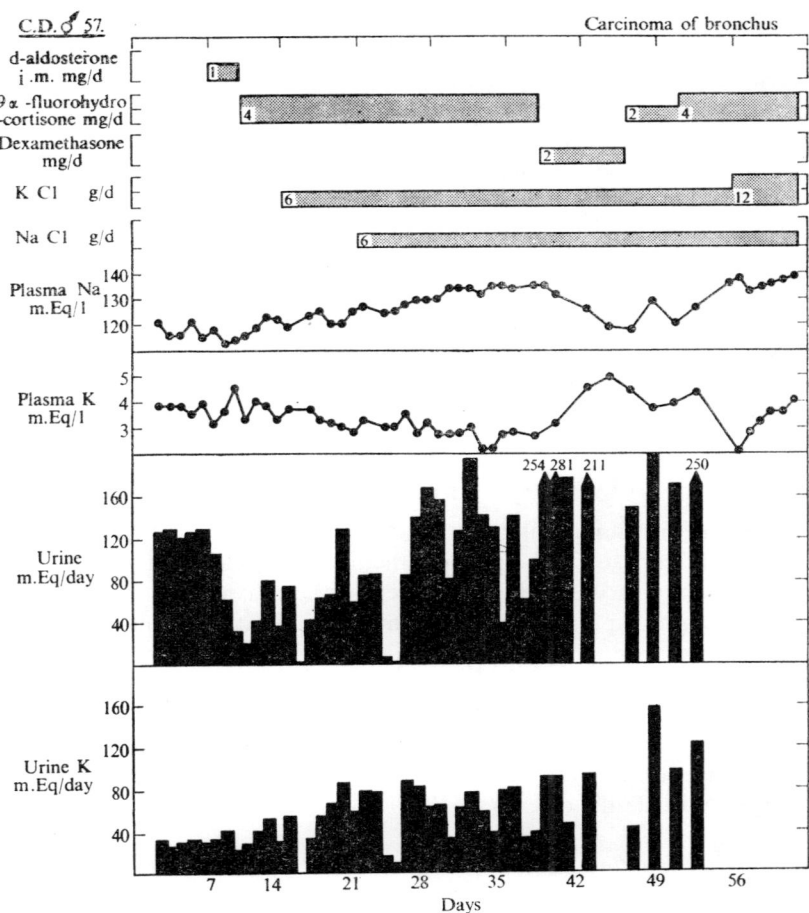

FIG. 2. Dilutional hyponatremia and renal tubular defect complicating carcinoma of the bronchus. Administration of 9α-fluorohydrocortisone failed to correct the hyponatremia until supplements of both NaCl and KCl were given. (From Ross, E., 1964, by permission of Pitman Medical Publishing Co. Ltd.)

by the large dose of mineralocorticoid, and potassium supplements may be necessary. If there is a proximal renal tubular defect in addition, large supplements of sodium and potassium are required as well as 9α-fluorohydrocortisone to restore plasma sodium and potassium to normal (Fig. 2). Treatment should also be directed to the tumor whenever possible and dramatic improvement may follow resection, chemotherapy or irradiation. It has been suggested that patients with bronchogenic carcinoma complicated by hyponatremia tend to have a better prognosis than might otherwise have been expected (Ross, 1964) but firm evidence for this impression is not yet available.

Preliminary observations in 23 patients with organic cerebral disease of neoplastic or other etiology and in four patients with non-pulmonary tumors without cerebral metastases suggest that injections of synthetic oxytocin, the release of which was retarded by addition of polyvinylpyrrolidone, in increasing doses along with ACTH resulted in clinical improvement (Bernard-Weil, 1966). Along with a rise in free water clearance there was an improvement in symptoms due to decreased cerebral edema and possibly in some patients an action on the tumor. Further studies are required to confirm these observations.

USE OF LYSINE VASOPRESSIN TO TEST PITUITARY-ADRENAL FUNCTION

Lysine vasopressin administration to patients causes a prompt rise in the level of cortisol in the plasma, mediated by release of ACTH from the anterior pituitary gland. Consequently the plasma cortisol response to lysine vasopressin has been used as a test of pituitary-adrenal function.

The present tests of pituitary-adrenal function depend on alterations in adrenocorticosteroid output to various stimuli. Hypothalamic, pituitary and adrenal abnormalities can be differentiated by different types of stimuli. Integrity of the adrenal cortex must be confirmed before it can be assumed that an impaired adrenal steroid response is due to pituitary-hypothalamic disease.

(1) *Adrenal function* can be tested directly by the steroid response to exogenous corticotrophin. (2) *Pituitary-hypothalamic function* can be tested in the presence of normal adrenals by: (a) Rise in plasma or urinary 17-hydroxycorticosteroid output in response to a metyrapone-induced fall in the plasma cortisol. This tests the so-called negative feed-back mechanism. (b) Rise in plasma cortisol in response to the stress of insulin-induced hypoglycemia or of pyrogen. (c) The fall in plasma or urinary

steroid output in response to high doses of synthetic steroids such as dexamethasone.

Tests that use corticotrophin as a stimulant evaluate only adrenocortical function while the corticotrophin-mediated adrenal response to stress or to alterations in the levels of circulating corticosteroids cannot be used to separate pituitary from hypothalamic lesions because they assess the integrity of the whole pituitary-adrenal axis. This complex situation has been well summarized by Cope (1965) who concludes that "the corticotrophin-release mechanism does not consist of a single center responding to stimulant, inhibitory or stressful stimuli but that a much more complex mechanism is involved in which each of these forms of influence is capable of exerting its own effect independently of the others and probably through a separate chain of events".

Mechanism of action of lysine vasopressin. The mechanism by which lysine vasopressin causes a rise in plasma cortisol in man is not yet fully understood. It could act on the hypothalamus or higher centers, on the pituitary or on the adrenal cortex. Its site of action certainly varies in different species and results obtained in animal experiments cannot necessarily be applied to man. In the dog, vasopressin acts directly on the adrenal causing a rise in the 17–OHCS levels in the adrenal veins of hypophysectomized animals (Hume, 1958) and after injections into the adrenal artery (Andersen and Egdahl, 1964). In man, however, lysine vasopressin is unlikely to act directly on the adrenal cortex since in patients who had received long-term adrenal steroid therapy and in whom adrenal responsiveness had been restored by corticotrophin, further administration of corticotrophin caused a sharp rise in plasma cortisol whereas no such effect could be produced by lysine vasopressin (Landon et al., 1965). Again Clayton et al. (1965) observed that prior administration of a single dose of dexamethasone abolished the response to lysine vasopressin, though not to corticotrophin (Gwinup, 1965). Further studies are required to give final confirmation that lysine vasopressin does not act directly on the adrenal cortex in man. These would include estimations of plasma ACTH levels after vasopressin administration and observations showing that vasopressin does not act in the acutely hypophysectomized patient. Experiments have already shown that in the rat hypophysectomy abolishes the effect of vasopressin (Vernikos-Danellis, 1964).

The claims of Landon et al. (1965) and of Gwinup (1965a and 1965b) that lysine vasopressin acts directly on the anterior pituitary in man warrant consideration. Release of corticotrophin from the anterior pituitary involves a humoral factor (or factors) designated corticotrophin-releasing factor (CRF) produced by the hypothalamus. The precise nature of CRF is not yet determined, though three such compounds have been isolated, they have been considered to be polypeptides, α_1 and α_2 types of CRF being related to α-M.S.H., and β-CRF to vasopressin. The ACTH-releasing activity of β-CRF is 50–100 times greater than that of α_1-CRF. Before accepting that a substance is a corticotrophin-releasing factor and is not acting as a trigger stimulating the release of endogenous CRF the following criteria should be satisfied (Leeman et al., 1962). The substance must: (a) Stimulate an increase in the rate of adrenal cortical secretion. (b) Fail to stimulate such an increase in recently hypophysectomized animals. (c) Fail to alter the response to exogenous ACTH. (d) Provoke an adrenal cortical response in animals in which the release of endogenous corticotrophin-releasing neurohumor has been impaired by a C.N.S. lesion or by a pharmacological agent. (e) The response in (d) would be identical with that in (a).

It has not yet been possible to apply all of these criteria to the study of the response to lysine vasopressin in man. There is general agreement that prior administration of morphine (McDonald et al., 1959; Gwinup, 1965) or of dexamethasone (Clayton et al., 1965; Gwinup, 1965) blocks the response to lysine vasopressin. These findings suggest that in man the site of dexamethasone and morphine inhibition is distal to or at the site of stimulation of vasopressin release in the CNS and that vasopressin does not itself act as a corticotrophin-releasing factor.

The bulk of the evidence available at present suggests that lysine vasopressin acts at some hypothalamic site. In rats, lysine vasopressin stimulates pituitary ACTH output while leaving the pituitary ACTH content unchanged, indicating stimulation of both synthesis and release of ACTH (de Wied, 1967). It is unlikely that the adrenal stimulation resulting from vasopressin administration is due to its hemodynamic effects. In animals there is no correlation between the vasopressin-induced rise in blood pressure and increased steroid output (de Wied et al., 1968) while in man there is usually no alteration in blood pressure with doses of lysine vasopressin sufficient to increase steroid output (Gwinup, 1965). It is also possible that the site or sites of action depends on the dose of vasopressin and the substance may act at multiple sites in the CNS including the hypothalamus and higher centers.

Landon et al. (1965) and Greenwood and Landon (1966) have compared the adrenal response to lysine vasopressin with other tests of pituitary adrenal function in patients with pituitary or hypothalamic disorders and in normal controls. Patients with pituitary tumors responded in three ways. In some of them all tests were normal, showing the integrity of the whole system. In others all tests were abnormal, since disturbance of function was enough to cause adrenal atrophy. A third group of patients had a normal response to lysine vasopressin and corticotrophin but not to metyrapone or insulin. In these patients there was evidence of suprasellar extensions of the tumor and they responded to the tests in the same way as patients with presumed hypothalamic lesions. This clinical evidence appears to support the view that a normal response to the lysine vasopressin test combined with abnormal responses to metyrapone or insulin indicates a lesion in the hypothalamus rather than in the pituitary. An alternative—and at present more likely—possibility is that lysine vasopressin acts on hypothalamic centers different from those involved in the other tests. It is of interest that lysine vasopressin stimulates growth hormone output in some normal subjects but the presence or absence of the response does not appear to be correlated with the changes in plasma cortisol or sugar levels (Greenwood and Landon, 1966). Figure 3 summarizes the tests used at present to determine pituitary-adrenal function.

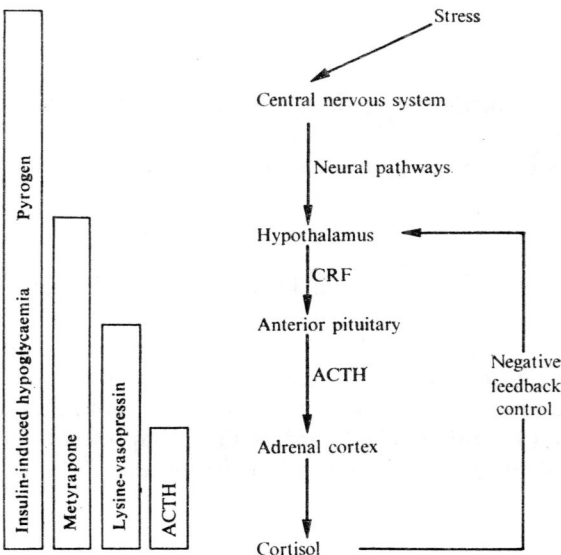

FIG. 3. Diagram of the tests of the mechanism controlling the secretion of cortisol. (From Greenwood and Landon, 1966, by permission of the *Journal of Clinical Pathology.*)

Methods of carrying out the lysine vasopressin test vary but all entail measurement of the baseline level of plasma cortisol usually by Mattingly's method for the determination of 11-hydroxycorticosteroids (Mattingly, 1962), followed by administration of lysine vasopressin and serial estimations of plasma "cortisol". The procedure recommended by Gwinup (1965) is satisfactory for routine use, synthetic [Lys^8]-vasopressin (Sandoz), 10 pressor units, being given intramuscularly (Gwinup, 1965). Venous blood specimens are taken immediately before and 30, 60, 90 and 120 min after injection of vasopressin and assayed for plasma "cortisol". Normal subjects had a prompt rise in plasma "cortisol" with a peak at 1 hr (mean value 36.2 μg/100 ml). All controls had levels above 23.6 μg/100 ml after 1 hr whereas patients with pituitary disease showed an impaired response. Nelson et al. (1966), however, reported that in 6 of 16 tests in control subjects a level of 23.6 μg/100 ml was not achieved in either 30 or 60 min specimens, so that impaired response to intramuscular lysine vasopressin must be interpreted with caution.

Landon et al. (1965) studied the plasma "cortisol" response at half-hourly intervals to the intravenous infusion of lysine vasopressin at a rate of 5 pressor units per hour for 2 hr in 19 control subjects. The maximum increase of plasma cortisol during the test ranged from 5.6 to 33.5 μg/100 ml with a mean rise of 13.1 ± 6.6 μg (S.D.). The intravenous infusion test is to be preferred if there is any possibility that the patient is suffering from ischemic heart disease since the infusion can be slowed or stopped at any time. Side effects have been slight including pallor, increased intestinal motility and uterine contractions. It would seem wise to avoid the test in patients with clinical evidence of ischemic heart disease and to check the electrocardiogram routinely before the test, since vasopressin may constrict coronary vessels (Ribot et al., 1961).

Further studies are required to localize the precise site of action of lysine vasopressin in man. The evidence is suggestive that it acts by way of pituitary corticotrophin release and not by direct stimulation of the adrenal cortex. Whether the present claims of a direct pituitary action are substantiated or not, it should prove a useful tool in the investigation of pituitary and hypothalamic disorders since it appears to act by mechanisms independent of those involved in existing tests.

REFERENCES

BOOKS, REVIEWS, AND MONOGRAPHS

BERDE, B. (1965). Les analogues synthétiques des hormones neurohypophysaires. Sont-ils une clef de l'étude des troubles de l'hormonogenèse de ce système. *Extrait de les troubles congénitaux de l'hormonogenèse. Rapports de la VIIIe réunion des endocrinologistes de langue française.*

BOWER, B. F. and GORDAN, G. S. (1965)^s. Hormonal effects of non-endocrine tumors. *Ann. Rev. Med.*, **16**: 83–118.

COPE, C. L. (1965). *Adrenal Steroids and Disease*, pp. 297. Pitman, London.

DALY, J. J., NELSON, M. A. and ROSE, D. P. (1963). Hyponatraemia with carcinoma of the bronchus, *Postgrad. Med. J.*, **39**: 158–159.

DE WIED, D., BOHUS, B., ERNST, A. M., DE JONG, W., NIEUWENHUIZEN, W., PIEPER, E. E. M., and YASUMURA, S. (1968). Several aspects of the influence of vasopressin on pituitary-adrenal activity. *Mem. Soc. Endocr.* **17**: 159–172.

HUME, D. M. (1958). *Pathophysiologia Diencephalica*, Curri, S. B., Martini, L. and Kovac, W. (eds.). Springer, Wien.

JAMES, V. H. T. and LANDON, J. (Eds.) (1968). The investigation of hypothalamic-pituitary-adrenal function. *Mem. Soc. Endocr.* **17**.

LIDDLE, G. W., GIVENS, J. R., NICHOLSON, W. E. and ISLAND, D. P. (1965). The ectopic ACTH syndrome. *Proc. 2nd Int. Congress of Endocrinology*, part 2, pp. 1063–1067. Taylor, S. (ed.). Excerpta Medica, London.

RODECK, H. (1955). Diabetes insipidus und primäre Oligurie. *Ergebn. Inn. Med. Kinderheilk.* **6**: 185–277.

ROSS, E. (1964). Hormonal syndromes in carcinoma of the bronchus. *Symposium on Advanced Medicine*. Compston, M. (ed.). Pitman, London.

ORIGINAL PAPERS

ANDERSEN, R. N. and EGDAHL, R. H. (1964). Effect of vasopressin on pituitary-adrenal secretion in the dog. *Endocrinology*, **74**: 538–542.

ARDUINO, F., FERRAZ, F. P. J. and RODRIGUES, J. (1966). Antidiuretic action of chloropropamide in idiopathic diabetes insipidus. *J. Clin. Endocr.*, **26**: 1325–1328.

BARLTROP, D. (1963). Diabetes insipidus treated with synthetic lysine vasopressin. *Lancet*, **ii**: 276–278.

BARRACLOUGH, M. A., JONES, J. J. and LEE, J. (1966). Production of vasopressin by anaplastic oat cell carcinoma of the bronchus. *Clin. Sci.*, **31**: 135–144.

BERNARD-WEIL, R. E. (1966). Effects of oxytocin on syndromes of inappropriate vasopressin secretion, in particular in cancer patients. *Schweiz. Med. Wschr.* **96**: 212–217.

BOWER, B. F., MASON, D. M. and FORSHAM, P. H. (1964). Bronchogenic carcinoma with inappropriate antidiuretic activity in plasma and tumor. *New Engl. J. Med.* **271**: 934–938.

CARTER, N. W., RECTOR, F. C. and SELDIN, D. W. (1961). Hyponatremia in cerebral disease resulting from the inappropriate secretion of antidiuretic hormone. *New Engl. J. Med.*, **264**: 67–72.

CLAYTON, G. W., LIBRIK, L., HORAN, A. and SUSSMAN, L. (1965). Effect of corticosteroid administration on vasopressin-induced adrenocorticotrophin release in man. *J. Clin. Endocr.*, **25**: 1156–1162.

CRAWFORD, J. D. and KENNEDY, G. C. (1959). Chlorothiazide in diabetes insipidus. *Nature, Lond.*, **183**: 891–892.

DASHE, A. M., CRAMM, R. E., CRIST, C. A., HABENER, J. F. and SOLOMON, D. H. (1963). A water deprivation test for the differential diagnosis of polyuria. *J. Amer. Med. Ass.*, **185**: 699–703.

DASHE, A. M., KLEEMAN, C. R., CZACZKES, J. W., RUBINOFF, H. and SPEARS, I. (1964). Synthetic vasopressin nasal spray in the treatment of diabetes insipidus. *J. Amer. Med. Ass.*, **190**: 1069–1071.

EARLEY, L. E. and ORLOFF, J. (1962). The mechanism of antidiuresis associated with the administration of hydrochlorothiazide to patients with vasopressin-resistant diabetes insipidus. *J. Clin. Invest.*, **41**: 1988–1997.

EDMUNDS, R. and WEST, S. P. (1962). A study of the effect of vasopressin on portal and systemic blood pressure. *Surgery Gynec. Obstet.*, **114**: 458–462.

EPSTEIN, F. H. and LEVITIN, H. (1959). "Cerebral salt-wasting": an example of sustained inappropriate release of antidiuretic hormone. *J. Clin. Invest.*, **38**: 1001.

GOLDBERG, M. and HANDLER, J. S. (1960). Hyponatremia and renal wasting of sodium in patients with malfunction of the central nervous system. *New Engl. J. Med.*, **263**: 1037–1043.

GOLDBERG, M. (1963). Hyponatremia and the inappropriate secretion of antidiuretic hormone. *Amer. J. Med.*, **35**: 293–298.

GREENWOOD, F. C. and LANDON, J. (1966). Assessment of hypothalamic pituitary function in endocrine disease. *J. Clin. Path.*, **19**: 284–292.

GWINUP, G. (1965a). Studies on the mechanism of vasopressin-induced steroid secretion in man. *Metabolism*, **14**: 1282–1286.

GWINUP, G. (1965b). Test for pituitary function using vasopressin. *Lancet*, **2**: 572–573.

HICKEY, R. C. and HARE, K. (1944). The renal excretion of chloride and water in diabetes insipidus. *J. Clin. Invest.*, **23**: 768–775.

HOBBS, C. B. and MILLER, A. L. (1966). Review of endocrine syndromes associated with tumours of non-endocrine origin. *J. Clin. Path.*, **19**: 119–127.

IVY, H. K. (1961). Renal sodium loss and bronchogenic carcinoma. *Archs Intern. Med.*, **108**: 47–55.

JADRESIC, A. and MAIRA, J. (1962). A simple test for the diagnosis of diabetes insipidus. *Lancet*, **i**: 402–403.

Lancet Leader, (1967). Hormones and histones? *Lancet*, **i**: 86–87.

LANDON, J., JAMES, V. H. T. and STOKER, D. J. (1965). Plasma cortisol response to lysine vasopressin. Comparison with other tests of human pituitary-adrenocortical function. *Lancet*, **ii**: 1156–1159.

LEBACQ, E. and DELAERE, J. (1965). Origine des substances antidiurétiques et explication de l'hypernatriurie dans le syndrome de Schwartz-Bartter. *Ann. Endocr.*, **26**: 375–382.

LEE, W. Y., GRUMER, H. A., BRONSKY, D. and WALDSTEIN, S. S. (1961). Acute water loading as a diagnostic test for the inappropriate ADH syndrome. *J. Lab. Clin. Med.*, **58**: 937.

LEE, J., JONES, J. J. and BARRACLOUGH, M. A. (1964). Inappropriate secretion of vasopressin. *Lancet*, **ii**: 792–793.

LEEMAN, S. E., GLENISTER, D. W. and YATES, F. E. (1962). Characterization of a calf hypothalamic extract with adrenocorticotropin-releasing properties: evidence for a central nervous system site for corticosteroid inhibition of adrenocorticotropin release. *Endocrinology*, **70**: 249–262.

MATTINGLY, D. (1962). A simple fluorimetric method for the estimation of free 11-hydroxycorticoids in human plasma. *J. Clin. Path.*, **15**: 374–379.

MCDONALD, R. K., EVANS, F. T., WEISE, V. K. and PATRICK, R. W. (1959). Effect of morphine and nalorphine on plasma hydrocortisone levels in man. *J. Pharmacol. Exp. Ther.*, **125**: 241–247.

MIGONE, L. and AMBROSOLI, S. (1965). Antidiuresis induced by saluretics in diabetes insipidus. *Minerva nefrol.*, **12**: 1–12.

NELSON, J. K., MACKAY, J. S., SHERIDAN, B. and WEAVER, J. A. (1966). Intermittent therapy with corticotrophin. *Lancet*, **ii**: 78–83.

PEPYS, J., JENKINS, P. A., LACHMANN, P. J. and MAHON, W. E. (1966). An iatrogenic autoantibody: immunological responses to "pituitary snuff" in patients with diabetes insipidus. *Clin. Exp. Immunol.*, **1**: 377–389.

PETERS, J. P., WELT, L. G., SIMS, E. A. H., ORLOFF, J. and NEEDHAM. J. (1950). A salt-wasting syndrome associated with cerebral disease. *Trans. Ass. Amer. Physns.*, **63**: 57–64.

RAPOPORT, S., WEST, C. D. and BRODSY, W. A. (1951). Salt losing conditions: renal defect in tuberculous meningitis. *J. Lab. Clin. Med.*, **37**: 550–561.

REES, J. R., ROSALKI, S. B. and MACLEAN, A. D. W. (1960). Hyponatraemia and impaired renal tubular function with carcinoma of bronchus. *Lancet*, **ii**: 1005–1009.

RIBOT, S., GREEN, H., SMALL, M. J. and ABRAMOWITZ, S. (1961). Cardiovascular effects of vasopressin. *Amer. J. Med. Sci.*, **242**: 612–619.

SCHWARTZ, W. B., BENNETT, W., CURELOP, S. and BARTTER, F. C. (1957). A syndrome of renal sodium loss and hyponatremia probably resulting from inappropriate secretion of antidiuretic hormone. *Amer. J. Med.*, **23**: 529–542.

SCHWARTZ, W. B., TASSEL, D. and BARTTER, F. C. (1960). Further observations on hyponatremia and renal sodium loss probably resulting from inappropriate secretion of antidiuretic hormone. *New Engl. J. Med.*, **262**: 743–748.

SIMS, E. A. H., WELT, L. G., ORLOFF, J. and NEEDHAM. J. W. (1950). Asymptomatic hyponatremia in pulmonary tuberculosis. *J. Clin. Invest.*, **29**: 1545–1557.

SKADHAUGE, E. (1963). Investigations into the thiazide-induced antidiuresis in patients with diabetes insipidus. *Acta Med. Scand.*, **174**: 739–749.

STORMONT, J. M. and WATERHOUSE, C. (1962). Severe hyponatremia associated with pneumonia. *Metabolism*, **11**: 1181–1186.

UNGER, R. H., LOCHNER, J. DE V. and EISENTRAUT, A. M. (1964). Identification of insulin and glucagon in a bronchogenic metastasis. *J. Clin. Endocr. Metab.*, **24**: 823–831.

UTIGER, R. D. (1966). Inappropriate antidiuresis and carcinoma of the lung: detection of arginine vasopressin in tumour extracts by immunoassay. *J. Clin. Endocr. Metab.*, **26**: 970–974.

VAN'T HOFF, W. and ZILVA, J. F. (1961). Chromophobe adenoma and hyponatraemia. *Clin. Sci.*, **21**: 345–354.

VERNIKOS-DANELLIS, J. (1964). Estimation of corticotropin-releasing activity of rat hypothalamus and neurohypophysis before and after stress. *Endocrinology*, **75**: 514–520.

WALKER, J. M. (1949). The effect of smoking on water diuresis in man. *Quart. J. Med.*, N. S. **18**: 51–55.

WINKLER, A. W. and CRANKSHAW, O. F. (1938). Chloride depletion in conditions other than Addison's disease. *J. Clin. Invest.*, **17**: 1–6.

AUTHOR INDEX

Aanning, H. L.   43, 57, 58, 179, 228
Abarbanel, A. R.   286, 292
Abel, J. J.   133, 144
Abrahams, V. C.   119, 123, 126, 127, 129, 144, 203, 212, 255, 257, 262, 267
Abramowitz, S.   442, 445
Abrash, L.   41, 42, 43, 51, 156, 165, 170
Acher, R.   5, 12, 25, 30, 32, 41, 49, 50, 51, 64, 65, 66, 67, 68, 69, 72, 76, 78, 90, 100, 106, 114, 133, 136, 141, 144, 145, 156, 168, 173, 178, 180, 182, 210, 212, 213, 215, 286, 292, 308, 314
Adams, C. W. M.   4, 12, 157, 171
Adams, J. Q.   183, 222
Adamsons, K. Jr.   112, 113, 115, 117, 142, 144, 173, 174, 175, 177, 178, 185, 190, 192, 194, 195, 199, 211, 213, 278, 298, 304, 305, 314, 401, 420, 422
Agishi, Y.   48, 50
Albergoni, V.   197, 222
Albers, R.   165, 169
Alcaraz, M.   300, 315
Aldrich, T. B.   5, 14, 62, 78, 178, 191, 221
Alexander, C. S.   240, 267
Ali, M. N.   262, 267
Allmark, M. G.   199, 222
Althabe, O. Jr.   198, 213, 307, 308, 315
Altman, J.   387, 395
Alvarado, R. H.   334, 335, 344
Alvarez, H.   414, 417, 420
Ambrosoli, S.   430, 445
Ames, R. G.   114, 118, 119, 127, 144, 183, 189, 208, 213, 227, 243, 250, 267, 278, 387, 393
Amiard, G.   27, 57
Anand, N.   35, 36, 51
Andersen, B.   358, 373
Andersen, R. N.   439, 443
Anderson, J.   332, 347, 362, 363, 374
Anderson, R. R.   197, 213
Andersson, B.   8, 12, 122, 126, 127, 128, 141, 144, 190, 213

Anselmino, K. J.   189, 213
Appelmans. F.   116, 144, 147
Aragon, G. T.   185, 218
Arduino, F.   431, 443
Arimura, A.   177, 182, 192, 213
Armstrong, D. A. J.   201, 202, 213
Arnott, D. J.   157, 171
Arnt, I. C.   198, 213, 307, 308, 315
Aroskar, J. P.   47, 52, 381, 388, 393
Assali, N. S.   230, 267
Assenmacher, I.   340, 344
Astwood, E. B.   133, 148, 165, 170
Atz, J. W.   324, 343
Au, W. Y. W.   254, 276
Audrain, L.   208, 213
Aujard, C.   201, 213, 388, 393
Austin, J. H.   183, 185, 186, 220
Austin, J. M.   242, 274
Aynedjian, H. S.   252, 267
Azimov, G. I.   312, 315

Bachinski, W. M.   199, 222
Baddeley, R. M.   300, 316
Baez, S.   126, 144
Bailey, P.   201, 227
Baird, S.   255, 257, 262, 267
Baïsset, A.   264, 265, 267
Bangham, D. R.   174, 213
Bank, N.   252, 267
Baratz, R. A.   127, 144, 188, 213
Barer, R.   4, 12 117, 118, 119, 120, 121, 125, 138, 139, 144, 156, 169
Bargmann, W.   3, 4, 12, 111, 133, 142, 144, 145, 156, 157, 169, 312, 315
Barltrop, D.   430, 443
Barnes, A. C.   407, 409, 412, 418, 421
Barnett, H. L.   246, 250, 251, 254, 267, 271
Barnett, R. J.   168, 170
Barondes, S.   159, 170
Barraclough, M. A.   264, 265, 267, 432, 433, 434, 443, 444

Barrett, J. F. 45, 56
Bartlett, M. F. 19, 28, 51
Bartos, J. 27, 57
Bartošek, I. 47, 50
Bartter, F. C. 249, 252, 264, 272, 274, 431, 434, 445
Barýshnikov, I. A. 296, 304, 313
Bashore, R. A. 48, 50
Bastide, F. 64, 76, 100, 101, 105
Bates, R. W. 177, 218
Bateson, R. 158, 171
Bauer, M. H. 7, 15
Bauman, J. W. Jr. 253, 267, 268
Bayo Bayo, J. 200, 218
Beasley, H. K. 253, 272
Beaulier, G. 4, 15, 117, 145, 156, 164, 170
Beaupain, D. 69, 76
Beauvillain, A. 200, 213
Beck, D. 252, 271, 275
Beleslin, D. 123, 124, 127, 128, 145, 208, 214
Bell, G. H. 201, 203, 214
Beller, F. K. 197, 214, 296, 315
Belugina, O. P. 312, 315
Bengtsson, L. Ph. 407, 408, 409, 420
Bennett, C. M. 231, 232, 233, 234, 235, 236, 240, 244, 245, 254, 268, 273, 275
Bennett, W. 431, 445
Benoit, J. 340, 346
Benson, G. K. 8, 12, 296, 311, 312, 313, 315, 379, 392
Bentley, P. J. 92, 94, 100, 106, 200, 204, 205, 206, 214, 217, 230, 273, 284, 287, 292, 322, 323, 324, 328, 329, 331, 332, 333, 334, 335, 336, 337, 340, 341, 342, 343, 344, 345, 346, 348, 371, 373
Berankova-Ksandrova, Z. 103, 104, 106, 189, 203, 207, 214, 305, 306, 309, 310, 315
Bercu, B. A. 387, 393
Berde, B. 36, 48, 53, 57, 81, 86, 87, 88, 89, 92, 97, 98, 99, 105, 106, 108, 174, 175, 194, 201, 203, 204, 206, 210, 211, 214, 215, 220, 226, 260, 268, 288, 290, 292, 296, 298, 305, 307, 308, 309, 313, 315, 339, 342, 401, 404, 405, 418, 420, 435, 443
Bergmann, F. 183, 224
Berkeley, H. J. 2, 12
Berliner, R. W. 190, 221, 231, 232, 233, 234, 235, 236, 240, 245, 246, 250, 254, 266, 268, 273, 274, 275
Berlyne, G. M. 239, 268, 371, 373
Bern, H. 111, 130, 142, 156, 169
Bernard–Weil, R. E. 260, 268, 438, 443
Berne, R. M. 127, 153, 163, 181, 227
Berrifield, M. 73, 74, 78
Berthet, L. 372, 373
Bespalova J. D. 36, 50
Beuzeville, C. F. 380, 382, 386, 387, 388, 393, 394, 395
Beyer, C. 300, 315, 318
Beyerman, H. C. 27, 50
Bhagavan, N. V. 160, 170
Biesold, B. 117, 148
Bilek, J. 302, 315
Birkhimer, C. A. 30, 32, 50
Birnie, J. H. 183, 185, 214
Bisset, G. W. 89, 90, 103, 104, 105, 106, 123, 124, 126, 127, 128, 145, 165, 170, 178, 186, 187, 189, 191, 192, 196, 199, 201, 203, 207, 208, 211, 214, 215, 257, 268, 298, 305, 306, 309, 310, 315, 410, 418
Black, M. D. 412, 422
Blackmore, K. E. 126, 152, 183, 185, 220
Blackmore, W. P. 188, 215
Blackshaw, J. K. 201, 219
Blair Bell, W. 9, 12, 399, 420
Block, R. J. 137, 145
Bloom, R. S. 129, 145
Blythe, W. B. 251, 278
Bocanegra, M. 378, 379, 380, 381, 382, 383, 384, 387, 388, 394, 395
Bodanszky, M. 27, 29, 30, 32, 39, 50, 51, 89, 106, 207, 217
Boissonnas, R. A. 6, 27, 28, 29, 30, 32, 36, 38, 50, 53, 54, 57, 81, 86, 87, 88, 90, 91, 96, 97, 98, 99, 105, 106, 107, 108, 174, 175, 204, 210, 215, 290, 292, 296, 307, 308, 309, 313, 339, 342
Bonjour, J. Ph. 229, 240, 243, 258, 261, 266, 268
Bontekoe, J. S. 27, 50
Boris, A. 248, 268
Borrero, L. M. 358, 374
Boss, W. R. 183, 214
Böttcher, D. 70, 78
Botting, J. H. 206, 215
Bouckaert, J. H. 128, 152

Author Index

Boura, A. 186, 187, 215
Bourguet, J. 323, 325, 331, 332, 333, 345, 348
Bourne, A. 9, 12
Bower, B. F. 433, 434, 435, 443
Bowers, C. Y. 47, 55, 180, 225
Boyd, E. M. 324, 345
Bradley, J. 252, 273
Branda, L. A. 34, 35, 36, 39, 46, 47, 50, 91, 99, 106, 108, 198, 213, 307, 308, 315
Brandt, J. L. 248, 268
Braude, R. 302, 315
Bray, G. A. 246, 268
Brecht, J. P. 244, 278
Brenneman, A. R. 311, 315
Brenner, W. E. 415, 421
Breslow, E. 41, 42, 43, 44, 50, 51, 156, 165, 170
Brest, A. 371, 375
Bricker, N. S. 254, 268
Brightman, M. 165, 169
Brimacombe, R. 73, 74, 78
Brodsky, W. A. 254, 276, 431, 445
Brokaw, H. 251, 268
Bromwich, A. F. 178, 215, 257, 268
Bronsky, D. 432, 444
Brook, A. H. 381, 394
Brooks, C. 128, 150
Brooks, F. P. 255, 262, 268
Brotánek, V. 310, 317
Brovetto, J. 8, 12, 182, 215, 411, 420
Brown, E. 372, 373
Brown, J. H. U. 116, 145
Brown, L. M. 118, 127, 142, 148, 242, 272
Brown, S. 163, 169
Broytman, A. J. 239, 272
Brunn, F. 6, 12, 329, 330, 345
Brunner, H. 230, 247, 255, 258, 260, 261, 264, 265, 268, 269, 272
Buchborn, E. 206, 215
Buck, A. S. 91, 107
Bucy, P. C. 2, 12, 201, 227
Bugbee, E. P. 5, 14, 62, 78, 178, 191, 221
Bundschuh, E. 255, 260, 274
Burack, W. R. 230, 274
Burg, M. B. 238, 240, 272
Burgess, W. W. 323, 324, 336, 338, 345
Burn, I. 126, 145

Burn, J. H. 9, 12, 126, 145, 173, 183, 185, 199, 215
Burstin, C. 381, 395
Buschmann, H. J. 264, 277
Butcher, R. W. 334, 344, 372, 373
Butler, A. M. 246, 271
Buzalkov, R. 190, 226, 242, 277
Byrom, F. B. 263, 269

Cabot, H. M. 8, 12, 182, 196, 197, 215, 222, 298, 306, 318, 406, 411, 419, 420
Cafruny, E. J. 248, 278
Cajal, S. R. Y. 2, 12
Calcagno, P. L. 250, 269
Caldeyro-Barcia, R. 8, 12, 196, 197, 198, 202, 213, 217, 222, 228, 298, 306, 307, 308, 313, 315, 318, 403, 405, 411, 414, 415, 417, 418, 419, 420
Callamand, D. 324, 345
Campbell, B. J. 44, 51
Campbell, J. 9, 16, 399, 410, 412, 422
Čapek, K. 238, 269
Carballo, M. A. 406, 419
Carlson, A. J. 3, 12
Carlson, I. H. 327, 345
Carlsson, L. 47, 51
Carone, F. A. 252, 271
Carroll, K. K. 178, 220
Carter, N. W. 431, 443
Carter, W. H. 180, 225
Cash, W. D. 91, 98, 99, 107, 108, 109
Casteels, R. 280, 292
Castleman, L. 248, 268
Cerletti, A. 88, 105, 175, 194, 203, 211, 214, 260, 268, 298, 305, 315, 405, 420
Chalmers, T. C. 253, 274
Chalmers, T. M. 247, 269
Chambers, G. H. 3, 12, 183, 185, 219
Chan, D. K. O. 323, 325, 327, 341, 345, 349
Chan, W. Y. 47, 53, 90, 91, 99, 107, 108, 200, 215, 231, 255, 259, 262, 264, 269, 276, 285, 287, 288, 289, 291, 293, 302, 307, 315, 317, 333, 339, 345, 346, 381, 388, 391, 392, 393, 395, 396
Chang, H. C. 127, 129, 145
Chartièr-Baraduc, M. M. 326, 348
Chaudhury, M. R. 126, 145, 303, 315
Chaudhury, R. R. 118, 123, 126, 127, 128, 145, 192, 215, 253, 257, 269, 303, 315, 384, 387, 390, 391, 394

Chauvet, J. 25, 30, 32, 41, 49, 50, 51, 64, 67, 68, 69, 72, 76, 78, 90, 100, 106, 114, 133, 144, 145, 173, 180, 184, 212, 213, 215, 286, 292, 308, 314
Chauvet, M. T. 30, 32, 49, 64, 67, 68, 69, 72, 76, 90, 106, 180, 212, 215, 286, 292, 308, 314
Chen, C. C. H. 39, 55
Chern, D. M. 248, 275
Chester, H. T. 188, 215
Chester Jones, I. 323, 325, 327, 341, 345, 349
Chia, K. F. 127, 129, 145
Chien, S. 127, 145, 153, 378, 387, 397
Childs, W. A. 206, 221
Chimiak, A. 35, 51, 105, 107
Cho, K. B. 340, 347
Chomety, F. 229, 240, 243, 268
Chow, B. F. 41, 57, 65, 77, 111, 133, 147, 156, 165, 171, 180, 207, 227, 304, 319
Christ, J. F. 112, 142, 158, 169
Christensen, M. L. 232, 277
Christman, D. R. 47, 52, 91, 92, 106, 371, 373, 391, 394
Chu, F. S. 44, 51
Churchill, P. 245, 271
Chuttani, H. K. 253, 269
Civan, M. M. 363, 365, 373
Clapp, J. R. 236, 269
Clark, B. J. 127, 146, 214
Clarke, D. L. 372, 373
Clarke, N. P. 127, 154, 187, 215
Clausen, H. J. 338, 345
Clauser, H. 208, 213
Clayton, G. W. 439, 440, 444
Cleugh, J. 201, 210, 216
Cleverley, J. D. 296, 298, 315
Coba, E. 123, 148
Cobo, E. 257, 271, 303, 317
Coch, J. A. 8, 12, 182, 215, 411, 420
Coda, H. 182, 215
Coffinet, B. 27, 57
Coggins, C. H. 245, 269
Cohen, J. 311, 315
Cohen, S. I. 252, 269
Cohn, M. 23, 51
Collin, R. 3, 12
Condliffe, P. G. 5, 12, 178, 216
Condon, N. E. 191, 216
Coon, J. M. 198, 199, 216, 339, 345

Cooper, W. D. 192, 227, 305, 319
Cope, C. L. 439, 443
Corcoran, A. C. 251, 271
Cort, J. H. 262, 263, 269
Coulson, R. A. 336, 342
Coussens, R. 123, 128, 152, 303, 318
Coutinho, E. M. 201, 216
Cowie, A. T. 8, 12, 114, 142, 194, 211, 296, 311, 313, 315
Crabbé, J. 244, 245, 250, 269
Craig, L. C. 20, 32, 40, 51, 56, 179, 216
Cramm, R. E. 426, 444
Crankshaw, O. F. 431, 445
Crawford, J. D. 183, 188, 216, 246, 269, 383, 386, 394, 430, 444,
Crepy, D. 30, 32, 49, 64, 68, 69, 72, 76, 90, 106, 180, 212, 286, 292, 308, 314
Crichton, E. C. 405, 420
Crist, C. A. 426, 444
Cross, B. A. 8, 11, 123, 126, 127, 128, 142, 146, 149, 193, 194, 216, 257, 269, 296, 301, 302, 303, 304, 305, 314, 315, 316, 402, 420
Cross, R. B. 235, 260, 262, 269, 270
Croxatto, H. 178, 202, 208, 211, 216, 255, 260, 270
Croxatto, R. 208, 216
Csanyi, E. 201, 213, 388, 393
Csapo, A. 201, 216, 282, 292, 407, 409, 419
Cullen, B. M. 407, 420
Curelop, S. 431, 445
Curtis, J. R. 242, 270
Cushing, H. 1, 3, 11, 12
Czaczkes, J. W. 187, 188, 216, 378, 380, 381, 382, 384, 385, 389, 394, 430, 444
Czakes, I. W. 243, 270
Czakes, J. W. 250, 270
Czakes, W. J. 242, 250, 277

Dahl, L. K. 384, 385, 396
Dahlstrom, A. 132, 146
Dale, H. H. 5, 6, 9, 13, 173, 190, 199, 215, 216, 279, 292, 385, 394, 405, 420
Daly, J. J. 435, 443
Daniel, A. 117, 118, 119, 120, 121, 122, 123, 125, 131, 132, 138, 139, 146, 168, 170
Dantzler, W. H. 230, 270, 336, 337, 338, 341, 345, 346
Darmady, E. M. 237, 270

Author Index 451

Darwin, C. 332, 343
Dashe, A. M. 426, 430, 444
Dasme, A. M. 249, 272
David, M. A. 263, 274
Davidson, D. G. 190, 221, 245, 246, 250, 253, 268, 274, 275
Davis, J. O. 249, 264, 270
Davoll, H. 21, 46, 55
Davy, M. J. 401, 420
Dean, R. C. 136, 146
Deane, H. W. 299, 316
Debackere, M. 128, 146, 198, 212, 216
De Beer, G. R. 7, 14
De Bodo, R. C. 126, 145
Debons, A. F. 384, 385, 396
De Duve, C. 116, 144, 147
Deetjen, P. 7, 15, 235, 277
Deis, R. P. 401, 420
Dekanski, J. 191, 216
Delaere, J. 431, 444
De la Maza, J. 208, 216
Dellman, H. D. 112, 146
Demonte, H. 264, 265, 267
Dempsey, E. F. 362, 363, 374
Demunbrun, T. W. 259, 270, 401, 402, 420
Denamur, R. 114, 128, 146, 151, 296, 298, 300, 301, 312, 314, 316, 318, 402, 419
Denning, G. S. Jr. 90, 91, 107
DeNuccio, D. J. 300, 316
De Robertis, E. 3, 13, 118, 129, 132, 143, 148, 157, 163, 167, 169, 171
Dettelbach, H. R. 186, 188, 216
de Weid, D. 126, 127, 153, 154, 187, 188, 216, 228, 440, 443
Dewey, R. R. 254, 268
Dexter, D. 126, 146
Dicker, S. E. 46, 51, 114, 115, 118, 119, 123, 127, 131, 146, 147, 186, 187, 215, 217, 232, 239, 245, 250, 252, 260, 270, 287, 292, 371, 373, 389, 390, 392, 394, 401, 420
Dieckmann, W. J. 391, 394
Diepen, R. 112, 142, 146
Dignam, W. J. 230, 267
Dingman, J. F. 48, 50, 182, 213
Dingwall, M. 324, 345
Dixon, W. E. 8, 13
Dlouha, H. 250, 270
Dobrowolski, J. 253, 268

Dodd, J. M. 230, 266, 322, 323, 324, 327, 335, 343
Dodd, M. H. I. 69, 78, 230, 266, 322, 323, 324, 343
Doepfner, W. 94, 106, 201, 203, 214, 288, 292
Donaldson, W. 179, 217
Donker, J. D. 296, 316
Douglas, W. W. 119, 131, 141, 147, 242, 270
Downes, J. C. 201, 219
Doyle, A. P. 246, 269
Drabarek, S. 34, 35, 39, 50, 51, 90, 91, 107, 308, 315
Driscoll, W. J. 9, 16, 399, 410, 412, 422
Duchen, L. W. 118, 147
Dudley, H. W. 5, 13, 62, 77
Duff, W. M. 255, 264, 266, 274
Duke, H. N. 126, 129, 147
Dumm, M. E. 189, 224
Durant, J. 236, 270
Dustan, H. P. 251, 271
Dutta, A. S. 35, 36, 51
du Vigneaud, V. 5, 6, 11, 12, 13, 16, 19, 20, 21, 22, 23, 24, 25, 26, 27, 28, 29, 30, 31, 32, 34, 35, 36, 37, 38, 39, 40, 42, 43, 44, 46, 47, 49, 50, 51, 52, 53, 54, 55, 56, 57, 58, 62, 65, 66, 67, 76, 78, 79, 87, 89, 90, 91, 92, 95, 99, 105, ,106, 107, 108, 109, 133, 136, 137, 143, 173, 175, 177, 178, 180, 207, 208, 213, 217, 221, 222, 224, 225, 227, 285, 291, 293, 307, 308, 309, 314, 315, 317, 333, 339, 345, 346, 381, 392, 393, 395
Dyball, R. E. J. 123, 127, 128, 147, 187, 189, 217

Earley, L. E. 430, 444
Eayrs, J. T. 300, 316
Edelman, I. S. 356, 375
Edelmann, C. M. Jr. 246, 250, 251, 254, 271
Eden, M. 246, 268
Edery, H. 303, 316
Edmunds, R. 429, 444
Edström, J. 163, 167, 169
Edwardson, J. A. 300, 316
Egami, N. 327, 346
Egdahl, R. H. 439, 443
Egenolf, G. F. 391, 394

Eggleton, M. G. 239, 270, 371, 373, 389, 394
Ehrental, K. 264, 277
Eichner, D. 163, 167, 169
Einstein, A. 356, 372
Eisentraut, A. M. 434, 445
Eisler, K. 35, 52, 88, 105, 107, 308, 309, 316
Eliakim, M. 250, 270
Elliot, G. M. 311, 314
Elmquist, A. 41, 55, 66, 78, 179, 198, 217, 221
Ely, F. 7, 13, 298, 302, 316
Embrey, M. P. 290, 293
Endroczi, E. 201, 217
Engel, S. L. 112, 113, 115, 117, 142, 144, 173, 174, 175, 177, 178, 185, 190, 192, 194, 195, 199, 211, 213, 278, 298, 304, 305, 314, 401, 420, 422
Engelhardt, F. 112, 142, 147
Epstein, F. H. 189, 221, 246, 249, 252, 254, 271, 273, 275, 431, 444
Erspamer, V. 183, 217
Eser, S. 389, 394
Evans, D. H. L. 406, 420
Evans, F. T. 440, 445
Eversole, W. J. 126, 127, 148, 183, 185, 206, 214, 221
Ewer, R. F. 329, 332, 346, 352, 373

Fairweather, D. V. I. 401, 417, 420
Fang, H. S. 126, 147, 190, 217
Farah, A. 246, 275
Farini, F. 6, 10, 13
Farner, D. S. 67, 77, 338, 340, 343, 346, 348, 350
Fawcett, C. P. 140, 152, 156, 165, 166, 171
Fear, R. 285
Feigelson, L. 116, 149
Fekete, K. 391, 394, 406, 420
Feldberg, W. 129, 130, 147, 302, 316
Fendler, K. 201, 217
Ferguson, D. R. 65, 67, 70, 72, 77, 114, 147, 181, 217, 333, 334, 345, 346
Ferguson, J. K. W. 126, 128, 147, 149, 402, 420
Ferraro, J. J. 34, 36, 52
Ferraz, F. P. J. 431, 443
Ferrell, C. B. 388, 396

Ferreri, E. 72, 77, 204, 205, 220, 336, 346
Ferrier, B. M. 34, 36, 39, 40, 47, 52, 54, 91, 92, 107, 108, 180, 217, 308, 317
Fichman, M. P. 249, 271
Fielitz, C. A. 8, 12, 182, 202, 216, 217, 228, 411, 420
Findlay, A. L. R. 299, 317
Fisch, L. 241, 271
Fischbach, H. 235, 276
Fitch, F. 251, 277
Fitt, P. S. 27, 51, 207, 217
Fitzgerald, M. G. 252, 269
Fitzpatrick, R. J. 8, 9, 11, 13, 94, 107, 128, 142, 148, 175, 178, 179, 182, 194, 195, 196, 200, 202, 211, 217, 296, 305, 311, 312, 313, 314, 317, 340, 343, 379, 392, 411, 419
Flatters, M. 200, 217
Fleischhauer, K. 312, 315
Fliegner, J. R. 405, 420
Flodin, P. 179, 224
Flouret, G. 34, 35, 39, 46, 51, 52, 291, 293
Follenius, E. 133, 142
Follett, B. K. 64, 67, 68, 69, 70, 71, 77, 90, 107, 114, 148, 181, 200, 204, 217, 286, 293, 322, 323, 333, 338, 340, 343, 345, 346
Folley, S. J. 8, 13, 114, 128, 142, 148, 179, 194, 195, 196, 211, 218, 296, 301, 306, 311, 312, 313, 314, 315, 317, 379, 384, 393, 394, 402, 410, 411, 419, 421
Fong, C. T. O. 46, 47, 52, 371, 373, 375, 384, 385, 391, 394, 396
Fontaine, M. 324, 343, 345, 346
Forbes, A. 299, 316, 317
Forbes, A. P. 299, 317
Forsham, P. H. 433, 434, 443
Forsling, M. L. 188, 218
Fosker, A. P. 35, 52
Fourman, P. 252, 269, 271
Fox, S. 299, 317
Fraga, A. 182, 215
Frank, H. S. 355, 356, 373
Frank, W. 34, 39, 52
Frankland, B. T. B. 41, 52, 53, 133, 134, 137, 148, 150, 180, 218
Franz, J. 48, 53
Franze, J. 206, 220
Fraser, A. M. 5, 16, 201, 208, 218, 255, 261, 271

Frazier, H. S.   365, 373
Friberg, O.   128, 148
Frick, A.   241, 274
Friedberg, V.   388, 394
Friedman, C. L.   127, 148, 250, 271
Friedman, E. A.   197, 218, 305, 310, 317
Friedman, S. M.   127, 148, 250, 271
Friesen, H. G.   133, 148, 165, 170
Fromageot, C.   41, 49, 114, 133, 136, 141, 156, 168, 178, 210
Fuchs, A. R.   128, 148, 203, 211, 218, 296, 317, 417, 421
Fuchs, F.   417, 421
Fuchs, G.   237, 238, 240, 269, 277
Fugo, N. W.   126, 148, 185, 218
Fuhrman, F. A.   331, 346
Fusco, M.   245, 271
Fuxe, K.   132, 146

Gabe, M.   4, 13
Gaddum, J. H.   176, 177, 198, 199, 200, 201, 202, 209, 210, 211, 216, 218
Gaines, W. L.   7, 13, 192, 218, 298, 317
Gaitan, E.   123, 148, 257, 271, 303, 317
Gamble, J. L.   246, 271
Gange, P. D.   9, 16, 399, 422, 410, 412
Garcia de Jalon, M.   200, 218
Garcia de Jalon, P.   200, 218
Garcia Romeu, F.   326, 348
Gardner, K. D. Jr.   238, 272
Gauer, O. H.   183, 187, 188, 189, 206, 218, 226, 243, 277, 381, 396
Gaunt, R.   183, 185, 214
Geesey, C.   129, 150
Geltinger, A.   235, 276
Gerlough, T. D.   177, 218
Gerschenfeld, H. M.   118, 129, 148
Gersh, J.   2, 3, 13
Gertz, G. C.   237, 271
Gessner, H.   117, 148
Gianetto, R.   116, 147
Giarman, N. J.   126, 148
Gibbs, O. S.   185, 218
Giebisch, G.   251, 254, 271
Giere, F. A.   126, 127, 148
Gill, J. R. Jr.   252, 272
Gillessen, D.   34, 37, 38, 44, 57, 58
Gilliland, P. F.   48, 53, 206, 218
Gilman, A.   118, 127, 148, 179, 218, 387, 394

Ginetzinsky, A. G.   239, 240, 272, 370, 373
Ginsburg, M.   4, 7, 13, 41, 42, 53, 111, 118, 121, 123, 127, 129, 133, 134, 135, 136, 137, 138, 139, 140, 141, 142, 143, 148, 149, 153, 156, 165, 166, 169, 170, 178, 180, 183, 185, 194, 203, 218, 219, 226, 242, 247, 257, 272, 310, 313, 317, 319, 378, 379, 380, 381, 382, 383, 384, 386, 387, 388, 391, 392, 393, 394, 395, 396
Gioia de Coch, M. N.   182, 215
Gish, D. T.   6, 13, 19, 29, 30, 32, 51, 53, 54
Givens, J. R.   435, 443
Glaubach, S.   185, 219
Glendening, M. B.   392, 395
Glenister, D. W.   440, 444
Glick, S. M.   48, 56
Goetsch, E.   3, 12
Gogan, F.   340, 346
Goldberg, M.   431, 433, 444
Goldblatt, E. L.   248, 272
Goldsmith, C.   253, 272
Golubow, J.   47, 53, 307, 317, 339, 346, 392, 395
Gomez, E. T.   8, 13
Gomori, G.   3, 13
Gonzalez-Panizza, V. H.   194, 202, 211, 217, 378, 382, 389, 393, 406, 419
Goodfriend, T. L.   311, 317
Goodman, A.   242, 272
Goodman, L.   118, 127, 148, 179, 218, 387, 394
Goodwin, R. F. W.   296, 315
Gorbman, A.   112, 150, 322, 328, 347, 348
Gordan, G. S.   435, 443
Gordon, S.   5, 13, 19, 20, 27, 39, 46, 52, 53, 55
Göres, E.   91, 105
Gottschalk, C. W.   232, 236, 237, 240, 252, 272, 274, 275, 277
Graber, J. W.   340, 346
Graham, A.   9, 16, 399, 410, 412, 422
Grantham, J. J.   238, 240, 272
Green, H.   126, 146, 442, 445
Green, J. D.   3, 13, 111, 129, 142
Greenbaum, A. L.   46, 51, 390, 394
Greene, J. A.   10, 14
Greenwood, F. G.   440, 441, 444

Greep, R. O. 41, 57, 65, 77, 111, 133, 147, 156, 165, 171, 180, 207, 227, 304, 319
Greving, R. 2, 14
Griffiths, W. J. 252, 269
Grinnell, E. H. 255, 264, 266, 274
Grollman, A. 182, 219
Gross, F. 261, 272
Grosvenor, C. E. 128, 149, 300, 301, 316, 317
Grote, I. W. 5, 14, 62, 78, 178, 191, 221
Grumer, H. A. 432, 444
Guerné, J. M. 200, 219
Guggenheim, K. 252, 272
Guggenheim, M. A. 103, 109
Guillemin, R. 45, 56, 66, 79, 180, 225, 227, 335, 343
Gulland, J. M. 208, 219
Gunther, M. 8, 14
Guttmann, S. 27, 30, 36, 37, 50, 53, 54, 87, 88, 91, 106, 108, 110, 174, 175, 215, 296, 307, 308, 313
Guyot-Jeannin, C. 253, 268
Gwinup, G. 439, 440, 442, 444

Habener, J. F. 249, 272, 426, 444
Haeger, K. 404, 421
Haempel, O. 327, 346
Hagemann, I. 262, 263, 269
Haigh, A. L. 401, 421
Haldar, J. 123, 124, 127, 128, 145, 201, 203, 208, 211, 214
Hall, C. E. 3, 16
Haller, E. W. 140, 152, 156, 162, 165, 169, 171
Hallowell, D. S. 249, 264, 270
Ham, G. C. 179, 185, 189, 219
Hamburger, C. 199, 219
Hamilton, H. C. 191, 219
Hammond, J. 298, 314
Handler, J. S. 240, 266, 275, 334, 348, 372, 373, 374, 431, 433, 444
Handley, C. A. 259, 272
Hara, T. J. 112, 150, 328, 347
Hare, K. 3, 14, 183, 185, 188, 219, 248, 250, 267, 272, 426, 444
Hare, R. S. 3, 14, 183, 185, 188, 219, 248, 250, 267, 272
Harfenist, E. J. 40, 46, 51, 53, 179, 216
Hargitay, B. 232, 278
Harkness, M. L. R. 407, 421

Harkness, R. D. 407, 420, 421
Harman, J. W. 116, 149
Harrah, J. 381, 395
Harrington, A. R. 232, 273
Harris, G. W. 8, 14, 114, 122, 126, 142, 146, 149, 193, 194, 216, 257, 273, 296, 314, 315
Hart, P. D. 183, 219
Hartley, B. S. 82, 105
Hartmann, A. 30, 54
Harvey, A. M. 323, 324, 336, 338, 345
Hasselbach, C. H. 138, 149
Hastings, A. B. 201, 205, 227, 286, 287, 293
Haterius, H. O. 126, 149
Hauser, D. 253, 275
Havran, R. T. 58
Hawker, R. W. 194, 201, 208, 211, 219
Hawkins, D. F. 202, 219, 407, 421
Haynes, R. C. 372, 373
Hays, R. L. 197, 209, 227, 297, 298, 299, 306, 319, 402, 422
Hays, R. M. 249, 273, 334, 343, 352, 353, 354, 358, 359, 360, 361, 362, 363, 374
Hearn, I. C. 180, 225
Heaton, G. S. 44, 53
Hebb, C. O. 301, 302, 317
Hedwall, P. R. 254, 276
Hegsted, D. M. 253, 272
Heidenreich, O. 258, 259, 262, 273
Heinbecker, P. 245, 278
Held, U. 251, 278
Heller, H. 4, 6, 7, 11, 12, 13, 14, 15, 32, 53, 62, 64, 65, 66, 67, 68, 69, 70, 72, 75, 77, 90, 91, 98, 100, 107, 111, 113, 114, 115, 116, 117, 118, 125, 126, 127, 129, 139, 142, 143, 144, 147, 148, 149, 151, 156, 164, 166, 169, 170, 175, 177, 179, 180, 181, 183, 185, 189, 194, 201, 204, 205, 211, 217, 218, 219, 220, 223, 230, 239, 242, 250, 251, 252, 260, 266, 270, 273, 286, 293, 322, 323, 324, 328, 329, 332, 333, 334, 335, 336, 341, 343, 345, 346, 379, 380, 381, 383, 384, 385, 386, 387, 390, 391, 392, 393, 394, 395, 401, 420
Heller, J. 188, 209, 220, 240, 273, 381, 396
Henderson, L. J. 355, 372
Hendricks, C. H. 403, 404, 405, 409, 414, 415, 419, 421

Hendrikx, A.   246, 249, 254, 271, 273
Herdan, G.   189, 220, 242, 273
Hermann, P.   37, 53
Hernandez, T.   336, 342
Herring, P. T.   3, 7, 10, 14, 16
Herxheimer, A.   249, 270
Hess, G. P.   19, 29, 30, 32, 51, 53, 54
Hewer, T. F.   252, 270
Heymès, R.   27, 57
Hibbard, B. M.   405, 420
Hickey, R. C.   3, 14, 188, 219, 426, 444
Hierholzer, K.   242, 244, 273, 278
Hild, W.   3, 4, 14, 71, 77, 111, 123, 133, 149, 157, 170
Hilton, S. M.   126, 145, 165, 170, 178, 215
Hindson, J. C.   410, 421
Hinke, J. A. M.   127, 148
Hirano, T.   117, 150, 337, 340, 346, 347
Hirata, K.   371, 375
Hobbs, C. B.   436, 444
Hochster, G.   371, 375
Hoerner, J. K.   399, 421
Hofbauer, J.   9, 14, 399, 421
Hoffman, J. F.   361, 375
Hoffmann, F.   189, 213
Hofmann, L.   248, 273
Hogben, L. T.   7, 14, 190, 198, 220
Holland, R. C.   127, 149
Holländer, L. P.   48, 53, 206, 220
Hollander, W. Jr.   251, 252, 273, 275, 278
Hollenberg, M. D.   41, 52, 53, 133, 134, 135, 136, 137, 148, 149, 150, 156, 165, 170, 180, 218
Holliday, M. A.   251, 275, 381, 395
Holmes, R. L.   129, 149, 323, 325, 346
Holmes, W. N.   323, 325, 327, 345, 346, 347
Holton, P.   200, 201, 205, 210, 216, 220
Homiller, R. P.   21, 57
Hong, S. K.   249, 278
Honzl, J.   27, 56, 88, 104, 108
Hope, A. B.   133, 136, 137, 143
Hope, D. B.   37, 39, 41, 42, 44, 49, 52, 53, 87, 107, 133, 134, 135, 136, 137, 146, 148, 149, 150, 156, 165, 170, 180, 218, 392, 393
Hoppe, W.   181, 224
Horan, A.   439, 440, 444
Horster, F. A.   255, 258, 262, 273

Horster, M.   235, 276
Horton, E. W.   202, 211
Houghton, E. M.   10, 14
Hourdry, J.   323, 325, 348
Houssay, B. A.   327, 329, 347
Howard, B.   245, 275
Howard, J. D.   37, 103, 109
Howarth, A. T.   401, 421
Howell, W. H.   2, 14
Hruby, V.   34, 35, 46, 50
Hsü, C. M.   127, 129, 145
Huang, J. J.   127, 145
Hubbard, S.   44, 51
Hughes, F. B.   202, 220
Huguenin, R. L.   28, 29, 30, 32, 35, 36, 37, 38, 50, 53, 54, 57, 86, 96, 97, 98, 99, 100, 106, 107, 108,
Hume, D. M.   439 443
Hyatt, R. E.   249, 264, 270

Ibayashi, H.   181, 189, 210, 228
Illanes, G.   208, 216
Ingraham, R. C.   127, 144, 188, 213
Ireland, M.   4, 13, 41, 42, 53, 133, 134, 135, 136, 138, 139, 141, 148, 156, 165, 170, 180, 219, 380, 394
Irving, G. W. Jr.   23, 51
Ishii, S.   117, 130, 150, 153, 327, 340, 346, 347
Ishikawa, T.   128, 150
Island, D. P.   435, 443
Isselbacher, K. J.   230, 274
Ito, E.   160, 170
Ivanova, L. N.   239, 272
Ivy, H. K.   434, 444

Jacobsohn, D.   8, 14, 296, 315, 404, 421
Jacobson, H. N.   260, 264, 265, 273
Jadresic, A.   427, 444
Jaenike, J. R.   190, 220, 238, 264, 273
James, V. H. T.   439, 440, 442, 443, 444
Jamison, R. L.   233, 273
Jancsó, N.   329, 330, 343
Janovský, M.   302, 315
January, L. E.   10, 14
Jaquenoud, P.-A.   27, 30, 36, 50, 54, 86, 90, 91, 108, 175, 215
Jard, S.   230, 247, 273, 274, 275, 328, 330, 332, 333, 337, 343, 347, 348, 365

Jarvis, D. 34, 39, 40, 52, 54, 92, 108, 180, 217, 308, 309, 317
Jasinski, A. 112, 150, 328, 347
Jayasena, K. 121, 133, 134, 136, 137, 138, 141, 148, 156, 165, 170, 180, 219
Jeffers, W. A. 183, 185, 186, 220, 242, 274
Jenkins, P. A. 429, 445
Jenkins, R. 185, 214
Jepson, J. B. 201, 213
Jeronimus, S. C. 200, 223, 286, 289, 293
Jessup, D. C. 178, 182, 220
Jewell, P. A. 119, 150
Jick, H. C. 253, 274
Jinks, R. 126, 154, 183, 226
Jöhl, A. 19, 28, 30, 51, 54
Johnson, S. R. 334, 335, 344
Jones, A. M. 192, 201, 220, 384, 385, 395
Jones, J. J. 188, 189, 190, 218, 221, 432, 433, 434, 443, 444
Jones, N. F. 252, 264, 265, 267, 272, 274
Jones, R. C. 198, 221
Jones, R. V. H. 232, 245, 274
Jongkind, J. F. 246, 274
Joplin, G. F. 192, 215
Jørgensen, C. B. 331, 335, 343, 347
Jošt, K. 27, 33, 34, 39, 54, 56, 81, 90, 92, 103, 104, 105, 106, 108, 189, 203, 207, 214, 305, 306, 308, 309, 310, 315, 320
Jung, H. 281, 292, 401, 409, 419
Jungmannová, Č. 310, 317

Kabayashi, H. 117, 150
Kalliala, H. 123, 128, 150, 190, 221, 303, 317, 318
Kamemoto, F. I. 340, 348
Kamm, D. E. 253, 274
Kamm, O. 5, 14, 62, 78, 178, 191, 221
Kao, C. Y. 280, 282, 283, 284, 292
Kaplan, S. A. 232, 278
Kar, K. 35, 36, 51
Kardos, Z. 115, 152
Karvonen, M. J. 123, 128, 150, 190, 221, 262, 264, 274, 303, 317, 318
Kasafírek, E. 34, 36, 54, 104, 108, 308, 309, 320
Kastin, A. J. 127, 150
Katchalsky, A. 362, 367, 374

Katsoyannis, P. G. 5, 6, 13, 19, 26, 27, 29, 30, 31, 32, 51, 52, 53, 54, 62, 78, 88, 95, 96, 97, 108, 173, 208, 217, 221
Kaurov, O. A. 36, 50
Kauz, G. 117, 151
Kazda, S. 310, 317
Kedem, O. 362, 363, 367, 373, 374
Keele, C. A. 201, 213
Keller, A. D. 259, 270, 272, 401, 402, 420
Kelley, N. 285, 287, 288, 291, 293
Kellog, R. H. 230, 260, 264, 265, 274
Kelsall, A. R. 126, 150
Kelsey, H. A. 410, 422
Kennedy, G. C. 237, 271, 430, 444
Kennedy, W. P. 189, 213
Kerr, T. 327, 335, 343
Kestranek, W. 185, 221
Kimbrough, R. D. Jr. 37, 52, 54, 99, 108
King, B. C. 157, 171
King, L. S. 114, 154
Kinsky, S. C. 368, 370, 374
Kirkensgaard, T. 254, 268
Kitchin, A. H. 260, 270, 401, 421
Kiyoi, R. 27, 56
Klauker, M. L. 248, 272
Kleeman, C. R. 187, 188, 189, 216, 221, 241, 243, 246, 271, 378, 380, 381, 382, 384, 385, 389, 394, 430, 444
Klein, L. A. 48, 56
Klevay, L. M. 389, 395
Klieger, E. 32, 35, 54
Klingler, L. Jr. 253, 278
Klose, R. M. 254, 271
Knaggs, G. S. 8, 13, 126, 128, 142, 148, 153, 179, 195, 196, 211, 217, 296, 301, 302, 303, 304, 306, 308, 309, 314, 317, 319, 379, 384, 393, 394, 395, 410, 411, 419, 421
Knaus, H. H. 8, 11, 15, 399, 405, 421
Knoop, A. 4, 12, 312, 315
Knowles, F. G. W. (Sir F.) 4, 11, 15, 111, 130, 142, 156, 163, 169, 324, 327, 347
Knowlton, F. P. 10, 15
Knudsen, P. J. 241, 277, 371, 375
Kobayashi, H. 130, 151, 153, 340, 347, 350
Koch, A. C. 27, 50
Koefoed, J. 241, 277, 371, 375
Koefoed-Johnsen, V. 331, 347, 351, **358**, 374

Koelle, G. B.   129, 132, 150
Koenig, E.   158, 170
Koenig, M.   187, 188, 216, 243, 270, 381, 385, 389, 394
Koizumi, K.   128, 150
Kolc, J.   37, 58, 97, 98, 99, 109
König, A.   70, 78
Konigsberg, W. H.   40, 51
Konzett, H.   87, 88, 89, 94, 105, 106, 108, 174, 175, 201, 203, 211, 214, 215, 288, 292, 296, 308, 313
Kook, Y.   258, 259, 262, 273, 340, 347
Kordon, C.   340, 346
Korr, I.   338, 347
Kovács, K.   263, 274
Kraft, A.   8, 16
Kramar, J.   255, 264, 266, 274
Kramer, K.   7, 15, 235, 277
Kraus, M.   250, 270
Krecek, J.   250, 270
Krejčí, I.   89, 94, 103, 104, 105, 106, 109, 189, 200, 203, 207, 211, 214, 221, 224, 285, 293, 304, 305, 306, 309, 310, 315, 318
Krestinskaya, T. V.   371, 373
Krogh, A.   332, 343
Kroon, D. B.   246, 274
Krumholz, K. H.   197, 214, 296, 315
Kuchárová, M.   262, 278
Küchel, D.   262, 278
Kuehn, E.   264, 274
Kühn, E.   198, 212
Kühn, W.   232, 233, 274, 278, 356, 374
Kullander, S.   303, 318
Kumar, D.   407, 421
Kumaresan, P.   197, 213
Kunkel, H. G.   23, 54, 57
Kupkova, B.   94, 105, 207, 221
Kuriyama, H.   280, 292
Kuroda, R.   388, 395
Kuschinsky, C.   127, 150
Kuschinsky, G.   230, 247, 255, 258, 260, 262, 264, 265, 268, 269, 273, 274

Labarca, E.   255, 260, 270
LaBella, F.   4, 15, 116, 117, 145, 156, 164, 170
Lachmann, P. J.   429, 445
Lahlouh, B.   323, 325, 345, 348
Laidlaw, P. P.   173, 190, 199, 216, 405, 420

Laken, B.   189, 224
Lambdin, E.   189, 221, 358, 359, 361, 374
Landgrebe, F. W.   191, 221, 324, 344
Landis, E. M.   179, 185, 189 219
Landon, J.   439, 440, 441, 442, 443, 444
Lane, G. J.   187, 189, 217
LaPointe, J. L.   72, 78, 205
Larsen, L. O.   335, 343
Larson, E.   385, 386, 389, 395
Lassiter, W. E.   236, 241, 274, 278
Laszlo, F. A.   127, 154
Lauber, J. K.   206, 221
Lauryssens, M.   198, 212
Lauson, H. D.   166, 169, 174, 179, 211, 378, 379, 380, 381, 382, 383, 384, 386, 387, 388, 389, 390, 392, 393, 394, 395
Law, H. D.   33, 34, 35, 49, 52, 207, 221
Lawler, H. C.   5, 6, 13, 16, 21, 22, 24, 25, 51, 55, 56, 67, 78, 208, 221
Laws, D. F.   340, 348
Lazo-Wasem, A. E.   6, 15
Leach, E.   210, 216
Leaf, A.   238, 240, 245, 249, 264, 266, 269, 273, 274, 332, 333, 334, 343, 347, 352, 353, 354, 358, 359, 360, 361, 362, 363, 364, 365, 366, 368, 369, 370, 371, 372, 374
Leatherland, J. F.   328, 347
Leathers, D. H. G.   72, 77, 204, 205, 220, 336, 346
LeBacq, E.   431, 444
Le Breton, E.   201, 213, 388, 393
Le Brie, S. J.   336, 337, 347
Lechêne, C.   236, 275
Leder, P.   73, 74, 78
Lederis, K.   3, 4, 6, 11, 12, 14, 15, 65, 67, 70, 75, 77, 111, 112, 113, 114, 115, 116, 117, 118, 119, 120, 121, 122, 123, 125, 130, 131, 132, 133, 138, 139, 143, 144, 146, 149, 150, 151, 156, 168, 169, 170, 175, 177, 181, 182, 201, 205, 220, 221, 257, 266, 327, 347, 381
Lee, A. K.   329, 341, 345
Lee, J.   178, 188, 189, 190, 215, 218, 221, 257, 268, 432, 433, 434, 443, 444
Lee, W. Y.   432, 444
Leeman, S. E.   440, 444
Leeson, P. M.   252, 271
Legait, H.   133, 151
Lenci, M. T.   32, 41, 50, 51, 67, 68, 76, 78, 100, 106, 133, 145, 173, 180, 212, 215

Leppänen, V. 128, 150, 190, 221, 262, 264, 274, 303, 318
Leslie, S. H. 189, 224
Leveque, T. F. 117, 151
Lever, A. F. 233, 274
Levi, H. 331, 347
Levinsky, N. G. 190, 221, 245, 246, 250, 268, 253, 254, 274, 329, 347
Levitin, H. 242, 252, 271, 272, 275, 431, 444
Levitskaya, E. S. 299, 318
Levitt, M. F. 253, 275
Levkoff, A. H. 259, 270, 401, 402, 420
Levy, B. 405, 421
Levy, M. N. 127, 152
Levy, M. S. 253, 275
Lewin, J. E. 201, 203, 211
Lewis, A. G. 183, 221, 247, 269
Lewis, D. 3, 15
Lewis, G. P. 104, 106, 189, 192, 201, 214, 215, 302, 303, 316
Li, C. H. 75, 98, 108
Librik, L. 439, 440, 444
Lichardus, B. 262, 263, 269
Lichtenstein, N. S. 333, 347, 368, 369, 370, 374
Liddle, G. W. 435, 443
Liebau, G. 235, 276
Liebert, P. 127, 150
Light, A. 5, 12, 65, 66, 67, 76, 78, 180, 213
Lilienfield, L. S. 7, 15, 235, 266
Lim, R. K. S. 127, 129, 145
Lin, Y. 339, 342, 349
Lindner, E. B. 41, 55, 66, 78, 179, 221, 224
Lindquist, K. M. 185, 221
Ling, V. 258, 259, 262, 273
Linzell, J. L. 193, 197, 222, 298, 299, 300, 301, 302, 303, 304, 306, 317, 318
Lipscomb, H. S. 180, 225
Lissak, K. 201, 217
Little, J. B. 127, 151, 188, 227, 243, 278, 389, 395
Liu, H. M. 126, 147, 190, 217
Livermore, A. H. 20, 55, 178, 222
Livezey, M. M. 183, 185, 186, 220, 242, 274
Livingston, A. 130, 131, 132, 151
Livingston, L. M. 33, 34, 37, 49, 81, 105, 333, 344, 391, 393

Lloyd, S. 260, 270
Lochner, J. de V. 434, 445
Lockett, M. F. 401, 420
Lojda, Z. 240, 273
Longo, L. 230, 267
Louie, D. D. 46, 52
Low, B. W. 39, 55
Lowry, O. H. 372, 374
Lozano, R. 251, 271
Lu, F. C. 126, 145, 303, 315
Lü, V. M. 127, 129, 145
Lübke, K. 33, 34, 49
Lubowitz, H. 254, 268
Lundborg, R. A. 401, 415, 421, 422
Luse, S. A. 368, 374

Macalister, A. 2, 11
Macaulay, M. H. I. 191, 221
Macdonald, A. D. 190, 220
MacDowel, M. 251, 275
Macfarlane, W. V. 245, 275
Mach, B. 160, 170
Mackay, J. S. 442, 445
Mackay, M. E. 324, 348
Mackenzie, K. 192, 222, 225
Mackler, B. 254, 276
Maclean, A. D. W. 435, 445
MacRobbie, E. A. C. 365, 374
Maetz, J. 32, 50, 64, 68, 76, 77, 78, 91, 100, 106, 107, 108, 180, 201, 204, 205, 212, 220, 222, 230, 273, 323, 324, 325, 326, 331, 332, 333, 343, 345, 347, 348
Maffly, R. H. 238, 271, 358, 359, 361, 374
Maganzini, H. G. 7, 15, 235, 266
Magnus, R. 10, 15, 255, 275
Magoun, H. W. 3, 11
Mahaffey, L. M. 91, 107
Mahon, W. E. 429, 445
Main, A. R. 329, 332, 341, 345, 348
Main, I. H. M. 202, 211
Maira, J. 427, 444
Malamed, A. 117, 153
Malamed, S. 4, 17, 156, 171
Malnic, G. 126, 152
Malvin, R. L. 245, 271
Manitius, A. 252, 271, 275
Manning, M. 34, 35, 36, 55
Mansour, T. E. 372, 374
Manunta, G. 197, 222, 387, 395

Marc-Aurele, J. 91, 92, 100, 101, 102, 103, 104, 106, 108, 333, 349, 391, 393
Marongiu, A. 387, 395
Marsh, D. J. 232, 233, 275
Marshall, E. K. 323, 324, 336, 338, 345
Marshall, F. H. A. 8, 13
Marshall, J. M. 194, 197, 227, 281, 282, 283, 284, 293, 306, 319, 409, 410, 419, 422
Marshall, S. 246, 275
Martin, L. M. 3, 12
Martin, P. J. 207, 222, 284, 293, 304, 318
Martinet, J. 114, 128, 146, 151, 296, 298, 300, 301, 316, 318
Martinov, V. F. 36, 50
Mason, D. M. 433, 434, 443
Massie, E. 387, 393
Mathé, G. 387, 395
Matthews, E. R. 236, 270
Mattie, L. R. 126, 148
Mattingly, D. 442, 445
Maurer, S. 3, 15
Mauro, A. 358, 375
Maxwell, A. L. I. 192, 193, 222
Maxwell, D. J. 111, 129, 142
Mayer, F. S. 182, 222, 388, 395
Mayer, H. 33, 57
Mayer, N. 326, 348
Mazur, A. 126, 144
McArthur, C. G. 133, 151
McBean, R. L. 323, 325, 347
McCann, S. M. 123, 126, 144
McCreary, A. B. 183, 222
McDonald, R. K. 440, 445
McDonald, S. J. 250, 275
McDowell, R. J. S. 202, 220
McGandy, R. B. 389, 395
McKhann, C. F. 246, 271
McNaught, M. L. 313, 317
McWatters, S. 68, 78
Meienhofer, J. 29, 32, 34, 49, 50, 55
Meites, J. 312, 314
Mellett, L. B. 248, 278
Melville, E. V. 183, 185, 219
Melville, K. I. 178, 222
Mena, F. 300, 315, 318
Menczel, J. 242, 250, 277
Mendez-Bauer, C. J. 195, 196, 197, 211, 222, 298, 306, 318, 378, 382, 389, 393, 406, 419

Menzel, H. 258, 259, 262, 273
Merrill, C. H. 10, 14
Mertz, D. P. 260, 275
Meyer, W. C. 2, 15
Michl, H. 5, 16, 23, 57
Migone, L. 430, 445
Miles, B. E. 232, 275
Miller, A. L. 436, 444
Miller, L. H. 241, 271
Miller, T. B. 246, 275
Mills, E. 126, 127, 151
Miltenberger, F. W. 187, 222
Mirsky, I. A. 183, 206, 222, 226, 322, 340, 348
Mitchell, A. A. 201, 216
Mitchell, K. G. 302, 315
Mizrachi, M. 123, 148, 257, 271, 303, 317
Moawad, A. H. 403, 421
Mohun, G. 392, 395
Molitor, H. 185, 219, 221
Montastruc, P. 264, 265, 267
Moore, D. H. 119, 127, 144, 208, 213, 387, 393
Moore, R. D. 197, 209, 222, 298, 304, 306, 318
Moore, S. 20, 55
Moran, W. H. 187, 222
Morel, F. 32, 50, 64, 68, 76, 77, 78, 91, 100, 101, 105, 106, 107, 108, 127, 151, 180, 201, 204, 205, 212, 220, 222, 230, 236, 237, 240, 247, 274, 275, 328, 330, 332, 333, 337, 343, 347, 348
Morley, B. 391, 394
Morosi, H. J. 253, 278
Morrell, C. A. 199, 222
Morris, A. 196, 217
Morris, L. 339, 349
Morris, R. G. 187, 189, 217
Morris, R. J. H. 245, 275
Morrison, R. S. 253, 274
Moses, A. M. 127, 151, 165, 168, 170
Mossinger, M. 3, 16
Motais, R. 326, 343
Motohashi, K. 181, 189, 210, 228
Motzfeldt, K. 126, 151
Moyle, C. L. 248, 275
Mueller, J. M. 21, 46, 55
Muirhead, J. M. B. 410, 422
Müller, H. 117, 148
Münchow, O. 247, 255, 260 268

Munsick, R. A.   5, 15, 62, 63, 67, 68, 70, 72, 78, 79, 92, 100, 108, 109, 180, 181, 190, 200, 201, 204, 205, 222, 223, 225, 286, 287, 288, 289, 293, 337, 339, 348, 349
Murti, V. V. S.   37, 39, 44, 47, 52, 53, 87, 107, 381, 388, 393
Muscholl, E.   191, 223
Mussett, M. W.   174, 213
Mylle, M.   232, 236, 237, 240, 252, 272, 274, 275, 278

Nagel, W.   235, 276
Nakajo, S.   339, 349
Nakashima, M.   250, 271
Nalbandov, A. V.   338, 340, 346, 349
Namara, H. M.   250, 267
Nambu, M.   327, 346
Natochin, J. V.   36, 50, 371, 373
Needham, D. M.   280, 292
Needham, J.   431, 445
Negreiros de Paiva, C. E.   406, 419
Nelson, E. E.   185, 223
Nelson, J. K.   443, 445
Nelson, M. A.   435, 443
Némethy, G.   355, 374
Nesvadba, H.   47, 57, 88, 104, 108, 392, 396
Nettleton, D. E. Jr.   91, 107
Neugebauerova, L.   250, 276
Newton, M.   200, 224
Newton, W. H.   417, 422
Neyland, M.   299, 317
Nibbelink, D. W.   164, 170
Nicholson, W. E.   435, 443
Nicoll, C. S.   312, 314
Niedrich, H.   91, 105
Nielson, A. T.   174, 175, 177, 189, 212, 223
Nirenberg, M.   73, 74, 78
Nixon, W. C. W.   407, 421
Noble, R. L.   113, 143, 178, 182, 183, 220, 223, 388, 395
Nobuhara, Y.   27, 56
Noddle, B. A.   313, 318
Novelli, A.   329, 330, 348
Nunn, J.   114, 115, 118, 127, 147, 250, 270

O'Connell, M.   27, 51, 200, 207, 215, 217, 289, 293

O'Connor, W. J.   189, 190, 223
O'Dell, R.   236, 277
Odell, W. D.   47, 55
Okinaka, S.   181, 189, 210, 228
Oksche, A.   340, 343, 348
Olhaberry, J.   182, 215
Olivecrona, H.   164, 170
Oliver, G.   2, 6, 15
Oliver, J.   251, 252, 273, 275
Olivereau, M.   324, 345
Olivry, G.   41, 50, 114, 133, 144, 180 182, 213
Olofson, R. A.   33, 57
Ondetti, M. A.   30, 32, 50
O'Neal, C.   73, 74, 78
Oota, Y.   117, 130, 150, 151
Opel, H.   339, 340, 348
Orloff, J.   240, 245, 266, 275, 334, 348, 372, 373, 374, 430, 431, 444, 445
Orlov, A. F.   239, 240, 275, 312, 315
Orr, J.   181, 223
Ortmann, R.   3, 15, 114, 117, 151
Osborn, C. M.   183, 214
Osinchak, J.   163, 167, 170
Ôta, K.   301, 312, 313, 318, 320
Otani, S.   160, 170
Ott, I.   6, 15, 192, 223
Ottolenghi, A.   183, 217
Overman, R. R.   183, 222
Overweg, N. I. A.   86, 97, 107, 309, 319, 391, 397
Oyaert, W.   128, 152
Øye, I.   334, 344
Oztan, N.   322, 348

Pacheco, P.   300, 315
Page, E. W.   392, 395
Page, I. H.   179, 183, 212, 251, 271
Page, L. B.   332, 347, 362, 363, 374
Paladini, A. C.   40, 51, 179, 216
Palay, S. L.   114, 129, 143, 151, 156, 169
Panigel, M.   338, 348
Pappenheimer, J. R.   358, 374
Papper, S.   253, 278
Pardoe, A. U.   4, 15, 116, 117, 152, 164, 171
Parker, C. W.   48, 55, 206, 223
Pasqualini, R. Q.   330, 349
Passoneau, J. V.   372, 374
Paton, A.   232, 275

Paton, D. N. 6, 16, 198, 199, 223
Paton, W. D. M. 200, 223
Patrick, R. W. 440, 445
Pauling, L. 355, 372
Pawan, G. L. S. 247, 269
Peachey, L. D. 365, 366, 375
Peeters, G. 123, 128, 146, 152, 198, 212, 216, 264, 274, 296, 302, 303, 318
Pehling, G. 236, 277
Pepys, J. 429, 445
Pereda, T. 178, 202, 211
Peric, B. 127, 145, 153
Perisutti, G. 206, 222
Perks, A. M. 32, 55, 69, 78, 230, 266, 322, 323, 324, 343
Perlmutt, J. H. 264, 276
Permutt, M. A. 48, 55, 206, 223
Persson, N. 190, 213
Peters, G. 229, 230, 235, 236, 240, 242, 243, 246, 247, 249, 253, 254, 255, 256, 258, 260, 261, 262, 264, 265, 266, 268, 269, 273, 276
Peters, J. P. 431, 445
Petersen, M. J. 48, 56
Petersen, W. E. 7, 13, 192, 223, 298, 302, 316, 402, 419
Photaki, I. 27, 35, 55, 90, 108
Pick, E. P. 185, 221
Pickering, B. T. 32, 53, 64, 66, 67, 68, 69, 77, 78, 91, 98, 100, 107, 108, 180, 181, 201, 204, 220, 223
Pickford, G. E. 69, 79, 324, 327, 343, 348, 349
Pickford, M. 67, 77, 119, 123, 126, 127, 129, 144, 147, 152, 183, 189, 190, 203, 207, 212, 224, 247, 255, 257, 259, 260, 262, 267, 268, 270, 276, 296, 302, 303, 318, 342, 343, 400, 401, 419, 420, 421
Pierce, J. G. 20, 21, 39, 46, 55, 57, 91, 109, 173, 178, 224, 227
Piguet, A. R. 136, 149
Pines, I. L. 2, 16
Pinkham, B. 183, 188, 216, 383, 386, 394
Pitkänen, M. E. 262, 264, 274
Pliška, F. 47, 50
Pliška, V. 99, 103, 104, 106, 110, 186, 187, 188, 189, 193, 203, 214, 224, 250, 270, 305, 306, 309, 310, 315
Poisner, A. M. 119, 126, 131, 145, 147, 165, 170, 178, 215

Polacek, E. 250, 276
Poláček, I. 94, 105, 200, 207, 211, 221, 304, 318
Polak, R. L. 123, 124, 127, 128, 145, 208, 214
Polimeros, D. 253, 275
Pomeroy, S. R. 200, 215, 289, 293
Popenoe, E. A. 5, 6, 13, 16, 21, 24, 25, 28, 46, 47, 51, 52, 55, 56, 67, 78
Porath, J. 5, 16, 41, 55, 66, 78, 179, 221, 224
Portanova, R. 41, 56, 162, 169, 180, 224
Potick, D. 329, 347
Pottinger, R. E. 391, 394
Pratt, O. E. 263, 269
Prescott, A. S. 239, 275
Pressman, B. C. 116, 147
Prestcott, K. F. 126, 145
Preston, A. S. 246, 268
Primavesi, L. 3, 13
Probst, J. H. 246, 269
Prout, T. E. 48, 53, 206, 218
Pursel, S. 246, 271
Purser, R. M. Jr. 259, 270, 401, 402, 420

Rabasa, S. L. 183, 224
Rábek, V. 36, 54, 104, 108
Race, B. 100, 108, 204, 222
Radford, E. P. Jr. 127, 151, 188, 227, 243, 278, 389, 395
Raffy, A. 324, 345, 346
Raisz, L. G. 189, 224, 254, 276
Rall, T. W. 372, 373
Ralli, E. P. 189, 224
Ralph, C. L. 338, 349
Ramalingaswami, V. 253, 269
Ramel, A. 233, 274
Randall, S. S. 208, 219
Rankin, J. C. 323, 325, 349
Ranson, S. W. 3, 11
Rapoport, S. 254, 267, 431, 445
Rasmussen, H. 32, 56, 91, 92, 100, 101, 102, 103, 104, 105, 108, 333, 349, 365, 366, 371, 375, 391, 393, 396
Razabeck, K. 99, 110
Rector, F. C. 253, 272, 431, 443
Rees, J. R. 435, 445
Reeves, J. L. 187, 215
Regoli, D. 229, 240, 243, 258, 261, 266, 268

Reiffenstein, R. 4, 15, 117, 145, 156, 164, 170
Reindel, F. 181, 224
Relman, A. S. 251, 276
Renkin, E. M. 358, 374
Rennels, M. L. 165, 171
Ressler, C. 5, 13, 19, 21, 22, 26, 27, 29, 45, 46, 52, 56, 67, 79, 92, 109, 173, 175, 208, 217, 224, 291, 293
Retzius, G. 2, 16
Riad, A. M. 392, 395
Ribot, S. 442, 445
Rich, E. 160, 170
Richardson, K. C. 193, 224, 298, 296, 299, 306, 315, 318
Rinderknecht, H. 182, 183, 223, 388, 395
Rink, H. 30, 54
Ritchie, A. E. 259, 276
Rivera, M. J. 252, 271
Robbins, E. 358, 375
Roberts, C. W. 5, 13, 19, 26, 27, 29, 52, 173, 208, 217
Roberts, G. S. 336, 349
Roberts, J. 165, 171
Roberts, V. S. 201, 219
Robertson, P. A. 194, 201, 219
Robinson, C. V. 356, 375
Robinson, R. R. 236, 269
Robson, J. M. 201, 203, 214, 224
Rocha e Silva, M. 126, 127, 146, 152, 214
Roch-Ramel, F. 229, 235, 236, 246, 249, 255, 258, 261, 266, 268, 276
Rodeck, H. 114, 149, 443
Rodrigues, J. 431, 443
Roeske, R. 28, 52
Roffman, F. 73, 74, 78
Rokaw, S. N. 387, 393
Rolleston, Sir H. D. 1, 11
Romas, C. 91, 107
Romeis, B. 2, 11
Rorie, D. 200, 224
Rosalki, S. B. 435, 445
Rose, D. P. 435, 443
Rosenfeld, J. B. 371, 375
Rosenfeld, M. 133, 152
Ross, E. 436, 437, 438, 443
Roth, G. B. 176, 224
Roth, J. 48, 56
Roth, K. 392, 395
Rothballer, A. B. 168, 171
Rothen, A. J. 41, 57, 65, 77, 111, 133, 147, 156, 165, 171, 180, 207, 227, 304, 319
Rothera, A. C. H. 192, 193, 222
Rott, D. 385, 396
Rouffignac, C. de 236, 275
Roussy, G. 3, 16
Roux, V. 372, 373
Rowe, L. W. 5, 14, 62, 78, 178, 185, 191, 219, 221
Roy, B. P. 69, 77
Rubin, M. E. 189, 221
Rubin, M. I. 250, 269
Rubin, R. P. 119, 147
Rubini, M. E. 251, 276
Rubinoff, H. 430, 444
Ruch, W. 181, 224
Rudinger, J. 6, 27, 33, 34, 35, 36, 37, 39, 51, 52, 54, 56, 58, 81, 88, 89, 90, 91, 92, 94, 103, 104, 105, 107, 108, 109, 189, 200, 203, 207, 211, 214, 221, 224, 262, 263, 269, 285, 293, 304, 305, 306, 308, 309, 310, 315, 316, 317, 318, 320, 371, 375
Rumrich, G. 237, 238, 241, 269, 277, 274
Ruskin, H. D. 248, 268
Russell, J. J. 407, 421
Rutledge, D. I. 10, 16
Rychlík, I. 47, 49, 50, 103, 104, 106, 186, 187, 188, 189, 193, 203, 207, 214, 224, 305, 306, 309, 310, 315, 391, 393
Rydén, G. 197, 209, 210, 224, 225, 298, 306, 318
Rydin, H. 126, 127, 152, 183, 224
Rydon, H. N. 44, 53
Rynearson, E. H. 10, 16

Saameli, K. 201, 203, 214, 288, 289, 290, 292, 293, 405, 411, 412, 421, 422
Sachs, H. 4, 17, 41, 56, 57, 112, 115, 117, 127, 140, 152, 153, 156, 158, 159, 160, 161, 162, 164, 165, 166, 169, 171, 180, 181, 182, 208, 224, 226, 227, 390, 396
Sacks, B. 402, 421
Saito, Y. 160, 170
Sakakibara, S. 27, 28, 56
Sakota, N. 180, 224
Sala, N. L. 298, 300, 318, 319
Salvestrini, H. 208, 216

Samaan, A. 185, 225
Sanderson, P. H. 252, 276
Santorini, G. D. 1, 11
Santos, R. F. 249, 264, 274
Sanwal, M. 117, 145
Sasai, T. 180, 224
Sawyer, C. H. 127, 149
Sawyer, M. K. 336, 349
Sawyer, W. H. 5, 6, 15 32, 55, 62, 64, 67, 68, 69, 70, 72, 75, 78, 79, 81, 85, 86, 88, 96, 97, 100, 101, 107, 109, 111, 143, 174, 175, 181, 188, 189, 190, 191, 192, 201, 204, 205, 212, 223, 225, 227, 230, 231, 243, 255, 259, 261, 262, 264, 266, 269, 276, 286, 292, 307 309, 314, 319, 323, 324, 327, 328, 329, 330, 333, 336, 337, 338, 339, 344, 347, 348, 349, 350, 378, 380, 382, 388, 391, 393, 396, 397
Sax, M. G. 371, 373
Schachter, B. A. 41, 52, 53, 133, 134, 137, 148, 150, 180, 218
Schaechtelin, G. 261, 272
Schäfer, E. A. 2, 6, 7, 10, 15, 16, 192, 193, 225, 255, 275, 298, 314
Schally, A. V. 45, 47, 55, 56, 179, 180, 224, 225
Scharrer, B. 3, 11, 111, 157, 169
Scharrer, E. 3, 4, 11, 12, 16, 111, 117, 145, 151, 157, 163, 169
Scheer, R. L. 254, 276
Scheraga, H. A. 355, 374
Schiebler, T. H. 4, 16, 116, 152
Schild, H. O. 198, 200, 201, 207, 209, 222, 224, 225, 284, 293, 304, 318, 406, 420
Schlapp, W. 190, 192, 201, 220, 384, 386, 395
Schmidt-Nielsen, B. 117, 144, 236, 277, 336, 337, 346, 349
Schmidt-Nielsen, K. 117, 144
Schneiden, H. 126, 152
Schneider, C. H. 38, 47, 52, 56, 381, 388, 393
Schneider, W. 200, 225
Schnermann, J. 235, 276
Schoessler, M. A. 47, 52, 371, 375, 391, 396
Schofield, B. M. 407, 410, 421, 422
Schofield, J. A. 44, 53
Schor, N. 163, 167, 169
Schröder, E. 32, 33, 34, 35, 49, 54, 227

Schröder, R. 264, 277, 385, 396
Schroeder, H. A. 188, 227
Schroeder, S. A. 392, 395
Schulz, H. 34, 56
Schwartz, I. L. 32, 34, 36, 37, 47, 49, 52, 57, 81, 91, 92, 100, 101, 102, 103, 104, 105, 106, 108, 109, 333, 344, 349, 371, 373, 375, 384, 385, 391, 393, 394, 396
Schwartz, W. B. 251, 276, 431, 434, 445
Scott, J. C. 6, 15, 192, 223
Sealock, R. R. 20, 25, 44, 46, 56, 208, 225
Sebkova, M. 250, 276
Segar, W. E. 251, 275
Seldin, D. W. 253, 272, 431, 443
Selye, H. 3, 16, 312, 319
Semm, K. 406, 419
Senay, L. C. Jr. 232, 277
Sexton, A. W. 323, 325, 349
Shakhmatova, E. I. 36, 50
Shannon, J. A. 166, 171, 245, 259, 277
Share, L. 127, 152, 162, 165, 166, 169, 171, 181, 188, 208, 225, 257, 277, 378, 381, 382, 384, 394, 396
Sharpey-Schäfer, E. 10, 11
Sheridan, B. 442, 445
Sherman, G. H. 372, 373
Sherrington, L. A. 235, 270
Shimonishi, Y. 27, 28, 56
Shinde, Y. 312, 318
Shirley, H. V. 338, 340, 349
Shoenberg, C. F. 280, 292
Shorr, E. 126, 144
Sica-Blanco, Y. 195, 211, 378, 382, 389, 393
Siddiqi, S. 127, 152, 202, 225
Sidel, V. W. 361, 375
Sierens, G. 302, 318
Silver, I. A. 194, 216, 296, 298, 301, 302, 304, 316, 319
Silver, L. 46, 47, 52, 118, 127, 153, 177, 208, 226, 371, 373, 375, 380, 384, 385, 391, 394, 396
Silver, M. 302, 318
Silverman, A. C. 10, 15
Simon, A. 115, 152
Sims, E. A. H. 431, 445
Sjöholm, I. 47, 51, 56, 197, 209, 210, 224, 225, 298, 306, 318
Skadhauge, E. 128, 137, 153, 186, 188, 190, 225, 226, 238, 242, 277, 336, 338, 349, 430, 445

Slater, S. 392, 395
Sloper, J. 4, 12, 156, 157, 158, 169, 171
Small, M. J. 442, 445
Smart, D. 417, 420
Smart, E. 417, 420
Smirk, F. H. 126, 149
Smith, B. L. 98, 107
Smith, H. W. 255, 259, 266
Smith, M. W. 121, 123, 127, 128, 134, 137, 149, 153, 178, 179, 180, 186, 188, 197, 200, 201, 202, 203, 212, 216, 219, 225, 226, 242, 257, 272, 277, 304, 306, 310, 313, 317, 319, 379, 380, 381, 384, 386, 389, 390, 391, 395, 396
Smith, R. B. Jr. 198, 199, 226
Smith-Agreda, V. 112, 147
Smithies, O. 134, 153
Smyth, C. N. 414, 422
Smyth, D. G. 44, 56, 88, 90, 109
Snaith, A. H. 181, 223
Snyder, J. G. 253, 274
Sokol, H. W. 70, 75, 79, 117, 153, 164, 171, 188, 227
Soliman, A. A. I. 202, 220
Solomon, A. K. 358, 373
Solomon, D. H. 249, 272, 426, 444
Solomon, S. 233, 275
Šorm, F. 6, 34, 35, 36, 37, 47, 50, 52, 54, 58, 88, 97, 98, 99, 103, 104, 105, 106, 107, 108, 109, 110, 189, 203, 207, 214, 305, 306, 308, 309, 310, 315, 316
Špačkova, M. 262, 278
Spargo, B. 251, 277
Spears, I. 430, 444
Speidel, C. C. 111, 153
Spickett, S. G. 6, 11, 72, 75, 114, 149
Starling, E. H. 390, 396
Staverman, A. J. 361, 375
Stedman, R. J. 30, 53
Steggerda, F. R. 349
Stehle, R. L. 5, 16
Stein, M. 183, 226
Stein, W. H. 20, 55
Stelter, E. 230, 260, 277
Stephens, G. 339, 349
Stephenson, W. F. 126, 148
Sterba, G. 4, 16, 117, 148
Stevenson, R. H. 248, 268
Stewart, G. A. 199, 201, 226
Stewart, J. W. 201, 202, 213
Stewart, W. C. 330, 349

Stoker, D. J. 439, 440, 442, 444
Stokes, J. 254, 268
Stoklasa, E. 392, 396
Stolte, H. 244, 273, 278
Stone, M. L. 197, 228, 298, 319
Stoner, H. B. 126, 146
Stormont, J. M. 431, 445
Stormorken, H. 128, 152, 296, 303, 318,
Stouffer, J. E. 42, 47, 49, 52, 133, 136, 137, 143, 381, 388, 393
Strahan, R. 199, 226
Stranack, F. 236, 270
Strauss, F. 251, 277
Streefkerk, J. G. 133, 143
Strominger, J. 160, 170
Studer, R. O. 30, 56, 57, 98, 109
Štulc, J. 188, 209, 220
Stumpf, C. 200, 225
Sturkie, P. D. 339, 342, 349
Stürmer, E. 36, 57, 86, 97, 98, 106, 203, 226
Stutinsky, F. 200, 219
Styles, P. R. 201, 226
Sullivan, T. J. 201, 226
Sussman, L. 439, 440, 444
Sutherland, E. W. 334, 344, 372, 373, 374,
Sutherland, I. D. W. 336, 337, 347
Swain, R. W. 47, 55
Swan, J. M. 5, 13, 19, 22, 26, 27, 29, 52, 55, 173, 208, 217

Tabor, M. 235, 276
Taira, N. 284, 293
Takabatake, Y. 41, 56, 112, 115, 152, 159, 161, 162, 164, 166, 171, 180, 226
Tanaka, A. 117, 150
Tanaka, K. 339, 349
Tassel, D. 434, 445
Tata, P. S. 183, 187, 188, 189, 190, 206, 218, 226, 243, 277, 381, 396
Tatum, E. L. 160, 170
Taylor, N. B. G. 126, 153, 182, 183, 220, 223
Taylor, S. P. Jr. 22, 23, 54, 55, 57, 180, 226
Tello, F. 2, 16
Tennent, R. A. 412, 422
Theobald, G. W. 9, 16, 123, 128, 153, 183, 185, 226, 296, 319, 399, 401, 402, 403, 407, 408, 409, 410, 412, 413, 415, 416, 419, 420, 421, 422

Thesleff, S. 406, 420
Thomas, P. J. 121, 133, 134, 136, 137, 138, 148, 153, 156, 165, 171, 180, 219
Thomas, P. L. 30, 32, 50
Thompson, R. E. 198, 199, 226
Thomson, J. 250, 277
Thomson, W. B. 260, 277
Thorn, N. A. 118, 121, 127, 128, 134, 137, 139, 141, 153, 174, 177, 180, 186, 188, 208, 212, 226, 241, 242, 277, 371, 375, 380, 381, 387, 389, 390, 396
Thorp, R. H. 174, 199, 212
Thurau, K. 7, 15, 235, 236, 276, 277
Thürkauf, M. 356, 374
Tindal, J. S. 126, 153, 194, 196, 226, 297, 298, 303, 305, 312, 315, 319
Titov, M. I. 36, 50
Titova, L. K. 239, 272, 371, 373
Titus, M. I. 391, 395
Toennies, G. 21, 57
Topper, Y. J. 311, 315, 317
Towbin, E. J. 388, 396
Traeger, J. 232, 278
Tramezzani, J. H. 118, 129, 148
Trippett, S. 21, 22, 52, 56, 67, 79
Troupkou, V. 246, 250, 251, 254, 271
Truelove, L. H. 126, 145
Trupin, J. 73, 74, 78
Tsakhaev, G. A. 300, 319
Tsukuda, T. 180, 224
Tuppy, H. 5, 16, 23, 47, 57, 67, 79, 208, 212, 227, 392, 393, 396, 406, 407, 419, 422
Turner, C. B. 410, 421
Turner, C. W. 128, 149, 192, 197, 213, 227, 305, 319
Turner, R. A. 20, 21, 46, 57, 91, 109, 178, 227
Turvey, A. 126, 153, 303, 319
Tuthill, E. 246, 271
Tuyttens, N. 198, 216
Tüzünkam, P. 389, 394
Tverskoĭ, G. B. 300, 319
Tyler, C. 114, 147

Uemura, H. 130, 153
Ullmann, T. D. 242, 250, 270, 277
Ullrich, K. J. 237, 238, 241, 269, 271, 274, 277
Unger, R. H. 434, 445

Uranga, J. 330, 349
Urban, F. F. 385, 395
Usami, S. 127, 145, 153, 378, 387, 397
Ussing, H. H. 100, 109, 240, 278, 326, 331, 344, 346, 347, 351, 358, 365, 373, 374
Utiger, R. D. 48, 55, 206, 223, 434, 435, 445

Vaamonde, C. A. 253, 278
Vaamonde, L. S. 253, 278
Valtin, H. 70, 75, 79, 117, 153, 164, 171, 188, 190, 225, 227, 232, 235, 243, 245, 258, 267, 273, 276, 278
van Arman, C. G. 229, 278
van Deenen, L. L. M. 368, 374
van Demark, N. L. 402, 422
van Dongen, C. G. 193, 197, 209, 227, 297, 298, 299, 306, 319, 410, 422
van Dyke, H. B. 5, 6, 8, 11, 16, 41, 57, 62, 65, 67, 68, 69, 70, 72, 77, 78, 79, 86, 97, 100, 109, 111, 112, 113, 114, 115, 117, 118, 119, 127, 133, 137, 142, 144, 145, 147, 156, 165, 171, 173, 174, 175, 177, 178, 180, 181, 183, 189, 190, 192, 193, 194, 199, 201, 204, 205, 207, 208, 211, 213, 216, 223, 225, 227, 231, 243, 267, 276, 278, 286, 287, 293, 298, 304, 305, 309, 314, 319, 337, 339, 348, 349, 387, 391, 393, 396, 397, 401, 402, 420, 422
Vaneček, J. 262, 278
Vanschoubroek, F. 128, 152, 296, 303, 318
Van't Hoff, W. 431, 445
van Wagenen, G. S. 417, 422
Vávra, I. 207, 221
Vechetova, E. 250, 276
Velluz, L. 27, 57
Verney, E. B. 7, 16, 17, 118, 119, 126, 127, 152, 153, 183, 189, 190, 219, 223, 224, 390, 396, 397
Vernikos-Danellis, J. 439, 445
Versteeg, D. H. G. 72, 79
Vierling, A. F. 188, 227, 243, 278
Vieussens, R. 1, 11
Vliegenhart, J. F. G. 72, 79
Vogel, J. 250, 276
Vogt, M. 158, 171, 112, 117, 129, 130, 147, 153, 181, 191, 208, 223, 227

Vogt, W. 202, 212
Vollrath, L. 327, 347
von den Velden, R. 6, 10, 17
von Haller, A. 1, 11
von Schlichtegroll, A. 113, 152, 181, 227
Vorherr, H. 198, 247, 278, 305, 319, 227, 388, 394
Vos, B. J. Jr. 198, 226, 227

Wagner, G. 128, 148, 203, 218, 296, 317
Wagner, H. N. Jr. 245, 275
Waldstein, S. S. 432, 444
Walker, A. M. 179, 185, 227
Walker, J. M. 118, 123, 126, 127, 145, 152, 153, 178, 201, 202, 215, 225, 257, 269, 384, 387, 390, 391, 394, 427, 445
Waller, H. 128, 153
Waller, J.-P. 27, 50, 175, 215
Walmsley, C. F. 8, 11, 13, 128, 148, 175, 178, 179, 182, 187, 194, 195, 196, 201, 211, 212, 217, 219, 379, 392, 411, 419
Walter, R. 31, 34, 35, 36, 37, 39, 46, 51, 57, 91, 92, 109
Wang, C. C. 127, 129, 145
Wang, J. W. 356, 375
Wang, K. L. 127, 129, 145
Wang, S. C. 126, 127, 147, 151
Wang, S. M. 190, 201, 217, 227
Ward, D. N. 66, 79, 180, 227
Wardener, H. E. de 232, 242, 245, 249, 250, 252, 269, 270, 274, 275
Waring, H. 191, 199, 221, 226, 228, 324, 339, 344, 349
Waterhouse, C. 190, 220, 264, 273, 431, 445
Watson, A. 6, 16, 198, 199, 223
Watson, B. P. 399, 420, 422
Watt, J. A. 126, 129, 147, 152
Wattiaux, R. 116, 144, 147
Weatherall, M. 4, 15, 116, 117, 152, 164, 171
Weaver, J. A. 442, 445
Weinstein, H. 4, 17, 117, 127, 153, 156, 171, 181, 227
Weintraub, D. H. 250, 269
Weise, V. K. 440, 445
Weisel, G. F. 6, 15
Weiss, P. 157, 169

Welt, L. G. 252, 272, 273, 275, 278, 431, 445
Werle, E. 202, 212
West, C. D. 232, 254, 276, 278, 431, 445
West, S. P. 429, 444
Whalley, P. J. 253, 272
White, H. L. 245, 278
Whittaker, V. P. 130, 153, 201, 216
Whittlestone, W. G. 193, 198, 227, 296, 298, 302, 305, 319
Wiederholt, M. 242, 244, 273, 278
Wiederman, J. 197, 228, 298, 319
Wiegershausen, B. 91, 105
Wilhelmi, A. E. 327, 349
Williams, F. T. 251, 275
Williams, P. C. 182, 183, 223, 388, 395
Williams, T. F. 252, 273
Willis, T. 1, 11
Willumsen, N. B. S. 390, 396
Wilson, F. E. 340, 350
Wilzbach, K. E. 47, 57
Windhager, E. E. 254, 271
Winestock, G. 37, 47, 52
Winkler, A. W. 431, 443, 445
Winslow, J. B. 1, 11
Winters, R. W. 252, 272, 273, 275
Wintersberger, E. 208, 227, 392, 393, 396
Wiqvist, I. 202, 228
Wiqvist, N. 202, 228
Wirz, H. 232, 234, 236, 267, 278
Wise, J. H. 246, 274
Wislocki, G. B. 114, 154
Wolff, H. S. 410, 421
Wolfson, A. 340, 350
Wood, C. 407, 422
Woods, B. 182, 219
Woods, G. G. 185, 223
Woodward, R. B. 33, 57
Woolley, P. 199, 228, 335, 337, 339, 350
Wrong, D. 249, 264, 274

Yamaguchi, T. 177, 192, 213
Yamanoi, T. 160, 170
Yamashiro, D. 28, 34, 37, 38, 43, 44, 57, 58, 66, 79, 179, 228
Yasamasu, I. 117, 150
Yates, F. E. 440, 444
Yokoyama, A. 194, 196, 226, 297, 298, 301, 305, 312, 313, 318, 319, 320

Yoon, M. C. 249, 278
Yoshida, S. K. 181, 189, 210, 228
Young, R. 100, 101, 102, 103, 104, 108, 333, 349
Yun, K. O. 340, 347
Yuniband, P. 251, 278

Zaidi, S. M. A. 189, 220, 242, 273, 379, 390, 395
Zaks, M. G. 239, 272, 296, 299, 314, 320
Zambrano, D. 163, 167, 171
Zamorano, B. 178, 202, 211
Zaoral, M. 27, 29, 36, 37, 53, 56, 58, 97, 98, 99, 106, 109, 110
Zarrow, M. X. 197, 209, 222, 298, 304, 306, 318
Zedeck, M. S. 248, 278
Zeininger, K. 197, 214, 296, 315
Zerahn, K. 100, 109
Zetler, G. 3, 4, 14, 71, 77, 111, 123, 133, 149, 157, 170
Zhuze, A. L. 308, 320, 309
Zilva, J. F. 431, 445
Zuckerman, S. 248, 268
Zuidema, G. D. 127, 154, 187, 215
Zumoff, B. 248, 268

SUBJECT INDEX

Where a reference occurs on a number of consecutive pages, only the first page number is given

Acetone-lysine-vasopressin 43
Acetone-oxytocin 43, 179
N-Acetyl-O-acetyloxytocin 90
Acetylcholine
  action on mammary tissue 306, 410
  effect on isolated rat uterus 202
  interference
    in milk-ejection assay 196
    in vasopressor assay 192
  occurrence in neurohypophysis 129
    subcellular particles associated with 130
    vasomotor function 132
  role in release of vasopressin and oxytocin 126, 129
N-Acetyloxytocin 87, 88
Actinopterygians 66
  see also Chondrostei, Holostei, Teleostei
Active transport *see* Sodium transport
Adenohypophysis
  effect of neurohypophysial hormones on 327, 335, 340, 342
  stimulation by coitus 402
Adenosine 3′,5′ monophosphate *see* Cyclic AMP
Adenosine triphosphate
  interference with milk ejection assay 196
  release of neurohypophysial hormones by 126
Adrenaline
  action on mammary tissue 197, 302, 306
  effect
    on avian blood pressure 199
    on isolated rat uterus 202
Adrenergic blocking drugs
  effect in teleost fishes 327
  use in vasopressor assays 191, 192
Adrenocorticotrophic hormone (ACTH) *see* Corticotrophin
Agnatha, arginine vasotocin in 71
[1-Alanine, 6-alanine]-arginine-vasopressin *see* Dethio-arginine-vasopressin
[1-Alanine, 6-alanine]-lysine-vasopressin *see* Dethio-lysine-vasopressin
[4-Alanine]-oxytocin 310
[4-β-Alanine]-oxytocin 35
[8-Alanine]-oxytocin 36
[9-Alanine]-oxytocin 36
[9-β-Alanine]-oxytocin 36
Aldosterone
  effect
    on flounders (*Platichthys flesus*) 326
    on renal medullary sodium 244
    on sodium excretion 244
    on vasopressin action 244, 250
  secretion in dilutional hyponatremia 432
Alligator, effect of Pitressin in 336
Ambystoma, effect of neurohypophysial hormones in 334
Ameiurus, effect of neurohypophysial hormones on water metabolism in 323
[8-α-Aminobutyric acid]-oxytocin 36
[8-[3(2-Aminoethyl)thio]-alanine]-vasopressin *see* [8-Thialysine]-vasopressin
2-*p*-Aminophenylalanine-oxytocin 263
Amphibians
  effect of neurohypophysial hormones in 329
  in Anura
    on bladder
      comparison of *Rana* and *Bufo* 333
      sodium transport 332
      water movement 100, 327, 333
    on kidney 230, 330
    on skin 330
  in Urodela 334
    on isolated oviduct 336
  hormonal mole ratios in 71
  neurohypophysial hormones present in 66, 68

Subject Index

Amphotericin B, effect on toad bladder 368
Anesthesia, effect on milk-ejection response 304
Analogues of neurohypophysial hormones 6, 34, 59
  activity 88, 89
  of oxytocin 86, 87, 308
    inhibitory action on galactokinetic effect 310
    milk ejection activity 87, 307
  of vasopressin 95
  synthesis of 32, 37
  use of magnesium ratios in identification of 87
  see also individual names
Angiotensin 104
  effect
    on isolated rat uterus 201
    on uterus *in situ* 203
  interference with milk-ejection assay 196, 302
  milk ejection activity 302
  natriuretic effects 261
    compared with oxytocin 261
    compared with vasopressin 265
  role in sodium excretion 258
Anguilla
  effect
    of neurohypophysial hormones in 323, 325, 327, 341
    of prolactin on 326
  sodium balance in 326
Antibodies
  to lysine vasopressin 48, 206
  to oxytocin 48
Anticholinesterases, release of neurohypophysial hormones by 126
Antidepressants, vasopressin antagonism 249
Antidiuretic assays *see under* Vasopressin
Antidiuretic hormone (ADH) *see* Arginine vasopressin, Lysine vasopressin, Vasopressin
Anura *see under* Amphibians *and individual species*
[8-Arginine]-oxytocin *see* Arginine vasotocin
Arginine vasopressin ([3-phenylalanine, 8-arginine]-oxytocin) 64

action of bromine water on 22, 46
activity, specific 85, 96, 97, 99, 101, 176, 308
amino acid constitution 20
assays for 174, 184, 190
  block of rat vasopressor response 207
  comparison with lysine vasopressin 175, 189
  interference of oxytocin with 174
  see also Vasopressin
biosynthesis 155
  effect of puromycin on 161, 162
  isotope techniques in 159
  precursor model 163
  rate of 166
  site of 158, 160
  see also Neurosecretory cells, Neurosecretory granules
calciuretic effect 241
clearance 377, 388
complex with neurophysin 41, 133
  effect of calcium on 138
deficiency *see* Diabetes insipidus
desulfurization 46
determination of structure 5
duration of antidiuresis due to 391
effect
  of drugs on release of 126
  in *Ambystoma* 334
  in *Bufo bufo* 329, 335
  on ACTH release 335
  on fowl oviduct 339
  on milk-ejection response to oxytocin 303
  on reptilian oviduct 337
  on toad bladder 101, 353
enzymic degradation 47
evidence for production in hyponatremia 433
extraction from biological tissues and fluids *see* Vasopressin
genetic relationship to lysine vasopressin 72
half-life in plasma 7, 383
  in urine 387
inappropriate secretion of 431, 433
isoelectric point 23
methods of identification 62
molecular weight 21
natriuretic effect 255, 263

Subject Index

Arginine occurrence 176
  oxidation 23
  plasma concentration of 382
  plasma protein binding of 380
  reduction of 46
  separation from lysine vasopressin 181
  stability 176
  storage 155, 165
  structure 23, 24, 60, 84
  synthesis 6, 19, 29
  tritium-labelled 47, 385
[8-D-Arginine]-vasopressin 37, 97, 98, 99
Arginine vasotocin ([8-arginine]-oxytocin) 61
  activity, specific 62, 96, 173, 176, 286, 289, 308
  assays 204
    antidiuretic effect in hen 190
    chicken depressor 199
    frog water balance 204
    hen oxytocic 205
    isolated frog bladder 205
    isolated frog skin 204
    turtle 205
    viviparous reptiles 205
  effects
    in amphibians 100, 101, 329, 334
    in birds 237, 338
    in bony fishes 323, 327
    in *Lampetra fluviatilis* 323
    in lungfish 323
    in reptiles 230, 337
    on blood glucose concentration in toads 206
    on oviposition in chickens 339
  evolutionary role of 72
  inhibition by related peptides 247
  isolation from *Pollachius virens* 66
  natural occurrence 32, 61, 67, 176, 204
  potency ratios 63, 64, 101
  separation from oxytocin 64
  structure 31, 60, 102
Artiodactyls, mole ratios of neurohypophysial hormones in 70
[4-Asparagine, 5-glutamine]-oxytocin 91
[4-Asparagine, 8-lysine]-vasopressin 37, 99
[4-Asparagine]-oxytocin 90, 101, 289, 308
  effect on frog and toad bladders 101, 103

[5-D-Asparagine]-oxytocin 36
Assays *see under substances assayed*
Axolotl see *Ambystoma*

Basal meningitis as a cause of diabetes insipidus 424
Bichir (African) see *Polypterus senegalus*
Biossay *see individual substances*
Biosynthesis of neurohypophysial hormones *see* Neurohypophysia hormones, *individual hormones*
Birds
  effect of neurohypophysial hormones in 338
  hypothalamic control of pars distalis 340
  neurohypophysial hormones in 66, 67
Blood
  anomalous oxytocic effects of 201
  clearance of neurohypophysial hormones from *see* Plasma clearance
  extraction of neurohypophysial hormones from 178
  neurohypophysial hormones in 123
  oxytocin concentration in 382
  physical state of oxytocin and vasopressin in 379
  see also Plasma
Blood–brain barrier in hypothalamus 113
Boston hake, neurohypophysial hormones in 69
Brachiopterygii, neurohypophysial hormones in *Polypterus senegalus* 69
Bradykinin 104
  activity, specific 104
  effect
    on isolated rat uterus 201
    on uterus *in situ* 203
  interference with milk ejection assays 196
  milk ejection activity 302
  release of neurohypophysial hormones by 126
Brattleboro strain of rats 75, 117
  effect of dehydration on 245
  neurophysins in 165
  sensitivity to vasopressin 188, 243
  use in antidiuretic assays 188, 243

Bufo arenarum, effect of oxytocin and vasopressin on 330
Bufo bufo
  effect of neurohypophysial hormones on 329
  mesotocin in 68
Bufo marinus 100, 329

Calcium
  effect
    on binding of hormones by neurophysin 121, 137
    on bound vasopressin 380, 390
    on proximal tubule permeability 241
  renal disturbances
    due to hypercalcemia 252, 424
    due to hypercalciuria 252
  role
    in antidiuresis 241
    in release of hormones 121, 140
  vasopressin antagonism 252
N-Carbamyloxytocin 88
  membrane diffusion of 41
  preparation of 44
Carboxypeptidases, effect on oxytocin and vasopressin 209
Carcinoma 423, 431, 433, 435
  see also Tumors
Cerebrospinal fluid
  anomalous oxytocic effect of 201
  oxytocic activity in 8
Chelonids 336
Chicken
  effect of neurohypophysial hormones in 338
  neurohypophysial hormones in 67
Chicken depressor assay *see* Oxytocin
p-Chloromercuribenzoate, effect on vasopressin 390
Choline acetylase, occurrence in neurohypophysis 129, 130
Cholinergic neurons, involvement in hormone release 120, 129
Cholinesterases in neurohypophysis 129
Chondrostei, neurohypophysial hormones in 61, 69
Chronic renal failure as a cause of polyuria 425
Chymotrypsin effect on oxytocin and vasopressin 208, 388

Cirrhosis of the liver associated with dilutional hyponatraemia 253
[8-Citrulline]-oxytocin 86, 101, 309, 310
[8-Citrulline]-vasopressin 97, 101
Cod, neurohypophysial hormones in 69
Colostrum, oxytocic kinins in 202
Corticosteroids
  effect on oxytocin natriuresis 257
  plasma "cortisol"
    after insulin-induced hypoglycemia or pyrogen 438
    in dilutional hyponatremia 433
    measurements in lysine vasopressin test 438, 442
Corticotrophin (ACTH)
  associated with tumors 435
  release 335, 438
  species-specific differences in 75
Counter-current distribution, separation of oxytocin and vasopressin by 5, 20, 178
Counter-current multiplier system in kidney 234, 244, 251
Creatinine, effect of oxytocin on renal clearance of 260
Cyclic AMP 334, 372
[3-Cyclohexylglycine]-oxytocin 35, 88
[3-D-Cyclohexylglycine]-oxytocin 35
[3-Cyclopentylglycine]-oxytocin 35, 87, 88
Cyclostomes
  effect of neurohypophysial hormones on 322
  neurohypophysial hormones in 61, 66, 70
Cytostatic drugs 248

4-Deamido-oxytocin ([4-glutamic acid]-oxytocin) 35, 90
9-Deamido-oxytocin ([9-glycine]-oxytocin) 36, 91
Deamino-[8-alanine]-oxytocin ([1-β-mercaptopropionic acid, 8-alanine]-oxytocin) 35
Deamino-[8-alanine]-vasopressin ([1-β-mercaptopropionic acid, 8-alanine]-vasopressin) 37
Deamino-arginine-vasopressin ([1-β-mercaptopropionic acid, 8-arginine]-vasopressin) 36

Subject Index

"Deamino-1-carba-oxytocin", synthesis of 33, 38, 93
Deamino-4-decarboxamido-oxytocin ([1-β-mercaptopropionic acid, 4-α-aminobutyne acid]-oxytocin) 34, 308
  crystallization of 39
Deamino-deoxy-arginine-vasopressin ([1-β-mercaptopropionic acid, 2-phenylalanine, 8-arginine]-vasopressin) 36
Deamino-deoxy-4-decarboxamido-oxytocin ([1-β-mercaptopropionic acid, 2-phenylalanine, 4-α-aminobutyric acid]-oxytocin) 34
Deamino-deoxy-[ornithine]-oxytocin ([1-β-mercaptopropionic acid, 2-phenylalanine, 8-ornithine]-oxytocin) 35
Deamino-deoxy-[ornithine]-vasopressin ([1-β-mercaptopropionic acid, 2-phenylalanine, 8-ornithine]-oxytocin) 37
Deamino-deoxy-[8-ornithine]-vasopressin ([1-β-mercaptopropionic acid, 2-phenylalanine, 8-ornithine]-vasopressin) 37
Deamino-deoxy-oxytocin ([1-β-mercaptopropionic acid, 2-phenylalanine]-oxytocin) 309
Deamino-dethio-arginine-vasopressin ([1-propionic acid, 6-alanine, 8-arginine]-vasopressin) 36
Deamino-dethio-lysine-vasopressin ([1-propionic acid, 6-alanine]-lysine-vasopressin) 37
Deamino-[6-hemi-selenocystine]-oxytocin 34, 39
Deamino-[2-isoleucine]-oxytocin ([1-β-mercaptopropionic acid, 2-isoleucine]-oxytocin) 34
Deamino-isotocin ([1-β-mercaptopropionic acid, 4-serine, 8-isoleucine]-oxytocin) 35
Deamino-lysine-vasopressin ([1-β-mercaptopropionic acid, 8-lysine]-vasopressin) 40, 43, 101
Deamino-[8-ornithine]-oxytocin ([1-β-mercaptopropionic acid, 8-ornithine]-oxytocin) 35
Deamino-[8-ornithine]-vasopressin ([1-β-mercaptopropionic acid, 8-ornithine]-vasopressin) 37
Deamino-oxytoceine ([1-β-mercaptopropionic acid]-S, S'-dihydro-oxytocin) 34, 44
Deamino-oxytocin ([1-β-mercaptopropionic acid]-oxytocin) 33, 40, 87, 89, 101, 180, 288, 289, 307, 308, 339
  crystallization of 39
  effect on frog and toad bladders 101, 333
  inhibition of antidiuretic action of vasotocins 247
  X-ray crystallographic data on 39
[1-Deamino-penicillamine]-oxytocin 34, 285
Deamino-[7-D-proline]-oxytocin ([1-β-mercaptopropionic acid, 7-D-proline]-oxytocin 34
Deamino-[1,6-selenocystine]-oxytocin 34
Deamino-[2-D-tyrosine]-oxytocin (1-β-mercaptopropionic acid, 2-D-tyrosine]-oxytocin) 34
Deamino-[4-valine]-oxytocin ([1-β-mercaptopropionic acid, 4-valine]-oxytocin) 34, 46
Deamino-[5-valine]-oxytocin ([1-β-mercaptopropionic acid, 5-valine]-oxytocin) 34
4-Decarboxamido-oxytocin ([4-α-aminobutyric acid]-oxytocin) 89, 90, 91, 288, 308, 310
5-Decarboxamido-oxytocin ([5-alanine]-oxytocin) 89
9-Decarboxamido-oxytocin 36, 89, 91
Deoxy-arginine vasopressin ([2-phenylalanine, 8-arginine]-vasopressin) 98
Deoxy-4-decarboxamido-oxytocin ([2-phenylalanine, 4-α-aminobutyric acid]-oxytocin) 35
Deoxy-lysine vasopressin ([2-phenylalanine, 8-lysine]-vasopressin) 98
Deoxy-[8-ornithine]-oxytocin ([2-phenylalanine, 8-ornithine]-oxytocin) 35, 98
Deoxy-[8-ornithine]-vasopressin ([2-phenylalanine, 8-ornithine]-vasopressin) 37, 98
Deoxy-oxytocin ([2-phenylalanine]-oxytocin) 89, 90, 101, 263, 309, 310

Deoxy binding to neurophysin 42
cupric ion complex with 44
Desamino-oxytocin see Deamino-oxytocin
Dethio-arginine-vasopressin ([1-alanine, 6-alanine, 8-arginine]-vasopressin) 36, 46
Dethio-lysine-vasopressin ([1-alanine, 6-alanine-lysine]-vasopressin) 36, 46
Dethio-oxytocin ([1-alanine, 6-alanine]-oxytocin) 46, 89
Diabetes insipidus 75
 in birds 338
 causes 423, 424
 clinical features 424
 congenital, in rats see Brattleboro strain of rats
 diagnosis 424
 effect of bicarbonate on response to vasopressin in 250
 glomerular filtration rate in 245, 259
 nephrogenic 424, 430
 renal vascular effect of oxytocin in 259
 tests for absence of vasopressin in 425
 treatment 428
 urinary hyaluronidase activity in 371
 use of posterior pituitary extract in 7, 10, 429
Diabetes mellitus
 polyuria in 425
 use of chlorpropamide in 431
[8-(2:4-Diaminobutyric acid)]-vasopressin 37, 97, 99
[8-D-(2:4-Diaminobutyric acid)]-vasopressin 37, 97, 99
Diastereoisomers, separation of 38
N,O-Dicarbamyl oxytocin 44, 90
[3-Diethylalanine]-oxytocin 35, 87, 308
S,S'-Dihydro-oxytocin see Oxytoceine
S,S'-Dihydrovasopressin see Vasopresseine
S,S'-Dihydro-analogues 37
Diisopropylphosphofluoridate, effect on vasopressin 390
Dilutional hyponatremia 248, 249, 431, 432, 433, 435, 437
Dimers of oxytocin and the vasopressins 45
Diodone, effect of oxytocin on renal clearance of 260

Diphenylhydantoin, vasopressin antagonism 249
Dipnoi 66, 72
effect
 of arginine vasotocin in 328
 of oxytocin in 328
Diuretics 248
 in treatment of diabetes insipidus 430
[1,6-Djenkolic acid 8-lysine]-vasopressin 37, 103
[1,6-Djenkolic acid]-oxytocin 37
Dogfish, neurohypophysial hormones in 69

Eel see Anguilla sp.
Elasmobranchs
 effect of neurohypophysial hormones on 323
 neurohypophysial hormones in 61, 66, 69
Electrophoresis
 separation of oxytocin and vasopressin by 5, 184
 identification of arginine vasopressin in urine by 388
Enzymic degradation of oxytocin and vasopressins 47, 208
Epinephrine see Adrenaline
Ergometrine (Ergonovine) 400
Ergot 279, 404
Estradiol, effect on uterine activity 407
Estrogen
 effect
  on uterine activity 281, 409
  on vascular action of oxytocin 401
  interaction with oxytocin on uterus 8, 289
Ethanol, effect on vasopressin secretion 189, 242, 425
Ethylenediamine-tetraacetate, effect on vasopressin 390
Ethyleneimine, vasopressin antagonism 248
[2-p-Ethylphenylalanine]-oxytocin 90, 263, 309
[2-O-Ethyltyrosine]-oxytocin 90, 263
Euryhaline teleosts, sodium balance in 326
Evolutionary pathways of neurohypophysial hormones 71

Fanconi's syndrome as a cause of polyuria 425
Ferritin, release of neurohypophysial hormones by 126
Fluid deprivation tests 426
Frog see *Rana* sp.
Fundulus sp.
  effect of neurohypophysial hormones on 326
  isotocin in 69

Galactobolic effects *see under* Oxytocin
Galactokinetic effects *see under* Oxytocin
Galactopoietic effects *see under* Oxytocin
Glial cells in neurohypophysis 2
β-Globulins, binding of vasopressins to 380
Glomerular filtration rate
  effect
    of diuretics on 430
    of 5-hydroxytryptamine on 230
    of hypophysectomy on 259, 401
    influence of neurohypophysial hormones on 230, 244, 259, 322, 325, 330, 335, 336, 338, 341, 401
Glumitocin ([4-serine, 8-glutamine]-oxytocin) 72, 90, 286, 308
  evolutionary role 72
  genetic pathway to relationship to other peptides 73
  occurrence 30, 61
  potency ratio 64
  in *Raia clavata* 69
  structure 31
[4-Glutamic acid]-oxytocin *see* 4-Deamido-oxytocin
[4-D-Glutamine, 5-D-asparagine]-oxytocin 35
[4-D-Glutamine]-oxytocin 35
[5-Glutamine]-oxytocin 91
"Glutathione-oxytocin transhydrogenase" 391
[3-Glycine]-oxytocin, binding to neurophysin 42
[4-Glycine]-oxytocin 35
  binding to neurophysin 42
[8-Glycine]-oxytocin 36, 101, 309
[9-Glycine]-oxytocin *see* 9-Deamido-oxytocin

Glycylglycylglycyl-lysine-vasopressin 36
Glycylglycyl-lysine-vasopressin 36
Glycylglycyl-oxytocin 34, 309
Glycyl-lysine-vasopressin 36
Glycyl-[2-O-methyltyrosine, 8-lysine]-vasopressin 36
Glycyloxytocin 309
  inhibition of assay response of oxytocin 207
Glycylprolyl-[8-lysine]-vasopressin 36
Gomori stain 3

[1-Hemi-D-cystine]-oxytocin 34, 38, 40
[6-Hemi-D-cystine]-oxytocin 36
[1-Hemi-homocystine]-oxytocin 40, 42
[6-Hemi-selenocystine]-oxytocin 36, 39
Henle's loop 232, 233, 251, 252
"Herring bodies" 3
Hippopotamus, lysine vasopressin in 67
Histamine
  effect
    on mammary tissue 302
    on isolated rat uterus 202
  interference with milk-ejection assay 196
  release of neurohypophysial hormones by 126
[8-Histidine]-vasopressin, membrane diffusion of 40
Holostei, neurohypophysial hormones in 61, 69
Hormonogens 103, 309, 310
Hyaluronidase
  role in antidiuresis 239, 371, 390
  urinary excretion 239
11-Hydroxycorticosteroids 433, 442
17-Hydroxycorticosteroids 438, 439
[7-Hydroxyproline]-oxytocin 36
5-Hydroxytryptamine
  effect
    on glomerular filtration rate 230
    on isolated rat uterus 202
    on mammary tissue 303
    on superfused uterus 202
    on uterus *in situ* 203
  in antidiuretic assays 185
  interference with milk-ejection assay 196, 197
Hyperglycemia, induction by neurohypophysial hormones 321

Hyperparathyroidism, renal disturbances due to 252
Hyponatremia see Dilutional hyponatremia
Hypothalamo-neurohypophysial system 4, 117
Hypothalamus
  acetylcholine, acetylcholinesterase and choline acetylase in 130
  action of acetylcholine on cell bodies in 129
  blood–brain barrier in 113
  control of pars distalis by 340, 438
  hormone content of, in mammals 112
  hormone synthesis in 112, 155
  mole ratios of hormones in 70, 112
Hypothalamus-median-eminence (HME) tissue, use in biosynthesis experiments 159, 161, 167

Ichthyotocin see Isotocin
Insulin
  effect on carbohydrate metabolism in mammary parenchyma cells 311
  species-specific differences of 75
Inulin clearance 260, 388
Ion-exchange chromatography 5, 66, 180
[2-Isoleucine]-oxytocin 35
  binding to neurophysin 42
[3-*allo*-Isoleucine]-oxytocin 88, 101, 309, 310
[8-Isoleucine]-oxytocin see Mesotocin
Isoprenaline (Isoproterenol) 400
Isotocin (Ichthyotocin, [4-serine, 8-isoleucine]-oxytocin) 76, 90, 101, 286, 289, 307, 308, 325
  evolutionary role 72
  in teleost fishes 69, 325
  occurrence 30, 61
  potency ratio 64, 101
  structure 31, 60
  synthesis 30
  vasopressor effect in eels 327
Isotope techniques
  in biosynthesis experiments 158
  in milk secretion and resorption 312
  in renal permeability studies 236
  in toad bladder 352, 359, 365

Kidney
  collecting ducts
    lesions in 252
    permeability of 232, 237, 254
    comparison with toad bladder 240
    concentrating action 234; see also Urine
  effect
    of dehydration on 232
    of hypercalcemia on 252
    of vasopressin on 232, 235
  hyaluronidase activity in distal nephron 371
  medullary blood flow 235
  medullary sodium concentrating system 244
  medullary sodium concentrations 235, 244, 251
    effect of aldosterone on 244
  medullary urea 246
  receptor sites for vasopressin 364
Kinins
  effect
    in rat antidiuretic assay 189
    on isolated rat uterus 201
  interference in vasopressor assays 192

Labor, induction of
  by amniotomy 412
  by buccal oxytocin 414
  by intravenous oxytocin drip 399, 412
[3-Leucine]-oxytocin 88
[des-8-Leucine]-oxytocin 100
[3-D-Leucine]-oxytocin 38, 40, 309
[8-Leucine]-vasopressin 97
Leucylglycylglycyloxytocin 309, 310
Leucylleucyl-[8-lysine]-vasopressin 36
Leucylleucyloxytocin 34, 309
Leucyl-[8-lysine]-vasopressin 36
Leucyloxytocin 309
D-Leucyloxytocin 34, 310
[8-Lysine]-oxytocin see Lysine vasotocin
Lysine vasopressin
  action of bromine water on 22, 46
  activity on various preparations 64 85, 96, 97, 99, 101, 176, 308
  amino acid constitution 21
  antibodies to 48, 206
  as a test of pituitary-adrenal function 438

Lysine vasopressin mechanism 439
    side effects and contra-indications 442
  assay *see under* Vasopressin
  blockade of action by drugs 439
  calciuretic effect 241
  comparison with arginine vasopressin 175
  complex with neurophysin 42, 134
    effect of calcium on 137, 138
  cupric ion complex 43
  desulfurization of 46
  dimer 45
  duration of antidiuresis due to 175, 391
  effect
    on adrenocorticotrophic hormone release 440
    on anura 101, 330, 331
    on growth hormone release 441
    on milk-ejection response to oxytocin 303
    on patients with pituitary or hypothalamic disorders 440
    on urodela 334
  enzymic degradation of 47
  extraction from biological tissues and fluids *see* Vasopressin
  genetic relationship to arginine vasopressin 72
  half-life in plasma 384, 391
  inactivation by pregnancy serum 392
  in pig-like animals (Suiformes) 67
  in Pitressin 382
  molecular shape 40
  molecular weight 21
  occurrence 67, 85, 94, 176
  oxidation of 46
  reaction with acetone 43
  reduction of 46
  stability 177
  structure 5, 25, 60, 84
  synthesis 19, 28
  plasma clearance of 382
  tritium-labelled 47
  urinary clearance 388
  see also Vasopressin
[8-D-Lysine]-vasopressin 37, 97, 99, 286, 288
Lysine vasotocin 40, 95, 96, 101, 247, 258, 330, 339

Mammals, neurohypophysial hormones in 66
Mammary gland
  action of oxytocin on *see* Oxytocin
  action potentials in 299
  carbohydrate metabolism of parenchyma cells in 311
  contractile tissue in *see* Myoepithelial cells
  during pregnancy and lactation 300
  effect of adrenaline and noradrenaline on 302
  engorgement 402
  inhibition of milk-ejection *see* Milk ejection
  oxygen requirement 304
  retardation of involution 312
  in vitro
  as assay method for oxytocin *see* Oxytocin
  effect
    of adrenaline on 197, 306
    of cations on 304
    of thioglycollate on 304
  sensitivity 197, 297
Marsupials, mole ratio of neurohypophysial hormones in 70
Methoxy progesterone acetate (Provera) 407
Melanocyte-stimulating hormone (MSH) 75, 324
[1-Mercaptoacetic acid, 4-β-alanine]-oxytocin 34
[1-Mercaptoacetic acid]-oxytocin 34, 309
[1-β-Mercaptobutyric acid]-oxytocin 34
[1-D-β-Mercaptobutyric acid]-oxytocin 34
[1-γ-Mercaptobutyric acid]-oxytocin 34, 92
  crystallization of 39
  X-ray-crystallographic data 39
[1-β-Mercaptopropionic acid]-oxytocin *see* Deamino-oxytocin
[1-β-Mercaptopropionic acid, 8-alanine]-oxytocin *see* Deamino-]8-alanine]-oxytocin
[1-β-Mercaptopropionic acid, 4-α-aminobutyric acid]-oxytocin *see* Deamino-4-decarboxamido-oxytocin

[1-β-Mercaptopropionic acid, 8-arginine]-vasopressin *see* Deamino-arginine-vasopressin

[1-β-Mercaptopropionic acid]-S,S'-dihydro-oxytocin *see* Deaminooxytoceine

[1-β-Mercaptopropionic acid, 2-isoleucine]-oxytocin *see* Deamino-[2-isoleucine]-oxytocin

[1-β-Mercaptopropionic acid, 8-ornithine]-oxytocin *see* Deamino-[8-ornithine]-oxytocin

[1-β-Mercaptopropionic acid, 8-ornithine]-vasopressin *see* Deamino-[8 ornithine]-vasopressin

[1-β-Mercaptopropionic acid, 2-phenylalanine]-oxytocin *see* Deaminodeoxy-oxytocin

[1-β-Mercaptopropionic acid, 2-phenylalanine, 4-α-aminobutyric acid]-oxytocin *see* Deamino-deoxy-4-decarboxamido-oxytocin

[1-β-Mercaptopropionic acid, 2-phenylalanine, 8-arginine]-vasopressin *see* Deamino-deoxy-arginine-vasopressin

[1-β-Mercaptopropionic acid, 2-phenylalanine, 8-ornithine]-oxytocin *see* Deamino-deoxy-[8-ornithine]-oxytocin

[1-β-Mercaptopropionic acid, 2-phenylalanine, 8-ornithine]-vasopressin *see* Deamino-deoxy-[8-ornithine]-vasopressin

[1-β-Mercaptopropionic acid, 7-D-proline]-oxytocin *see* Deamino-[7-D-proline]-oxytocin

[1-β-Mercaptopropionic acid, 4-serine, 8-isoleucine]-oxytocin *see* Deamino-isotocin

[1-β-Mercaptopropionic acid, 2-D-tyrosine]-oxytocin *see* Deamino-[2-D-tyrosine]-oxytocin

[1-β-Mercaptopropionic acid, 4-valine]-oxytocin *see* Deamino-[4-valine]-oxytocin

[1-β-Mercaptopropionic acid, 5-valine]-oxytocin *see* Deamino-[5-valine]-oxytocin

Mesotocin ([8-isoleucine]-oxytocin) 72, 86, 101, 286, 289. 308
  evolutionary role of 72
  effects on lungfish 328
  genetic pathway to 72
  inhibition of vasotocins by 247
  occurrence 30, 61, 68
  potency ratio 64, 65, 101
  structure 31, 60
  synthesis 30
N-Methyloxytocin 310
[2-p-Methylphenylalanine]-oxytocin 90, 309, 310
[3-O-Methylthreonine]-oxytocin 35, 309
[2-O-Methyltyrosine, 8-lysine]-vasopressin 99, 263
[2-O-Methyltyrosine]-oxytocin 263
  inhibition of assay responses of neurohypophysial hormones 89, 207
Micropuncture techniques 245
Milk ejection 7
  effect of suckling on 402
  inhibition of 301, 302, 303, 304, 309, 310
  oxytocin concentration necessary for 195, 404
  role of neurohypophysial hormones in 7, 295
  role in milk removal 300
  use in assay of oxytocin *see* Oxytocin and Vasopressin
Mitochondria, association of neurohypophysial hormones with 111, 116
Morphine 440
  release of neurohypophysial hormones by 126
Myoepithelium
  action of adrenaline on 302
  contraction during milk ejection 194, 295, 301
  effect
    of anesthetics on 304
    of oxytocin on 193, 295, 402
  function 194
  morphology 299
Myometrium
  effect of oxytocin on strips of 406
  electrophysiological properties of cells
    action potentials 281
    effect
      of oxytocin on 282
      of sex steroids on 282
    resting potential 280

Myometrium
  functions 280
  response to oxytocin 282, 305, 406, 415

"Natriuresis"
  definition 229
  see also Neurohypophysial hormones, Oxytocin and Vasopressin
Nephrogenic diabetes insipidus
  clinical features 424
  effect of vasopressin in 239
  treatment with diuretics 430
  urinary excretion in 389
  urine hyaluronidase activity in 239, 371
Neurohypophysial hormones
  antidilutional effect
    definition 229
    mechanism 232
    site of action 232
    see also Vasopressin
  antinatriuretic effects 247
  assay methods for characterization 62, 63
  biological and chemical characteristics of 19, 82
  biosynthesis 111
    control of 166
  biosynthesis of neurophysin with 157, 165
  complex with neurophysin see Oxytocin and Vasopressin
  content of neurohypophysis 114
  differential secretion of oxytocin and vasopressin 71, 255
  effect
    in lower vertebrates see individual groups
    of magnesium ions on 62, 87
    of sodium thioglycollate on 59
    on ACTH release in *Bufo bufo* 335
    on ion transport 321
  evolution 66, 71
  extraction from biological tissues and fluids see individual hormones
  in blood 123
  in urine see individual hormones
  mammary action 294
  mode of action on toad bladder 371
  mole ratios 70, 114
  natriuretic effects 229, 255, 259, 263
    definition 229
  phyletic distribution 61
  plasma clearance of see individual hormones
  potency ratios 6, 62, 63, 64, 65
  precursors of 112, 162
  receptor sites for 81, 284
  release 119
    acetylcholine in 129
    by calcium chloride injection 128
    by carotid sinus receptor stimulation 127
    by coitus and ejaculation 128
    by drugs 126
    by electrical stimulation of CNS (supropticohypophysial tract) 122, 126
    by hemorrhage 122, 123, 125, 127
    by osmotic stimulation 127
    by parturition dilatation of birth canal and cervical stimulation 128
    by stressful stimuli and anesthetics 118, 122, 125, 126
    by suckling or mammary stimulation 128
    by vagal stimulation (peripheral and central) 127
    by vagotomy and carotid occlusion 127
    role of calcium in 119
    separate release of oxytocin and vasopressin 117, 122, 123
  storage 112, 156, 164
  structure 23, 24, 25, 60
  subcellular particles associated with 116
  see also individual hormones
Neurophysin 66
  binding capacity of 41, 133
  binding to analogues 42
  biosynthesis of 157, 165
  bovine 134
  complex with neurohypophysial hormones 41, 133, 180
    effect of calcium on 121, 137, 138
    "extragranular pool" 139
    in elementary granules 134
    mechanism of binding 42, 136
    staining reactions 138

Neurophysin fractions 41, 134, 136
  function 136, 165
  in circulating blood 141, 380
  molecular weight 134, 135, 136
  ovine 133
  porcine 134
  role in release of hormones 136, 156, 165
  separation from peptide hormones 65
  subcellular distribution 4, 165
  use in extraction of hormones 5, 41, 165, 180
Neurosecretory cells
  biosynthesis in 111, 155, 159
  see also Neurosecretory granules
Neurosecretory granules (NSG) 4
  formation 163
  function 156
  occurrence 156
  separate granules for oxytocin and vasopressin 164
  size 156, 158
  synaptic granules 4, 129
  see also Neurosecretory cells
Neurosecretory material (NSM) 117
  axoplasmic flow 157
  depletion 118, 340
  microscopic studies
    during ether anesthesia 118
    Gomori-stainable material 3, 112, 328
  production 158
Nicotine
  effect on blood oxytocin and vasopressin concentrations 257
  release of neurohypophysial hormones by 126, 427
  test 427
Noradrenaline (Norepinephrine)
  action on mammary gland 302, 306
  effect on isolated rat uterus 202
  in neurohypophysis 133
  interference with milk-ejection assay 197
Norepinephrine see Noradrenaline
[3-Norleucine]-oxytocin 88
[3-Norvaline]-oxytocin 88, 309

[8-Ornithine]-oxytocin 86
[8-Ornithine]-vasopressin 97, 98, 99

Osmoreceptor center 119, 425
Osmotic diuresis 254, 425
Oviposition, role of neurohypophysial hormones in 327, 339, 342
Oxypressin ([3-phenylalanine]-oxytocin) 31, 95, 96, 101
  half-life in plasma 387
Oxytoceine (S,S'-dihydro-oxytocin) 27, 34, 44, 391
Oxytocin 64
  action of bromine water on 21, 46
  action on cell membranes in uterus 282
  activity, specific 64, 65, 85, 89, 96, 177
  amino acid constitution 20
  analogues see Analogues of neurohypophysial hormones, also individual names
  antibodies to 48, 206
  assay of
    antidiuretic effect 173
    chicken vasodepressor 198
    clinical aspects 287
    comparison of in vitro and in vivo assays 287
    immunochemical 206
    inhibitors 207, 284, 291
    interference of arginine vasopressin with 174
    milk ejection 192
    statistical treatment of results 209
    uterus in vitro 63, 199
      effect of ions on 286
      of estrous cycle on 289
      of pH on 287
      superfused uterus 202
      use of magnesium ratios 92, 201, 286
    uterus in vivo 94, 203, 287
  biosynthesis 155, 164
  calciuretic effect 241
  carbamylation of 44
  chemical functional groups in 87
  clearance from blood 377, 389, 390
  complex with neurophysin 41, 133
    effect of calcium on 137, 138
    nature of binding in 42
    "oxytocin neurophysin" 136
  concentration in plasma 382, 410
  crystalline salts of 39
  cupric ion complex of 43
  desulfurization 21, 46, 91

Oxytocin determination of structure 5
  dimer 40, 45
  distinction from vasotocin 204
  effect
    on Amphibia
      anura 101, 329
      urodela 334
    on birds 338
    on carbohydrate metabolism 206, 295, 311
    on *Lampetra fluviatilis* 322
    on non-pregnant uterus 86, 407
    on *Protopterus aethiopicus* 328
    on reptiles 336
    on teleosts fishes 324, 325
      vasopressor effect in eels 327
  elucidation of structure 22
  extraction from body tissues and fluids 178
  genetic pathway to 73
  half-life in plasma 384
  hepatic clearance of 385
  inactivation 47, 207, 208, 391
    by pregnancy serum 391, 406
  induction of labor by 399
  inhibitors 88
  intravenous drip 399, 401
  in treatment of hyponatremia 438
  in urine 388
  iodination 48
  isoelectric point 23
  mammary action
    action potentials 299
    dose for milk-ejection response 296, 305
    dose-response relationships for various species 298
    effect on intramammary pressure (galactokinetic or galactobolic effect) 295, 403
      on mammary engorgement 404
      on mammary involution 300, 312
    galactopoietic effect 295, 311
    inhibition of milk ejection *see* Milk ejection
    mammary clearance of 386
    mammary uptake 313
    resorption of milk constituents 312
    role in milk removal 7, 300
    sensitivity changes in mammary gland 300
    species difference in milk removal 300
    species difference in pressure response 296
  mode of action on uterus 282, 406, 411
  molecular shape 40
  molecular weight 20
  natriuretic effects
    comparison with vasopressin 255
    dosage 255
    effect of corticosteroids on 257
    in dehydration 258
    renal vascular effects 259
    tubular effects 260
  occurrence 61, 66, 177
  oxidation of 21, 46
  "oxytocinergic" neurons 117
  physical state in blood 177, 379
  precursor 112
  purification 20
  reaction with acetone 43
  reduction of 20, 46
  release
    experimental *see* Neurohypophysial hormones
    role of acetylcholine in 129
    separate release from vasopressin 117, 123, 164
    stimuli for 126
  renal clearance 385
  reverse uterine peristalsis due to 402
  role in parturition 8, 411
  separation from vasopressin 5, 64
  stability 176
  standardization 174, 400
  storage 41, 112, 164
  structural requirements for activity 86, 285, 290
  structure 19, 22, 23, 60, 82
  subcellular particles associated with 116, 124
  synthesis 6, 19, 25
  tritium labelled 47
  use in post partum hemorrhage 404
  use with ergometrine 400
  vascular effects 259, 401
  vasopressin: oxytocin ratios *see* Neurohypophysial hormones
D-Oxytocin 35, 38, 291
Oxytocinase 47, 178, 198, 208, 307, 383, 392, 406

Paper chromatography, separation of neurohypophysial hormones by 6, 65, 181, 388
Paraventricular nuclei 2, 4, 112, 120, 158, 164, 338
Pars intermedia 324, 327
Partition chromatography, purification of oxytocin analogues by 5, 28, 66
Peccary, vasopressins in 67
[1-Penicillamine]-oxytocin 34, 285
[1-D-Penicillamine]-oxytocin 34
Pepsin, effect on oxytocin and vasopressin 209
Perissodactyla, mole ratio of neurohypophysial hormones in 70
Petromyzon marinus
  effect of neurohypophysial hormones on 322
  neurohypophysial hormones in 70
[2-Phenylalanine, 4-α-aminobutyric acid]-oxytocin *see* Deoxy-4-decarboxamido-oxytocin
[3-Phenylalanine, 8-arginine]-oxytocin *see* Arginine vasopressin
[2-Phenylalanine, 8-ornithine]-oxytocin *see* Deoxy-[8-ornithine]-oxytocin
[2-Phenylalanine, 8-ornithine]-vasopressin *see* Deoxy-[8-ornithine]-vasopressin
[2-Pehylalanine]-oxytocin *see* Deoxyoxytocin
[3-Phenylalanine]-oxytocin *see* Oxypressin
Phenylalanyl-[8-lysine]-vasopressin 36
Phenylalanyl-oxytocin 34
Phenyl-pyrimidine compounds as vasopressin antagonists 248
Pig, neurohypophysial hormones in 67, 85
Pigeon
  effect of oxytocin in 339
  neurohypophysial hormones in 67
[7-Pipecolic acid]-oxytocin 36
Pitressin
  clearance 386
  effect on reptilian kidney 336
  half-life in plasma 383, 385
  natriuretic effects 264
  see also Vasopressin
Pituicytes 2
Pituitary-adrenal function, use of lysine-vasopressin as a test for 438
Pituitary tumors 431, 440
  see also Tumors
Plasma
  clearance of hormones from 377, 382
  concentration of hormones in 255, 382
  "cortisol" *see* Corticosteroids
  electrolytes
    hypercalcemia as a cause of polyuria 424
    in diabetes mellitus 425
    in dilutional hyponatremia 432
    in fluid deprivation tests 426
  osmolality
    during administration of vasopressin 426
    in dilutional hyponatremia 432
    in fluid deprivation tests 425
Poliomyelitis, associated with dilutional hyponatremia 431
Pollachius virens (Pollack), isolation of neurohypophysial hormones from 66, 69
Polydipsia, psychogenic 425
Polydon, neurohypophysial hormones in 69
Polypterus senegalus, neurohypophysial hormones in 69, 73
Polyuria 423
  in birds 338
  see also Urine
Posterior pituitary extract 2, 6, 9
  see also individual hormones
Posterior pituitary hormones *see* Neurohypophysial hormones
Postpartum hemorrhage, treatment 9, 400, 404, 418
Potassium depletion
  as a cause of polyuria unresponsive to vasopressin 424
  as a cause of proximal renal tubular defects 432
  effect on urinary concentration in kidney 251
  in thiazide therapy 431
Preoptic nucleus 2, 4
"Pressin" ring 31
Progesterone
  blood level in menstrual cycle 409
  effect of oxytocin on kidney after treatment with 263

Progesterone
  effects on uterus 8, 409
Prolactin 312, 326
[7-D-Proline]-oxytocin 36
Prolyl-[8-lysine]-vasopressin 36
Prolyloxytocin 34, 309
[1-Propionic acid, 6-alanine, 8-arginine]-vasopressin see Deamino-dethio-arginine-vasopressin
[1-Propionic acid, 6-alanine, 8-lysine]-vasopressin see Deamino-dethio-lysine-vasopressin
[2-O-Propyltyrosine, 8-lysine]-vasopressin 37
Prostaglandins, effect on isolated rat uterus 202
Protein deficiency, renal defects due to 252
Protein synthesis
  amino acid code for neurohypophysial hormones 72
  correlation with evolutionary pathways 73
Propterus aethiopicus
  effect of neurohypophysial hormones in 323, 328
  neurohypophysial hormones in 68
Puromycin
  effect on vasopressin biosynthesis 160
  inhibition of effect of oxytocin on mammary carbohydrate metabolism 311
Pyrogen
  vasopressin antagonism 248

Rana sp.
  effect of neurohypophysial hormones
    on bladder of 332, 351
    on kidney of 330
    on skin of 239, 330, 351, 365
  neurohypophysial hormones in 68
Receptor sites for neurohypophysial hormones
  for vasopressin in kidney 371
  for vasotocins in amphibian kidney 330
  in amphibian skin 331
  in toad bladder 364
  inhibitors 88, 284
  nature of 91, 94, 372

Reflection coefficient 361, 362
Renal disease 252, 424, 425, 432
  see also Chronic renal failure
Renal plasma flow
  after hypophysectomy 259, 401
  effect of oxytocin on 259, 401
Renin, role in sodium excretion 258
Reptiles
  effect of neurohypophysial hormones
    on kidney 230, 336
    on oviduct 72, 337
  neurohypophysial hormones in 62, 66, 67
Reserpine, release of neurohypophysial hormones by 126
Ruminants, mole ratio of neurohypophysial hormones in 70

Salamandra maculosa (Salamander) 334
"Salt-losing nephritis", associated with dilutional hyponatraemia 433
Sarcoidosis, as a cause of diabetes insipidus 424
[9-Sarcosine]-oxytocin 91, 309
Sarcosyl-glycyl-[8-lysine]-vasopressin 36
Sarcosil-oxytocin 310
Selenium in analogues of oxytocin and deamino-oxytocin 39, 92, 285
[1,6-Selenocystine]-oxytocin 34, 39
[4-Serine, 8-glutamine]-oxytocin see Glumitocin
[3-Serine, 8-isoleucine]-oxytocin 32, 35
[4-Serine, 8-isoleucine]-oxytocin see Isotocin
[2-Serine, 8-lysine]-vasopressin 103
[4-Serine]-oxytocin 308
Sheep, oxytocin in 67
Sick e-cell anemia, renal defects associated with 253
Sodium balance, effect of neurohypophysial hormones on 325, 328, 329, 337
Sodium transport
  across Henle's loop 233, 244, 251
  across toad bladder 362
Substance P
  effect
    on avian blood pressure 199
    on isolated rat uterus 201
Suiformes, [8-lysine]-vasopressin in 67

Supraoptic nuclei 2, 4, 112, 122, 158, 167, 338
Sympathomimetic amines
 effect
  in rat antidiuretic assay 189
  in vasopressor assay 199
 see also Adrenaline and Noradrenaline
Syntometrine, use in post-partum hemorrhage 405
Syphilis as a cause of diabetes insipidus 424

Teleost fishes (Teleostei)
 effect of neurohypophysial hormones on sodium balance 325
 effects of neurohypophysial hormones on water metabolism 323, 324
 euryhaline teleosts 324
 induction of spawning by neurohypophysial hormones 327
 neurohypophysial hormones in 61, 69
 mole ratios of hormones in 71
 vasopressor effects of neurohypophysial hormones in 327
Testosterone, effect on isolated rat uterus 409
Theophylline, effect on toad bladder 372
[8-Thialysine]-vasopressin ([8-(3-(2-aminoethyl)thio)-alanine]-vasopressin) 37
Thiazides 248, 430
Thin-layer chromatography, separation of neurohypophysial hormones by 65
α-Thioglycerol inhibition of oxytocin 207
Thioglycollate inactivation of oxytocin and vasopressin 207, 303
Toad bladder
 effect of neurohypophysial hormones
  on sodium transport 332, 362
  on solute transport 358
  on water permeability 332, 352
 site of action 364
 structure 332, 352
"Tocin" ring 31
Tranquillizers, vasopressin inhibition 248
Trout
 effect of vasopressin in 325
 hormone depletion in 327

Tryptophyl-[8-lysine]-vasopressin 36
Trypsin, effect on oxytocin and vasopressin 208, 388
[3-Tryptophan]-oxytocin 88
Tumors, hormone production by 433
Turkey, neurohypophysial hormones in 67
Tylopoda 67
 mole ratio of neurohypophysial hormones in 70
Tyrosinase effect on oxytocin and vasopressin 208
[2-D-Tyrosine]-oxytocin 35, 42
[3-Tyrosine]-oxytocin 88
Tyrosyl-[8-lysine]-vasopressin 36

Urea
 in blood in renal disease 254
 in blood in dilutional hyponatremia 432
 role in urine concentration 238, 245, 254
 role in potassium deficient rats 251
 transport across toad bladder 358
Urine
 aminoaciduria in dilutional hyponatremia 432
 anomalous oxytocic effects in 202
 antidiuretic material in 184
 assay parameters for vasopressin 188
 concentration mechanism 232, 236
  effect of
   adrenalectomy on 253
   cirrhosis of the liver on 253
   hypophysectomy on 253
   protein deficiency on 253
   salt deprivation on 253
   sickle cell anemia on 253
   vasopressin on 236, 239, 244
   vasopressin antagonists on 247
  in newborn 250, 254
  role of urea in 251, 254
 hypercalcuria 425
  in oral sodium chloride test 427
 osmolality 241, 245
  after vasopressin administration 230, 428
  effect of sodium bicarbonate on 242
  in dilutional hyponatremia 432

Urine
  in protein deficiency 252
  oxytocin in 388
  rate of flow
    effect
      of oxytocin on 247, 261
      of vasopressin antagonists on 246
  sodium and chloride in
    effect
      of oxytocin on 260
      of vasopressin on 264
  specific gravity of 425, 426
  total solute in, effect of oxytocin on 260
  vasopressin in 387
  volume
    after vasopressin administration 428
    in diabetes insipidus 424
    in nicotine test 428
    in oral sodium chloride test 427
Urodela see Amphibians
Uterus
  during pregnancy and parturition 8, 409
  effect of oxytocin on 94
    amount required for uterine activity 410
    in non-pregnant state 405
    mode of action 282, 406
  interaction of oxytocin and ovarian hormones on 8, 199
  intrauterine pressure 404, 417
  post partum hemorrhage 404
  sensitivity to neurohypophysial peptides 287
  see also Myometrium

[5-Valine]-angiotensin-II-amide, effect on glomerular filtration rate 229
[3-Valine]-oxytocin 87, 88, 101, 289, 308, 310, 333
  half-life in plasma 384, 387
  inhibition of vasotocins 247
  retardation of mammary involution 312
[4-Valine]-oxytocin 35
[5-Valine]-oxytocin 36, 91
[8-Valine]-oxytocin 86
Van Dyke protein 41, 65

Vasopresseine (S,S'-dihydrovasopressin) 27, 44
  in synthesis of lysine vasopressin 29
Vasopressinase in pregnancy serum 392
Vasopressin
  amino acid composition 20
  antagonism to antidiuresis by
    antidepressants 248
    bicarbonate 250
    cystostatic drugs 248
    diphenylhydantoin 248
    ethyleneimine 248
    old age 250
    overhydration 249
    oxytocin 247
    phenylpyrimidine compounds 248
    pyrogens 248
    tranquillizers 248
  antagonism to concentrating effects 245
  antidilutional effects see below and Neurohypophysial hormones
  assay methods 63, 173, 182
    antidiuretic 184
    inhibition of responses 207
    statistical treatment of results 209
    vasopressor 190
  biosynthesis 112, 115, 155
  calciuretic effect 240
  chemical inactivation 207
  clearance from blood 377
  clearance studies
    in isolated organs 389
    in isolated tissues 390
  complex with neurophysin 121, 133
    "vasopressin neurophysin" 136
  concentration in plasma 382
  determination of structure 5
  effect
    in chicken depressor assay 199
    in psychogenic polydipsia 425
    of acid load on response to 242
    of adrenalectomy on response to 253
    of aldosterone on response to 244, 245
    of dehydration on response to
    of ethanol anesthesia on response to 242
    of potassium deprivation on response to 251

Vasopressin
- of salt deprivation on response to 253
- of season on sensitivity to 242
- on anura 329
- on carbohydrate metabolism of mammary parenchyma cells 311
- on chickens 338
- on countercurrent multiplier system 235
- on frog skin 351
- on intramammary pressure 296
- on *Lampetra fluviatilis* 322
- on protein-deficient rats 252
- on proximal guinea-pig colon 206
- on renal tubular permeability 236
  - collecting ducts 234, 236
  - effect of glucocorticosteroids 242, 251
  - mechanism 239
- on sodium concentrations in renal medulla 235
- on teleost fishes 324
- on toad bladder 352
  - permeability barrier 367
    - effect of Amphotericin B 368
  - site of action 367
- enzymic inactivation 47, 208
- extraction from biological tissues and fluids 178
- gland content 114
- hepatic clearance of 385
- inactivation 391
- inappropriate secretion 431
- inhibition of galactokinetic action of oxytocin 303
- in lymph 381
- in urine 387
- mammary clearance of 386
- milk ejection 193, 197
- natriuretic effects 258, 263
  - comparison with angiotensin 264
  - comparison with oxytocin 255
  - factors affecting 265
  - in water loaded mammals 264
  - see also Neurohypophysial hormones
- oxytocin : vasopressin ratios in blood 257
- physical state in blood 177, 379
- pressor effect in frogs and toads 335
- purification of 41
- release of 115, 126
  - acetylcholine in 129
  - separate release of oxytocin and vasopressin 117, 123, 164
  - "stimulus secretion coupling" 119, 137
- renal clearance 385
- repletion 115
- retardation of mammary involution 312
- sensitivity of mammary gland to 296
- sensitivity in newborn 250
- sodium transport 362
  - stimulation by Amphotericin B 368
- solute transport 358
- storage 41, 112
- subcellular particles associated with 116
- tumor production of 431
- vascular action 7
- vasopressin : oxytocin ratios see Neurohypophysial hormones
- vasopressinergic neurons 117
- water transport 352

Vasotocin see Arginine vasotocin
Vitamin D intoxication, renal disturbances due to 252

Warthog, vasopressins in 67
Water intoxication in psychogenic polydipsia 425
Water metabolism
- effect of neurohypophysial hormones on
  - amphibians 329, 334
  - birds 338
  - lungfish 328
  - reptilians 336
  - teleost fishes 324
Water transport across amphibian bladder see Amphibians
Whale, oxytocin in 67
Wild boar (European), vasopressins in 67

Xenopus laevis, effect of neurohypophysial hormones in 329, 333

Yohimbine 126